TEXTBOOK OF HEALTHFUL LIVING

TEXTBOOK OF
Healthful Living

HAROLD S. DIEHL, M.A., M.D., Sc.D.

Professor of Preventive Medicine and Public Health, and Dean of the Medical Sciences, University of Minnesota; Vice-Chairman, Health Resources Advisory Committee, U.S. Office of Defense Mobilization; Former Director, Health Studies, American Youth Commission; Member, National Advisory Health Council, U.S. Public Health Service; Member Governing Council, American Public Health Association; President, American Student Health Association

FIFTH EDITION

McGRAW-HILL BOOK COMPANY, INC.

New York   Toronto   London

1955

TEXTBOOK OF HEALTHFUL LIVING

Library of Congress Catalog Card Number 54-11754

IV

*To those
who prefer facts to fads,
sanity to superstition,
understanding to belief*

PREFACE

SOME years ago, at the request of Dr. Morris Fishbein, editor of the Whittlesey House Health Series, I wrote a book for the general reader entitled "Healthful Living." In so doing I attempted not to plead any cause, point any moral, or promote any health fad, but to set forth for the consideration of the intelligent reader the more significant available information concerning the preservation and improvement of health.

The progress which has been made in the conquest of disease and the improvement of health is a dramatic and fascinating story, and my years of teaching in this field have convinced me that this is a subject that can be presented in a manner that is interesting as well as medically and scientifically accurate.

It was not my thought originally that this book would be used as a textbook, but after its publication several colleges and universities immediately, and an increasing number subsequently, adopted it as a textbook for their courses in personal hygiene. In view of this, the publishers requested that I revise the book, giving special consideration to its use as a college textbook. The first edition of this book represented my response to that request.

As a basis for this revision the publisher invited suggestions from teachers who had used this book most extensively in their classes. Many suggestions were received, but the one request that stood out above all others was that we avoid the usual textbook style. I have tried to do this and at the same time incorporate such additional scientific information and detail as seemed desirable for a textbook.

Subsequent editions in response to requests from teachers using the book have been expanded to include a number of chapters on Community Health and Organized Health Services. The purpose of these added chapters is to present information of interest and value to college men and women as they assume their responsibilities as citizens of the communities in which they live.

This fifth edition of the Textbook of Healthful Living not only incorporates the most recent information and data concerning the length of life and the causes of death, of illness, and of physical and emotional disabilities, but also adds new sections or material on drowning, on the prevention of poliomyelitis, on cancer of the lung, on Rh incompatibilities, on hormones, on antibiotics, on the treatment of drinking water and milk for personal use, on rehabilitation of the disabled, and on the World Health Organization.

In addition, a new Appendix B has been included which presents a complete and easily used table of Food Values in Common Portions; and Appendix D has been revised to include the 1955 revision of the American Public Health Association's Manual on the Control of Communicable Diseases in Man.

An important adjunct to the previous edition was the five sound motion pictures and five silent filmstrips specifically correlated with selected chapters of the text. Individual films cover such subjects as recommended routines for developing desirable personal health habits; description of the structure and function of body organs shown in animation sequences; the counterbalances to human disease; the reproductive systems of men and women and the process of normal human birth; and the establishment of psychiatric techniques as normal treatment for persistent emotional upsets. As a supplement to this fifth edition two additional motion pictures have been prepared. One of these presents the more important effects of the endocrine glands upon normal life processes and day-to-day living. The other deals with the heart and circulatory system and some of the things that go wrong with them.

For their assistance in the preparation of this edition the author wishes to acknowledge his indebtedness to the following friends and colleagues who have reviewed and contributed to various sections of the manuscript: Miss Mary Switzer, Director, United States Office of Vocational Rehabilitation; Dr. Howard Rusk and Eugene Taylor of the New York Institute for Physical Medicine and Rehabilitation; Dr. Stewart Thomson, Professor of Preventive Medicine and Public Health, University of Minnesota; Dr. Alan Treloar, Professor and Director of the Division of Biostatistics, University of Minnesota; Dr. Gaylord Anderson, Professor and Director of the School of Public Health, University of Minnesota; Dr. L. R. Boies, Professor and Director of the Department of Otolaryngology, University of Minnesota; Miss Gertrude Thomas, Associate Professor of Dietetics and Director of Nutrition, University of Minnesota Hospitals; Herbert Bosch, Professor of Public Health Engineering, University of Minnesota; Dr. Francis Lynch, Associate Professor of Dermatology, University of Minnesota; Dr. James E. Perkins, Managing Director, Dr. Lloyd Feldman, Assistant Director, and Dr. Edward Sierks, Consultant in Health Education, of the National Tuberculosis Association; Dr. Ruth Boynton, Professor of Public Health and Director of the Students' Health Service, University of Minnesota; Dr. Ruth Grout, Professor of Health Education, University of Minnesota; Dr. Robert Bush, Instructor in Psychiatry, University of Minnesota; Dr. William P. Shepard, Second Vice-President, Metropolitan Life Insurance Company; Dr. Reginald Atwater, Executive Secretary, American Public Health Association; and Dr. Hans Kraus, Assistant Clinical Professor of Rehabilitation and Physical Medicine, New York University College of Medicine.

The author also wishes to express his appreciation to the users of this textbook who have made valuable suggestions for revision and to the several authors and publishers who have graciously granted permission to reproduce copyrighted material.

HAROLD S. DIEHL

[ix]

CONTENTS

[xi]

CONTENTS

[xii]

Illumination. Glare. Color Blindness. Care of the Eyes and Prevention of Eyestrain.

[xiv]

CONTENTS

[XV]

CONTENTS

TEXT-FILMS ON HEALTH EDUCATION

THE following is a list of the McGraw-Hill Text-Films, 16-mm sound motion pictures and 35-mm silent filmstrips available for use with this book. A brief description of each motion picture is given at the end of the chapter with which it is correlated.

The Body Fights Bacteria (motion picture 17 min). Correlated with Chapters II, XII, and XIII.

Emotional Health (motion picture 20 min). Correlated with Chapter III.

The Nose, Throat, and Ears (motion picture 11 min). Correlated with Chapter XIV.

Body Care and Grooming (motion picture 17 min). Correlated with Chapters XVI and XVII.

Human Reproduction (motion picture 21 min). Correlated with Chapters XVIII, XIX, and XX.

Hormones and the Endocrine Glands (motion picture about 15 min, available spring, 1955). Correlated with Chapter XVIII.

Diseases of the Heart and Circulatory System (motion picture about 15 min, available spring, 1955). Correlated with Chapters II and XXI.

Chapter I

POSSIBILITIES OF LONGER LIFE
AND BETTER HEALTH

EXCEPT for conditions attributable to war, human life today is longer and healthier than ever before in the history of the world. Science has unraveled the mystery of one disease after another and the application of science has led to disease control until we can almost proclaim that anyone may have good health if he will follow the established rules of hygiene. Certain illnesses, accidents, psychological situations, and social and economic conditions are as yet not within our control. But the health of most of us could be materially improved and our pleasure of living increased if we would only live a little more intelligently.

But can people be induced to be intelligent concerning health? There is abundant evidence that they will blindly follow fads which promise health of body or mind and that they will pour fortunes into the laps of unscrupulous charlatans who offer them panaceas for everything under the sun. But will they think? Have they the strength of mind to look critically at their health prejudices, hobbies, and fads? If so, they will find that living is fascinating and that the maintenance of health is much less difficult and mysterious than they have believed.

Some are fearful that the public may be told too much concerning health, and that people will be led to worry unnecessarily about themselves. But we rarely worry about the things we understand. It is the unknown that fills us with apprehension. On every hand we are confronted with suggestions that if we do not eat this food, take these vitamins, drink this tonic, gargle with this antiseptic, or use these nose drops, health may be forever lost. The instilling of fear is the objective of much of the advertising in the health field. Unless one secures authoritative information on the subject, one is likely to follow the admonitions of the best salesman.

I recently learned from a reliable source that the gasoline which I have been using in my car is one of the poorest gasolines that I could buy, that it dilutes the crankcase oil, leaves a sticky residue in the motor, and is relatively difficult to ignite in cold weather. I had been buying this gasoline because advertisements assured me that it was the best gasoline available. Many products promoted in the name of health do much more damage to the human body than poor gasoline could do to my motor. Is it sensible for intelligent persons to remain in ignorance concerning matters of such vital importance? This does not imply that one need become a health prig or a health crank. Such deluded persons make life miserable for themselves and are a nuisance to friends and associates. Nor is it necessary that people become timid, shrinking creatures who go through life with a thermometer in one hand and a bottle of antiseptic gargle in the other. Intelligent people follow a different course. They acquaint themselves with the facts, face their problems with intelligence, and proceed to get the most out of life.

Man cannot live forever, nor can he enjoy perfect health always; but of both life and health every normal person would like his full share. Predicting what this amounts to is stock in trade for the fortuneteller. We shall try to arrive at a more intelligent prediction by analyzing the problems involved.

This analysis necessitates the raising of several related questions. First, what are the possibilities, biologically and statistically, of adding to the length of human life? Second, what are the causes of untimely deaths, and what hope is there of reducing them? And, third, what are the physical and mental handicaps and disabilities which detract most from our efficiency and enjoyment of life, and what, if anything, can be done to avoid, correct, or minimize these?

Health and the National Welfare

Health is such a personal matter that in normal times few persons think of it as being of national importance. Yet Disraeli, Queen Victoria's renowned and beloved Prime Minister of England, stated, "The public health is the foundation upon which reposes the happiness of the people and the strength of the nation. Care of the public health is the first duty of the state."

In times of national emergencies, on the other hand, everyone realizes that good health is essential for the national welfare and even for national existence. Illness destroys the effectiveness of the armed forces, hampers industrial production, undermines morale, and places an enormous burden of medical care upon a weakened populace.

Illustrative of the serious effects of illness upon national production is the report of the U.S. Public Health Service, which estimates that approximately 350,000,000 man-days are lost annually on account of illness and accidents among industrial workers in this country. This loss corresponds to the total working time of more than a million workingmen for a whole year. Translating this into terms of national defense production, the Surgeon General of the U.S. Public Health Service said:

Not all of this can be prevented; but suppose we prevent 10% of this—a conservative estimate—what would be the result in defense production? Based on data from the Bureau of Labor Statistics, showing the man-hours required to produce various kinds of war material, I have calculated that a 10% reduction in industrial manpower losses from disability would build 12 cantonments of average size, 5 battleships, or 16,407 combat tanks. Representative McCormack, of Massachusetts, made another comparison. He estimates that man-days lost to industry last year on account of disability were 50 times as great as those lost on account of strikes and lock-outs. We hear much about the latter but little of the former.[1]

Other extensive surveys of illness among industrial workers show that the average loss of time on account of illness is 8 days

[1] Parran, Thomas, "The Function of Public Health in Defense," *Journal of the American Medical Association*, vol. 117, p. 186, July 19, 1941.

per year for men and 12 days per year for women. The sum of these individual disabilities makes the staggering total referred to above. Fortunately, though also tragically, much of this is preventable.

Length of Life

There is no more brilliant achievement of man than the progress he has made in the prevention of disease and the prolongation of life. From superstition, ignorance, and early death man has advanced in a few centuries to an understanding and solution of most of his health problems.

Physicians can never eradicate death from the face of the earth; their function is to prolong life and to relieve pain. Death is not preventable, but some deaths are postponable. As more deaths are postponed to higher ages, the number of deaths per year will tend to increase. Therefore, the success of medical care and public health programs must be measured by the number of years the average person lives, not by the number of deaths that occur in any year.

In the sixteenth century the average length of life in western Europe is said to have been 19 years; in the seventeenth century, 25 years; in the eighteenth century, 32 years. In the nineteenth century in this country life averaged approximately 40 years; at the beginning of the present century this average had increased to 49 years; and by the end of the first quarter of the twentieth century to approximately 57 years for boys and approximately 60 years for girls. By 1950 this increase in life expectancy at birth in the United States had extended to 66.6 years for white males and 72.4 years for white females (Fig. 1).

An increase in life expectancy, or in the average length of life, occurs when there has been a decrease in the diseases or conditions which tend to destroy life prematurely; in other words, a reduction in the death rate. The increase in the length of life, however, is not necessarily proportionate to the decrease in death rate, for a reduction in the death rate of children has a much greater effect on the average length of life than a similar reduction in the death rate of older people.

Between 1900 and 1952, when the decrease in the death rate for people of all ages in this country was 44 per cent, there was a drop of 80 per cent in the rate among children under 1 year of age. Among adults the reductions became less with advancing age until the reduction was only 30 per cent in the age group

FIG. 1. TREND IN THE EXPECTATION OF LIFE AT BIRTH

MALES	YEAR	FEMALES
34.9	1800	36.1
38.9	1850	40.5
41.7	1880	43.5
46.1	1900	49.5
59.3	1930	62.6
66.6	1950	72.4

Each figure represents 5 years expectation of life at birth

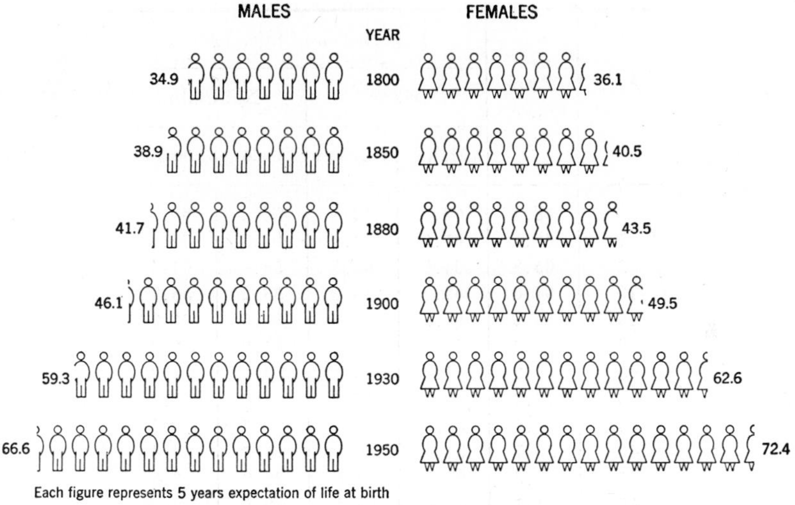

Data for 1790–1930, Massachusetts; 1950 for United States.

fifty-five to sixty-four, and 25 per cent in the age group seventy-five to eighty-four.

Changes in Life Expectancy with Age

As a result of smaller reductions in death rates, the life expectancy for older persons shows but little increase. In other words, the chances of long life for an older person today are very little greater than they were a generation ago. Today, however, many of us reach older age who, in an earlier period, would have died in childhood or early adult life.

The changes in life expectancy with age by 5-year periods are shown in Table 1. As this table shows, the average life expectancy of children at 1 year of age is greater than that of newborn babies. This is true because of the high death rate during the first year of life. This table shows also that the life expectancy of a boy of 20 is 49.7 years and of a girl of 20, 54.9 years; and that the average remaining expectancy for men of 65 is 13.0 years and for women of 65 is 15.3 years.

TABLE 1

EXPECTATION OF LIFE IN THE UNITED STATES AT SPECIFIED AGES BY COLOR AND SEX, 1950*

| Age, Years | Total Persons | Expectation of Life, Years | | | |
| | | White | | Nonwhite | |
		Males	Females	Males	Females
0	68.4	66.6	72.4	59.2	63.2
1	69.5	67.6	73.1	61.3	64.8
5	65.8	64.0	69.5	58.0	61.4
10	61.0	59.2	64.6	53.2	56.7
15	56.2	54.4	59.7	48.5	51.9
20	51.5	49.7	54.9	44.0	47.3
25	46.9	45.2	50.1	39.7	42.9
30	42.2	40.5	45.4	35.5	38.5
35	37.6	35.9	40.6	31.5	34.4
40	33.1	31.4	36.0	27.5	30.4
45	28.8	27.1	31.5	23.8	26.6
50	24.7	23.0	27.1	20.5	23.2
55	20.9	19.3	22.9	17.6	20.2
60	17.3	15.9	19.0	15.2	17.7
65	14.1	13.0	15.3	12.7†	14.6†
70†	11.3	10.4	12.1	10.8	12.7
75†	8.6	7.8	8.6	8.7	10.5

* *Statistical Bulletin*, Metropolitan Life Insurance Company, July, 1953.
† Estimates by author.

Another interesting analysis (Table 2) shows that the life expectancy at birth of persons born in a group of the North Central States is very close to the highest found anywhere in the world. For 1939–1941, the expectation of life at birth for white males ranged from 66.25 years in Nebraska to 56.83 years in Arizona, and for white females from 70.04 years in Nebraska to 60.96 years in New Mexico.

The expectation of life is the obverse of the death rate and is calculated from it; hence, the life expectancy in states which are

TABLE 2

EXPECTATION OF LIFE AT BIRTH IN EACH OF THE UNITED STATES, 1939–1941*

State	Expectation of Life at Birth Years		Rank by Expectation of Life at Birth	
	White Males	White Females	White Males	White Females
Nebraska	66.25	70.04	1	1
South Dakota	66.09	69.99	2	2
Minnesota	65.97	69.74	3	3
Iowa	65.81	69.70	4	4
North Dakota	65.71	69.31	5	7
Kansas	65.58	69.67	6	5
Wisconsin	65.22	68.75	7	9
Arkansas	64.24	67.96	8	18
Oregon	64.09	69.49	9	6
Connecticut	64.00	68.19	10	16
Oklahoma	63.87	68.32	11	13
Washington	63.62	68.95	12	8
Missouri	63.50	67.82	13	19
New Hampshire	63.48	67.54	14	22
Idaho	63.45	68.23	15	15
Michigan	63.45	67.36	16	25
Indiana	63.36	67.10	17	32
Delaware	63.33	67.32	18	28
Rhode Island	63.31	67.36	19	26
Massachusetts	63.25	67.62	20	21
Ohio	63.25	67.33	21	27
Utah	63.21	68.60	22	12
New Jersey	63.09	67.10	23	33
Vermont	63.05	66.99	24	36
Wyoming	62.90	68.09	25	17
New York	62.90	67.03	26	35
Illinois	62.86	67.46	27	23
UNITED STATES	**62.81**	**67.29**	**28**	**29**
Montana	62.69	67.69	29	20
Maine	62.62	66.44	30	40
Tennessee	62.48	66.76	31	38
Florida	62.39	68.65	32	11
North Carolina	62.32	67.28	33	30
Mississippi	62.26	67.17	34	31
Pennsylvania	62.20	66.24	35	44
District of Columbia	62.19	68.69	36	10
Maryland	62.00	66.86	37	37
California	61.90	68.27	38	14
Alabama	61.77	66.28	39	42
Georgia	61.72	67.46	40	24
West Virginia	61.71	66.00	41	46
Colorado	61.61	66.28	42	43
Kentucky	61.57	65.62	43	48
Virginia	61.28	66.73	44	39
Louisiana	61.18	67.09	45	34
Texas	61.07	65.96	46	47
South Carolina	60.01	66.12	47	45
Nevada	58.98	66.42	48	41
New Mexico	57.20	60.96	49	50
Arizona	56.83	63.74	50	49

* *Statistical Bulletin*, Metropolitan Life Insurance Company, vol. 29, p. 6, September, 1948.

[7]

considered health resorts and so have a high invalid population would be adversely affected. Climate at once suggests itself as another possible factor in the differences in life expectancy among the states, but industrialization is clearly a much more important factor. The highly agricultural states as a group have a high life expectancy, while the typically industrial states have a correspondingly low life expectancy. Related to industrialization also is the racial composition of the population which may influence longevity unfavorably. The adequacy of the organized public health program bears an obvious relationship to illness and death rates in both urban and rural communities.

It has been suggested that the safeguards which are being placed about the health of children may lead to the development of a physically inferior adult population; that modern public health work is interfering with nature's plan to improve the race by eliminating the weak and permitting only the fit to survive. Yet no one would suggest that we expose children to communicable diseases, inadequate diets, or other hazards in order that only those of superior vitality might survive. A better plan is to improve health and vitality by intelligent living so that the degenerative processes of advancing age may be postponed.

International Differences in Longevity[2]

Great differences exist in the longevity, that is, the average age at death, of the people in the various countries of the world. In general, where social and economic conditions are good and health standards are high, longevity is high; while in countries where social and economic conditions are poor and health standards low, longevity is little better today than it was in ancient times.

New Zealand reports the best longevity record in the world, with Australia, the United States, Canada, Great Britian, and the Scandinavian countries not far behind. The poorest record is

[2] Data from *Statistical Bulletin*, Metropolitan Life Insurance Company, March, 1950; and Ancel Keys, "Diet and the Incidence of Heart Disease," *Bulletin of the University of Minnesota Hospitals*, February 20, 1953.

found in Asia and most of Africa; with most European and Latin American countries in an intermediate position.

For example, in 1940, when the life expectancy at birth in the United States was 63 years, it was 68 in New Zealand; 66 in Australia, the Netherlands, Denmark, and Sweden; well under 40 in Mexico; 35 in Chile; 30 in Peru; and 27 in India.

The relatively favorable position of the United States in longevity or life expectancy at birth is obviously due to the saving of lives in infancy and childhood since death rates in this country between the ages of 40 and 65 are higher than in any other English-speaking country and with one or two exceptions in any western European country. This is particularly disturbing since these high death rates fall in man's most productive years.

An analysis of the causes of death in these countries shows that the excess number of deaths in the United States is due primarily to cardiovascular diseases. Why this is true and why women live longer than men are questions of major importance. Let us hope that the researches under way will provide answers upon which we can base future health programs.

Is Long Life Desirable?

During the Middle Ages in Europe the average length of life was less than 20 years. Today in the United States, owing largely to reduction in the death rates of infants and children, life expectancy at birth has increased to approximately 68 years. What an enormous difference this makes in the welfare of the race and the possibilities of human progress! With an average life span of 20 or 30 years, many of the potential leaders in every field die in childhood and the average person has relatively few years of maturity in which to contribute to the progress of the race. Under such circumstances an occasional genius will stand out, but the life of most men will be cut short before they can make their more modest contributions to society.

Sir William Osler is frequently, though somewhat incorrectly, credited with saying that by the age of 40 man's constructive work usually has been completed and that not later than 60 he should take a peaceful departure by chloroform. In recent years students of this question have shown that the greatest period of productive leadership is after, rather than before, the age of 40 has been reached.

Thorndike finds that what he calls the "masterpiece age" for authors, artists, scientists, and scholars averages just under 50. Darwin was 50 when he published his greatest work, "Origin of Species," and William James, foremost of American psychologists, had not published a single book and few articles by the age of 40. Michelangelo and Titian painted their greatest masterpieces after the age of 80, and Harvey discovered the circulation of the blood at 72. Sorenson reports that most scholars and scientists do their best intellectual work at about 50 years of age but with a considerable variability within 10-year periods before and after 50. During the late forties there seems to be a slight downward trend in the curve of individual accomplishment, but the average drop is so slight that at the age of 60 the curve has dropped little from its greatest peak of 10 years before. In view of such studies it is easy to understand that a civilization with an average length of life less than half what it is today could be hardly other than backward.

Biological Limits to the Span of Life

In spite of these increases in the average length of life and the expectancy of life at birth, the span of life, that is, the time from birth to life's upper biological limits, has changed little or not at all from remote antiquity. Although a greater proportion of people live to relatively advanced ages, the occasional person does not attain any greater age today than in the past. Our grandparents, and to a greater extent their grandparents, lost many of their children from diphtheria, smallpox, typhoid fever, and other diseases which constitute comparatively little hazard for children today. Consequently, many more persons are now passing through the dangers of infancy and childhood and reaching adult life.

The number of persons who reach the venerable age of 100

years is certainly small, yet a person living at any age still has some life expectancy, small though it may be, beyond that age. There are authoritative records of persons who have attained the age of 120 years, and possibly one who lived to be 140. Whether such cases represent the upper biologic limit for the race or whether they are merely "freaks" of nature we do not know.

Studies of tissue cells suggest that under ideal conditions individual cells from the animal body may continue to live indefinitely. For example, although the normal life span of a chicken is 3 to 7 years, the late Dr. Alexis Carrel was able to keep the heart of an embryo chick alive in his laboratory for over 20 years. To do this he supplied the food which it needed, removed waste products, and regulated environmental conditions of temperature and moisture.

Unfortunately the communities of cells which constitute the human body are not provided with such ideal conditions of existence. They are exposed to the weakening influence of imperfect diets, the wear and tear of activity, the toxins of infections, the burden of overeating, and the poisons of alcohol and tobacco. No matter how great the biologic possibilities of life may be, the practical upper limit for the average person probably is not much beyond the age attained by a reasonable percentage of the population. This is not, however, conclusive evidence that the efforts of scientific medicine and public health may not, at some future time, succeed in extending this span of human life beyond its present biologic limits.

Is the Prolongation of Life Possible?

The possibility of science leading to an increase in the span of life makes interesting speculation, but for the present we must look elsewhere for practical possibilities of prolonging life. Fortunately we need look only at the average length of human life today to see opportunities for improvement. While the gain in the average length of human life, or life expectancy at birth, has been enormous, it is apparently still on the increase (Fig. 1). That this increase will continue at its present rate much longer is improbable; for as the number of deaths of young persons approaches the minimum, gains become more difficult to attain and tend to be offset by increases in the deaths of older people.

Today the expectancy of life at birth of approximately 68 years is still 2 years short of the Biblical "three score and ten" and 20 years short of the age attained by approximately 15 per cent of our population. In 1908 Professor Irving Fisher of Yale University estimated that it should be possible to extend the average duration of life by at least 13 years. This much was realized in a quarter of a century. How much more is possible there is no way of knowing; but it is conservative to estimate that if people will make reasonable use of the scientific knowledge now available, not only will 5 to 10 years be added to the average length of life, but greater relative gains may be made in individual health and happiness.

Preventable Causes of Death

Since, theoretically at least, it should be possible to extend the life of the average individual, the specific question arises as to just how this can be accomplished. The answer requires definite information as to the diseases and conditions which in the main are responsible for destroying life before its biologic limit has been reached.

Mortality reports for the United States show that in 1952 the leading causes of death for all ages, in order of importance, were heart disease, cancer, apoplexy, accidents, diseases of early infancy and congenital malformations, influenza and pneumonia, arteriosclerosis, diabetes, tuberculosis, etc. At the beginning of the century the list of our favorite executioners was quite different, with tuberculosis in the lead and pneumonia, diarrhea and enteritis, and heart disease following in order (Table 3).

The shifts in the relative importance of these diseases have been the result primarily of two factors: first, the reduction of the communicable diseases of infancy and childhood; and, second, the increase in the average age of our population. Men and women who have escaped the hazards of infancy and childhood are entering upon a period of life when they are confronted by

TABLE 3
CHANGES IN THE LEADING CAUSES OF DEATH IN THE UNITED STATES SINCE 1900

1900		1952	
Cause of Death	Death Rate per 100,000 Population, All Ages	Cause of Death	Death Rate per 100,000 Population, All Ages
Tuberculosis................	194.4	Diseases of the heart........	351.3
Pneumonia.................	175.4	Cancer....................	143.9
Diarrhea and enteritis.......	139.9	Apoplexy*.................	108.9
Diseases of the heart.........	137.4	Accidents.................	63.2
Nephritis*.................	88.7	Diseases of early infancy and congenital malformations.	53.8
Diseases of early infancy and congenital malformations..	89.3	Influenza and pneumonia...	30.5
Apoplexy*..................	72.0	Arteriosclerosis*..........	20.0
Accidents.................	66.6	Diabetes mellitus..........	16.2
Cancer....................	64.0	Tuberculosis...............	16.1
Bronchitis.................	45.3	Nephritis*.................	13.3
Meningitis.................	40.6	Suicide....................	10.3
Diphtheria.................	40.3	Cirrhosis of liver..........	10.2
Typhoid fever..............	31.3	Hypertension without mention of heart.............	8.2
Influenza..................	26.7		
Paralysis..................	26.2	Ulcers of stomach and duodenum.................	5.8
Convulsions...............	24.4		
Diseases of stomach (exclusive of cancer)............	23.9	Gastritis and enteritis (diarrhea)...................	5.5
Peritonitis.................	13.8	Homicide.................	5.3
Diseases of pregnancy.......	13.4	Prostate enlargement.......	4.0
Measles...................	13.3	Syphilis...................	3.7
Syphilis...................	12.7	Poliomyelitis..............	2.1
Cirrhosis of liver...........	12.5	Bronchitis.................	1.8
		Appendicitis..............	1.7
		Diseases of pregnancy......	1.6

* "Apoplexy," also called "stroke," is the medical term for hemorrhage into the brain; "nephritis," also called "Bright's disease," for inflammation of the kidney; and "arteriosclerosis," for hardening of the arteries.

hazards of a different character. This change is introducing new problems.

Only two of the leading causes of death today are communicable, namely, tuberculosis and pneumonia. Of the entire group it is only these two which show a downward trend, and of the two the downward trend is by far the more rapid in tuberculosis, whose communicable character is considerably greater than that of pneumonia.

Most of the other leading causes of death—heart disease, cancer, apoplexy, arteriosclerosis, and nephritis—present a radically different public health problem from that of the communicable diseases, for these are degenerative diseases. They represent the disintegration of the individual's vital machinery before the insidious accumulation of the relatively minor injuries of previous illnesses, of hereditary factors, and of personal habits, the total effect of which is too great for the individual to withstand. Man is mortal, and though life is prolonged by evading acute illness, death must come, then, through some form of wearing out or degenerative process.

Individual Causes of Death. It has already been indicated that degenerative processes are chiefly involved in these leading causes of death. In only one, tuberculosis, is there a single causative agent specifically isolated and of communicable nature. Tuberculosis is now well understood, and there is a steady diminution in the number of deaths from it. Pneumonia, like tuberculosis, is a germ disease, but far less is known concerning it. There are a number of different germs which may cause pneumonia, and these produce diseases of varying severity and varying responses to treatment.

Of the remaining leading causes of death, accidents are a purely artificial and man-made hazard and by man can be reduced. Cancer is still largely a mystery.

There remain the heart diseases, apoplexy, arteriosclerosis, and nephritis. These represent to a large degree the breakdown of one vital system of the body, the circulatory or so-called "cardiovascular" system. Since it is weakened in many instances from birth by poor heredity, suffers throughout its entire existence from improper diets and from toxins produced by the infectious diseases, and is subjected to the demands which high-pressure modern living places upon it, it is small wonder that this system should break down and that it should come to occupy, as it has, a position of chief importance in present-day mortality. Diseases of early infancy and congenital malformations have decreased but with proper prenatal and obstetrical care can be reduced still more. Suicide should be preventable.

The Breakdown of Tissues. The various tissues of the body are continually defending themselves against injury, whether that injury be chemical, toxic, inflammatory, mechanical, or what not. In most cases this defense is adequate and the individual survives, but almost always the body is a little weaker afterward than it was before, because tissues which have been injured are replaced, not by the identical tissue which has been destroyed, but by scar tissue, by fibrous change.

It so happens that practically all the vital structures of the body are generously constructed, so that even though much of them be gradually replaced by nonfunctioning scar tissue, there will nevertheless be enough left to carry on life. For example, much of the lung, liver, or kidney tissue may be totally lost to the body and yet enough remain so that the functions of these organs may be adequately carried on.

Since these diseases represent to a large extent the terminal phase of a series of degenerative processes, it is obvious that they are amenable only to preventive measures and to such alterations in the hygiene of the individual as will permit him to live and function with a radically altered amount of vital tissue in his body. It becomes overwhelmingly apparent that for age to attempt to simulate youth is a folly which can have only one conceivable result—an early death. Some authors dismiss the whole subject fatalistically as nature's method of removing individuals no longer of biologic value, namely, individuals no longer capable of reproduction. The poet contemplates this gradual change of tissues from another standpoint:

> My candle burns at both its ends;
> It will not last the night;
> But ah, my foes, and oh, my friends.
> It gives a lovely light!
> —*Edna St. Vincent Millay.*[3]

Regardless of how the individual may react to his changing

[3] From "A Few Figs from Thistles," published by Harper & Brothers. Copyright, 1922, by Edna St. Vincent Millay.

physical capacities, they must be met. Much can be done to postpone degenerative processes, but this must come through the utilization of available scientific knowledge and not through the transplantation of "monkey glands," the consumption of vitamin capsules, or the adoption of health fads.

Health Hazards of Infancy and Childhood

What about the possibilities of preventing the deaths of children and young people, when the saving of life means so much more than it does to postpone for a short while the death of the aged? At no other period of life does the relative importance of the various diseases change so rapidly as in childhood. From 1 to 14 years of age, accidents, influenza and pneumonia, cancer, congenital malformation, poliomyelitis, and meningitis head the list. Ten years later in life, accidents, cancer, heart diseases, and tuberculosis are the leading killers (Table 4).

These major health problems of childhood and youth are for the most part acute conditions. Accidents are an unnecessary hazard and should be eliminated. Their continuance at the present high rate is disgraceful. Tuberculosis is no longer inevitable. Influenza, pneumonia, and meningitis usually can be cured if treated promptly and properly. Cancer and diseases of the heart present more difficult problems, but much can be done against them. Past gains have been greatest in the control of communicable diseases. Future progress will be more difficult but certainly is possible.

Causes of Illness and Disability

Just as desirable as the prolongation of life is the maintenance of health throughout life. All too frequently one's usefulness and joy of living are seriously impaired years before life is ended. The conditions and diseases chiefly responsible for disability and lowered vitality are well shown in a study by the U.S. Public Health Service of the illnesses in approximately 9,000 families in eighteen states over a period of 12 months. Altogether there were 39,185 individuals in these families, with an age distribution corresponding quite closely to that of the general population. When more

[16]

TABLE 4

LEADING CAUSES OF DEATH UNDER 45 YEARS OF AGE*

Age, Years	Cause of Death	Deaths	Death Rate†
Under 1‡	Certain diseases of early infancy..............	64,580	1924.5
	Congenital malformations.....................	14,590	435.3
	Influenza and pneumonia.....................	8,980	267.9
	Gastritis, enteritis, colitis§....................	4,120	122.9
	Accidents...................................	3,870	115.1
	Meningitis..................................	1,200	35.8
	Hernia and intestinal obstruction..............	1,000	29.8
	Bronchitis..................................	610	18.2
1–14	Accidents...................................	11,390	28.1
	Influenza and pneumonia.....................	3,560	8.8
	Cancer.....................................	3,180	7.8
	Congenital malformations.....................	2,560	6.5
	Poliomyelitis...............................	1,430	3.5
	Meningitis..................................	1,260	3.1
	Tuberculosis................................	950	2.3
	Rheumatic fever............................	450	1.1
15–24	Accidents...................................	12,860	60.9
	Cancer.....................................	1,910	9.1
	Heart diseases..............................	1,320	6.3
	Tuberculosis................................	1,290	6.1
	Homicide...................................	1,270	6.0
	Suicide.....................................	880	4.2
	Pregnancy and childbirth.....................	700	3.3
	Poliomyelitis...............................	660	3.1
25–34	Accidents...................................	12,360	51.7
	Heart diseases..............................	4,690	19.6
	Cancer.....................................	4,600	19.2
	Tuberculosis................................	2,650	11.1
	Homicide...................................	2,480	10.4
	Suicide.....................................	1,950	8.2
	Pregnancy and childbirth.....................	1,200	5.0
	Influenza and pneumonia.....................	1,140	4.8
35–44	Heart diseases..............................	18,920	85.7
	Cancer.....................................	13,700	62.1
	Accidents...................................	11,090	50.2
	Apoplexy...................................	3,900	17.7
	Tuberculosis................................	3,640	16.5
	Suicide.....................................	2,780	12.6
	Cirrhosis of liver...........................	2,240	10.1
	Homicide...................................	1,980	9.0

* For rates of higher age groups see Table 26.
† Estimated rates per 100,000 population in each age group for the United States as a whole in 1952.
‡ Note that the deaths for this age group are for a single year; the next group for a 14-year period and subsequent groups for 10-year periods.
§ Formerly called diarrhea and enteritis.

[17]

FIG. 2. TOTAL ANNUAL INCIDENCE OF SPECIFIC CONDITIONS IN 8,758 SURVEYED FAMILIES IN 18 STATES

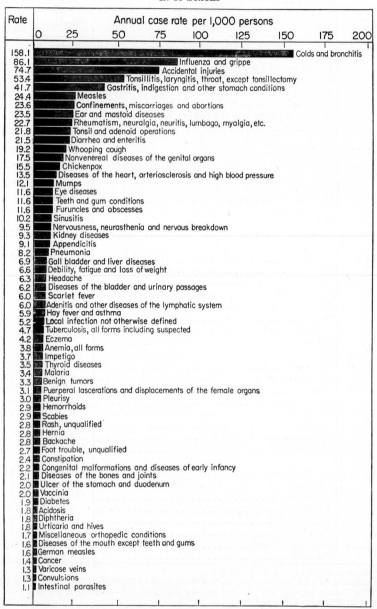

Rate	Annual case rate per 1,000 persons
	0 25 50 75 100 125 150 175 200
158.1	Colds and bronchitis
86.1	Influenza and grippe
74.7	Accidental injuries
53.4	Tonsillitis, laryngitis, throat, except tonsillectomy
41.7	Gastritis, indigestion and other stomach conditions
24.4	Measles
23.6	Confinements, miscarriages and abortions
23.5	Ear and mastoid diseases
22.7	Rheumatism, neuralgia, neuritis, lumbago, myalgia, etc.
21.8	Tonsil and adenoid operations
21.5	Diarrhea and enteritis
19.2	Whooping cough
17.5	Nonvenereal diseases of the genital organs
15.5	Chickenpox
13.5	Diseases of the heart, arteriosclerosis and high blood pressure
12.1	Mumps
11.6	Eye diseases
11.6	Teeth and gum conditions
11.6	Furuncles and abscesses
10.2	Sinusitis
9.5	Nervousness, neurasthenia and nervous breakdown
9.3	Kidney diseases
9.1	Appendicitis
8.2	Pneumonia
6.9	Gall bladder and liver diseases
6.6	Debility, fatigue and loss of weight
6.3	Headache
6.2	Diseases of the bladder and urinary passages
6.0	Scarlet fever
6.0	Adenitis and other diseases of the lymphatic system
5.9	Hay fever and asthma
5.2	Local infection not otherwise defined
4.7	Tuberculosis, all forms including suspected
4.2	Eczema
3.8	Anemia, all forms
3.7	Impetigo
3.5	Thyroid diseases
3.4	Malaria
3.3	Benign tumors
3.1	Puerperal lacerations and displacements of the female organs
3.0	Pleurisy
2.9	Hemorrhoids
2.9	Scabies
2.8	Rash, unqualified
2.8	Hernia
2.8	Backache
2.7	Foot trouble, unqualified
2.4	Constipation
2.2	Congenital malformations and diseases of early infancy
2.1	Diseases of the bones and joints
2.0	Ulcer of the stomach and duodenum
2.0	Vaccinia
1.9	Diabetes
1.8	Acidosis
1.8	Diphtheria
1.8	Urticaria and hives
1.7	Miscellaneous orthopedic conditions
1.6	Diseases of the mouth except teeth and gums
1.6	German measles
1.4	Cancer
1.3	Varicose veins
1.3	Convulsions
1.1	Intestinal parasites

(*Collins, S. D., "Causes of Illness in 9,000 Families. Based on Nation-wide Periodic Canvasses, 1928–1931," Public Health Reports, vol. 48, p. 283, Mar. 24, 1933.*)

than one diagnosis was reported for an illness, the one which seemed of major importance was considered the primary cause of the illness. Figure 2 shows the relative frequence of the illnesses, mild or severe, which were reported. Further tabulations which show bed confinement and loss of time from work indicate practically the same relative importance of the various illnesses as is shown in this figure.

From this as well as numerous other studies it is apparent that most of the illnesses, minor as well as disabling, from which people suffer are colds, bronchitis, influenza, tonsillitis, and other acute infections of the upper respiratory tract. Clearly these constitute a major health problem of today. The present status of our knowledge concerning these illnesses and the possibilities of reducing them will be considered in a subsequent chapter.

Accidents are a major cause of disability as well as of death. "Stomach disorders" rank as the fifth cause of illness. Although many of the conditions included under this term are of minor importance as far as mortality is concerned, others are the first warnings of serious disease. The significance, prevention, and correction of these disorders will be considered. Of the other illnesses reported, some are caused by specific infections, others by abnormal physiological processes. Still others are the direct result of unhygienic living. It is within our power to prevent or reduce most of these.

Lowered Vitality and Physical Efficiency

Records of death and illness are the best index we have of individual and community health, but they do not tell the entire story. There are many people who are not disabled and could not be classed as ill but whose physical efficiency is lowered and whose joy of living is seriously impaired by fatigue, nervous exhaustion, irritability, emotional frustration, defective vision, impaired hearing, or other physical or emotional handicaps. In a study of employed and unemployed workers, conducted by the Employment Research Stabilization Institute of the University of Minnesota, it was found that a close relation existed between the physical condition and the employment status of professional men and women, clerical workers, and skilled and unskilled laborers. These individuals either were employed or were applicants for employment and considered themselves in at least reasonably good health. In spite of this there was not only a definite relationship between employment status and physical handicaps but also a surprisingly high incidence of correctible physical handicaps among the employed as well as the unemployed groups.

The Health of Our Armed Forces

In times of war vigorous physical health both of the armed forces and of the supporting civilian population is of vital importance. Physical weaklings and the physically handicapped are liabilities to combat forces. Campaigns and even wars have been lost as a result of the ravages of disease.

Among our own armed forces reports show a remarkably low incidence of illness during the Second World War and the war in Korea. For the first time in history during the mobilization of troops no serious epidemics of disease occurred in the training camps.

This is a splendid record, but reports of the physical examinations under the Selective Training and Service Act present a different picture. During the war in Korea the rejection rate was 35 per cent, with ranges for the different states from lows of 19 per cent in Kansas, 20 per cent in North Dakota, and 21 per cent in Minnesota to highs of 52 per cent in Georgia, 54 per cent in Louisiana, 55 per cent in Mississippi, and 61 per cent in South Carolina.

An analysis of the conditions responsible for these rejections shows that they include mental deficiencies of various types as well as failure to meet minimum intelligence standards; also that many of the physical defects listed are not serious and are of little, if any, handicap in civilian life. In interpreting the results of examinations for military service it must be kept in mind that the purpose of these examinations is to select young men who can be trained for military combat under grueling conditions. Furthermore, standards for acceptance for service change in relation to the urgency of the need for manpower. It was said that in the early days of the Second World War only those in perfect physical condition were accepted, but that toward the end of the war anyone who could tell night from day and had two teeth that matched was "in."

Table 5 shows the causes of rejection for military service during the first year of the war in Korea. Commenting on the large percentage of young men unfit for military service, Major General Lewis B. Hershey, Director of Selective Service, stated: "This is indicative of a general physical condition of this country's youth, of which we nationally should be thoroughly ashamed."

Although an analysis of the causes of rejection for military service shows that many are little, if any, handicap to a normal civilian life and that others are conditions which medical science does not know how to prevent or to correct, there is still sufficient truth in General Hershey's statement to make every loyal American resolve, in the interest of national strength, to do everything possible to improve the health and efficiency of our youth.

During the Second World War and the war in Korea our Army and Navy health and medical records were such as would not have been believed possible a few years ago. Troops lived and fought in areas of the world previously considered uninhabitable for white men. They were able to do this because new insecticide sprays, new antimalarial drugs, and modern sanitary engineering methods prevented the malaria which previously had infected every human in the area; because vaccines and DDT protected them against typhus fever which had always before accompanied the devastation of major wars; because modern methods of food processing, food sanitation, and transportation assured adequate and safe nutrition from the arctic to the tropics; because new vaccines and new drugs, such as the sulfonamides and the antibiotics, helped to prevent and combat infections and infectious diseases; and because blood plasma and whole blood were flown to the battlefields in the most remote corners of the globe.

The result of these improved health programs was less illness among our military forces than ever before. During the First World War there were 852 hospital admissions per 1,000 troops per year. This was the best record ever attained. Yet in the

TABLE 5

MEDICAL CAUSES OF REJECTION OF SELECTIVE-SERVICE REGISTRANTS, JULY, 1950 TO JUNE, 1951

Principal Disqualifying Defect	Number Disqualified	Per Cent
Total	245,358	100.0
Psychiatric disorders	30,322	12.4
Psychosis	1,475	0.6
Psychoneurotic disorders	15,571	6.4
Mental deficiency	328	0.1
Character and behavior disorders	12,948	5.3
Neurological diseases	5,900	2.4
Epilepsy	2,622	1.1
Other neurological diseases	3,278	1.3
Infective and parasitic diseases	8,031	3.3
Tuberculosis	4,425	1.8
Venereal diseases	164	0.1
Other infective and parasitic diseases	3,442	1.4
Neoplasms	6,064	2.5
Malignant neoplasms	164	0.1
Nonmalignant neoplasms	5,572	2.3
Other neoplasms	328	.1
Allergic diseases	13,112	5.3
Asthma	12,292	5.0
Other allergic diseases	820	0.3
Endocrine system diseases	4,098	1.7
Diabetes mellitus	1,803	0.7
Other endocrine system diseases	2,295	1.0
Metabolic and nutritional diseases	328	0.1
Blood and blood-forming organic diseases	328	0.1
Eye defects	19,504	8.0
Defective vision	12,784	5.2
Inflammatory and other eye defects	6,720	2.8

TABLE 5 (*Continued*)

Principal Disqualifying Defect	Number Disqualified	Per Cent
Ear and mastoid process diseases......................	15,734	6.4
Defective hearing.....................................	1,967	0.8
Otitis media, with or without impaired hearing..........	12,292	5.0
Inflammatory and other diseases of the ear and mastoid process..	1,475	0.6
Circulatory system diseases............................	39,172	16.0
Rheumatic fever......................................	656	0.3
Heart diseases, organic and valvular...................	19,832	8.1
Heart disease, functional.............................	3,278	1.3
Hypertensive diseases................................	13,112	5.4
Other diseases of the circulatory system...............	2,294	0.9
Respiratory system diseases...........................	3,278	1.3
Digestive system......................................	27,043	11.0
Insufficient serviceable teeth.........................	7,867	3.2
Other teeth and supporting-structure diseases...........	1,475	0.6
Hernia of the abdominal cavity.......................	13,276	5.4
Other diseases of the digestive system.................	4,425	1.8
Genitourinary-system and breast diseases............	2,294	0.9
Skin and cellular-tissue diseases.......................	5,245	2.1
Bones and organs of movement diseases and defects........	34,583	14.1
Arthritis...	1,475	0.6
Ankylosis..	1,147	0.5
Limitation of motion.................................	2,622	1.1
Musculoskeletal diseases.............................	11,473	4.7
Flatfoot...	5,409	2.2
Deformities..	10,654	4.3
Amputations of extremities...........................	1,803	0.7
Congenital malformations.............................	10,490	4.3
Miscellaneous diseases and defects.....................	19,832	8.1
Failure to meet height and weight standards.............	6,884	2.8
Other miscellaneous diseases and defects................	12,948	5.3

Second World War it was further reduced to 588 and in the Korean War to 468 per 1,000.

In medical care, too, the record was unbelievable, for only 4.5 per cent of the wounded men who received medical care died during the Second World War as compared to 8.0 per cent during the First World War. During the war in Korea this was further reduced to 2.3 per cent, yet the weapons of warfare were the most destructive and deadly ever known.

These excellent results are due, according to the Surgeon Generals of our armed forces, not alone to new scientific discoveries but even more to the excellent quality of the professional medical service which was available to the wounded. This service extended from the beachheads and battlefields through emergency dressing stations and field hospitals to the large general hospitals where long-time definitive treatment was received. This high quality of medical care in turn was due to the excellence of medical education and hospital training in this country and was rendered by the same physicians who in peacetime serve our civilian population.

DISCUSSION SUGGESTIONS

1. Discuss the more important reasons for the great increase which has occurred in the average length of life over the past several centuries.
2. Why has it been possible for the average length of life to increase so greatly even though the span of life has remained unchanged?
3. Has the life expectancy of persons above 50 years of age increased? Give reasons.
4. Discuss the reasons for the differences in the average life expectancy in different parts of this country.
5. Can one expect that the mortality rate will continue to decline much longer? Discuss.
6. It has been said that public health work interferes with natural processes for improving the race. Is there any justification for this opinion?
7. At what ages are the peaks of physical and intellectual achievement reached?
8. Discuss the reasons for the changes which have occurred in the leading causes of death in the United States over the past 50 years.
9. What relation do the infectious and degenerative diseases have to the length of life?

10. What is your own life expectancy and the life expectancy of the other members of your family?
11. What are the chief causes of death in your age group and in the age groups of the other members of your family?
12. Discuss the reasons for the differences in morbidity and mortality. Which gives the more accurate picture of the health problems of a community? Why?
13. What are the more common physical defects discovered in physical examinations?
14. What possibility is there of increasing still more the average length of life? Of increasing the length of life of a particular individual?
15. What are the major causes of rejection for military service?

REFERENCES AND READING SUGGESTIONS

1. Cohn, Alfred E., and Claire Lingg: "The Burden of Diseases in the United States," Oxford University Press, New York, 1950.
2. Collins, S. S.: "Trends in Illness and Mortality," *Public Health Reports*, vol. 67, p. 487, May, 1952.
3. Dickinson, F. G., and E. L. Walker: "Mortality Trends in the United States, 1900–49," American Medical Association, Chicago, 1952.
4. Dublin, Louis I.: "The Facts of Life from Birth to Death," The Macmillan Company, New York, 1951.
5. ———, A. J. Lotka, and Mortimer Spiegelman: "Length of Life: A Study of the Life Table," rev. ed., The Ronald Press Company, New York, 1949.
6. Galdston, Iago, ed.: "The Epidemiology of Health," Health Education Council, New York, 1953.
7. Lehman, H. C.: "Age and Achievement," Princeton University Press, Princeton, N.J., 1953.
8. Maxcy, K. F., ed.: "Rosenau's Preventive Medicine and Hygiene," 7th ed., Appleton-Century-Crofts, Inc., New York, 1951.
9. Newsholm, H.: "Story of Modern Medicine," The Williams & Wilkins Company, Baltimore, 1929.
10. Spiegelman, Mortimer: "Our Increasing Longevity and What It Means," *Analysts Journal*, May, 1952.
11. Wiehl, Dorothy G.: "Mortality and Social-Environmental Factors," *Milbank Memorial Fund Quarterly*, vol. 26, p. 335, October, 1948.
12. Committee on Interstate and Foreign Commerce: "Health Inquiry. The Toll of Our Major Diseases; Their Causes, Prevention and Control. Preliminary Report." Government Printing Office, Washington, D.C.

Chapter II

MAJOR HEALTH PROBLEMS

IN PLANNING a campaign, the military strategist surveys the
entire field of action, appraises its strong points and its weaknesses, and then concentrates his efforts where the dangers seem
greatest and the possibilities of success brightest. Tables 3 to 7
give us a composite view of our major health problems. As shown
by Table 4, these change with age and, as shown in Table 6, they
are of various degrees of importance in cutting short life expectancy and in reducing working years. Let us examine these
and then direct our attention to those conditions which offer the
greatest possibilities of improvement.

Accidents

The importance of accidents as a preventable cause of death
and disability demands that they be given first place in the consideration of our specific health problems. In 1952 one person
in the United States was injured accidentally every $3\frac{1}{3}$ seconds
—9,600,000 persons in all. Of these, 300,000 were permanently
disabled and an accidental death occurred approximately every
$5\frac{1}{2}$ minutes. The total economic loss from these accidents is
estimated as $8,700,000,000. The 96,000 deaths in this one year
exceeded the number of combat fatalities in the U.S. Army in
any of the wars in which this country has engaged, except for
the Civil War and the Second World War. During the Revolu-

tionary War, 4,044 American soldiers were killed or died from
wounds; during the War of 1812, 1,956; during the Mexican
War, 1,549; during the Civil War, 114,757 among the Northern
armies and 95,000 among the Southern forces; during the
Spanish-American War, 1,443; and during the First World War,
51,259. In the Second World War, which lasted for almost four
years, 237,049 combat deaths occurred among all of our armed
forces. During the invasion of France the number killed and

TABLE 6

AVERAGE AGE AT DEATH, AVERAGE LIFE YEARS LOST, AND WORKING YEARS LOST
PER DEATH FROM EACH OF SEVEN LEADING CAUSES IN 1945*

	Heart Disease	Cancer	Apoplexy	Accidents	Nephritis	Pneumonia	Tuberculosis
White Males:							
Average age at death	66.6	64.7	69.6	43.3	67.8	48.8	49.3
Average life years lost	13.5	14.4	12.0	30.6	13.5	27.9	24.4
Average working years lost	4.1	4.8	2.8	19.9	4.3	14.7	14.7
White Females:							
Average age at death	70.9	62.6	70.9	55.9	68.8	49.9	42.1
Average life years lost	13.3	17.8	13.1	26.1	14.8	30.8	33.9
Average working years lost	3.0	6.5	2.7	13.5	4.3	15.6	21.8

* Dickinson, Frank G., and E. L. Walker, *Bulletin* 64, Bureau of Medical Economic Research, American Medical Association, Chicago, 1948.

wounded was very large. Yet, the total casualties during the first
10 days of the Normandy invasion were less than the number of
casualties from automobile accidents for an average 10-day
period in 1952. In the three years of rugged fighting in Korea
33,660 Americans were killed or died from wounds, a little more
than one-third the number killed by accidents in 1952.

Home Accidents. Accidents are of major importance at all
ages but, relatively at least, they take their greatest toll of life in
childhood, ranking as the first cause of death in every age group
from 1 to 35 years of age. Most accidents to children occur in or
about the home and are due to carelessness or poor housekeeping.
In 1952, 29,000 people lost their lives in home accidents, 125,000
were permanently disabled, and 4,200,000 were less seriously

[27]

injured. Approximately 50 per cent of these fatalities were the result of falls; 18 per cent, of burns; 5 per cent, of suffocation; 4 per cent, of poisoning; 3 per cent each from gas and from fire-arms; and 17 per cent, of various other causes. Of fatal falls, 39 per cent occur on the stairs; 19 per cent, in the yard; 18 per cent, in the kitchen; 7 per cent, in bedrooms; 7 per cent, on the porch; and 6 per cent, in the basement.

TABLE 7

DEATH RATES FROM CERTAIN CAUSES BY AGE GROUPS
(Per 100,000 population, United States, 1952)

Age, Years	Acci- dents	Tuber- culosis	Pneu- monia	Heart Disease	Cancer	Diabetes	Suicide
Under 1	115.5	6.9	244.0	9.5	8.9	0.9	0
1–14	28.1	2.3	7.7	1.1	7.8	0.4	0
15–24	60.9	6.1	2.5	6.3	9.1	1.1	4.2
25–34	51.7	11.1	4.3	19.6	19.2	1.8	8.2
35–44	50.2	16.3	7.8	85.7	62.1	3.6	12.6
45–54	56.8	27.5	17.1	293.2	172.4	12.7	18.6
55–64	72.5	34.3	32.8	783.0	407.8	43.8	23.5
65–74	113.7	50.6	75.2	1763.1	703.3	95.2	29.5
75–84	304.8	50.0	227.9	4218.2	1157.4	163.4	27.4
85 and over	829.2	51.2	671.6	8144.3	1431.5	148.7	32.4
All ages	63.2	16.2	26.6	351.3	143.9	16.2	10.3

Material reduction of these various types of home accidents can be accomplished if people will take the following precautions:

1. Provide adequate lighting and hand rails for stairways and use stepladders for reaching objects beyond their grasp.

2. Avoid the storage of objects on stairways and the accumulation of ice and snow on porches and steps.

3. Guard against slippery floors, loose rugs, and toys on the floor.

4. Be certain that electric cords are kept in good condition and that electric fans and heaters are adequately protected.

5. Avoid the use of inflammable cleaning fluids indoors.

6. Keep knives, garden tools, broken glass, boiling water, open fires, matches, and medicines out of the reach of children.

7. Be certain that poisons are kept in distinctly marked containers.

8. Be careful of doors that stand ajar and of blind swinging doors.

9. Guard against gas stoves or plates with leaky or rubber tubing.

10. Do not smoke in bed or start automobiles in the garage with the doors closed.

FIG. 3. TREND IN ACCIDENTAL DEATHS, 1911–1950
(Exclusive of deaths from enemy action)

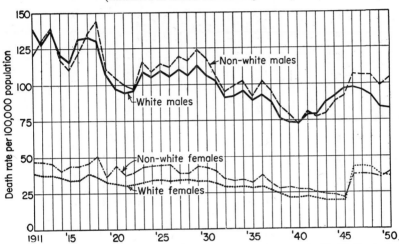

(*Data from National Office of Vital Statistics, United States Public Health Service.*)

It seems almost trite to enumerate such commonplace and homely precautions, but carelessness in regard to them was responsible for most of the fatal and nonfatal home accidents each year.

Industrial Accidents. Industrial or occupational accidents were responsible for 15,000 deaths in 1952. This is far too many, but it represents a vast improvement over the 35,000 deaths from this cause in 1913. One of the nation's large industries reported in 1952 that its employees had worked 28,132,583 consecutive man-hours without a disabling injury. Had their accident rate been that of American industry in general, they would

[29]

Fig. 4. Accidental Deaths by Color, Sex, and Age

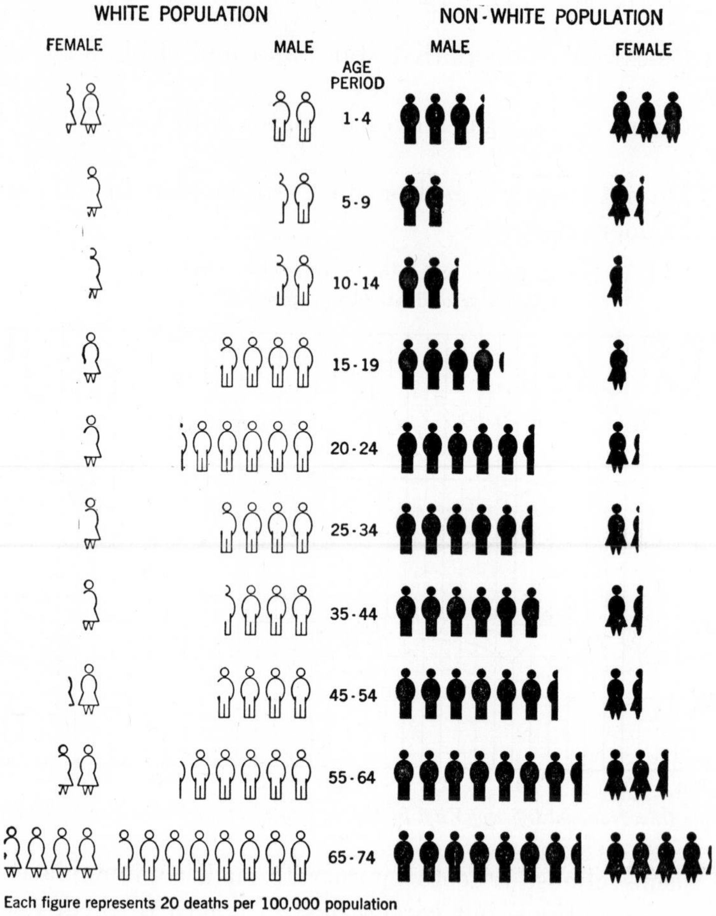

Each figure represents 20 deaths per 100,000 population

Averages of annual death rates per 100,000 persons by color, sex, and age. Ages 1 to 74 years. (*Data from National Office of Vital Statistics.*)

have had 55 disabling injuries. In 1907, 4,500 railroad employees and 610 passengers were killed in accidents. In 1952 this total was reduced to 384 employees and 14 passengers. In 1943, 115 passengers were killed and 316 injured in two railroad accidents, both of which were reported to have been preventable.[1]

[1] Brecher, Ruth, and Edward Brecher, "These Railroad Accidents," *Harper's Magazine*, June, 1944.

[30   ]

Such marked reduction in occupational accidents is the result not of chance but of an organized effort on the part of most of the larger and some of the smaller industries. In many states the passage of industrial compensation laws has given effective impetus to the prevention of industrial accidents. Many companies and corporations have made their plants such safe places to work, and have instructed their employees so well in safety measures,

Fig. 5. Trends in Deaths from Automobile Accidents

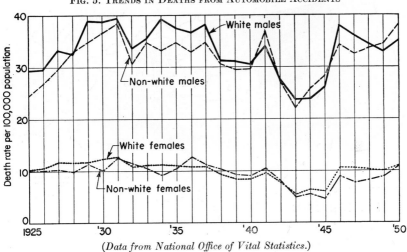

(*Data from National Office of Vital Statistics.*)

that their accident records are almost perfect. Unfortunately, there are still thousands of small and medium-sized plants all over the country that make little or no effort to prevent accidents to their employees and so as a group have disgraceful accident rates (see also page 201).

Automobile Accidents. The development of the modern automobile has introduced the most serious accident problem of all time; in fact, the increase in automobile accidents has more than offset the gain made by the reduction of industrial accidents. During 1952, 38,000 deaths were due to motor vehicle accidents and 1,350,000 persons were injured severely enough to be disabled beyond the day of the accident.

The importance of this problem can be better comprehended

when we realize that, if the present rate of slaughter continues, one out of every twenty-five persons in the United States will be injured or killed in a motor vehicle accident within the next 5 years. An even more startling prophecy is that unless some drastic means of combating traffic accidents is instituted, two out of

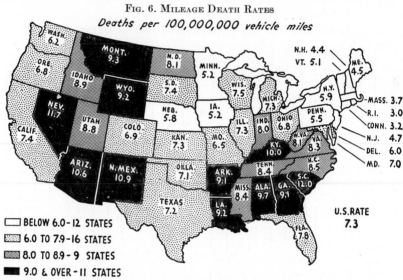

FIG. 6. MILEAGE DEATH RATES

Deaths per 100,000,000 vehicle miles

☐ BELOW 6.0 - 12 STATES
▨ 6.0 TO 7.9 - 16 STATES
▦ 8.0 TO 8.9 - 9 STATES
■ 9.0 & OVER - 11 STATES

Data for 1952. Deaths per 100 million vehicle miles. (*Courtesy National Safety Council, Chicago, Ill.*)

every three children under ten years of age now living will be injured in a motor vehicle accident in their lifetime.

According to the National Safety Council almost 18 per cent of drivers and 26 per cent of adult pedestrians involved in fatal accidents had been drinking. Alcohol dulls the senses, interferes with judgment, slows reactions, and reduces muscular control. Clearly, one who has been drinking does not belong behind the wheel of an automobile (see also page 201).

Exceeding the speed limit or driving too fast for existing conditions was reported in one out of three fatal accidents. Unsafe driving practices of other kinds, such as passing on a hill or curve, driving on the wrong side of the road, changing a tire on a high-way, failure to yield the right of way, turning without proper signal, etc., were factors in approximately half the fatal accidents.

Occasionally, a mechanical defect of the car or a blowout of a tire results in an accident. Physical defects of the driver, obstructions to vision, bad weather or road conditions, and unsafe pedestrian acts, such as crossing between intersections, are also important factors in many accidents. Important also is the fact that almost two-thirds of fatal accidents occur after dark. Accident rates for drivers 16 to 20 years of age are five times as high as for drivers 45 to 50 years old.

Passenger-miles flown by commercial airlines in the United States during 1952 are reported to have had a passenger death rate of 0.35 per 100,000,000 miles. This is about one-eighth the death rate from automobile traffic accidents computed on a passenger mileage basis.

That many automobile accidents can be prevented by community action is evidenced by the following facts:

In one group of cities, each with a million or more population, one city has a traffic accident record of 16.8 fatalities per 100,000 population, while another city in the same group has a loss ratio of 37. In another group of cities each with a population of 250,000 to 500,000, one city has a record of 7.8 fatalities per 100,000 population, and another has a loss ratio of 32. Or again, in a group of cities, each with a population of 100,000 to 250,000, one city has a record of 6.1 fatalities per 100,000 population, while another has a loss ratio of 46.

Must we admit, then, that we do not sufficiently *want* to save lives? The real trouble is that old weakness of the human creature. . . . He is not only ignorant and stupid, but a fatalist and entirely reckless of accidents. Sometimes he seems to grow quite mad when he gets into the seat of a powerful machine capable of doing 100 miles an hour. He is lawless, too, when the public welfare interferes with his personal desires. We are extremely fortunate, therefore, that our accident records of highway disasters show that, after all, only a small percentage of all motor vehicle drivers cause the very great majority of all the accidents. There is in traffic deaths and injuries the same "accident prone" type of person that we have found in industry and in transportation.[2]

[2] Rohweder, A. V., "What Shall We Do about Accidents?" address delivered at the Conference of State and Provincial Health Authorities of North America, Washington, D.C., 1937.

[33]

Drowning

In 1952, 6,800 persons died by drowning in the United States. The great majority of these were young people, with the largest number (1,600) 15 to 25 years of age and the next largest (1,350) 5 to 14 years old. This is a terrific toll of young people, particularly from a cause of death that one can so easily avoid. In fact, following the American Red Cross "Ten Tips on Water Safety" would save most of these lives:

1. Learn to swim before you go beyond your depth, either in the water or in a canoe or small boat.
2. Limit your stay in the water.
3. Make sure the water is deep enough and free of obstruction before attempting to dive.
4. Stay out of the water when you are overheated or overtired.
5. Wait about one and one-half hours after eating a meal before going in the water.
6. Learn how to swim with a qualified instructor.
7. Avoid long swims after a season of inactivity; train gradually.
8. Take a boat along for distance swimming.
9. Every swimmer needs a water buddy to help him, or to give the alarm in case of accident. Don't swim alone.
10. The back-pressure arm-lift method is a most effective means of reviving a drowning person Do not wait for a doctor or machine—go to work at once.

Tuberculosis

Tuberculosis, long called the "captain of the men of death," is classed today as a preventable disease. It has been pointed out that, of the leading causes of death, the tuberculosis rate is falling most rapidly. When it is recalled that for many years tuberculosis was the leading cause of death, this drop to approximately one-tenth of the rate at the beginning of this century becomes impressive. The change came in response to improved standards of living, to a definite plan of attack on the disease, to an extensive educational campaign for its prevention, and to other factors (see Tables 3, 4, 6, 7, and Figs. 7 and 8).

If the death rate of 1900 had prevailed in 1952, not 25,000 but 300,000 persons in this country would have died from tuberculosis. This miraculous improvement suggests that tuberculosis is rapidly becoming an unimportant disease. Unfortunately, this is not true, for the number of new cases is declining very slowly and the number of known cases is showing some increase. In 1952 a total of 109,837 new cases of tuberculosis was reported in the United States, of which 85,807 were active or probably

FIG. 7. TUBERCULOSIS DEATH RATES AMONG WHITES AND NONWHITES IN THE UNITED STATES, 1910–1950

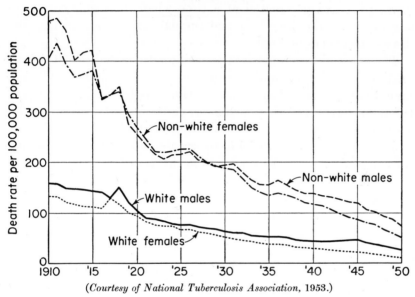

(*Courtesy of National Tuberculosis Association,* 1953.)

active. It is estimated that approximately half a million persons in the United States have active tuberculosis.

In recent years a number of significant changes have come about in the occurrence of tuberculosis. It is no longer a disease which takes its toll primarily among young adults, particularly women. In 1924 the median age at death was 33; in 1934, 38; in 1944, 43; and in 1950, 50 years. Today more than half the deaths from tuberculosis are of men 40 years of age and older. Death rates are highest also among persons of poor social-economic status. The tuberculosis death rate among patients in mental institutions is nineteen times the rate among the general population.

[35]

A few years ago we believed and taught that by the age of 20 practically everyone was infected with tuberculosis. Today we know that this is not true; according to examination of college and university students by the thousands, approximately four out of five have had no infection with tuberculosis whatsoever. By means of these examinations we also determine whether or not those who have been infected have active disease. If they have, they can be treated at a time when their chances of recovery are of the very best and the danger of transmitting the disease to others negligible.

The cause of tuberculosis is a specific germ called the "tubercle bacillus," the bovine and the human strains of which may infect man. Some years ago milk was a serious mode of transmission of the bovine strain of this bacillus to children, but with the widespread adoption of the pasteurization of milk and the effective program for the eradication of tuberculosis among cattle, bovine infection of man has become rare in this country.

In the control of human tuberculosis, unfortunately, we have made much less progress than the veterinarians have made in the control of the disease among animals. Yet all of the scientific information necessary eventually to eradicate this disease is available. All that we need to do is to apply it.

We know, for example, that a person who becomes infected has taken into his body, usually through inhalation, living tubercle bacilli and that these tubercle bacilli have been discharged relatively recently, usually by means of coughing, from the body of someone else. Hence, if we can discover the individuals who are disseminating tubercle bacilli and can isolate or treat them so that they will be no longer infectious, the chain of continuing infection will be broken.

That raises the question as to how the disseminators of infection can be identified. This can be accomplished in two ways. One is by the widespread use of the tuberculin test to determine what individuals have been infected. This test is usually performed by the injection into the skin of the forearm of a minute amount of tuberculin—the so-called "Mantoux test." If the area of injection becomes red, it indicates that the person has been infected at some time or other with tubercle bacilli. This infection may be active at the time or it may have occurred long ago and be completely healed; in fact, it may have been overcome without ever gaining any real foothold in the body. The Mantoux

FIG. 8. TUBERCULOSIS DEATH RATES AMONG WHITE AND NONWHITE MALES AND FEMALES BY AGE IN THE UNITED STATES, 1950

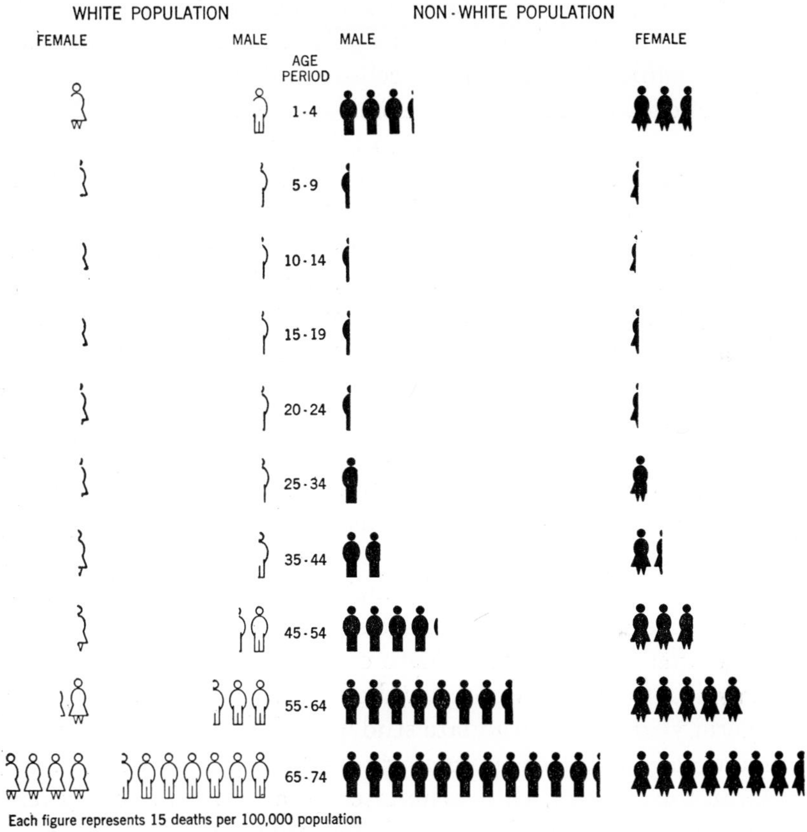

Each figure represents 15 deaths per 100,000 population

(*Courtesy of National Tuberculosis Association, 1953.*)

test does not distinguish between an active, a quiescent, and a healed infection.

The next step, obviously, is to have a more thorough examination of those individuals who react to the tuberculin test. This requires, first of all, an x-ray of the chest and then a careful appraisal of x-ray findings and physical condition by a physician. Most of those who react to tuberculin show no evidence of active tuberculosis; some show findings which make frequent reexamination desirable; and a few are found to have definitely active disease. These are either infectious or potentially infectious and should be treated as such.

Most colleges and universities now include tuberculin tests and/or chest x-rays of students as a part of their routine entrance physical examinations. This procedure is discovering each year in the colleges of this country some students who would have been active sources of infection to others if these tests had not been performed. An example of what can happen if students with active tuberculosis live in close association with other students is contained in the following reports of actual occurrences:

In early February a few years ago, a young man reported to the Students' Health Service for examination. He was found to have extensive pulmonary tuberculosis involving both lungs. Tubercle bacilli were abundantly present in the sputum. He stated that he would go to his home physician immediately to arrange for treatment. Instead of doing so he continued in the university until the school year ended in June. These facts did not come to light until eight months later, when another young man reported for examination because of recent symptoms and was found to have active pulmonary tuberculosis. There had never been any clinical tuberculosis in his family, but the year before he had been the roommate of the first student, who had advanced disease and who later died of tuberculosis.

Several years ago a graduate student in her thirties was found to have far advanced pulmonary tuberculosis with tubercle bacilli in the sputum. Her roommate was examined but physical and x-ray film examinations revealed no evidence of disease. Five years later this roommate showed evidence of tuberculosis in the right lung. The following year, she had extensive disease with cavity formation.

Dr. Stiehm of the University of Wisconsin has reported the case of a girl who in her senior year lived in a sorority house. She had had a persistent cough for three months before she consulted a physician. Examination revealed evidence of far advanced pulmonary tuberculosis and her sputum contained large numbers of tubercle bacilli. Of fifteen sorority sisters who were given the tuberculin tests, eleven had been found negative to the test on entrance examinations or in high school. All of these girls after exposure to this sorority sister reacted positively to the test. Of the remaining four girls who had not previously been tested, three now reacted positively to the test. The only one who was negative had lived in the sorority house only two weeks.

Nine students of the University of North Dakota died from tuberculosis within 10 years after they had lived in a fraternity house with another student who had an active case of this disease.

Tragedies such as these rarely occur today but they could be repeated if active tuberculosis is not discovered in even an occasional college student who lives in close association with other students.

The tuberculin test is a valuable procedure to determine whether or not an individual has been infected with tuberculosis. If the original test indicates that the person has not been infected, the test should be repeated periodically, preferably each year if the person seems well, and whenever he exhibits any symptoms which suggest the possibility of tuberculous infection. If the Mantoux test is positive, indicating past infection, but the x-ray and physical examination show no evidence of active disease, the test does not need to be repeated because in all probability it will continue to be positive, but an x-ray examination of the chest should be made periodically to see if there is evidence of the infection becoming active. One might ask why not wait until symptoms suggestive of tuberculosis occur. The answer is that evidences of beginning activity of a tuberculous infection of the lungs may be seen in an x-ray plate $2\frac{1}{2}$ years, on the average, before symptoms appear, and by the time that recognizable symptoms bring the patient to the physician 85 per cent of cases are moderately or far advanced. Since the results of treatment of tuberculosis depend to a great extent upon the stage at which treatment is begun, these months of delay may be of vital importance in determining the final outcome of the disease. X-ray examinations of men for military service in the Second World War led to the discovery of more than 100,000 cases of tuberculosis.

Some patients with early active tuberculosis can be successfully treated at home but most persons with tuberculosis should be treated in a tuberculosis hospital. Rest and good food, together with the use of antituberculosis drugs and in some instances a temporary collapse of the infected lung so as to put it at complete rest, make it possible for certain patients to be satisfactorily treated at home. However, those patients who can be treated at home should be under careful medical and nursing supervision.

Collapse of the lung is accomplished by the introduction of air into the pleural cavity, called artificial pneumothorax, or into the abdominal cavity, pneumoperitoneum. This air is gradually absorbed by the tissues and so must be replaced periodically until the lung has become sufficiently healed to permit it to function normally again.

Patients with more advanced disease, and particularly those who are infectious to others, need hospital care. Some of these can be rendered noninfectious and their recovery hastened by surgery or by artificial pneumoperitoneum.

The antibiotic drug streptomycin, as well as isoniazid and para-aminosalicylic acid, are proving of value in the treatment of tuberculosis. When used they should be part of an over-all plan of treatment, including institutional care, and for some patients other forms of treatment.

A second line of approach to the control of tuberculosis is to search for the source of infection whenever an infected individual is discovered. When an adult is infected, it frequently is difficult to find the source, but when children react positively to the tuberculin test, the source of infection can usually be discovered. The tuberculin testing of school children is becoming increasingly widespread and its chief value is to lead to the discovery of "open cases" in the community. Usually the open case which is serving as a source of infection is in the home, although numerous instances have been reported in which teachers have been responsible for the infection of large numbers of school children.

The disseminators of infection can be identified not only by the use of the tuberculin test but also by x-ray examination of the chest. Routine x-rays are particularly valuable in special groups such as hospital and clinic patients, military recruits, college students, and employee groups. Mass x-rays of whole communities, including one city of 500,000 population, have revealed undiagnosed cases in sufficient numbers to justify the effort and the expense involved.

The great reduction which has occurred in tuberculosis and the demonstrated effectiveness of control measures justify the hope that in another generation or two tuberculosis may become a rare disease. Persons who have been infected can know their exact condition and can obtain treatment if necessary. Beds in carefully controlled institutions are now available for actively contagious cases. The tremendous hazard of the open, contagious case of tuberculosis in the community is being gradually diminished. When all patients with active disease are treated and those who are a danger to others are isolated, our children can grow up without even that first infection which seemed unavoidable a generation ago.

Everyone who develops tuberculosis has been exposed to some person or some animal with the disease. And when a child becomes infected, this person is most likely within the family—a parent, possibly, or a grandparent with "chronic bronchitis," or an older brother or sister, or a nursemaid or cook. A recent study in Cattaraugus County, New York, shows that the risk of death from tuberculosis is nine times greater for children in tuberculous families than for children in the general population.

How long will it be before we protect our children from tuberculosis by being certain that the adults with whom they have intimate contact are not exposing them to infection?

Vaccination against Tuberculosis. Approximately 25 years ago scientists at the Pasteur Institute in Paris produced a vaccine against tuberculosis. This vaccine, which is called "BCG,"

(Bacillus Calmette-Guerin) consists of a strain of tuberculosis germs from cattle. The germs have been grown in the laboratory so long that they are no longer able to produce disease. They do, however, produce a mild and harmless infection which results in an increase in a person's resistance to tuberculosis. In this country BCG vaccine is being used and the results carefully observed in persons who are closely and continuously exposed to patients with active tuberculosis. Vaccination of large population groups, however, shows no evidence of value.[3]

On the other hand, results reported from Europe suggest that this vaccine may have a role to play in the control of tuberculosis among persons who are intimately exposed to active infection. BCG vaccination, however, should be regarded as only one of many procedures to be used in tuberculosis control and not as a substitute for hygienic measures or public health practices designed to prevent or minimize tuberculous infection and disease.

Tuberculosis eradication, not just control of tuberculosis, is being urged as a reasonable goal for the quarter century just ahead. Clearly, the measures for its eradication are in our hands. Unfortunately, however, tuberculosis still causes approximately 25,000 deaths a year in this country and ranks as the fourth or fifth cause of death between fifteen and forty-five years of age. The slow onset of this disease frequently hinders its early diagnosis; arrested cases may again become open, and the public is thus still exposed to an unnecessarily large risk of infection. The war against tuberculosis is by no means over!

Pneumonia

Pneumonia is really not a single disease, for it may be caused by various germs and it acts differently at different periods of life. Although always serious, pneumonia is rarely fatal to persons in the prime of life. In infancy and old age pneumonia is largely a terminal process; that is, it is the actual method by which death comes to a large number of individuals previously weakened by infectious disease, by injury, or by the lowered

[3] Palmer, Carrol, and Lawrence Shaw, *American Review of Tuberculosis*, vol. 68, p. 462, September, 1953.

FIG. 9. PNEUMONIA DEATH RATES BY COLOR, AGE, AND SEX

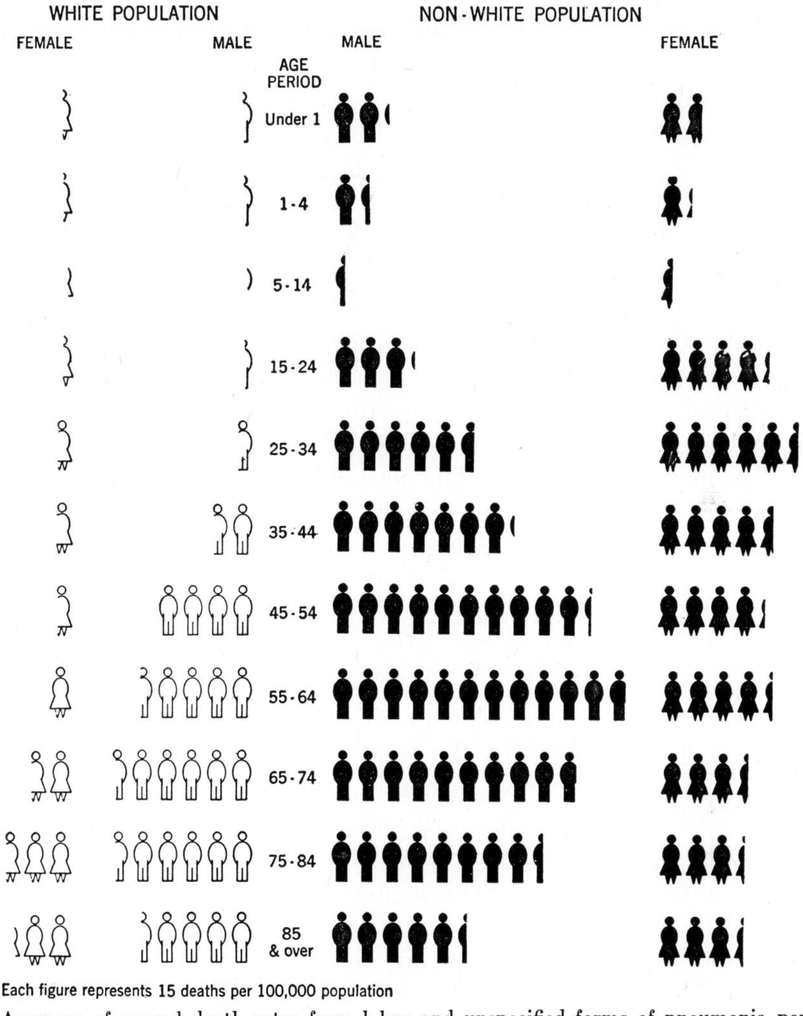

Each figure represents 15 deaths per 100,000 population

Averages of annual death rates from lobar and unspecified forms of pneumonia per 100,000 persons by color, sex, and age. Ages 1 to 74 years. (*Data from National Office of Vital Statistics.*)

vitality characteristic of extreme youth or extreme age (see Tables 3, 4, 7, and 23). Osler says of it: "Pneumonia may well be called the friend of the aged. Taken off by it in an acute, short, not often painful illness, the old escape those 'cold gradations of decay' that make the last stage of all so distressing."

Pneumonia is an inflammatory process of the lungs which causes a portion of one or both lungs to be filled solidly with serum, red blood cells, and leucocytes. The cause of pneumonia is a germ—most commonly a virus or the pneumococcus or the streptococcus, although the tubercle bacillus, the staphylococcus, or other germs may occasionally be responsible.

Pneumonias caused by the streptococcus are usually secondary to some other disease, such as measles, whooping cough, or influenza, and produce small areas of inflammation scattered throughout the lungs. These areas of infection begin around small branches of the bronchi and the condition is frequently spoken of as "bronchopneumonia." The prevention of such pneumonias depends primarily upon the prevention or, failing that, the early and adequate care of the primary disease. The experience during the First World War showed that the pneumonia rate with influenza was much higher among soldiers in the field than among those who were promptly hospitalized. Children with measles or whooping cough should be carefully protected from all contact with persons who have colds and from conditions which tend to lower their resistance. In the treatment of streptococcic pneumonia, the sulfonamides, penicillin, and other antibiotic drugs give excellent results in most cases. All pneumonia patients should have adequate medical and nursing care.

Pneumonias caused by the pneumococcus, of which there are a considerable number of different types, frequently involve one or two lobes of the lungs at a time and so are called "lobar pneumonias." Bronchopneumonias, however, also may be caused by the pneumococcus. These pneumococcic pneumonias are considered as primary pneumonias, although patients usually report having had a cold before the onset of the pneumonia. It seems that, even with virulent pneumococci present in the nose and throat, some temporary lowering of the resistance from fatigue, alcohol, chilling, malnutrition, or a cold is frequently necessary for an actual pneumonia to develop.

Pneumococci are disseminated with the nose and throat discharges of patients and of healthy carriers. In fact, during seasons of pneumonia prevalence there are many more healthy persons carrying pneumococci in their noses and throats than there are actual cases of the disease.

In recent years most cases of pneumonia have been so-called viral pneumonias, that is, caused by a filtrable virus. Drugs have but little effect upon the course of these pneumonias but, fortunately, most of them are relatively mild. Little is known about the transmission of viral pneumonia.

One attack of pneumonia does not confer a permanent immunity against subsequent attacks. On the contrary, there seems to be an increased susceptibility to the disease after one attack. Vaccines have been tried at various times for the prevention of pneumonia, but no definite value for them has as yet been established.

Really dramatic progress, however, has been made in the treatment of pneumonia since the discovery of the antibiotics and the sulfonamides. Penicillin, other antibiotics, and to a lesser extent, the sulfonamide drugs are saving the lives of most of the victims of this disease, many of whom could not possibly have survived a few years ago.

For the prevention of pneumonia one can suggest only general measures for the avoidance of anything which tends to reduce vitality, such as dissipation, loss of sleep, fatigue, overwork, worry, poor or insufficient food, alcohol, colds, and excesses of all kinds. More care than is usual should be given to acute minor respiratory infections such as colds, influenza, bronchitis, and sore throats. Persons with these infections should be confined to bed during the acute stage and at least as long as there is fever. Pneumonia should be considered a communicable disease and patients with pneumonia should be isolated in order to reduce the spread of infection to others.

Cancer

In his message to Congress in January, 1954, President Eisenhower stated that last year there were in this country 224,000 deaths from cancer and that cancer will claim the lives of 25,000,000 people of our present 160,000,000 population unless the present cancer death rate is lowered.

Cancer as a cause of death has a natural tendency to increase as more people reach the cancer age; but so rapidly have cancer deaths mounted that it seems that there must be an absolute as well as a relative increase in cancer. This increase in cancer deaths, however, may be checked to a certain extent as more and more people present themselves for medical care at the first onset of symptoms such as the following which could be due to cancer:

1. A sore that does not heal normally, particularly about the tongue, mouth, or lips.

2. A lump or thickening, especially in the breast, lips, or tongue.

3. Bloody discharge from the nipple or abnormal bleeding from any of the body openings.

4. Progressive change in the size or color of a mole or wart.

5. Persistent indigestion.

6. Persistent hoarseness, unexplained cough, or difficulty in swallowing.

7. Any pronounced change in usual bowel habits.

Improvements in cancer treatment are giving encouraging results. Surgery and, in carefully selected cases, x-ray and radium are proving increasingly effective. Reliable clinics report that 20 to 30 per cent of the cancer patients whom they treat are living and well after five years or more. In no disease is early diagnosis more vital to successful treatment (see also Tables 3, 4, 6, 7, and page 451).

Heart Disease

Some years ago heart disease assumed first place as a cause of death for people of all ages and in 1952 took a toll of 817,000

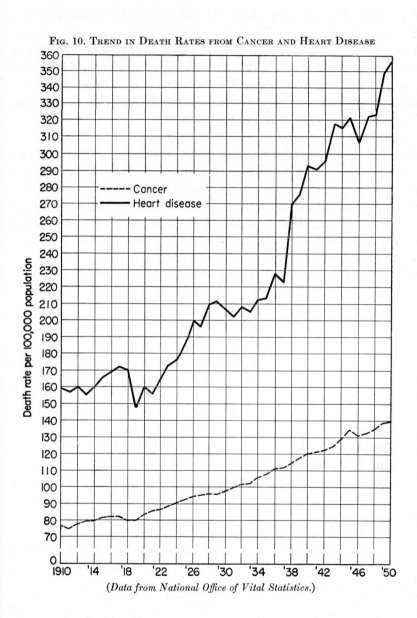

Fig. 10. Trend in Death Rates from Cancer and Heart Disease

(Data from National Office of Vital Statistics.)

lives. In spite of better diagnosis and treatment this death rate is still on the increase. This is discouraging but not quite so hopeless as it might appear on first thought. Approximately 35 per cent of heart disease is due to infections involving the heart muscles and valves, 45 per cent to degenerative processes, 10 per cent to syphilis, and 10 per cent to a variety of other causes (see Tables 3, 4, 6, 7, and 23, and Fig. 10).

Rheumatic Heart Disease. Rheumatic fever, or so-called "inflammatory rheumatism," is an infectious disease of the body as a whole but with a tendency to affect most severely the joints and the heart. Rheumatic fever contracted in childhood is responsible for 25 per cent of deaths from heart disease up to the age of 50 years. Between the ages of 10 and 14 years acute rheumatic fever and rheumatic heart disease combined cause more deaths than any other disease. Between the ages of 15 and 24 years, it is outranked only by cancer and tuberculosis.

Rheumatic fever occurs only in human beings, with first attacks most common in children between 5 and 10 years of age. It is most frequent in cool climates and in urban communities, more prevalent in whites than in Negroes, slightly more in females than in males. It is responsible for much of the heart disease of later life and in the United States as a whole affects more than a million persons, young and old.

There seems to be a definite familial susceptibility to rheumatic fever and a significant relationship between its occurrence and malnutrition and poor living conditions. Rheumatic-fever rates are almost twice as high in crowded as in noncrowded homes; higher in Northern than in Southern States and particularly high in the Rocky Mountain area and in the Middle Atlantic States (Fig. 11).

Surveys indicate that approximately 1 to 5 per cent of school children have rheumatic fever at some time or other and approximately 60 per cent of children infected give evidence of heart involvement, permanent damage being most frequent to the heart valves. Repeated attacks occur in about half of those who have had first attacks, and about one-fourth of the patients, particularly girls, develop chorea, so-called "St. Vitus's dance," as a complication.

The cause of rheumatic fever is a type of hemolytic streptococcus. The initial attack usually is preceded by tonsillitis, scarlet fever, or some other acute respiratory infection. Transmission is from person to person either directly or indirectly by way of hands, drinking glasses, etc. Individual susceptibility varies widely. Most persons are resistant to rheumatic fever even

Fig. 11. Geographic Distribution of Mortality from Rheumatic Fever

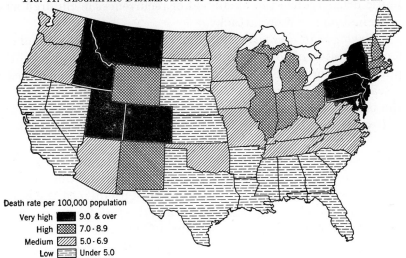

Death rate per 100,000 population

Very high	■	9.0 & over
High	▨	7.0 - 8.9
Medium	▨	5.0 - 6.9
Low	▤	Under 5.0

White persons, ages 5 to 24 years, in the United States. Includes chronic rheumatic heart disease. (*Data from Metropolitan Life Insurance Company.*)

though they get throat infections with the strain of streptococcus that causes this disease.

Efforts to control this serious and widespread disease still depend, primarily, upon general measures such as isolation, the adequate care of patients during the acute stages of the disease, a properly safeguarded and regulated convalescence, attention to problems of poor housing and malnutrition, and the discovery early in life of children whose hearts have been damaged. This means the widespread careful examination of school children.

Existing damage to the heart cannot be repaired but the functional condition of the heart can be determined and future lives planned with intelligent consideration of the physical limits which damaged hearts impose. Under proper conditions most persons who have had rheumatic fever can live normal or relatively normal lives.

Studies in army and navy camps suggest that sulfadiazine may be useful in controlling the spread of the streptococcus which causes rheumatic fever. Other studies indicate that certain antibiotic drugs reduce the likelihood of recurrences in children who have had one or more attacks.

Valvular heart disease, other than rheumatic, usually occurs as a complication of some infection such as scarlet fever, tonsillitis, pneumonia, or abscesses at the roots of teeth. This type of heart disease can be reduced; in fact, it is being materially reduced by the prevention and better care of these infections.

Degenerative Heart Disease. Less encouraging is the outlook for the heart disease which, like apoplexy and certain types of kidney trouble, is an end result of the stress, strain, and degenerative processes which have been slowly undermining the circulatory system. Over many years our most useful measure in the treatment of these diseases has been rest—rest from the stress and strain of worry, of overeating, of physical activity—rest which the individual failed to provide until his body's reserves were exhausted. The hope for a reduction of these degenerative processes is not entirely a forlorn one, since the American people seem to be taking a more sane and intelligent attitude toward living. Many are beginning to ask themselves whether the mad race for material success and "keeping up with the Joneses" is worth the price. As more and more decide that it is not, they will get more joy out of living and will postpone senescence with its disintegration of vital tissues (see page 445).

Syphilitic heart disease is a complication of syphilis, which is considered in Chapter XIX.

Disabling Disabilities

Recognized today as one of our major health problems is the rehabilitation of persons disabled by illness, accidents, war wounds, birth injuries, and congenital disabilities. The First and Second World Wars focused attention upon the importance of this problem and produced effective programs and strong leadership to get something worthwhile done about it, not only for war casualties but also for the general population.

The enormity of this problem is apparent from the following figures. The number of children in this country with handicapping conditions according to recent estimates are cerebral palsy, 285,000; epilepsy, 270,000; rheumatic fever and its after-effects, 675,000; cleft palate and harelip, 64,000; eye defects needing care, 7,500,000, of whom 60,000 need special educational help; handicapping hearing loss, 250,000 to 500,000; speech handicaps, 320,000; orthopedic defects of bones, joints, muscles of sufficient severity to need medical care, 3 per cent of children 5 to 17 years of age.[4] The U.S. Bureau of Labor Statistics estimates that approximately 8 million males of working age have disabilities which make it difficult or impossible to find employment. The U.S. Office of Vocational Rehabilitation states that 2,000,000 disabled persons could be made employable by proper medical and vocational rehabilitation and that about 250,000 persons become disabled as a result of accidents or diseases each year.

Chronic disease is responsible for 88 per cent of disabilities requiring rehabilitation; congenital conditions, 2 per cent; occupational accidents and injuries, 5 per cent; other accidents, another 5 per cent.

Effective programs of rehabilitation begin with a thorough examination and good medical and surgical care. Coordinated with this is a program of physical and occupational therapy planned to meet the needs of the particular patient. Vocational training or retraining then follows as soon as the patient is ready for it. A complete rehabilitation program thus involves teamwork on the part of physicians with various specialized abilities, such as physiatrists, internists, orthopedic surgeons, neurologists, and psychiatrists; physical therapists; occupational therapists; psychologists; vocational counselors; teachers and social workers.

[4] Lesser, Arthur, and Eleanor Hunt, "The Nation's Handicapped Children," *American Journal of Public Health*, vol. 44, p. 166, February, 1954.

The rehabilitation of disabled persons is an involved and time-consuming process that requires skill and patience of the highest order. The results, however, more than justify the cost and the effort involved.

At the Minneapolis Veterans Hospital a few years ago one building was devoted to the care of eighty patients who the physicians in charge believed would have to spend the rest of their lives in bed. This meant that the Veterans Administration would have to provide for them many years of medical, nursing, and hospital care. Even more important for the patients themselves it meant a hopeless and seemingly endless existence for the rest of their lives. At the end of one year of an active rehabilitation program half of these men had gone home, and half of these had some type of remunerative employment. The others were able to care for themselves and do certain things about the home. Of those who remained in the hospital half were able to be up and about and to a considerable extent take care of themselves. Only twenty of the group were still bed patients and some of these were making progress toward self-care. This particular program in the space of one year saved the taxpayers millions of dollars and made life once more worth living for these veterans and their families.

The personal human side of rehabilitation is illustrated by the following case report: Glen Cunningham, who until 1954 had run the fastest mile on record, was crippled in childhood in a schoolhouse fire. The doctor said that only a miracle would enable him to walk again; he was out of luck. He began walking by following a plow across the fields, leaning on it for support; and then went on tireless experimentation to see what he could do with his legs until he broke all records for the mile run.[5]

A physician's daughter broke her back in an automobile accident twelve years ago. For more than five years she remained in bed completely paralyzed from the waist down and without bladder and bowel control. Rehabilitation training enabled her to control her bladder and bowels and to walk on braces and crutches. After six months she took on a full-time job in New

[5] Fosdick, H. E., "On Being a Real Person," Harper & Brothers, New York, 1943.

York City. The only time that she has missed from work in six years was from a fractured femur, at which time she was off six weeks. The usual time off from work from this condition is three months. She lives in an apartment, travels everywhere in New York, is taking postgraduate work in a University, has made one trip to Europe, and is a completely integrated, self-supporting, dignified citizen.

A physician with five years' training in medicine and neurology was shot in the back by a psychotic policeman and her cord was severed about the middle of her back. She remained in a large teaching hospital for 14 months and was led to believe she could never practice medicine again. Her physicians neglected to remember that locomotion is not an essential in the practice of medicine. Medicine is practiced with eyes, ears, hands, voice, mind, and spirit. She was put in a combined program of training and patient care, training herself half the day and patients the other half; within three months she was able to return to her home city alone, walking on her braces and crutches. She has now finished her training and will continue to teach and practice in the field of medical rehabilitation.

A young woman of thirty had contracted poliomyelitis at two years of age, with paralysis of both legs and deformity of the back. Over the years she had 26 surgical procedures, including operations on her spine in the hope of improving her condition. She could walk a slow gait on crutches but could not get up or down curbs. She was homebound for 28 years, graduated from high school with a home teacher, could type accurately and rapidly but could not get a position because she could not walk and travel. After five months of training, she was able to take a full-time job and has now been at work five years, during which time she has never missed a day or been late a morning, but she waited 28 years because there was an 8-inch wall around her home. Meticulous training was the answer to her problem.

Throughout the country, general hospitals, nursing homes, and other types of institutions are providing custodial care for many thousands of persons who could be home with their families, many of them mothers and fathers of young children,

[53]

and could be productive members of society if adequate rehabilitation services were available to them. To provide such services requires more personnel trained in rehabilitation and community interest and support for the conduct of these programs.

Acute Respiratory Infections

The acute respiratory infections are a major cause of illness at all ages but take an exceptionally heavy toll of life in infancy. Pneumonia has been considered. Colds will be discussed in a special chapter. Influenza is still unsolved. Each of these diseases is especially serious in infants and presents problems of control distinct for this age period. Exposure to respiratory infections transmitted from one person to another through the air or by means of the hands can hardly be avoided by older children and adults. But not so with infants. Infections must be carried to them. This is usually done by well-meaning parents, brothers, sisters, or other relatives. If possible, persons with colds should not be permitted to go into the rooms of infants, nor should they prepare or handle their food or drink. The danger of infection can be reduced also by thorough washing of the hands with soap and hot water before touching the child or its food and, if one has a cold, by covering the nose and mouth with a piece of gauze, linen, or muslin. A specific immunizing agent against these diseases may some time be developed. Until then we must rely upon general measures for their control.

Other Major Health Problems

Other major health problems which are responsible for a large amount of illness and disability as well as for premature deaths will be considered in subsequent chapters. Mental illnesses and mental health in the following chapter; apoplexy and nephritis, which are end results of degenerative processes in the cardiovascular system, in the chapter on Health Problems of Advancing Years; the diseases of early infancy, in the chapter on Modern Parenthood; diabetes, in the chapter on Glands of Internal Secretion; suicide, which is a result of mental disturbance, in the chapter on Mental Health; etc.

A study of our major health problems cannot fail to convince one there is much that we can do individually and collectively to reduce them or to alleviate their effects. Further substantial accomplishments are clearly possible; but they will come about only when we clearly understand the problems and then proceed with determination to do something about them.

DISCUSSION SUGGESTIONS

1. How do accidents compare in importance with other causes of disability and death? What are the most frequent types of accidents?
2. Discuss measures which you would advocate for the reduction of automobile accidents; home accidents; industrial accidents.
3. Do people get tuberculosis from being "run-down"? Give reasons. What are the usual sources from which man contracts tuberculosis?
4. Explain and discuss the program for the control of tuberculosis in your college; in your state.
5. Discuss the changes which have occurred in the death rate from tuberculosis in the past 50 years and the factors which you think have been chiefly responsible for this.
6. What program would you advocate for the further reduction of tuberculosis?
7. What measures have been found most effective in the treatment of tuberculosis?
8. Pneumonia is frequently secondary to what other diseases?
9. What measures are suggested for the prevention of pneumonia?
10. What is meant by "heart disease" and how does this rank as a cause of death? What types of heart disease are on the increase?
11. What do you understand by rheumatic fever and what is its relation to heart disease?
12. What are the most important causes of deaths in terms of working years lost for white males? For white females?
13. Why was rehabilitation urged by President Eisenhower as a major national program in his message to Congress in 1954?

REFERENCES AND READING SUGGESTIONS

1. American Red Cross: "First Aid Text Book," The Blakiston Company, New York, 1947. Supplement 1, 1953.
2. "Accident Handbook," Children's Medical Center, Boston, 1950.
3. Blakeslee, Howard: "TB—The Killer Cornered," Public Affairs Pamphlets, New York, 1952.
4. ———: "Know Your Heart," Public Affairs Pamphlets, New York.

5. Bliven, Bruce: "How to Save Lives in Traffic," *Harper's Magazine*, p. 87, January, 1950.
6. Bolton, William: "What to Do until the Doctor Comes," The Reilly & Lee Co., Chicago, 1953.
7. "Civil Defense Supplement to the American Red Cross First Aid Textbook," The Blakiston Company, New York, 1951.
8. Dickinson, Frank, and E. L. Walker: "What Is the Leading Cause of Death? Two New Measures," *Bulletin* 64, American Medical Association, Chicago, 1948.
9. Dubos, René, and Jean Dubos: "The White Plague," Little, Brown & Company, Boston, 1952.
10. Gray, George W.: "The Advancing Front of Medicine," McGraw-Hill Book Company, Inc., New York, 1941.
11. Jacobziner, Harold, and Herbert Rich: "Home Safety and Accident Prevention in a Child Health Conference," *American Journal of Public Health*, vol. 44, p. 83, January, 1954.
12. Kessler, Henry H.: "Rehabilitation of the Physically Handicapped," Columbia University Press, 1953.
13. Myers, J. A.: "Tuberculosis among Children and Young Adults," 3d ed., Charles C Thomas, Publisher, Springfield, Ill., 1951.
14. National Safety Council: "Accident Facts," Chicago, 1953.
15. Perkins, James E., and Floyd M. Feldmann: "You and Tuberculosis," Alfred A. Knopf, Inc., New York, 1952.
16. Rusk, Howard A., and Eugene Taylor: "New Hope for the Handicapped," Harper & Brothers, New York, 1949.
17. ―――― and ――――: "Living with a Disability—At Home—At Work—At Play," The Blakiston Company, New York, 1953.
18. Switzer, Mary E., and Howard A. Rusk: "Doing Something for the Disabled," Public Affairs Pamphlets, New York, 1953.
19. Wilmer, Harry A.: "Huber the Tuber—A Story of Tuberculosis," National Tuberculosis Association, New York, 1942.
20. Yahraes, Herbert: "Rheumatic Fever—Childhood's Greatest Enemy," 3d ed., Public Affairs Pamphlets, New York, 1948.

Text-Films

The following McGraw-Hill Text-Films on Health Education are recommended for use with this chapter of the text:

The Body Fights Bacteria (motion picture 17 min). For description see listing on p. 283.

The Heart and Circulatory System (motion picture about 15 min, available spring, 1955). For description see p. 466.

Chapter III

MENTAL HEALTH[1]

MENTAL illnesses have long been a major cause of death and disability in this country. Federal and state governments maintain almost half a million hospital beds for patients with mental illnesses. One out of every twelve children born in the United States this year at some time in life will suffer a mental illness severe enough to justify hospitalization.

Reasonable estimates as to the numbers of the mentally ill run as high as 10,000,000. This includes the problem drinkers, of whom there are estimated to be nearly 4,000,000, three-quarters of a million of these being chronic alcoholics. It includes a good share of the 50,000 who are addicted to narcotics and of the 275,000 children under seventeen who are brought into the juvenile courts each year. It includes the 16,000 Americans who in an average year commit suicide. And finally, it accounts for a substantial part of the divorces (one for every four marriages), of crime, of absenteeism, and of accident proneness in industry. At the present time the mentally ill constitute about half of all patients in the hospitals of the United States. Of all separations from military service, 51 per cent are for personality problems. From 50 to 60 per cent of all patients who consult doctors do so for complaints due primarily to emotional disorders. Many pro-

[1] Prepared in collaboration with Dr. E. M. deBerry, formerly psychiatrist of the Students' Health Service, University of Minnesota.

[57]

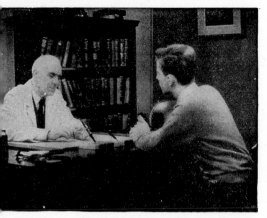

This boy, concerned about recurrent chest pains, consults his medical doctor.

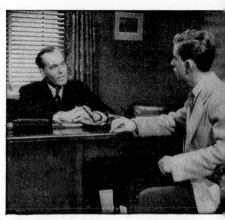

With no physical cause apparent, the do suspects a mental upset and recommen psychiatrist.

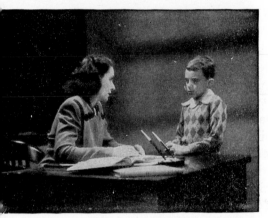

Subsequent visits bring out the fact that poor school grades were often the cause of unpleasant scenes.

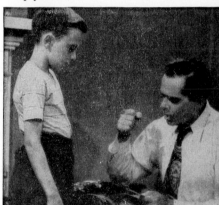

Conflicts in early life often manifest t selves in emotional disturbances in later

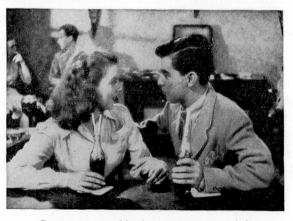

Competent psychiatric treatment can help restore social and emotional balance.

(From Emotional Health, a McGraw-Hill Text-Film)

ductive persons continuously maintain a chronically neurotic adjustment to life. And most individuals have minor emotional disturbances, often not recognized but of medical significance.

In spite of all this the average person has a curious attitude toward mental health. He admits the importance of physical health, realizes that not everyone who is up and about is physically well, and may even go so far as to take some elementary precautions against disease. If not exactly intelligent about physical health, he is at least interested and will seek advice from physicians, quacks, or advertisements. But in regard to his mental health his attitude until recently has been strangely indifferent. If he thinks about it at all, he regards it as something quite foreign to him, much as he might give passing attention to the antics of a foreign bandit. He considers his friends and associates as in perfect mental health; when his attention is forced to this subject by the "sudden" onset of a mental illness in someone he knows, he is surprised and shocked. If the afflicted person is a member of his own family, he attributes the disease to overwork, to worry about finances, to physical illness, or to some other socially acceptable factor. If the afflicted person is merely an acquaintance, he is likely to consider heredity, alcohol, and syphilis as probable causes. Only rarely does he try to think intelligently as to why these things happen or attempt to inform himself by reading or by consulting specialists in the field. This attitude seems particularly strange when one considers the horror with which mental illness is generally regarded.

But even when one does try to inform oneself, one meets with difficulties. In unguided reading, one finds discrepancies and confusion which may seem completely baffling.

Definite instructions for avoiding mental illness cannot be given, but a general understanding of the problems and processes involved frequently helps in the handling of minor emotional distresses. And psychiatrists deal not only with actual insanities but also with all those borderline conditions and maladjustments which are not ordinarily regarded as belonging in the category of mental illnesses. Fortunately, this type of service is rapidly expanding.

Types of Mental Disorders

Among the mental disorders are conditions so grave that even the untrained person recognizes that the patient is "insane." These illnesses or psychoses, however, usually go unrecognized until they are so far advanced that treatment becomes exceedingly difficult. Rarely does mental illness come suddenly out of the blue. The symptoms are present for months or years but are usually disguised as nervous breakdown, neurasthenia, or physical illnesses.

A second group comprises persons who are not considered insane by their associates but who present various peculiar symptoms of almost any degree of severity. Morbid fears, compulsions, and obsessions, generally diagnosed as psychoneuroses with some modifying term, are particularly characteristic of this group. With these also might be placed chronic invalidism, in which the disability is on a psychological rather than a physical basis.

The third group consists of individuals who are apparently neither mentally nor physically sick, but who fail to make a socially adequate adjustment. It includes certain types of alcoholics, delinquents, vagrants, and persons of unusual sexual behavior. In this group we might include also those persons who, while apparently making a good social adjustment, nevertheless are tremendously hampered by feelings of inadequacy, emotional instability, fears, and other personality disturbances which interfere with efficiency and happiness.

Problem children constitute a fourth group. It is now generally recognized that difficulties of training, poor habits, school problems, temper tantrums, enuresis, and childhood delinquencies are evidences of emotional disturbance which may be corrected by proper investigation and treatment.

Feeble-mindedness is an incurable congenital deficiency with a strong hereditary basis and, as such, has little relation to mental or emotional disorders. It is primarily a problem of eugenics and sociology.

Even such an incomplete listing of psychiatric problems forces us to recognize that we can no longer regard mental illness or insanity as the only field for psychiatric investigation. Emotional disturbances and personality problems, which may be regarded as lesser forms of mental illness, constitute ever-present problems, touching all of us.

Theory of Mental Illness

From the scientific data at hand, we have no reason to conclude that heredity is a major factor in the causation of mental illnesses. In spite of this, heredity is commonly believed to be the most important cause of mental illness. This belief is unfortunate, for the assumption that mental illness is caused by heredity leads to the conclusion that it cannot be prevented or cured.

To assume that a mental illness is hereditary because it "runs in a family" is erroneous, since it is impossible to separate the effects of environment, or so-called "social heredity," from those of physical heredity. By social heredity is meant the transference of traits of character or types of behavior by contact with and imitation of those persons with whom one lives, while physical heredity implies the transmission of characteristics or types of behavior through the reproductive cells. One has only to consider the abnormal environment which exists in a family in which there is a mentally ill person, to realize the great possibility of a child in such a family becoming mentally unbalanced, even though no hereditary factors are active at all. In order to establish the hereditary character of a disease one must demonstrate that the disease was not caused by environmental factors and that it follows recognized laws of inheritance. Neither of these requirements has been met in the case of most mental diseases. Furthermore, it does not follow that, even if a hereditary factor were present, the development of the disease could not be avoided by the manipulation of environmental factors. Hence, we shall do well to turn our attention from the heredity theory of mental illness to what may be more profitable approaches.

Certain mental illnesses have a definite physical basis. For example, the psychoses of general paresis,[2] arteriosclerosis, senility,

[2] A type of mental disease due to syphilis.

injury, brain tumor, etc., are due directly to destruction of brain tissue.

Furthermore, hallucinations, fears, compulsions, or other emotional disorders may be due to disturbances in the functioning of the glands of internal secretion; to infectious processes, the toxins of which give rise to states of delirium; to the action of drugs; or to actual destruction of brain tissue. Such conditions may, and do, give rise to strange thinking and behavior. Their prevention and cure depend upon meeting the physical and emotional needs of the patient.

On the other hand, ideas and emotional attitudes are usually a product of the social environment. A man may let his hair grow to shoulder length because his thinking has been deranged by the activity of the spirochete of syphilis in the cortex of his brain; or he may wear his hair long because he has been taught a religious belief in which long hair is worn as a symbol of the Christlike life. In the first case, we explain and treat his unusual behavior on a physical basis. In the second, we explain it in psychological and social terms.

In the investigation and treatment of the abnormal emotional reactions which constitute the material of poor mental health, it is necessary both to investigate those physical disturbances which may interfere with the complex functions of behavior and belief and to recognize those factors in the environment which may disturb these same functions. There is no real conflict in these approaches. In some cases physical disturbances predominate, while in others mental and social situations are of major importance.

Psychological Mechanisms of Mental Ill-health

The behavior of the mentally ill patient is not qualitatively different from that of healthy persons or from his own behavior before his illness developed. In fact, the behavior and the thinking of the mentally ill are strange only because they are exaggerated or inappropriate to particular situations. Moreover, when the history of a mental patient is carefully studied, it is found that his illness is the logical and inevitable outgrowth of his experiences and his interpretation of those experiences in reaction to the situation confronting him, and to his physical make-up and condition at the time. The illness then presents itself as the only way left for that particular individual to solve the problems which have arisen as the result of his interpretation of and reaction to his experiences. It is found, moreover, that the solution, that is, his mental illness, is not a new one but is an exaggeration of methods which he has used before and which everybody uses to greater or lesser degree. But because he uses these methods at the expense of more healthy and efficient ones, the patient accumulates dissatisfaction and a poor equipment for handling this dissatisfaction. This may be illustrated by the example of the chronic invalid who avoids uncomfortable duties or responsibilities, or acquires attention, by becoming ill. This procedure accounts for a large number of the so-called "neurotics" and "psychoneurotics" who crowd the hospital clinics and the consulting rooms of physicians and who manage, quite unconsciously, to make the lives of their families and friends, as well as their own lives, unhappy.

Avoidance of Unpleasant Situations. A boy, aged ten, wakes one morning with a cold. He is not very sick but is kept in bed as a precautionary measure. During the course of the morning his condition improves. His mother lets him get up and play about the house and entertains him with stories and games. He is not in the habit of getting so much attention and he enjoys it. He particularly enjoys it at this time because he has been having difficulty at school. He is slightly nearsighted, but this defect has not been noticed. It makes it difficult for him to see what is written on the board. For this and various other reasons he is behind in his school work. He doesn't try hard to catch up because he feels hopeless about it. He makes small troubles in the classroom instead. The teacher doesn't like him, or at least he thinks that she doesn't, which amounts to the same thing.

After being out a day or so with his cold, he returns to the classroom even farther behind than he was. He is punished for inattention and making a nuisance of himself. Things go from bad to worse. Even on the playground he can find no satisfaction.

He is small for his age; he has never acquired skill in the games that other boys play. He feels his inadequacy and allows himself to be bullied because he hasn't enough self-confidence to "stick up for his rights." Things go on like this for a week or two, getting steadily worse. Finally matters are about to reach a climax. His teacher has given him a note to his mother about his bad conduct. The boy has destroyed the note. There is a new bully on the playground who promises to "beat him up" the next time he catches him. He manages to elude the bully on his way home that afternoon; he stays safely in his own back yard. But the next morning he no sooner wakes than he realizes the disagreeable situation. He dreads going to school and wishes he could stay at home. He remembers the last time he stayed at home; he was sick that time. He asks himself if he is sick now. By the time he gets to breakfast he is really feeling unwell. He complains to his mother. He is not malingering, because by this time he really feels uneasy in his stomach. Remembering his illness of the week before, his mother is a little worried. She allows him to remain at home, intending to take him to see the doctor. But the boy has discovered a way of getting out of unpleasant things. It isn't a good way, and he gains nothing in the long run; in fact, he only makes matters worse. If the situation remains the same, he will get sick again and again until he becomes a chronic invalid.

But suppose his parents realize what he is doing and set about changing things in a rational way. His eye defect is correctible; he could be given special tutoring to catch up with his class or, if necessary, changed to another school where he could make a new start. His satisfaction in play could be improved if he were sent to a camp in the summer or were given instruction in sports. It usually is easy to correct the habit at this stage.

On the other hand, if this boy continues to be sick, he will keep on becoming sick in more critical situations all of his life, and when he gets to be an adult he will do it in the face of important situations. In this case he will become a chronic invalid and be diagnosed by one physician after another as a neurotic, a psychoneurotic, or a hysteric.

Parental Domination. Adolescence gives rise to an increasing urge for independence and personal responsibility on the part of all normal children. Parents should prepare themselves and their children for this by the development of an attitude of mutual helpfulness and respect. If this is not done, as occurs all too frequently, conflicts arise as a result of the efforts of parents to continue their domination and the struggle of their children for independence.

When this occurs, warping of the child's personality is likely to result. Either rebellion or submission is unfortunate. Rebellion, without self-discipline and training in the assumption of responsibility, may lead to serious antisocial acts, while submission, which continues during adolescence at childhood levels of dependence, may handicap the individual throughout his or her whole life.

Daydreaming. It is out of dreams of better things that ambition, inventions, scientific discoveries, and social movements are born. He who does not "dream dreams" is dull and unimaginative. Yet daydreaming may come to be a source of emotional satisfaction and a substitute for real accomplishment. It is easier to achieve success and to escape unpleasant situations in a world of make-believe than in a world of reality. For this reason excessive daydreaming is likely to occur in maladjusted individuals.

Most persons daydream occasionally; some daydream excessively; and a few, whom we know as patients with dementia praecox, live continuously in a world of phantasy. The solution for the daydreamer is to turn his dreams into reality and to seek opportunities for satisfaction in achievement.

Inferiority Complex. Every intelligent person experiences feelings of inferiority at certain times and in certain situations. Such feelings are not abnormal and need not be disturbing. No one can excel in everything and few reach the limit of their ambitions in anything.

If one has handicaps or limitations, they should be recognized and considered in relation to one's abilities and capacities. On the basis of such an appraisal one should turn his energies into those fields in which he has the greatest chance of achieving success and satisfaction.

Superiority Complex. It is just as natural for one to feel superior in certain situations as it is to feel inferior in others. Some persons feel and act superior because of wealth, good looks, athletic skill, etc. This usually leads to unpopularity and to an unhealthy mental and emotional state.

Many persons who seem to exhibit a superior attitude are really overcompensating for feelings of inferiority. The man whose daily work makes him feel inferior and the woman who is unsuccessful in her social contacts are apt to be tyrants with their families. A ruthless judge on the bench may be a "worm" at home.

No one is perfect. Everyone has his good points as well as his faults. Overattention to either is undesirable. In order to be in a contented and healthy state of mind one must accept oneself as he is, make the most of his capabilities and opportunities, and not be too discouraged with achievements which fall below one's aspirations.

Worry is an ineffectual expenditure of time and nervous energy upon uncertainties or upon situations beyond one's control. For the most part worry is confused and disorganized thinking, which interferes with both accomplishment and peace of mind. To avoid this common weakness, one must make decisions upon the best available information and be content with such decisions. At times additional information is needed before an intelligent decision can be made. In such instances the problem should be put out of mind until the necessary information has been obtained and a decision is possible. Otherwise indecision and procrastination lead to delay, confusion, and worry.

Worry over mistakes that one has made, uncertainties ahead, or situations beyond one's control obviously can be of no avail. Yet such worry is difficult to avoid. Concentration upon one's work or one's hobbies and participation in sports, particularly if this involves physical exercise, will help to replace worry with organized thinking and activity. The appropriate sharing of one's feelings and thinking with a friend or a friendly group is a satisfying experience that tends to reduce anxiety.

Refusal to face difficulties or unpleasant situations gives rise to emotional conflict and worry. Discussion of one's problems with an understanding physician or friend frequently provides relief from their burden and may lead to a solution. To many, religion or philosophy serves as a stabilizer and as an anchor in the storms of emotional conflict.

Poise is one of the most widely admired personal characteristics of young and old. It suggests easy self-assurance without conceit. The cultivation of poise depends primarily upon mastery of one's self, which in turn implies good mental health. "He that ruleth himself is greater than he that taketh a city."

Happiness. The attainment of happiness, with all that that implies, is the goal toward which most of our efforts in life are directed. Yet all too frequently we follow false beacons along life's highway leading to this goal. The modern Chinese philosopher Lin Yutang[3] says, "The only problem unconsciously assumed by all Chinese philosophers to be of any importance is: how shall we enjoy life, and who can best enjoy life? No perfectionism, no straining after the unattainable, no postulating of the unknowable; but taking poor, mortal human nature as it is, how shall we organize our life that all can work peacefully, endure nobly and live happily?" And he answers his own question by saying, "The ideal character best able to enjoy life is a warm, unafraid soul."

Add to this the ability to love deeply and to work effectively and satisfyingly and one has a basis for real and enduring happiness.

Psychoneuroses. Some persons, young and old, facing insecurity, failure, unpleasant tasks, or embarrassment find an acceptable escape through illness. This is usually entirely subconscious. Therefore, the patient is dissatisfied when his physician says that there is "nothing organically wrong with him." His pain is just as real to him as though it were caused by organic

[3] Lin Yutang, "The Importance of Living," The John Day Company, Inc., New York, 1937.

disease, and if his physician does not discover its cause and recommend appropriate treatment, he is likely to drift into the hands of anyone who promises to help him.

The symptoms which may accompany the psychoneuroses are legion: headaches, abdominal pain, diarrhea, nausea, vomiting, rapid heartbeat, shortness of breath, blurring of vision, paralysis, etc. Careful investigation of such a patient's symptoms, worries, and anxieties may reveal the basic cause of the trouble, although the services of a psychiatrist are frequently necessary for both diagnosis and treatment.

Sex Conflicts.

The whole subject of sex has too long been shrouded in mystery and fear— fear nourished by ignorance and misunderstanding (thus overstressing the sexual aspects of personality and living). Other fears of mankind have been dispelled by understanding. We have learned that many diseases are caused by bacteria and viruses and not evil spirits. Consequently we no longer feel an irrational terror of disease but try to control it by isolation, inoculation, and chemotherapy.

Perhaps the greatest obstacle to universally healthy sexual attitudes is the fact that although many parents realize the value of sex education, they feel inadequate and ill prepared to offer guidance to their children. They are still afflicted with inhibitions, embarrassment, and a feeling that sex is unclean. As a result the child gathers independently a distorted unhealthy collection of misinformation and misinterpretations.

The injudicious handling of sex curiosity in young children may have lasting effects. Many of the barriers that prevent a normal, healthy response in adolescents toward members of the opposite sex have their origin in such early encounters. A deep-seated fear of sex may lead to repressions that make the young girl or boy shrink within a shell of reserve that they cannot explain. Years of maladjustment and unhappiness may result from early mismanagement.

The most practical safeguard against the development of sex conflict in adolescence is a campaign of sound sex education for both parents and children. The guiding principle for parents should be honesty and an air of casual frankness. It is not necessary to attempt a full discussion of biology in one sitting, for such earnestness and overemphasis is as extreme as complete refusal to discuss the topic. In answer to the child's questions about other things it is not customary to sit down and give him a full lecture on each subject. A simple, honest answer to his question is all that is needed, and although the original question may be followed by others for elaboration, the subject is.

soon dropped and the youthful mind follows its natural course to other things. The child's interest may appear first in questions about his own origin and if the answers are supplied without emotional display or concern, the child accepts them matter-of-factly. These suggestions may seem obvious to us, but it is amazing how many of the children who come under observation at the clinic are totally ignorant of the scientific fundamentals of sex.[4]

Individual Problems Complicated.   Various types of emotional reactions, only a few of which have been discussed, are usually operative in producing the symptoms exhibited by a given individual. This is well illustrated by the following case report: The patient was a young man in college, who came to the psychiatrist with the following complaints. For four years he has tried in vain "to get control of himself" and has become thoroughly discouraged and about "at the end of his rope." He has had mastoid, sinus, and tonsil infections which he thinks have affected his mind. For the last three years he has been intensely unhappy— has made no friends, because "people despise him." He says that he is a physical coward and is "mentally tortured by bad habits." Ideas run through his head so that he cannot sleep. At times he has felt that people were reading his thoughts and watching him on the street; and occasionally he believes he is going insane and has resolved to commit suicide.

This young man's childhood was unhappy, owing both to unfortunate neighborhood conditions and to the incompatibility of his parents. During most of their married life his parents were kept together more by financial and religious considerations than by any regard for each other. Finally, the father decided that the only way out of the difficulty was to break up the home. Unable to talk it over reasonably with the patient's mother, and in order to avoid a painful scene, he sent the family to another city, where he had arranged a home for them. He also provided that the mother receive a certain sum of money each month for the support of herself and the two boys. At this point the father dropped out of the picture, as he went to another state to reestablish himself in business.

[4] Clarke, Eric K., "Mental Hygiene for Community Nursing," pp. 108–109, University of Minnesota Press, Minneapolis, 1942.

The boy's early social contacts were unfortunate. He had several prolonged illnesses, which affected him physically to such an extent that for a time he was unable to compete with other boys in physical things. Moving into a new community made this doubly hard. He was bullied unmercifully by other boys. Finally, he came under the domination of a boy who was living in the same apartment house—a boy somewhat older, rather stupid, but well developed physically. The latter assumed a sort of protective attitude toward the patient. It was from this boy that the patient had his first sex instruction. He was taught to masturbate and at the same time told that it would hurt him physically. He confessed his first experience to his mother, who was horrified and shocked. She told him that this was only a confirmation of her belief that he took after his father in his weaknesses. She told him that his father had always been sensual and impressed the boy with her disgust for masturbation and with her conviction that it was a great sin. He made a resolution to stop, broke the resolution, made another, and with each attempt became more and more convinced that he was unable to combat this evil. He felt that he must conquer it in order to prove to himself and his mother that he was not a weak character. It became for him a sort of symbol of his whole struggle against the idea of evil. If he could conquer this thing, it would mean that he could conquer the weakness he had inherited from his father, he would regain the respect and affection of his mother and be able to compete with his younger brother for her regard.

His idea about masturbation added to his difficulties with other boys. He felt that not only was he physically handicapped by the illnesses which he had had and his subsequent awkwardness but also that he was not equal morally to the other boys in his group. He heard from some of them that one could always tell a masturbator by the pimples on his face and the inability to look a man in the eye. He became even more self-conscious and developed a fear that his habit would be discovered. As a result, he avoided meeting other boys and stayed at home a great deal, neglecting physical exercise and recreation. About this time there were in the neighborhood several bullies. They were quick to recognize the patient's attitude, and on one or two occasions waylaid him on the way from school, challenging him to fight. He was frightened and ran. On the only occasion when he did put up a fight because he could not get away, he was severely beaten up by the two boys. This convinced him that he was a physical coward and added to his already growing disgust with himself.

In his university courses, this boy had shown an uncanny ability to pick out bits of information which tended to confirm certain things which worried him. He learned something of the biological theory of heredity and was strengthened in the belief that he had inherited his father's weakness of character. He learned something of scientific determinism, interpreting it to mean that man is in no way a free agent, and that it is impossible to develop one's will power if one does not already have it. He heard of the evils of the so-called "inferiority complex" and, having found a word under which he could sum up his problems, he was more than ever impressed by the magnitude of them. There had been only negative taboos and fear instilled with no suggestion of and emphasis on acceptable positive satisfactions and other forces of character as positive assets. Although he made good grades, success in this was of little value to him—not enough value, in fact, to act as a compensation for the other failures. He therefore lost interest and began to neglect his studies. Above all things he needed that recognition, friendship, social contact, which his own feelings prevented him from getting.

It was found at the outset that any simple explanation and advice would not be of any value to the patient. He had already had such explanations from various competent faculty advisers. What was required was a thorough emotional reeducation. It is obvious from the account of the patient's life that his problems were deep-seated and involved such fundamental relations as that of the patient toward his family, toward religion, and toward the problem of sex. The patient was unusually intelligent and cooperative throughout the procedure. He was seen at least

[71]

three or four times every week; and although there have been times when he showed great depression, on the whole his progress has been marked.

At present this boy is handling the family situation well. He is no longer irritable, quarrelsome, and seclusive at home. He has been able to make several valuable acquaintances on the campus. He is now quite able to apply himself consistently to his work, and his grades have improved. He has chosen a profession and, even though he is not yet ready to enter his professional training, he is exceedingly interested in it and has done a great deal of outside reading on related subjects. He has solved the sex problem satisfactorily and is not masturbating or doing any unusual amount of phantasying about sex things. He no longer believes himself a coward.

In military service, the problems of the emotionally unstable young man are greatly intensified. Kipling pictures it thus:

> I have a dream—a dreadful dream—
> A dream that is never done,
> I watch a man go out of his mind,
> And he is My Mother's Son.
>
> They pushed him into a Mental Home,
> And that is like the grave;
> For they do not let you sleep upstairs,
> And you're not allowed to shave.
>
> And it was *not* disease or crime
> Which got him landed there,
> But because they laid on My Mother's Son
> More than a man could bear.
>
> What with noise, and fear of death,
> Waking, and wounds and cold,
> They filled the cup for My Mother's Son
> Fuller than it would hold.
>
> They broke his body and his mind,
> And yet they made him live,
> And they asked more of My Mother's Son
> Than any man could give.

[72]

For, just because he had not died
　　Nor been discharged nor sick;
They dragged it out with My Mother's Son
　　Longer than he could stick—

And no one knows when he'll get well—
　　So, there he'll have to be;
And 'spite of the beard in the looking-glass,
　　I know that man is me!

The Logical Result.　The histories of mental illnesses make it impossible to escape the conclusion that the resultant mental condition is the logical and inevitable outgrowth of learned methods of behavior, that these methods, with variations, probably would have been adopted by almost anyone subject to similar situations, and that the final symptoms which appear to be so abnormal are essentially the reactions found in every normal person under certain circumstances. These things hold true not only for the simple types of cases described above but for most of the other mental illnesses. Thus the patients with certain forms of dementia praecox live in a dream so deep that it shuts them off from all contact with reality. They derive satisfaction from imaginary companions, activities, and achievements. This is precisely the same method used by child and adult when they daydream gratification they have been unable to derive from reality. Such a dementia praecox patient behaves like a child in getting pleasure from the infantile activities which the adult has so outgrown that they seem senseless and disgusting. This finds an exact parallel in the normal adult who, when meeting an obstacle which he is unable to overcome, exhibits childish temper or drops his work to indulge in play.

Suicide, which ranks as the sixth cause of death in every age group from fifteen to forty-five years of age, is one of the tragic consequences of mental ill-health. Suicide occurs in a number of kinds of emotional disturbances but is most frequent among persons who are severely depressed.

Physiological Effects of Emotions

The emotions affect, favorably or unfavorably, the functioning of practically every organ of the body. Excitement prepares the

[　73　]

body for emergency action and great exertion. Anger, particularly anger against oneself, can help to bring about ulcer of the stomach or duodenum. Resentment can prevent food from entering one's stomach. Disgust, even after one has forgotten all about it, can result in skin rashes. Feelings of guilt, not only about things which one has done but also about things which one may have thought of doing, can lead to distraction, carelessness, and accidents. Mental depression can lead to constipation. Anxiety often causes diarrhea, and can produce heart and blood pressure disorders. Emotion, stress, and tensions are also common causes of headaches.

The Basis of Prevention and Treatment

If we accept this explanation of mental and emotional disorders, the general trend of prevention and therapy is immediately obvious. If mental illnesses are the result of learned reactions, gradually acquired, therapy becomes a process of reeducation, during which the patient unlearns old unhealthy emotional and mental habits and acquires new and more efficient methods. This is a general principle that underlies all the modern therapeutic procedures, however varied these appear to be on casual inspection.

Freudian psychoanalysis consists primarily of the conscious recall and emotional reenacting of the infantile repressed memories, which are reinterpreted during the analytic procedure—essentially a reeducational process. Adler's attempt to redirect the patient to a better or more socially acceptable goal than that which had been acquired through previous maladjustment is likewise an educational procedure. Those who practice suggestion, persuasion, and similar methods are doing the same thing on a more superficial level. Even the rest cures, sea voyages, and changes of occupation so often recommended probably owe their effectiveness to removal of stresses and tensions inherent in old associations and activities.

Many methods have been found to be surprisingly effective, which substantiates the belief that mental illnesses are psychological phenomena, the result of experience and interpretations

of experience; and that treatment consists of corrective emotional experiences of one kind or another. Likewise, prevention
will be logically directed against environmental factors which
tend to produce or exaggerate unhealthy adaptation and toward
the correction of such reactions before they have become such
an ingrained part of the individual's equipment that he will use
them in serious matters and will fail to develop others.

The student who faces the college adjustment while still dependent on and
closely identified with his family—and most students are—has a special
handicap in all the phases of his development. Before he can fit into the college
environment altogether successfully he must complete the changes which are
expected to occur in the family relationship as the individual grows up. . . .
For detachment from the family is a necessary step toward the emotional
maturity of an individual; it is a prerequisite to the smooth development of
other growth process. . . . Detachment from the family does not imply
antagonism to it or a complete denial of its participation in the individual's
life. And in the achievement of detachment, parental guidance need not be
thrown off abruptly or ignored. As the phrase is used here, the development of
independence means not a severance of all relations between the growing
individual and his family but the gradual establishment by the individual of
habits of independence in choosing his goals, his values and his associates. [5]

Most emotional maladjustments have their basis in experiences of childhood, experiences which occur before the individual
has the power to control the forces that play upon him and before
he has learned to judge his reactions to these forces. By the time
the age of discretion is reached, most persons have developed certain emotional habits which are unhealthy. But this is nothing
to worry about unless the number of these habits is sufficiently
great or their use sufficiently frequent to interfere with happiness
and efficiency.

Occasionally one needs the advice of a physician trained in the
field of psychiatry to correct unhealthy emotional habits. But
more commonly one is able to work out one's own solution. On
the other hand, even the "average person" fairly well adjusted
to life, in whom there are no long-standing or deep-seated conflicts, may, by the neglect of a few relatively simple and self-

[5] Fry, Clements C., "Mental Health in College," Commonwealth Fund, Division of
Publication, New York, 1942.

evident principles, tangle his emotional life to the extent of completely incapacitating himself for happiness. It is not within the scope of this book to discuss these principles at length; but although they appear dogmatic when stated briefly and without modification, a few of them will be set down, in the expectation that the reader will realize their importance and supply for himself the necessary modifications and enlargement.

Emotional difficulties are not likely to become serious in a person who is thoroughly conscious of what he wants from life and is able to face the difficulties involved in getting it. This makes knowledge of the facts about oneself a fundamental necessity. One must accept one's physical and intellectual handicaps in order to plan a satisfactory life inside these limitations. There are thousands of people suffering from hopeless frustration because they set a goal for themselves which is beyond their abilities.

Ann Bridge expresses this well in a sentence from her book "Illyrian Spring":

> Freedom consists of two things; to know each one his limitations—that is the same thing as to know one's self and to accept one's self as one is, without fear, or envy or distaste; and to recognize and accept the conditions under which one lives, also without fear, or envy or distaste. When you do this you shall be free.[6]

On the other hand, it is equally dangerous to use one's handicaps as an excuse for not attempting some useful and satisfactory work. Everyone has his capabilities as well as his limitations. These assets he should take stock of so as to direct his efforts along lines in which he may expect the greatest degree of accomplishment and personal satisfaction.

The facts about oneself which one should understand include more than one's physical and intellectual endowments. Emotional attitudes, desires, and ambitions are equally a part of one's equipment. They must be recognized and given their proper weight. Satisfaction of emotional needs is a primary necessity for mental health, but such satisfaction requires evaluation, plan-

[6] Bridge, Ann, "Illyrian Spring," p. 252, Little, Brown & Company, Boston, 1935.

ning, and control. This means a plan of life in which the deepest emotional needs of the individuals are given the greatest attention and in which every precaution is taken against their frustration. The plan must make room also for lesser desires which, although subordinated to the major aims, will be given adequate expression. In general, these requirements are best met by the one who, in addition to his chief work, cultivates a taste for the arts, develops hobbies, enjoys friendships and play, and takes an interest in public affairs or other matters beyond the sphere of mere personal concern.

DISCUSSION SUGGESTIONS

1. Discuss the importance of mental diseases in the United States.
2. Explain the physical basis for certain mental illnesses.
3. What are the other more important types of mental disorders?
4. Discuss the relation of physical and social heredity to mental illness.
5. Define insanity, psychosis, neurosis, delusion, hallucination, delirium.
6. Discuss the mechanism of the development of mental ill-health.
7. What is the relation of syphilis to mental disease?
8. Discuss daydreaming and feelings of inferiority.
9. Discuss the prevention and treatment of mental ill-health.

REFERENCES AND READING SUGGESTIONS

1. Beers, Clifford: "A Mind That Found Itself," 7th ed., Doubleday & Company, Inc., New York, 1948.
2. Clarke, Eric Kent: "Mental Hygiene for Community Nursing," University of Minnesota Press, Minneapolis, 1942.
3. Gumpert, Martin: "The Anatomy of Happiness," McGraw-Hill Book Company, Inc., New York, 1951.
4. Fosdick, Harry Emerson: "On Being a Real Person," Harper & Brothers, New York, 1943.
5. Havighurst, Robert G., and Hilda Taba: "Adolescent Character and Personality," John Wiley & Sons, Inc., New York, 1949.
6. Healey, William: "Personality in Formation and Action," W. W. Norton & Company, Inc., New York, 1938.
7. Liebman, Joshua L.: "Peace of Mind," Simon and Schuster, Inc., New York, 1946.
8. Menninger, Karl: "The Human Mind," Alfred A. Knopf, Inc., New York, 1945.
9. Peale, Norman V., and Smiley Blanton: "The Art of Real Happiness," Prentice-Hall, Inc., New York, 1950.

10. Strecker, F. S., and K. Appel: "Discovering Ourselves," 2d ed., The Macmillan Company, New York, 1944.
11. Thorman, George: "Toward Mental Health," Public Affairs Pamphlets, New York.
12. Yost, O. R.: "What You Should Know about Mental Illness," Exposition Press, New York, 1953.
13. Pamphlets of National Committee for Mental Hygiene, New York.

Text-Films

The following McGraw-Hill Text-Film on Health Education is recommended for use with this chapter of the text.

Emotional Health (20 min sd MP).[7]   In following the progress of a case history of a single college freshman, this film aims at removing the stigma associated with emotional upsets and establishing psychiatric techniques as the *normal* treatment of persistent emotional disturbances.

Silent follow-up filmstrip based on material contained in the motion picture offers opportunity for review, testing, and further discussion.

[7] The running time (min), whether it is silent (si), or sound (sd), and whether it is a motion picture (MP) or filmstrip (FS), are listed with each title throughout the book. All the motion pictures are 16 mm; filmstrips are 35 mm.

Chapter IV

NUTRITION AND GROWTH

ADEQUATE nutrition is a prime requisite to vigorous health.
Every living thing, from the simplest form of plant life to
the most highly developed animal organism, must have food;
food for growth, food for energy, food to regulate body processes,
and food to replace worn-out tissues; food adequate in amount
and of proper composition.

To the average individual a plant or an animal appears to be a
unit, a single functioning mechanism. The scientist, on the other
hand, sees in the simple plant as well as in the animal body a multitude of individual cells of microscopic size, each living its own
existence, becoming more and more specialized, and functioning
cooperatively in the community of cells of which it is a part.
Each of these cells is a chemical machine for the conversion of
foodstuffs into energy or into new compounds for growth and
development. The various tissues and organs of the body are
composed of a seemingly infinite number of highly specialized
cells.

The process which we call digestion is the preparation of foodstuffs so that they can be utilized by these cells.

. . . Large chemical molecules are reduced in size to a sort of common de-
nominator, or at any rate, to particles beyond the limits of microscopic visi-
bility. No appreciable amounts of the food elements can pass through the
walls of the intestinal canal and enter the blood stream for use by the body

proper unless their particle size is smaller than one twenty-five-millionth of an inch in diameter. If such a particle were the diameter of a penny, 25 million of them side by side would be 252 miles long. Sugar and salt readily dissolve in water to form particles much smaller than this, but starches and fats and most proteins do not dissolve in water at all, and therefore require the chemical disintegration which we know as digestion.[1]

The products of digestion are taken up from the intestinal tract into the blood, which carries food, water, and oxygen to the cells and removes the waste products of their activity. The food needs of the body, then, become the food needs of its individual cells.

The foods which these cells must have and are able to utilize are divided by the chemist into the following groups: water, proteins, carbohydrates, fats, vitamins, and minerals. Although certain cells, such as those of the bones, hair, muscles, thyroid gland, and red blood corpuscles, need more of certain food elements than do other cells, the sum total of the needs of all these cells makes up the nutritional needs of the body as a whole (see Fig. 12 and Table 8).

Except for water and certain minerals, the real source of man's food supply is the plant kingdom. Even the food of the Eskimo, which consists almost entirely of animal tissues and animal products, comes indirectly from plants. Plants utilizing the energy of the sun, the oxygen, carbon dioxide, and nitrogen of the air, and the water and mineral salts of the soil, manufacture the carbohydrates, fats, proteins, and vitamins which serve as food for man and animals.

We welcome the first appearance of green in the grass and on the trees as a sign that winter is past. The verdant landscapes have been painted by artists and praised by poets. But the chemist sees in this green color more than the artist's picture or a poet's song. The chemist sees that nature is again starting the greatest of all chemical factories, one that manufactures products which are essential for the maintenance of life upon the earth. . . . When we burn sugar heat is evolved. Just as much heat, in the form of radiation from the sun, must first have been fixed in the sugar, through the agency of the green chlorophyll, as is later liberated when the sugar is burned. Therefore we have

[1] Palmer, Leroy Sheldon, "The Fundamentals of Nutrition," *Journal-Lancet*, vol 58, pp. 219–223, May, 1938.

FIG. 12. ALIMENTARY CANAL WITH DIGESTIVE GLANDS

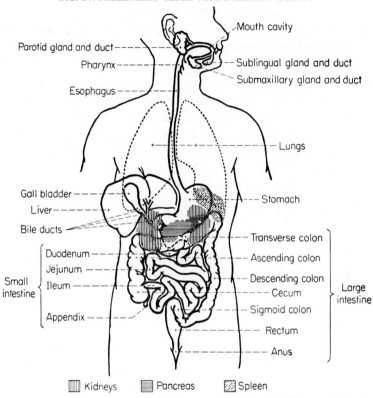

The parotid, sublingual, and submaxillary are salivary glands. (Schematic drawing.)

here, in the green leaf cells, a mechanism for storing up the sun's energy in a form which may be kept almost indefinitely.[2]

Nitrogen Cycle

All animals require carbon and nitrogen for the support of growth and activity. Yet they are unable to utilize these chemical elements unless they are combined with hydrogen and oxygen in the form of organic chemical compounds called "proteins," "fats," and "carbohydrates." Animals themselves are unable to build these compounds from pure chemical elements or inorganic

[2] Gortner, R. A., "Plants and Man as Seen by a Biochemist," *Minnesota Chats,* vol. 17, p. 1, December 24, 1934.

salts, but green plants have the capacity to do so. For this reason, animals are dependent upon plants for their existence.

The combining of carbon dioxide and oxygen from the air with water and nitrogen-containing salts from the soil to form proteins and carbohydrates takes place in green plants as the result of the action of sunlight upon the chlorophyll in their leaves and stems. When these plants are used as food by animals, either the proteins and carbohydrates are broken down into simple chemical forms within the digestive tract and absorbed and reconstructed to form tissues and supply energy to the animal, or they are eliminated as excreta. The tissues and much of the excreta of animals are chemically too complex to serve directly as plant foods; but in the process of decay they are broken down by the action of saprophytic (nondisease-producing) bacteria into simple chemical compounds which plants can utilize.

In addition, a small group of so-called "nitrogen-fixing" bacteria, found chiefly around the nodules or roots of leguminous plants, are able to take nitrogen out of the air and combine it with other chemical elements to form the nitrogen-containing salts needed for the growth of plants.

From this brief consideration of the "nitrogen cycle" it is apparent that there is a constant rotation of the various chemical elements which make up animal and plant tissues between the plant and animal kingdoms. In plants, with the aid of the energy of the sun, the simple chemical elements and compounds are synthesized (built up) into complex organic compounds which the animal body utilizes and eventually breaks down again into simpler chemical compounds. In this cycle between plants and animals, however, there are important gaps which, if unbridged by bacteria, would result in the cessation of life upon this planet.

The Need for Water

The body is a chemical machine which builds new tissues, replaces worn-out ones, and provides heat and energy. These chemical changes upon which life depends take place in solutions. In solution foods are digested, the products of digestion carried to the tissue cells, and the waste products taken away.

TABLE 8

DIGESTION AND ABSORPTION

Portion of Digestive Tract	Digestive Juice	Secretory Glands	Digestive Enzymes or Ferments	Foods Digested	Digestion Carried to Stage of	Absorption
Mouth	Saliva	Salivary	Ptyalin	Starches	Double sugars	None
Stomach	Gastric juice	Gastric	1. Pepsin 2. Rennin	1. Proteins 2. Milk	1. {Proteoses Peptones} 2. Casein	Practically none. Small amounts of alcohol and glucose
Duodenum, i.e., first part of small intestine	Pancreatic juice	Pancreas	1. {Trypsin Myopsin} 2. Steapsin 3. Amylopsin 4. Maltase	1. Proteins 2. Fats 3. Starches 4. Maltose	1. {Proteoses Polypeptides Amino acids} 2. Glycerine and fatty acids 3. Double sugars, maltose 4. Glucose	Some absorption of water, salts, vitamins, amino acids, single sugars, emulsified fats, fatty acids, and glycerine
	Bile	Liver	None	Fats	Emulsifies and so prepares for digestion and absorption	
Jejunum and ileum, i.e., second and third portions of small intestine	Intestinal juice	Glands in wall of intestinal tract	1. Erepsin 2. Maltase 3. Invertase	1. Proteins and split products (peptones, etc.) 2. Maltose 3. Cane sugar }	Amino acids Simple sugars	Major absorption of water, salts, vitamins, amino acids, single sugars, emulsified fats, fatty acids, and glycerine
Large intestine	None	None	Mainly bacterial enzymes	Fermentative and other actions on undigested foodstuffs		Water

Water makes up the major portion of every secretion of the body. It plays an important part in every healing process. It regulates body temperature. Truly, in the body we have "water, water everywhere." Hence, water may well be considered the most important single constituent of the living organism. A man may survive a month or longer without food but death will occur within a few days if he is deprived of water.

The proportion of the body weight which is due to water varies with age. At the sixth week of life the human embryo is 97.5 per cent water. At birth, water represents approximately 70 per cent of the body weight, while a little less than two-thirds of the weight of an adult is due to water.

The important sources of body water are water taken as drink, water contained in food, and water formed in the oxidation (burning) of foods in the body. Water is lost from the body in the urine, in the feces, in perspiration, and through evaporation from the skin and lungs.

The amount of water which the body requires varies with age, exercise, diet, temperature of the body, and temperature and humidity of the surrounding air. Under average conditions an adult requires approximately three quarts of water per day. An ordinary diet will provide two-thirds of this amount with the food (Table 9). The rest needs to be taken in the form of drink.

It is impossible to state exactly just how much water one should drink each day in order to provide optimum conditions for the various physiological processes of the body. In hot weather one needs more water than when it is cold and more when exercising than when inactive. Under average conditions six glasses of liquid per day, in addition to that contained in the food, is commonly recommended. This quantity is more than sufficient to replace the fluids lost from the body in 24 hours and hence will supply the needs of the body and leave a margin of safety.

Fortunately we do not need to rely on theoretical computations of the amount of water which the body needs, for nature has provided a mechanism to insure an adequate fluid intake. This mechanism is the sensation of thirst, which under normal conditions can be relied upon to prevent any serious deficiency of water in the tissues.

TABLE 9

WATER CONTENT OF SOME COMMON FOODS

Food Material	Water Content, Percentage by Weight
Tomatoes	94
Carrots or beets	87
Oranges	86
Egg white	86
Cow's milk	85
Spinach	83
Fish, halibut	75
Bananas	75
Potatoes	63
Apples	63
Veal, leg	60
40 per cent cream	58
Beef, sirloin	54
Egg yolk	49
Fresh ham	48
Bread, average white	36
Cream cheese	34
Butter	15

The taking of large quantities of water is advocated and practiced as a health measure by many people. Some drink the water as it occurs in nature; others add a small amount of salt. Water in excess of that needed by the body is promptly excreted by the kidneys unless it contains salt in approximately the same concentration as salt occurs in the blood. Although the excretion of excess water ordinarily is of little or no importance, the drinking of large quantities of water after excessive sweating may result in severe headache, abdominal discomfort, cramplike pains, and muscle tremors—"miner's cramp" or "stoker's disease." If salt is added to the water in the proportion of a level teaspoonful to a quart of water, greater retention of the fluid results and the likelihood of such symptoms is reduced.

The supposed ill effects of drinking water with meals has not been confirmed by physiological experiments, for it has been shown that the digestive ferments act just as efficiently in dilute as in more concentrated solutions. On the other hand, saliva is of great importance for the digestion of starches; hence, the drinking of water is no substitute for thorough mastication and salivation of food.

Large amounts of water are frequently advocated for the treatment of acute infections such as colds, tonsillitis, and influenza. The theory upon which this is recommended is that water aids in the elimination of toxic products produced by the infection. Whether this actually occurs has never been demonstrated, so one can only conclude that the value of this practice is based on assumption rather than on definite evidence. When infection is accompanied by fever, the rate of evaporation is increased and it becomes necessary to replace the fluids thus lost. Here again nature warns us of this need by increasing the thirst.

As practical generalizations concerning the body's needs for fluids, we may conclude that thirst is a safe and reliable criterion of the amount of water which is needed, that there is a greater likelihood of taking too little than too much fluid, and that six glasses of liquids a day, in addition to that contained in the food, is a reasonable estimate of the average desirable intake.

The Minerals of the Body

The body contains certain inorganic, or mineral, salts. In a newborn child these amount to about 3 per cent of the total body weight; in an adult to about 4½ per cent. The chief of these are calcium, 3.8 pounds, enough to make 7 pounds of lime; phosphorus, about 2 pounds; sodium, to make a shaker of table salt; iron, for a good-sized nail; iodine, about a tenth of a drop of the tincture; and small amounts of sulfur, potassium, chlorine, copper, manganese, etc. Although these minerals are absolutely essential to health, many of their functions in the body are not completely understood.

Calcium and Phosphorus. Most of these minerals are in the bones and teeth to which they give strength and hardness, but the regulation of the irritability of the nervous system is probably an equally important function of calcium in the body. In fact, if the amount of calcium in the blood falls much below its normal concentration of about 1 part in 10,000, muscular spasms result and generalized convulsions may occur. The requirement of calcium and phosphorus, although continuous throughout life, is greatest for the growing child and the pregnant or lactating woman. Fortunately, milk is sufficiently rich in both calcium and phosphorus so that a quart a day will supply the needs of infants for both of these elements. In older children and adults the relative amount of milk in the diet usually is smaller. Hence, the diet needs to contain other foods rich in these elements, such as cheese, green leafy vegetables, broccoli, nuts, and molasses. Dr. R. R. Spencer of the U.S. Public Health Service reports that

. . . in Southern China, where the population is so dense that milk production is extremely difficult, the custom is to present a pair of pig's feet to prospective mothers. These are boiled in the presence of an acid and the dish is consumed to obtain calcium; this custom is followed throughout pregnancy and lactation, and sufficient calcium is supplied to mother and child. Older children and adults must make up the deficiency by consuming enormous quantities of fresh vegetables—daily quantities that Americans would find it impossible to get away with.

Iron is utilized by the body primarily for the formation of hemoglobin. Hence, it is an important factor in determining the capacity of the blood to transport oxygen to the tissues. The amount of iron lost from the body per day averages about 1 milligram for men and 1.5 to 2.0 milligrams for women. Studies indicate that many infants, particularly those born prematurely, do better if their usual diets of milk and cereals are supplemented with iron or iron-containing foods. The addition of the yolk of one egg per day to the milk diet of infants has been estimated as adequate for ordinary requirements. Deficiency of iron in older children and adults is unlikely if their diets contain meat (liver, oysters, etc.), eggs, green leafy vegetables, prunes, molasses, raisins, soybeans, or other foods with a relatively high iron content. Of the iron contained in foods an average of only 10 to 20 per cent is absorbed from the intestinal tract into the blood and tissues. Ascorbic acid (vitamin C) greatly increases the absorption of iron. Most patients with the more common types of anemia are greatly benefited by large doses of iron salts.

[87]

Copper. The body needs copper for growth and health; but the amount required is exceedingly small. For example, nutritional studies indicate that experimental animals on a diet of raw milk, which usually has a low iron content, do not grow normally, even though this diet be supplemented with iron. However, if pasteurized milk is substituted for raw milk, normal growth results. The explanation offered is that copper aids in the utilization of iron by the body and that in the process of pasteurization infinitesimal but adequate amounts of copper are absorbed by the milk in its passage through the copper pipes of the pasteurizing machine. Any reasonably well balanced diet will supply the body's need for copper.

Iodine is another chemical element which, although necessary only in minute amounts, is essential to health. Its use in the body is primarily in connection with the function of the thyroid gland. If the iodine intake is insufficient, the thyroid gland enlarges and the condition known as "simple goiter" results. At times some stunting of growth accompanies this iodine deficiency.

Goiter and iodine deficiency are found chiefly in inland regions, from the soil of which for countless ages the iodine salts have been washed toward the sea. As a result of the low iodine content of the soil, the iodine content of water, of plants, and of animal tissues in these regions is low. Sea water, marine plants, and sea food, on the other hand, have a high iodine content. In recent years efforts have been made to assure to populations, and particularly to children, in goiterous regions the amount of iodine which the body requires. This amount is small, probably no more than 50 to 100 milligrams per year—0.0015 to 0.003 ounce. It may be administered daily, weekly, or at intervals of two or three months.

The methods usually advocated for supplying the necessary iodine are the use of foods rich in iodine, the use of iodized salt, the addition of iodine to the water supply, or the administration at regular intervals of tablets containing iodine. Any of these methods is satisfactory but the one which seems to reach the greatest number of people is the use of iodized salt. This is a simple, inexpensive method of administration which has been shown to be effective. In a city in Michigan 12.5 per cent of 89 children who had not been using iodized salt were found to have goiters, while only 0.1 per cent of 900 children who had been using iodized salt for three or more years had goiters. Persons with goiters should be under medical supervision and should not attempt self-medication, even with iodized salt.

Alkaline Foods. Alkaline foods, drinks, and drugs are constantly recommended through advertising channels because of their alleged health value. It is implied that acidosis in a mild degree is very common and that it is associated with susceptibility to infection and various forms of ill-health. Actually there is no scientific evidence to support these assertions. Acidosis may occur in the advanced stages of diabetes; but this is a distinctly abnormal condition in which the accumulation of acids in the tissues is the result of incomplete metabolism of fat. In healthy individuals on average diets it has not been demonstrated. In fact, neither of two subjects who lived on an exclusively meat diet for 12 months showed any evidence of acidosis. Certainly, then, there is no reason to be concerned about acidosis when one is using fruits, vegetables, cereals, milk, and dairy products.

The Need for Proteins

Proteins alone contain the nitrogenous compounds out of which new tissue can be built and worn-out tissue repaired. Hence, protein is a basic essential of the diet. Chemically, proteins differ from the other foods primarily in that proteins contain nitrogen. All proteins also contain carbon, hydrogen, and oxygen, and many contain sulfur, phosphorus, iron, and other minerals. Plants put these chemical elements together in various proportions and combinations to form nitrogenous compounds called "amino acids." Twenty-five of these amino acids are known to the biochemist. They constitute the building stones out of which all proteins, whether they be from plants or animals, are constructed.

Plants manufacture the amino acids which they need for growth. Animals are not so self-sufficient but are dependent upon plants for certain of these essential elements of tissue building.

[89]

Approximately half of these essential amino acids can be synthesized within the human body. The others must be obtained ready-made from plant or animal food products.

The so-called "complete" proteins contain all the amino acids that are necessary to health, while others, such as gelatin and the majority of vegetable proteins, are lacking in certain ones. In order that all the essential amino acids may be available, it is important that the proteins of the diet be derived from various sources.

In the process of digestion, proteins are broken down into the amino acids of which they are constituted. In this form, and only in this form, can they be utilized. If digestion fails to break them down to this stage, they will pass through the intestinal tract and be excreted as waste products. The amino acids are absorbed from the intestinal tract into the blood stream and carried by the blood to the tissue cells which are in need of them. Although a constant necessity, amino acids are not stored by the body. Hence, it is important that the diet supply each day the amount necessary to support growth and tissue repair.

Although the principal use which the body makes of proteins is for the growth and replacement of tissue, proteins may be oxidized to serve as a source of heat and mechanical or other energy. In fact, a gram of protein upon oxidation yields the same amount of heat as a gram of carbohydrate. However, the digestion and assimilation of proteins utilize more energy and produce more heat than the digestion and assimilation of carbohydrates. Hence, it is usual for the diet to contain a smaller proportion of protein foods in the summer than in the winter. Proteins also are less readily oxidized than carbohydrates and upon oxidation leave waste nitrogenous products to be excreted. For these reasons proteins are less desirable as sources of energy than are the carbohydrates and fats.

The protein requirements of the body vary with the rate of growth and with total energy intake. Approximately 10 per cent of the food of a nursing baby is protein. The diets of infants and nursing mothers should be planned so that 10 to 15 per cent of the total energy content will be derived from proteins. In older children and in adults 10 per cent, or about ½ gram of protein per pound of body weight, seems adequate. On the other hand, a diet without a reasonable content of the high-protein foods, such as meat and eggs, is unappetizing to many people, and there is no convincing evidence that moderate amounts beyond the minimum requirements are deleterious. Hence, the use of proteins up to 10 to 12 per cent of the diet is considered a reasonable protein allowance. In general terms, this means that one average portion of meat or meat substitutes per day, together with eggs, milk, and other protein foods, is adequate.

The Need for Carbohydrates

The carbohydrates, which occur in our foods chiefly as sugars and starches, are combinations of carbon, hydrogen, and oxygen, with the hydrogen and oxygen always in the same proportion as in water, that is, two parts of hydrogen to one part of oxygen. Carbohydrates can be absorbed into the blood stream and utilized by the tissue cells only as simple sugars, such as dextrose or glucose. Cane sugar and beet sugar, called "saccharose," are "double sugars." Starches contain multiple units of simple sugars, bound together in loose chemical combination. The digestion of carbohydrates reduces all of the double sugars and starches to simple sugars.

The first important step in the breaking down of starches occurs in the mouth as the result of a ferment contained in the saliva. There are no digestive ferments in the stomach which act upon starches or sugars. So if digestion is not started in the mouth, starches pass unchanged along the digestive tract until they reach the small intestine. For this reason thorough mastication even of soft, starchy foods is important.

After digestion, sugar is absorbed directly into the blood, from which the tissue cells withdraw it according to their needs. Any excess over current needs is stored in the liver and muscles as glycogen, converted into fat, or excreted through the urine. From the reserve supplies in the liver and muscles sugar is withdrawn according to the needs of the body. Then when these reserves are depleted, the body begins to burn its fats for energy.

[91]

If for any reason the amount of sugar in the blood falls below normal—a condition called "hypoglycemia"—various symptoms, such as weakness, nervousness, irritability, and a sensation of trembling, occur and eventually convulsions and death will follow unless sugar is administered (see also page 386).

In the tissue cells sugar is oxidized (burned) with the aid of insulin, and heat and energy are liberated. Just what part insulin, which is secreted by the pancreas and carried in the blood stream, plays in this oxidation of sugars is not completely understood. It is perfectly clear, however, that the body cannot burn sugar without it. The muscles may contain both sugar and oxygen, but without insulin to provide the "spark" no oxidation will occur. When the pancreas does not produce insulin in adequate amounts, diabetes mellitus results.

The oxygen for this burning of carbohydrates is carried from the lungs to the tissue cells by the hemoglobin of the blood. The end products of the process are carbon dioxide (carbonic acid gas) and water. The carbon dioxide is carried by the blood to the lungs, where it is given off into the air, while the water is available for use. The chemical changes involved in the oxidation of sugar in the body are the same as when sugar is burned in a flame, except that the body can regulate the rate of burning in accordance with its energy requirements.

The need of the body for carbohydrates depends primarily upon the amount of physical activity and the quantity of other energy foods, particularly fat, available. For example, the carbohydrate intake of a person engaged in physical labor may well be 50 to 100 per cent higher than that of a person in a sedentary occupation.

As a rule carbohydrates are relatively cheap foods. Hence, when economy is an important consideration in the selection of foods, there is a tendency to increase the proportion of carbohydrate in the diet. This is entirely safe, provided the diet also contains adequate amounts of the essential minerals, proteins, and vitamins.

The chief sources of carbohydrates in the average diet are potatoes, cereal grains, sugar, and certain starchy vegetables such as the legumes—peas, beans, lentils, etc. Wheat contains about 70 per cent carbohydrates and is useful as a food primarily for this reason. Whole-grain cereal foods, such as breakfast foods and bread, contain more minerals and proteins than the highly milled cereals, but even these are not complete foods. Evidences of dietary deficiency are frequently found where cereals make up a major portion of the diet. The reason is not that carbohydrates are deleterious but that other essential food elements are omitted.

The Need for Fats

Fats also are composed of the chemical elements carbon, hydrogen, and oxygen, but these exist in different proportions and combinations from those in carbohydrates. After digestion, fats are absorbed and then oxidized to produce energy, carbon dioxide, and water. Amounts in excess of current needs may be stored as body fat or converted into carbohydrate and stored as glycogen. As an energy-producing food, fat is exceptionally valuable, for the oxidation of 1 gram of fat yields approximately 9 calories,[3] while 1 gram of carbohydrate or 1 gram of protein yields 4 calories.

Fats used in cooking, salad dressings, etc., add to the palatability of food. Fat also decreases the motility of the stomach and the secretion of gastric juice, with the result that the stomach empties less rapidly and hunger contractions of the stomach are delayed.

The quantity of fat, like the quantity of carbohydrate, which should be included in the diet depends upon energy requirements and the quantity of other energy foods available. Fats of the diet are derived from both animal and vegetable sources. Among the foods with the highest fat content are vegetable oils, lard, butter, bacon, cream, nuts, and fatty meats.

The Need for Vitamins

The discovery of the vitamins and of the part which they play in growth and health is the most important contribution of recent years to our knowledge of nutrition. On the other hand,

[3] A calorie is a unit of heat (see p. 114).

much of the information which the public receives from commercial sources concerning vitamins is misleading. Actually, vitamins provide no heat, energy, or material for tissue building; yet they are essential for growth and health. The exact manner in which these substances influence nutrition is not known, but it is clear that minute amounts of them are adequate and that the lack of any one is deleterious to health.

The term "vitamin," which merely implies that it is something necessary for life, was adopted before the nature of vitamins was known. Some have been isolated in pure, crystalline form and their exact chemical structures determined. Several are now manufactured in the chemical laboratory. In time the nature of all vitamins probably will be known. Then the term will have lost much of its usefulness because the vitamins can be designated by the chemical names which describe their structure or nature.

Twenty-two substances having vitamin effects have been reported as occurring naturally in foods, but for practical purposes these may properly be reduced to about 14 different kinds of vitamins. This is because (1) in the case of vitamin A there are known to be four different but related yellow vegetable pigments which, when consumed in the diet, can be changed wholly or in part to vitamin A itself in the body and (2) because there are at least five different, closely related substances which occur naturally and which can cure or prevent rickets, in other words at least five different vitamin D's. Another helpful fact is that at least five kinds of vitamins are probably not of any importance for human nutrition. This leaves nine to consider for our welfare at the present stage of our knowledge. There are, according to the alphabet system, vitamins A, B, C, D, E, G, K, P, and the pellagra-preventive factor, also referred to as the P.P. factor.[4]

The best sources of vitamins for man are natural foods of vegetable and animal origin. Occasionally it may be desirable to supplement available natural foods with vitamin concentrates. There is, however, no evidence that growth can be promoted or health improved by adding to the diet more vitamins than it is possible to obtain from the *proper selection of natural foods*. In spite of this, the retail vitamin business in the United States increased from $1,000,000 in 1939 to $160,000,000 in 1952.

[4] Palmer, *loc. cit.*

The Individual Vitamins

Vitamin A is frequently called the "growth vitamin" or the "anti-infective vitamin." Both terms have some justification but tend to be misleading because neither is accurate. Vitamin A is essential for growth, but so also are proteins, carbohydrates, minerals, and several others of the vitamins. In animals a deficiency of vitamin A increases susceptibility to certain types of infection. On the other hand, there is no evidence that the addition of vitamin A to an average well balanced diet will increase resistance to infection.

The most specific effects of vitamin A deficiency are night blindness—that is, difficulty in seeing with dim illumination—and a disease of the eyes called "xerophthalmia." In 1913 McCollum demonstrated that this disease of the eyes could be prevented by the addition to the diet of a substance present in butterfat, egg yolk, and other foods. He later called this substance vitamin A. Many cases of this disease in children were observed in Denmark during the First World War. When local consumption of butterfat was increased, owing to regulations limiting exportation of dairy products, the disease disappeared. In Rumania, where the supply of dairy products was cut off, similar outbreaks of this disease were observed among children whose diets consisted largely of soups, cereals, and cereal products. The provision of cod-liver oil by the American Red Cross put an end to these outbreaks.

A study of the students in an Eastern medical school gave scientific evidence of relative vitamin A deficiency in 35 per cent of the group and symptoms of night blindness, photophobia, and dry skin in 12 per cent. These students reported difficulty in driving a car at night and in finding their seats in theaters or other darkened rooms, excessive discomfort from bright lights, and very dry skins and scalps. An analysis of their diets showed that they contained little or none of the foods containing vitamin A.

Other results of a deficiency of this vitamin in experimental animals are loss of appetite, retardation of growth, physical

[95]

weakness, susceptibility to infections (particularly of the eye, respiratory tract, and middle ear), secondary anemia, failure of reproduction, and formation of kidney stones.

Vitamin A is not destroyed by ordinary cooking, by pasteurization, or by canning. It is stored by the animal organism in the liver, in milk, and in eggs, so that once an animal has taken adequate amounts of this vitamin, symptoms of deficiency will not appear for a long time even though the vitamin be completely absent from the diet.

In the animal body vitamin A is formed from a chemical substance, called "carotene," which is the yellow pigment of certain vegetables and plants. In the leaves of most plants, in tomatoes, and in peas considerable amounts of carotene also occur, although the yellow color is covered up by other pigments.

The most reliable sources of vitamin A are fish oils (such as halibut-liver oil and cod-liver oil), egg yolk, codfish, liver and other glandular meats, butter, cream, cheese, carrots, sweet potatoes, squash, green peppers, tomatoes, various green leafy vegetables, apricots, cantaloupe, peaches, and prunes.

The requirements of the body for vitamin A have not been definitely established. Children need more than adults. In fact, most of the cases of xerophthalmia reported in Denmark were in children under six months of age and there were practically no cases in children over two years. No deleterious effects have been noted from the administration of reasonable amounts of this vitamin. Hence, until definite information is available as to the minimum amount necessary to maintain growth and health, the diet, particularly of the growing child, should contain liberal amounts of the foods rich in this vitamin. On such a diet there is no danger of deficiency and no need to supplement the diet with special vitamin concentrates or products. In fact, a study, which was concerned with the minimal vitamin A content of food that is safe for infants, concluded that the average diet of infants contains at least four times as many units as the minimum required to maintain nutritional status and resistance to infection.

Vitamin B Complex. In 1897 a Dutch physician discovered that by feeding pigeons nothing but polished rice he could produce a serious and widespread disease of the Orient called "beriberi." Having produced the disease, he found that he could cure it by adding to the diet of polished rice whole-grain cereals, milk, and certain fresh fruits and vegetables. The substance in these foods responsible for the prevention of beriberi was later named vitamin B. Subsequent and continuing investigations have revealed that vitamin B, instead of being a single vitamin as was first believed, is really a vitamin complex consisting of at least a dozen vitamins required by the body in small amounts and several other substances of which little is known. Best understood among the constituents of the B complex are thiamine, riboflavin, and niacin.

Thiamine, also called vitamin B_1, is concerned with the proper functioning of the nervous system and with carbohydrate metabolism. The results of a deficiency are nervous irritability, impairment of the appetite, digestive disturbances, growth failure, emaciation, weakness, anemia, impairment of lactation, multiple neuritis, and beriberi.

In this country the symptoms of B_1 or thiamine deficiency are usually mild. In other parts of the world, where polished rice and refined cereals are the chief articles of diet, symptoms of thiamine deficiency are much more common and severe. The amount of thiamine necessary for health is small. This normal requirement, however, is doubled during pregnancy and increases three- to fivefold during lactation. Growing children need more than adults.

The most reliable sources of this vitamin are yeast (especially brewers' yeast), whole-grain cereals, bread made from "enriched flour," fresh fruits, eggs, vegetables, legumes, and glandular organs, such as liver, sweetbreads, and kidney. Synthetic, chemically pure thiamine is also available. Certain amounts of both thiamine and riboflavin are produced by bacteria of the human intestinal tract.

Riboflavin is sometimes referred to as vitamin B_2 or vitamin G. Lack of adequate riboflavin in the diet may cause cessation of growth, loss of hair, soreness of the lips and tongue, and a type of blindness. The best sources of this vitamin are liver, yeast, kidneys, sweetbreads, lean meat, oysters, fish, milk and cream, eggs, whole-grain cereal products or enriched breads, peanuts, and green leafy vegetables. Riboflavin can also be prepared synthetically.

Niacin or Nicotinic Acid. A deficiency of niacin, or the "P.P. factor" as it was formerly called, causes pellagra. The symptoms of this deficiency are weakness, failure to grow, digestive disturbances, skin rashes, and, eventually, pellagra. In this country pellagra is more common in the South, particularly among the poorer classes, where it is said that it is due to a diet of the three M's: meal (cornmeal), meat (salt pork), and molasses. Pellagra occurs also in chronic alcoholics who take liquor instead of proper food. Foods rich in the pellagra-preventive factor are yeast, liver, and other glandular meats, lean meat, fowl, fish, oysters, eggs, milk, wheat germ, peanuts, and green leafy vegetables. There is no possibility of a deficiency of niacin, if one is on any reasonably balanced diet.

The requirements of thiamine, of riboflavin, and of niacin, according to present knowledge, are given in Table 11, page 115.

Among the other components of the B complex are *pyridoxin* (vitamin B_6), which has been tried with some apparent success in the treatment of certain types of anemia, muscular dystrophy, and neuritis, but no definite conclusions can yet be drawn as to its value; *pantothenic acid*, which seems to be necessary for normal growth of yeast, many bacteria, and certain animals; *choline*, which plays an important role in the nutrition of some animals; and B_{12} which has been shown to be effective in the treatment of pernicious anemia and some kinds of neuritis.

Vitamin C is called the "antiscorbutic vitamin" because its absence results in a disease called "scurvy." Adult scurvy, although rarely seen today, used to be very common, particularly among soldiers, sailors, and others cut off from regular supplies of fresh fruit. Infantile scurvy, which is said to be preeminently a disorder of modern times, is due largely to artificial feeding and to the use of commercially prepared foods for infants.

Almost all our domestic animals and household pets are more fortunately situated than we are with respect to vitamin C. They do not need dietary supplies, because they make the vitamin in their own bodies, out of what and by what process we do not yet know. There is evidence that we can store enough vitamin C to last a few months if need be, although we would probably know something was the matter before that time was terminated.[5]

Within the past few years vitamin C has been isolated in pure crystalline form and upon chemical analysis found to be hexuronic, or so-called "ascorbic acid." This may be prepared from adrenal glands or from citrus fruits, cabbage, paprika, and other plant materials. Recently it has been prepared synthetically in the laboratory.

The results of a deficiency of vitamin C in experiments with animals are lowered vitality, growth failure, capillary degeneration, spongy bleeding gums, anemia, hemorrhage, dental defects, fragility of the bones, degeneration of various organs, secondary infections, and scurvy.

Vitamin C is rapidly destroyed by oxidation. Heat accelerates the rate of oxidation and so hastens its destruction. Hence, pasteurized and boiled milk contain less vitamin C than raw milk. Cooking and canning, particularly if soda is added, reduce the vitamin C content of foods. The exclusion of air and the presence of salts or acids in cooking or canning reduce the rate of oxidation and so minimize the destruction of vitamin C.

Oranges, lemons, and grapefruit are the richest common source of vitamin C, while tomato juice contains approximately half as much as does orange juice. Strawberries, raspberries, cantaloupe, and various other fresh berries and fruits, as well as green peppers, cabbages, leafy vegetables, avocados, fresh lima beans, and liver are also rich sources of this nutritional factor. And potatoes, even when cooked, contain enough of this vitamin to afford much practical protection during the winter months.

Vitamin D is called the "antirachitic vitamin" because its absence from the diets of infants results in the disease rickets. Although rickets is usually considered a disease of the bones, because of the skeletal deformities which accompany it, it actually is a nutritional disease which affects the entire organism. The rachitic child is irritable, weak, restless, anemic, flabby, and susceptible to infections. The nervous manifestations seem to be

[5] Palmer, *loc. cit.*

due to a disturbance of calcium metabolism, while both calcium and phosphorus are involved in the faulty development of the bones. The function of vitamin D in this picture is to regulate the utilization of these minerals.

Another disease of children that is related to calcium metabolism and vitamin D is tetany. The symptoms of this disease, which involves also the parathyroid gland, are restlessness and intermittent or continuous contraction of certain groups of muscles, most frequently those of the neck, legs, and lower back.

The results of deficiency of this vitamin are muscular weakness, instability of the nervous system, enamel defects of the teeth, rickets, and possibly dental caries.

The distribution of vitamin D in nature is extremely limited. Egg yolk is its chief source in the average diet. Milk and dairy products contain very little unless enriched or irradiated. Liver and certain fish, particularly herring and salmon, contain considerable quantities, but the richest known source in nature is cod-liver oil.

For some years there was considerable confusion concerning the relation of this vitamin to rickets because it could be demonstrated that exposure to sunlight or ultraviolet light also would prevent or cure this disease. This apparent paradox was explained when it was discovered that the irradiation of certain oils, called "sterols," resulted in the formation of vitamin D. These sterols are present in certain oils, foods, and animal tissues, including the skin. Exposure of these to ultraviolet light produces vitamin D. Viosterol, an irradiated sterol, is the richest concentrate of vitamin D.

Various foods are now being irradiated to increase their content of this nutritional factor. Many of these have merit but the indiscriminate irradiation of foods and the exaggerated health claims made for some of them are entirely unjustified. At present considerable interest is being directed to increasing the vitamin D content of milk either by irradiation or by adding to the milk concentrates of this vitamin. This has great practical value as a convenient, dependable method of supplying vitamin D to children.

Just how much of this vitamin is necessary to maintain health we do not know, but it is clear that infants and growing children need a liberal supply of it. It has been estimated by some physicians that 50 to 75 per cent of the children of this country suffer some impairment of health as a result of an inadequate supply of vitamin D. Adults apparently need but little, but the nutritional status even of some adults probably would be improved by more liberal quantities of this vitamin in the diet.

Of all the vitamins, D is most likely to be deficient in the average well-balanced diet, at least during the winter, when but little ultraviolet radiation from the sun reaches the earth. During this period, October to April, cod-liver oil, a liberal number of eggs, or irradiated or vitamin-enriched milk should be included in the diet, particularly of children.

Vitamin E is concerned with the reproductive processes and functions. Its absence leads to sterility, muscular weakness, and, in the young, paralysis. It is found chiefly in whole-grain cereals, green vegetables, muscles, and glandular organs. Although a German physician reported recently that he had successfully treated seventeen out of twenty cases of habitual abortion with wheat-germ oil, there is little evidence that deficiency of this vitamin is a widespread problem as far as human health is concerned.

Vitamin K, until recently, was not regarded as important for human welfare. This vitamin is essential for certain blood-clotting principles and is thus concerned with blood coagulation. The vitamin appears to be formed in the digestive tract under normal conditions so that dietary supplies normally are not necessary.

Vitamin P, a newly discovered vitamin which accompanies vitamin K in nature, is concerned with some of the changes which occur in the blood vessels in scurvy, particularly with their fragility.[6]

Other vitamins, or vitaminlike substances, recently announced are vitamin L, which is essential to the proper lactation of rats; vitamin T, which is concerned with the formation of blood platelets; a "grass-juice factor," which influences the rate of

[6] *Ibid.*

growth of rats; and a "gizzard-erosion factor," the absence of which results in the development of ulcers in the lining of the gizzards of chicks. The importance of these in human nutrition is yet to be determined.

Multiple Vitamin Deficiencies

Diets that are markedly deficient in one vitamin are usually deficient also in others. Consequently, persons may develop several deficiency diseases simultaneously, although frequently the one producing the most prominent symptoms is diagnosed.

For this reason, the soundest treatment of patients with deficiency diseases is a diet that supplies liberal amounts of all the essential nutrients, supplemented with all the vitamins that are known to be essential for human nutrition.

Sprue. Among the deficiency diseases we should mention an interesting disease called sprue, long known in the tropics and recently diagnosed in various parts of the United States. Patients with fully developed sprue show great weight loss, weakness with muscular wasting, sores in the mouth and tongue, indigestion, and diarrhea with large, fatty, frothy, foul-smelling stools.

In the early stages treatment with liver extract, vitamins and a diet high in proteins and low in fats and carbohydrates is highly successful. Clearly this disease, which remained a mystery for so long, should now be classified as a dietary deficiency disease.

DISCUSSION SUGGESTIONS

1. Discuss the general purpose of digestion and its effects upon the various types of foods. What digestion takes place in the mouth, the stomach, the small intestine, and the large intestine?
2. What is meant by enzymes and what functions do they perform?
3. What happens to the various products of digestion? To the undigested portions of food?
4. Why does the body need water? How much is necessary and with what conditions does this vary?
5. What are the important minerals of the body? What are the chief functions which each performs in the body? From what dietary sources may each be obtained?
6. Discuss the geographical distribution of goiters.
7. Discuss the importance of alkaline foods.

8. Why is it essential that foods contain at least a minimum amount of protein? Why is it desirable that these be derived from various dietary sources?

9. Discuss the utilization of carbohydrates by the body. What does the body do with the excess quantities of sugar which are at times absorbed from the intestinal tract? What hormone is necessary for the utilization of sugar in the tissues? What do you understand by hypoglycemia and how may it be prevented?

10. How are fats utilized by the body? Upon what does the quantity of fat which should be included in the diet depend?

11. What do you understand by vitamins? From what sources may they be obtained? How many are known at the present time?

12. Discuss the need of the body for vitamin A; the possibilities and the symptoms of deficiency; the natural foods which are richest in this vitamin; and the artificial sources at present available.

13. Discuss vitamin B complex in the same manner.

14. Likewise vitamin C.

15. Likewise vitamin D.

REFERENCES AND READING SUGGESTIONS

1. DeKruif, Paul: "Hunger Fighters," Harcourt, Brace and Company, Inc., New York, 1928.

2. Fishbein, Morris: "Your Diet and Your Health," McGraw-Hill Book Company, Inc., New York, 1937.

3. Gerard, Ralph: "Food for Life," University of Chicago Press, Chicago, 1952.

4. Jensen, L. B.: "Man's Food," The Garrard Press, Champaign, Ill., 1954.

5. Kilander, H. F.: "Nutrition for Health," McGraw-Hill Book Company, Inc., New York, 1951.

6. McCollum, E. V., and J. E. Becker: "Food, Nutrition and Health," 5th ed., Lord Baltimore Press, Baltimore, 1948.

7. Roddis, Louis H.: "James Lind: Founder of Nautical Medicine," Henry Schuman, Inc., Publishers, New York, 1950.

8. Rose, Mary S.: "Foundations of Nutrition," 4th ed., The Macmillan Company, New York, 1944.

9. Sherman, H. C.: "Food and Health," The Macmillan Company, New York, 1948.

10. ———: "The Nutritional Improvement of Life," Columbia University Press, New York, 1950.

11. ——— and Caroline Sherman Sanford: "Essentials of Nutrition," 3d ed., The Macmillan Company, New York, 1951.

12. Wilson, Anna May: "The Conquest of Pellagra," *Today's Health*, vol. 30, p. 40, March, 1952.

Chapter V

THE CHOICE OF FOODS

AFTER the consideration of the nutritional requirements of the body, the next question is how one can make the best practical selection of foods to meet these requirements. Proteins, mineral salts, and vitamins may be essential, but what shall we eat, and how much of it? Nutritional requirements vary so enormously, even for persons of the same sex, age, and size, that a single answer to this question is impossible. Growing children and pregnant women need relatively large amounts of proteins, minerals, and vitamins; persons who are physically active need more energy foods than do those who lead a sedentary life; the same individuals need more heat-producing foods in winter than in summer. Furthermore, the quantity of certain foods in the diet modifies the body requirements for other foods; for example, if the diet contains plenty of carbohydrate and fat, the protein may be reduced to a minimum.

Some contend that the course to follow in the selection of foods is that suggested by the following verse:

Methuselah ate what he found on his plate
And never, as people do now,
Did he note the amount of the calorie count—
He ate because it was chow.
He wasn't disturbed as at dinner he sat
Destroying a roast or a pie,

To think it was lacking in lime or in fat
Or a couple of vitamins shy.
He cheerfully chewed every species of food,
Untroubled by worries or fears
Lest his health might be hurt by some fancy dessert,
And he lived over nine hundred years!

—*Anonymous.*

For such sentiments there is more justification than for the dietary fads which many people adopt. One may become so finicky about foods that one loses all pleasure in eating, and it is perfectly possible to avoid serious inadequacies of the diet by a *varied selection of natural foods.* On the other hand, the dietary problems of today, with our refined, preserved, and synthetic foods, are very different from what they were when most foods were consumed in their natural state. Then, too, scientific investigations in the field of nutrition have made it possible for us to select intelligently those foods which best meet the needs of the body under different conditions.

Basic Food Requirements

One-half of the people in the world went to bed hungry last night, will go to bed hungry tonight, will go to bed hungry tomorrow night, and every night for the rest of their lives. This is the dramatic language in which the following paragraph is often stated, "Only one-third of the world's people get enough of the right kind of food, and they consume three-fourths of the world's food supply. One-half of the human race actually goes hungry, and famine and starvation still stalk the earth, as in ancient times. Disease, low efficiency, social tensions, and political and economic crises, in many areas, reflect the scarcity of food."[1]

"Half the struggle for life is a struggle for food." The majority of the people of the world must spend as much of their earnings or time to provide themselves and their families with adequate food as they spend for all the other necessities of life combined. When any one necessity of life may consume so much of the total

[1] *American Journal of Public Health*, vol. 40, p. 797, July, 1950.

income, it is apparent that the food problems of some families may be great.

The family's food supply holds great potentialities for the health and advancement of the individual, the family, and society as a whole. Yet, studies by the U.S. Public Health Service indicate that more than one-third of American families subsist on diets which would not be rated better than "poor" by accepted standards.

Intelligent choice and use of foods, the formation of good food habits, and the use of the food allowance to provide the best possible diet for the family are an important part of a health education program. Food rationing in England during the Second World War resulted in better balanced diets for a large part of the population and in improved nutrition for the country as a whole.

The problem of health and nutrition begins with the pregnant woman in the nine months before the birth of her infant. A diet which provides adequately for the needs of the pregnant and nursing woman pays excellent health dividends for both herself and her child. An understanding of the value and use of foods adequate in kind and amount during these months is of prime importance to the health of both present and future generations. Nearly everyone appreciates the importance of food to the infant and growing child. Children whose diets are inadequate do not grow and develop normally. The responsibility of both the home and the school in providing and teaching good food habits to children at an early age is of paramount importance in building good health. The maintenance of positive health through a continuation of these good food habits all during life constitutes one of the newer and important phases of health education.

There are certain basic requirements for every diet whether it be for one who is old or young, large or small, active or inactive. These are water, vitamins, proteins, essential fatty acids, and inorganic salts. Thirst is a safe guide as to the amount of water which is necessary. Vitamins are essential, but the requirements cannot yet be defined in quantitative terms. Practically, however, fresh fruits, leafy vegetables, butter, milk, eggs, whole-grain cereals, and enriched bread, with cod-liver oil for infants and growing children, can be relied upon to provide adequate protection against vitamin deficiency.

The requirements for mineral salts—calcium, phosphorus, iron, copper, etc.—are supplied by milk, eggs, meat, fresh fruits, and leafy vegetables. In sections of the country removed from the seacoast it may be necessary to add iodine in some convenient form. The essential fatty acids are provided by the fats contained in any average diet.

TABLE 10

NUTRIENTS SUPPLIED BY THE BASIC SEVEN FOOD GROUPS

Food Group	Food Energy	Protein	Calcium	Iron	Vitamin A	Thiamine	Riboflavin	Niacin	Ascorbic Acid
Green and yellow vegetables			x	x	xx	x	x		x
Citrus fruits, tomatoes, raw cabbage					x	x			xx
Potatoes, other vegetables, fruits	x			x		x			x
Milk and milk products (liquid, dried, evaporated)	x	xx	xx		x	x	xx		
Meat, poultry, fish, eggs, dried beans, peas, nuts	x	xx		x		x	x	x	
Bread, flour, cereal (whole-grain or enriched)	xx	x		x		x	x	x	
Butter and fortified margarine	xx				x				

xx indicates an excellent source; x indicates a good source.

Proteins must be provided in sufficient quantities to supply the body's needs for growth and tissue repair. The smallest amount which will meet this requirement is approximately 2 calories of protein per day for each pound of normal body weight. In order that there may be a margin of safety, somewhat larger quantities are usually recommended. Meat once a day, in addition to eggs, milk, and vegetables, will adequately supply this need.

Are Excessive Amounts of Protein or Meat Harmful?

Certain religious sects and dietary faddists consider meat deleterious and so taboo it entirely. Dietitians usually limit its use to moderate amounts, because meat and protein foods are expensive sources of energy. It is believed that proteins favor intestinal putrefaction; and there is experimental evidence which suggests that animals kept on diets containing excessive amounts of proteins over a considerable period of time may show signs of kidney irritation and damage. Furthermore, studies on college students at Yale University indicate that young men on a low but adequate protein intake feel better and have more energy and physical endurance than those on diets of similar caloric value but with a higher proportion of proteins.

On the other hand, Eskimos live almost exclusively on a diet of meat, fish, fowl, and eggs and apparently enjoy the best of health. And Tobey reports that the physical strength of the Masai, an African tribe which lives mainly on meat, is 50 per cent greater than the strength of the Akikuyu, an adjacent tribe which lives chiefly on vegetables. Such diets, of course, are not exclusively protein because meat and fish contain large amounts of fat.

An interesting attempt to investigate the effect of a high-protein diet upon health was made a few years ago with the cooperation of two arctic explorers, Stefansson and Andersen. These men lived for twelve months in this country exclusively on meat. During this period, extensive physiological studies were carried out and careful records were kept of their condition. Some of the more interesting conclusions at the end of the year were that neither man showed any evidence of diminution of physical or mental vigor, that there was no tendency to constipation or to intestinal putrefaction, that there was no increase in blood pressure or demonstrable damage to the kidneys, that there was no evidence of deterioration of the teeth, and that both men appeared ruddier at the end of the experiment than at the beginning.

Another study suggests somewhat different conclusions concerning the effect of a meat diet upon blood pressure. This report is based upon the blood pressures of two groups of monks and friars. One group consisted of 115 Benedictines and Franciscans who followed an unrestricted diet; the other, of 110 Trappists, Carmelites, and Carthusians who abstained from meat, fish, butter, and eggs and observed fasting periods when only bread and water were taken. The study shows that at each age the average blood pressure of the meat eaters was higher than that of the vegetarians. After carefully weighing other factors, the author concludes that diet is the important cause of this difference. Concerning the hereditary factor in high blood pressure, he says that he recognizes its importance but believes that the tendency can be checked by external factors, the chief of which is the avoidance of meat in the diet.

Such apparently conflicting reports make generalizations difficult; but the consensus of medical opinion is that meats moderately in excess of protein requirements are not harmful to the normal person. If high blood pressure or kidney disease exists, the advice of a physician concerning diet should be followed.

Protective Foods

As scientific investigation indicated the basic nutritional needs of the body, Dr. E. V. McCollum of Johns Hopkins University, pioneer scientist in nutrition, applied the term "protective foods" to those foods which represent the richest sources of these basic nutritional needs. These are milk, milk products, eggs, fruits, and leafy vegetables.

Dr. H. C. Sherman, professor of chemistry at Columbia University, an eminent authority on nutrition, reported that it is possible to defer senility and to increase the average length of life of rats by approximately 10 per cent simply by increasing the proportion of protective foods in their diets.

Milk—The Perfect Food

Milk is nature's most nearly perfect food. Although deficient in iron and copper, it contains relatively large amounts of calcium and phosphorus, an assortment of other important mineral elements, several proteins of excellent quality, substantial amounts of carbohydrate and fat, a rich supply of vitamins A and B, and, if enriched or irradiated, an adequate amount of vitamin D. Such a complete food is rightly considered the most valuable food product available.

The quantity of milk which can profitably be included in the diet has been estimated as not less than a quart per day. This includes the milk taken as drink or beverage and that used in the preparation of cereals, soups, vegetables, desserts, bakery products, etc. In the diets of children from one to five years of age a quart of milk will constitute from 40 to 70 per cent of the total food requirement. In a child of fourteen this same quantity of milk will supply only about 25 per cent of the needs. For the diets of adults a pint of milk a day, including the milk used in cooking, is recommended. For any age group milk and milk products, such as butter and cheese, provide certain nutritive elements which may be lacking in other foods.

Skimmed milk contains just as much protein and calcium as whole milk but less vitamin A. Most of the vitamin A, being soluble in fat, is removed with the cream. If skimmed milk is used, it should be enriched or other sources of vitamin A, such as enriched foods, cod-liver oil, and vegetables rich in this vitamin should be included in the diet.

Cereal Grains—Inexpensive Foods

Plants store reserve supplies of food in their seeds for the nourishment of the young plants after the seeds have germinated. Man utilizes this rich source of energy as food for himself and his domestic animals.

Cereal grains and the food products, such as bread, derived from them make up a large proportion of the American dietary. They are valuable primarily because they constitute inexpensive, easily digestible sources of energy. These grains consist largely of starch, but in addition they contain small amounts of incomplete proteins and, if their outer coats are retained, certain minerals and vitamins.

Foods derived from cereal grains may safely constitute up to 30 per cent of the total energy requirements. With increased activity the relative as well as the actual cereal content of the diet may well be increased. When economy is an important consideration, the cereal grains are always freely used. However, if they make up more than 15 per cent of the total energy value, that is, the calories of the diet, attention should be given to the liberal use of other foods such as milk, citrus fruits, leafy vegetables, cabbage, and whole-grain cereals, for their mineral and vitamin content.

Fruits and Vegetables—Essential Foods

Because of their mineral and vitamin content, fruits and vegetables should constitute not less than 15 to 20 per cent of the diet. If not limited by cost, this proportion may well be increased to 25 per cent.

Oranges and tomatoes are the fresh fruits of greatest value, but all fruits and green leafy vegetables are of importance. The practice of eating some raw fruit and vegetable each day is very desirable. Potatoes, which are usually inexpensive, provide not only an excellent source of energy but also several mineral elements and vitamins B and C. The physical endurance at hard labor of a man who had been on an experimental diet of only potatoes and butter for several months was found to be greater than that of other laborers on ordinary diets. Potatoes are especially valuable for children and for people doing muscular work. The legendary health merit of the apple has received some scientific support through a study showing it to be of value as a home remedy for diarrhea in children.

The skins of vegetables contain valuable minerals and vitamins and should be used whenever convenient. In cooking, many of the minerals and vitamins go into solution, hence, *vegetables should be cooked in as little water as possible and this water utilized.*

Eggs and Meat—Expensive but Necessary

Eggs are such a rich source of several minerals and vitamins that they should be used liberally in the diet. Children need three or four eggs a week or, better still, an egg a day.

Although meat is appetizing and rich in proteins, phosphorus, and iron, it is an expensive source of energy and deficient in other minerals and vitamins. Many dietitians consider meat a luxury food to be used as supplementary to milk, eggs, butter, fruits, vegetables, and cereals. Liver is an unusually rich source of vitamins A and B and of iron and is a specific remedy for the formerly fatal disease, pernicious anemia. Many glandular meats are rich but inexpensive sources of essential food elements.

Fats—A Rich Source of Energy

Fats are useful in the body primarily as sources of energy and should be increased or decreased according to energy requirements. In infancy, fats are not easily digested but after the age of six they may well supply from 10 to 20 per cent of the total energy requirements.

Cod-liver oil, which contains both vitamins A and D, probably has the greatest nutritional value of any of the fats but can hardly be considered in the category of a regular food. Butter and cream not only contain fat but are among the best sources of vitamin A. Most nuts are rich in fat and are good sources of vitamin B. On the other hand, the nutritional value of most other animal and vegetable fats such as bacon, lard, suet, oleomargarine (unless enriched), and olive oil depends primarily upon the energy which they supply.

Sugar—Easily Available Energy

Sugars are useful in the diet only as a source of energy and as a means of improving the palatability of foods. Students of nutrition recommend that sugar be used sparingly in the diet because it tends to dull the appetite for foods which contain other nutritional elements. Most children on adequate, well-selected diets do not crave sweets. Sugars provide easily available energy, but even for this purpose foods which also supply other nutritional factors as well are to be preferred.

The Digestibility of Foods

Foods are frequently considered indigestible if they produce a sensation of fullness for a considerable time after eating. This sensation is a reflection of the rate at which foods pass out of the stomach and is not necessarily related to the ultimate nutritional value derived from them. Starches leave the stomach more rapidly than proteins, and proteins more rapidly than fats, while mixtures of proteins and fats remain in the stomach longer than either of these foods alone.

The preparation of food apparently has less influence upon digestibility than is generally believed, for careful studies have shown that fried potatoes, unless they have absorbed a great deal of fat, leave the stomach just as promptly and are just as digestible as boiled, baked, or mashed potatoes.

Enriched Foods

The refining of food products, which the public has come to demand, has had unfortunate effects upon the adequacy of the modern diet. Most serious among these are the loss of important food elements in the milling of white flour and other cereal grains and the substitution of sugar for other sources of energy. White flour contains only one-tenth to one-fifth as much thiamine as does whole wheat, and refined sugar contains no vitamins at all. Reports show that the parish poor in England in 1839 probably received about 650 to 850 international units of thiamine daily; one hundred years later supposedly good diets of persons in moderate circumstances supplied only about 450 to 550 units of this vitamin daily.

The best remedy for this situation would be to return to the use of whole-wheat flours and cereals. Unfortunately it is exceedingly difficult to convince the public that it should change its eating habits. Realizing this, authorities concerned with the nutrition of the nation have induced the milling industry of the country to "enrich" white flour by adding to it the approximate amounts of thiamine, riboflavin, and nicotinic acid which are removed in the milling process. Many mills are also adding calcium, phosphorus, and iron to their flours.

The soundness of this practice is obvious, and since enriched flour has become widely distributed and universally accepted it should make a material contribution to the national health.

[113]

Another "enriched" food which has been accepted by nutrition authorities is vitamin D milk. This is not a case of supplying a vitamin that has been removed from the diet but merely a convenient and inexpensive means of supplying the body's needs for vitamin D. Milk may be enriched with vitamin D either by exposure to ultraviolet light or by the addition of a cod-liver oil concentrate. The latter provides vitamin A as well as vitamin D, but either method is satisfactory.

The irradiation of certain other foods, such as cereals, increases their vitamin D content, but none of these is so satisfactory a vehicle as milk for supplying the vitamin D requirements of the body. In fact many advertised vitamin products and concentrates represent nothing more than the efforts of advertisers to exploit for their own profit the public interest in nutrition.

CONSERVING THE NUTRITIONAL VALUE OF FOODS[2]

1. Heat and air destroy some of the vitamins. In the preparation and serving of fresh fruits and vegetables exposure to air and heat should be kept at a minimum. Do not use soda.

2. Serve fruits and fruit juices fresh. If they must stand, keep covered and cold.

3. Wash vegetables quickly, do not soak, keep cool and in nature's covering until ready to cook.

4. Cut vegetables for salads just before using.

5. Cook vegetables quickly in small amounts of boiling water, stop when tender. Serve in own juice or use juice in sauce or soup.

6. Cook and serve vegetables whenever possible in nature's jacket.

7. Start cooking frozen vegetables while still frozen. Do not thaw first.

8. Keep milk cold. Do not let stand at room temperature.

9. Cool milk-egg dishes quickly after cooking; cover; keep cold; use soon. These dishes are ideal media for the germs which cause food poisoning.

10. Cook eggs slowly. Do not overcook. It makes protein tough.

Energy Requirements

In the planning of a diet, energy requirements as well as basic essentials need to be considered. These are usually expressed in units of heat, called "calories," a calorie being the amount of heat necessary to raise the temperature of 1 liter of water 1 degree centigrade (or 1 quart of water 1⅘ degrees Fahrenheit).

[2] Bureau of Home Economics, U.S. Department of Agriculture, Washington, D.C.

TABLE 11

FOOD AND NUTRITION BOARD, NATIONAL RESEARCH COUNCIL

RECOMMENDED DAILY DIETARY ALLOWANCES,* REVISED 1953

DESIGNED FOR THE MAINTENANCE OF GOOD NUTRITION OF HEALTHY PERSONS IN THE U.S.A.

(Allowances are considered to apply to persons normally vigorous and living in temperate climate)

	Age, Years	Weight, kg. (lb.)	Height, cm. (in.)	Calories	Protein, gm.	Calcium, gm.	Iron, mg.	Vitamin A, I.U.	Thiamine, mg.	Riboflavin, mg.	Niacin, mg.	Ascorbic Acid, mg.	Vitamin D, I.U.
Men	25	65 (143)	170 (67)	3,200†	65	0.8	12	5,000	1.6	1.6	16	75	
	45	65 (143)	170 (67)	2,900	65	0.8	12	5,000	1.5	1.6	15	75	
	65	65 (143)	170 (67)	2,600	65	0.8	12	5,000	1.3	1.6	13	75	
Women	25	55 (121)	157 (62)	2,300†	55	0.8	12	5,000	1.2	1.4	12	70	
	45	55 (121)	157 (62)	2,100	55	0.8	12	5,000	1.0	1.4	11	70	
	65	55 (121)	157 (62)	1,800	55	0.8	12	5,000	1.0	1.4	10	70	
Pregnant (3rd trimester)	..	......	......	Add 400	80	1.5	15	6,000	1.5	2.0	15	100	400
Lactating (850 ml. daily)		......	......	Add 1,000	100	2.0	15	8,000	1.5	2.5	15	150	400
Infants‡	0–½ §	6 (13)	60 (24)	kg. × 120	kg. × 3.5‡	0.6	6	1,500	0.3	0.4	3	30	400
	½–1	9 (20)	70 (28)	kg. × 100	kg. × 3.5‡	0.8	6	1,500	0.4	0.7	4	30	400
	1–2	10 (22)	75 (30)	kg. × 100	kg. × 3.5‡	1.0	6	1,500	0.5	0.9	5	30	400
Children	1–3	12 (27)	87 (34)	1,200	40	1.0	7	2,000	0.6	1.0	6	35	400
	4–6	18 (40)	109 (43)	1,600	50	1.0	8	2,500	0.8	1.2	8	50	400
	7–9	27 (59)	129 (51)	2,000	60	1.0	10	3,500	1.0	1.5	10	60	400
Boys	10–12	35 (78)	144 (57)	2,500	70	1.2	12	4,500	1.3	1.8	13	75	400
	13–15	49 (108)	163 (64)	3,200	85	1.4	15	5,000	1.6	2.1	16	90	400
	16–20	63 (139)	175 (69)	3,800	100	1.4	15	5,000	1.9	2.5	19	100	400
Girls	10–12	36 (79)	144 (57)	2,300	70	1.2	12	4,500	1.2	1.8	12	75	400
	13–15	49 (108)	160 (63)	2,500	80	1.3	15	5,000	1.3	2.0	13	80	400
	16–20	54 (120)	162 (64)	2,400	75	1.3	15	5,000	1.2	1.9	12	80	400

* In planning practical dietaries, the recommended allowances can be attained with a variety of common foods which will also provide other nutrient requirements less well known; the allowance levels are considered to cover individual variations among normal persons as they live in the United States subjected to ordinary environmental stresses.

† These calorie recommendations apply to the degree of activity for the reference man and woman described on page 3 of the text. For the urban "white-collar" worker they are probably excessive. In any case, the calorie allowance must be adjusted to the actual needs of the individual as required to achieve and maintain his desirable weight.

‡ The recommendations for infants pertain to nutrients derived primarily from cow's milk. If the milk from which the protein is derived is human milk or has been treated to render it more digestible, the allowance may be in the range of 2–3 gm. per kilogram. There should be no question that human milk is a desirable source of nutrients for infants even though it may not provide the levels recommended for certain nutrients. (See discussion in text.)

§ During the first month of life, desirable allowances for many nutrients are dependent upon maturation of excretory and endocrine functions. Therefore no specific recommendations are given.

SOURCE: National Academy of Sciences–National Research Council, Publication 302, Washington, D.C., 1953.

The energy values of various foods have been determined in terms of calories, and it has been found that 1 gram ($\frac{1}{30}$ ounce) of protein or of carbohydrate will yield 4 calories of heat and that 1 gram of fat will yield 9 calories.

Energy requirements vary with age, size, sex, activity, foods to be digested, clothing, temperature of the body and of the surrounding atmosphere, functioning of certain glands of internal secretion, etc. Hence, it is difficult to state exactly how much energy-producing food the body needs. It is possible, however, to estimate with reasonable accuracy the energy requirements of a normal person of a given size at complete rest. This is called the "basal metabolism." In terms of calories this basal requirement for a 24-hour period has been found to be about 11 calories per pound of normal weight, that is, 11 calories per pound of what one should weigh for one's age and height. The slight activity of a person in bed increases the requirement about 10 per cent. Walking uses up about a calorie per pound of body weight per hour.

An adult who is up and about, but relatively inactive, needs 20 to 30 per cent more calories than are required under basal conditions. For one engaged in a sedentary occupation, this extra energy requirement rises to from 30 to 40 per cent above basal; for one in moderately active muscular work, 40 to 80 per cent; and for one at hard muscular work, 80 to 200 per cent.

These are only approximations of energy requirements, but they provide a workable and reasonably satisfactory method of estimating what an individual's energy intake should be. For example, the energy requirement of a man in a sedentary occupation who takes little exercise, and whose ideal weight, according to age and height (see Chapter VI), is 160 pounds, is computed as follows: the basic energy requirement for a person weighing 160 pounds is 11 times 160, or 1,760 calories. Since the subject leads a relatively sedentary life, this requirement is increased by approximately 35 per cent, or 2,376 calories. In a similar manner, the approximate energy requirement for any adult may be estimated.

The menus in Tables 12 and 13 illustrate how the nutritional requirements of a moderately active adult may be supplied at a moderate cost. Innumerable substitutions and rearrangements can be made in such diets and still leave them entirely adequate in vitamins, proteins, and minerals as well as in calories (see table of food values in Appendix B).

Energy Requirements of Children. The rate of growth and the physical activity of children vary so enormously that it is difficult to estimate their energy requirements. Nutrition workers tell us that the best evidence that the nutritional requirements of children are being properly met is that they grow properly, feel well, sleep quietly, are mentally and physically active, and are not nervous. Give children each day an egg, four glasses of milk, some fresh fruit, two kinds of vegetables and all the bread, butter and potatoes they want, and there is little danger of inadequate nutrition. The appetite will take care of the quantity.

Energy Expenditure Decreases with Age. The basic food requirements are essentially the same at every age, but energy-producing foods should be reduced in accordance with the diminishing energy expenditure. The great dangers which accompany overweight with advancing age make it important that this be done before excess weight develops.

General Recommendations Concerning Diet

Diet Plans That Meet the Dietary Allowances. In following the recommended allowances given in Table 11 it should be emphasized that the amounts of the various nutrients provided for in these recommended allowances, with the exception of vitamin D, can be obtained through a good diet of natural foods plus enriched white flour and bread which have been improved according to recommendations of the Nutrition Board.

A simple way to insure that the dietary allowances are met is to include in the daily diet foods from each of the following seven basic groups: (1) Green and yellow vegetables—some raw, some cooked—frozen or canned; (2) oranges, tomatoes, grapefruit or raw cabbage or salad greens; (3) potatoes and other vegetables and fruits; (4) milk and milk products—enriched for children; (5) meat, poultry, fish, or eggs; (6) bread, flour, and cereals—

TABLE 12
SAMPLE MENUS OF MODERATE PRICE*
(Approximately 2,500 calories and adequate protective foods, proteins, minerals, and vitamins—standard portions)

1	2	3
Breakfast	**Breakfast**	**Breakfast**
Fruit in season	Canned or cooked fruit	Orange or grapefruit or tomato juice
Whole-grain cereal	Whole-grain cereal	Whole-grain cereal
Top milk	Top milk	Top milk
Sugar	Sugar	Sugar
Egg	Bacon (2 slices)	Waffles or griddle cakes
Whole-wheat rolls	Whole-wheat toast	Sirup or honey
Butter	Butter	Butter
Coffee	Cocoa	Milk
Cream		
Sugar		
Lunch	**Lunch**	**Lunch**
Cream of vegetable soup	Cream of vegetable soup	Hash with poached egg
Cracker	Cracker	Whole-wheat bread
Spanish spaghetti with ground meat or macaroni and cheese	Meat ball†	Butter
	Baked potato	Green vegetable salad
	Whole-wheat bread	Ice cream, sugar cooky
Whole-wheat bread	Butter	Coffee
Butter	Orange, grapefruit, or tomato salad	Cream
Lettuce salad		Sugar
Gingerbread	Cake	
Milk	Tea or coffee	
Dinner	**Dinner**	**Dinner**
Liver and bacon or roast lamb, mint sauce†	Tomato bouillon	Cream lima bean soup
	Cracker	Cracker
Parsley potatoes	Cubed steak†	Roast beef†
Peas in milk	Mashed potato	Stuffed potato
Green vegetable salad	String beans	Buttered carrots
Whole-wheat bread	Celery and carrot strips	Watercress salad
Butter	Whole-wheat bread	Whole-wheat bread
Fruit pie	Butter	Butter
Beverage‡	Raisin custard bread pudding	Apple crisp or fruit cobbler
	Beverage‡	Beverage‡

* The menus have been suggested by Miss Gertrude Thomas, Director of Nutrition, University of Minnesota Hospital.
† Occasionally sea food.
‡ Preferably milk.

natural whole grain, or enriched; (7) butter or "fortified" margarine.

College Students' Meals. Observation of the meals which college students choose at cafeterias and restaurants is convincing

TABLE 13
LOW-COST SUBSTITUTES IN SAMPLE MENUS*

For Canned Fruit		For Luncheon Meat
Prunes	Macaroni and cheese	Spaghetti and cheese
Apricots	Cheese sandwich	Asparagus with cheese
Dried peaches	Baked rarebit	sauce
Dried apples	Baked noodles and cheese	Creamed chipped beef on
	Cheese soufflé	toast
	Creamed eggs and cheese	Escalloped potatoes and
	Creamed eggs on toast	dried beef
	Rice and cheese	Escalloped potatoes and
		cheese
		Welsh rarebit on rice

For Roast Beef or Steak	For Vegetables, Peas, Beans, etc.	
Cubed steak	Rutabagas	Beets
Swiss steak	Cabbage	Squash (in season)
Meat balls	Carrots	
Pot roast	Turnips	
Meat pie	Parsnips	
Meat stew	Onions	

For Lettuce Salad	For Desserts	
Celery and/or carrot sticks	Bread pudding with raisins	Apple Betty
Cucumber, cabbage salad	Bread pudding with dates	Applesauce, other apple
Celery, cabbage	Corn-meal pudding with	desserts
Combination salad (lettuce,	molasses	In season:
radish, cucumber, green	Indian pudding	Bananas
pepper, in season)	Tapioca pudding with rai-	Prune desserts
Combination salad (lettuce,	sins	Rhubarb
carrots, cauliflower)	Tapioca pudding with dates	Watermelon and other
	Blancmange with raisins	low-cost fruits in or
	Blancmange with dates	as desserts

* Suggested by Miss Gertrude Thomas, Director of Nutrition, University of Minnesota Hospital.

evidence that many of them are either ignorant or negligent of their essential food requirements. Meat, potatoes, bread, coffee, and pie will supply calories but in time lack of energy, fatigue, nervousness, and other indefinite symptoms will reduce the individual's level of health and efficiency.

A student's daily food intake should include at least two glasses of milk or the equivalent in milk products; two squares of butter; one egg; one serving of meat or fish (cheese or legumes may be substituted twice a week); one raw orange, grapefruit, or tomato and one other fruit, raw or cooked; two servings of vegetables—besides potatoes—one of which should be leafy, raw, and green or yellow; some whole-grain cereal; and "enriched" or whole-wheat bread. The rest of one's food can safely be selected according to taste.

For students whose food budgets are exceedingly limited substitutions in these diets such as those shown in Tables 12 and 13 may be made with safety (see Appendix B).

The Practical Essentials. The Advisory Committee of the British Ministry of Health reported:

. . . the changes in the diet of the people which in the opinion of the Advisory Committee appear desirable . . . may be summed up in the words: more protective foods; more milk, more fresh vegetables and fruit, more eggs, more potatoes. And in view of the committee's general agreement with the recommendations of the Technical Commission of the League of Nations there may be added to these changes: less sugar, less white flour, and more lightly milled cereals.[3]

And Dr. McCollum says:

I am greatly annoyed and chagrined that so many false claims about proprietary foods are tolerated in this country, foods that are sold with medicinal claims. Mankind would be a great deal better off, and fishes a great deal worse off, if all these things were dumped into the ocean. It is still true, as I believed and as I said as far back as 1916, that the place to get your vitamins and your minerals and your proteins is in the market, in the grocery, and not in the drug store; but we see, year by year, an increasing promotion through the drug trade, of food principles and extravagant claims for them. . . . I believe there is a place in therapy for certain of the vitamins but for the general public, there is no need to buy anything out of a drug store for its food products.[4]

[3] Ministry of Health, Advisory Committee on Nutrition, *First Report*, H. M. Stationery Office, London, 1937.
[4] McCollum, E. V., "Nutrition a Public Health Problem," *Illinois Health Messenger*, vol. 9, p. 29, August 15, 1937.

Appetite and Nutrition

In a healthy, normal individual the appetite operates to assure good nutrition. When vitamins are deficient one craves fresh fruits and vegetables. Wild animals travel long distances for salt.

An interesting experiment was reported recently in which one group of young children was given a balanced and completely adequate diet; while the children in a second group, living under identical conditions, were offered an adequate diet but permitted to choose what they wished to eat. At first the latter group ate excessive amounts of candy and in general had a rather badly balanced diet. In a little while, however, they began to select foods which constituted an adequate diet. Over a period of several months the two groups showed no difference in growth or health.

Unfortunately appetite and eating habits are influenced by a variety of emotional and health factors.

Some babies, especially those breast fed, on a self-demand basis, may develop a feeling of enjoyment of eating which makes eating an occasion for gratification.

Other babies, compelled to accept a rigid feeding schedule which may ignore their individual needs and subject them to prolonged hunger, may develop strong feelings about food and eating which continue to operate, especially if reinforced by difficult weaning and "forced feeding." These babies may never develop a feeling of enjoyment toward eating, but rather they may learn to resist food, especially when the parents try to force them to eat. Some may learn to use food as a weapon to coerce their parents, refusing to eat unless they are cajoled and bribed, while others use food and digestion to fight their parents.[5]

DISCUSSION SUGGESTIONS

1. Discuss the basic requirements of diet and how they may be supplied.
2. What is the evidence for and against the idea that a "high protein" diet is harmful?
3. Why is milk called "the perfect food"?
4. Discuss the values and the shortcomings of cereals in the diet.

[5] Frank, Lawrence E., "Health Education," *American Journal of Public Health*, vol. 36, p. 357, April, 1946.

5. What is the dietary value of oranges? Of tomatoes? Of potatoes? Of green leafy vegetables?
6. What is the dietary value of meat? Of eggs? Of fats? Of starch? Of sugar?
7. Explain what is meant by "the protective foods."
8. Define calorie. What is meant by the caloric value of a certain food?
9. What is meant by metabolism? By basal metabolism?
10. Calculate your own energy requirements in accordance with the instructions given.
11. How do energy requirements vary with age?
12. Keep an accurate record of your diet for a week and estimate its adequacy or inadequacy in essential food elements and in caloric value.
13. Study the food table in Appendix B and list five foods that are good sources of calcium; of phosphorus; of iron; of vitamin A; of vitamin B_1; of vitamin C; of vitamin D; of carbohydrate; of protein; of fats.

REFERENCES AND READING SUGGESTIONS

1. Amidon, E. P., D. E. Bradbury, and V. Drenckhahn: "Good Food and Nutrition for Young People and Their Families," John Wiley & Sons, Inc., New York, 1947.
2. Bogert, L. Jean: "Nutrition and Physical Fitness," W. B. Saunders Company, Philadelphia, 1949.
3. Borsook, Henry, and William Huse: "Vitamins for Health," 3d ed., Public Affairs Pamphlets, New York, 1947.
4. Hambidge, Gove: "Your Meals and Your Money," McGraw-Hill Book Company, Inc., New York, 1934.
5. Kilander, H. F.: "Nutrition for Health," McGraw-Hill Book Company, New York, 1951.
6. McDougall, F. L.: "Food and Population," Columbia University Press, New York, 1952.
7. Nasset, C. S.: "Food for You," Charles C Thomas, Springfield, Illinois, 1951.
8. Rowntree, Jennie I.: "This Problem of Food," Public Affairs Pamphlets, New York.
9. Thomas, Gertrude: "The Dietary of Health and Disease," 4th ed., Lea & Febiger, Philadelphia, 1945.
10. Bulletins on Infant Feeding and on Preserving of Foods, U.S. Public Health Service, Department of Agriculture, and Children's Bureau, Washington, D.C.

Chapter VI

WEIGHT AND ITS CONTROL

A GLANCE at the advertising sections of magazines and newspapers leaves no doubt as to the interest of American people in their weight. The dictators of fashions have made us "weight-conscious." And now the writers of advertising copy are attempting to convince the thin and the fat alike that if they will only bathe in water containing this salt or eat this food or buy this exercising machine or take this or that drug preparation, a figure like that of the professional model pictured in the advertisement will follow in due time.

The desire for weight regulation is mostly to improve personal appearance. Scientifically there are better reasons why it is desirable, but this is sufficient justification. A recent study of employed and unemployed clerical workers indicates that both underweight and overweight are handicaps to employment, and that for women overweight is a greater handicap than underweight. This suggests that fat people may be less efficient than thin ones, but probably the employer's idea as to which makes the more pleasing appearance is of greater importance.

Life insurance companies are interested in the regulation of weight for the simple and practical reason that they find a definite relationship between weight and mortality. Young people who are underweight and persons over thirty-five who are overweight have death rates above the average. The payment of claims is expensive; therefore life insurance companies advise their policyholders to watch their weights. This is good advice, because if it is followed not only will the life insurance company make more money but the policyholder will live longer and enjoy better health and greater vitality.

Average Weight

On every hand one is confronted with charts and tables telling "what you should weigh" or what "normal weight" is for a person of your age, height, and sex. Actually these tables are nothing more than the average weights of large numbers of persons of the same age, height, and sex. The experience of life insurance companies indicates that, as a group, individuals of average weight, commonly called "normal weight," have a favorable mortality; but, except for the age period from thirty to forty-five, the lowest mortality does not occur among persons of exactly average weight. In the age group twenty to twenty-nine the lowest mortality is among persons 10 to 20 pounds *over average weight;* while in the age group forty-five to forty-nine the lowest mortality is among persons 10 to 15 pounds *under average weight;* and after fifty-five years of age the most favorable mortality occurs among persons who are 20 or more pounds *underweight.*

The most widely used tables of average weights are reproduced in Appendix A. From these the average weight for any age and height can be easily determined. Although the weights and heights given in these tables include shoes and ordinary clothing, they may also be used as standards for stripped heights and weights. This is permissible because the additional height due to the shoes puts the individual into the next taller group, the greater average weight of which is approximately equal to the usual weight of shoes and clothing. Age in these tables is taken as of the nearest birthday, whether it be past or future.

Ideal Weight. As pointed out, average weight is not necessarily the best weight because averages include overweights and underweights. On the basis of experience, therefore, life insurance companies have prepared tables of the weights which show the lowest mortality rates for various heights and for various types of body frames. One of these is reproduced in Table 14.

TABLE 14

BEST WEIGHTS AFTER TWENTY-FIVE YEARS OF AGE*

Men				Women			
Height Feet Inches	Small Frame	Medium Frame	Large Frame	Height Feet Inches	Small Frame	Medium Frame	Large Frame
5 2	116–125	124–133	131–142	4 11	104–111	110–118	117–127
5 3	119–128	127–136	133–144	5 0	105–113	112–120	119–129
5 4	122–132	130–140	137–149	5 1	107–115	114–122	121–131
5 5	126–136	134–144	141–153	5 2	110–118	117–125	124–135
5 6	129–139	137–147	145–157	5 3	113–121	120–128	127–138
5 7	133–143	141–151	149–162	5 4	116–125	124–132	131–142
5 8	136–147	145–156	153–166	5 5	119–128	127–135	133–145
5 9	140–151	149–160	157–170	5 6	123–132	130–140	138–150
5 10	144–155	153–164	161–175	5 7	126–136	134–144	142–154
5 11	148–159	157–168	165–180	5 8	129–139	137–147	145–158
6 0	152–164	161–173	169–185	5 9	133–143	141–151	149–162
6 1	157–169	166–178	174–190	5 10	136–147	145–155	152–166
6 2	163–175	171–184	179–196	5 11	139–150	148–158	155–169
6 3	168–180	176–189	184–202				

* From Metropolitan Life Insurance Co.
May be used either with shoes and ordinary clothing or for stripped heights and weights.

In the absence of standard tables an approximation of the "desirable weight" may be made as follows: consider the desirable weight of men 5 feet tall and twenty to thirty-five years of age as 100 pounds plus the age to the nearest birthday; and to this add 3 pounds for each inch in height over 5 feet. For example, the desirable weight of a man thirty-two years of age and 5 feet 10 inches tall would be 162 pounds. This is arrived at by allowing 100 pounds plus his age, or 132 pounds, for a person 5 feet tall. To this is added 30 pounds, 3 pounds for each of the 10 inches over 5 feet in height, making the total 162 pounds. In the interest of a low mortality there should be no increase in weight after thirty-five years. Hence, the computation for persons beyond this age is the same as for persons of thirty-five. This method of estimating "desirable weight" can be used for women by deducting 5 pounds from the weight which is desirable for men.

WEIGHT AND MORTALITY

A convincing analysis of the relationship of weight to the length of life and to the various causes of death was made a few

TABLE 15

RELATION OF WEIGHT TO MORTALITY*

A

Ages under Forty-five

Build Class	Death Rates per 100,000†	Percentage of Rate in "Normal" Weight Class
Underweights:		
15 to 34% underweight................	536	116
5 to 15% underweight................	487	105
Normal weights........................	463	100
Overweights:		
5 to 15% overweight.................	510	110
15 to 25% overweight.................	537	116
25% or more overweight................	682	147

B

Ages Forty-five and Over

Build Class	Death Rates per 100,000†	Percentage of Rate in "Normal" Weight Class
Underweights:		
15 to 34% underweight................	1,372	105
5 to 15% underweight................	1,255	96
Normal weight........................	1,308	100
Overweights:		
5 to 15% overweight.................	1,658	127
15 to 25% overweight.................	2,042	156
25% or more overweight................	2,436	186

* Dublin, Louis I., "The Influence of Weight on Certain Causes of Death," *Human Biology*, vol. 2, p. 159, May, 1930.
† All causes.

years ago by Dr. Louis I. Dublin of the Metropolitan Life Insurance Company. This study, the results of which are shown in Tables 15 and 16, covered almost 200,000 men twenty years of age and over.

The mortality among men of weights above or below normal

is strikingly excessive. Under forty-five years of age the hazard of overweight is relatively less than in later life, but, all ages taken together, overweights have a mortality nearly 40 per cent greater

TABLE 16

WEIGHT AND CAUSES OF DEATH*

Causes of Death	Death Rate per 100,000†		
	Under-weights‡	Nor-mals‡	Over-weights‡
All causes..	848	844	1,111
Circulatory diseases:			
Organic diseases of the heart.....................	65	80	121
Angina pectoris..............................	14	16	35
Diseases of the arteries.........................	17	23	38
Acute endocarditis and pericarditis..............	6	8	13
Nephritis, acute and chronic......................	63	82	141
Cerebral hemorrhage and apoplexy................	49	70	110
Paralysis..	12	14	17
Cancer..	62	61	68
Diabetes..	9	14	36
Tuberculosis, all forms..........................	126	64	30
Pulmonary tuberculosis........................	115	57	26
Respiratory diseases:			
Pneumonia, lobar and unspecified...............	70	63	59
Bronchopneumonia............................	5	6	7
Influenza.......................................	20	20	28
Diseases of the digestive system:			
Appendicitis..................................	15	17	20
Cirrhosis of the liver..........................	9	9	15
Typhoid fever...................................	28	29	39
General paralysis of insane......................	12	11	14
External causes:			
Accidents.....................................	55	60	67
Suicides.......................................	27	24	31

* Dublin, *loc. cit.*

† Standardized death rates per 100,000 for specified causes of death—all ages combined—by weight classes.

‡ The numbers of cases in these three weight classifications have been so adjusted that there is no age difference between them (Dublin).

than persons of normal weight. A moderate degree of under-weight is apparently advantageous, particularly in the older age groups.

As shown by Table 16, excessive mortality among persons of abnormal weight is due to a relatively few diseases.

The only disease which produces an excessively high mortality among underweight persons is tuberculosis. Overweight, on the other hand, is associated with an excessive mortality from diabetes, angina pectoris, diseases of the arteries, Bright's disease (nephritis), cerebral hemorrhage and apoplexy, organic disease of the heart, cirrhosis of the liver, and to a somewhat less degree with cancer, appendicitis, typhoid fever, and paralysis. The more important of these are degenerative diseases which represent the results of excessive wear and tear upon the system (see Table 16).

FACTORS WHICH INFLUENCE HEIGHT AND WEIGHT

The use of average weights as standards of normal is less satisfactory when applied to individuals than to groups, because various factors which may or may not be related to health are important influences in determining individual heights and weights. Of these the more important are racial characteristics, body build, diet, disease, heredity, and social and economic factors. In the final analysis, however, tables of average weights are useful, provided their limitations as standards for individual cases are recognized.

TYPES OF BODY BUILD

While it is difficult to define types of body build, some individuals are clearly of a "slight type," with small bony framework; while others are of a "heavy type," with large bony and muscular development. Such differences are largely hereditary and have little or no known relationship to health. In comparing the weights of individuals of such builds with the standard tables, a deviation of 10 to 15 per cent from the average weight is usually considered satisfactory.

HEREDITY

Certain racial or national groups, such as Jews, Italians, Chinese, Japanese, and Filipinos, are short of stature but frequently of stocky build. Doubtless both diet and heredity have contributed to the development of these characteristics. The effect of national dietary customs upon growth is shown by the observations of Holt that Australian-born children of English parents are heavier and taller than English children at home; that Japanese children born in America are bigger and heavier than the children of corresponding ages in Tokyo; and that American-born children of certain immigrants unless they retain their own national food habits tend to be several inches taller than their parents.

The common observation that tall, large parents frequently have tall, large children suggests that heredity influences growth. Palmer tested this thesis experimentally by a breeding experiment with rats from a single set of parents. All his rats received the same food, but matings in successive generations were controlled so that larger rats were mated together and smaller ones together. After the matings had been carried through nine generations, it was evident that the larger rats utilized food more efficiently than the small ones, and that the offspring of larger rats, followed through successive generations, were distinctly bigger and heavier than those of the smaller parents.

SOCIAL AND ECONOMIC FACTORS

The influence of social and economic factors upon growth is equally clear. Years ago, a survey of children in Glasgow showed that children in families which lived in a single room were, on the average, smaller and lighter than the children of families who occupied two rooms; and that the children of two-room families were smaller than those of three-room families, and that those of three-room families were smaller than those of four-room families. In other words, the poorer children were retarded in growth and nutrition. Likewise, children in an exclusive private school in Chicago were found to be taller and heavier than children of the same age in the public schools of that city.

Reports from England during the war indicated that, in spite of severe food shortages, the nutritional status of the higher as well as of the lower income groups improved as a result of the well-balanced diets provided by rationing.

[129   ]

THE PHYSICAL SUPERIORITY OF COLLEGE STUDENTS

An analysis of the heights and weights of 40,000 American college students[1] (23,000 men and 17,000 women) shows that as a group college students are taller and heavier than men and women of corresponding ages in the general population. At eighteen years of age college men are approximately 2 inches taller than applicants for life insurance and army recruits, while college women of the same age are an inch taller than applicants for life insurance.

In weight also the college men surpass the young men of any of the other groups, at eighteen averaging approximately 6 pounds heavier than army recruits and applicants for life insurance. College women, on the other hand, are heavier than applicants for life insurance only at sixteen years of age. At seventeen years of age the groups are of approximately the same weight; but from eighteen to twenty-one years the college women fall progressively farther behind in weight.

Another notable difference between college students and other groups is that during childhood the college students have grown the more rapidly in both height and weight; as a result of which they attain full growth several years before any of the others. For example, college men have practically completed their growth in height by eighteen years of age, while the men in the other groups continue to grow in height until at least twenty-one years of age; and college women show no increase in either height or weight after sixteen years, while women who are examined for life insurance increase in both height and weight until nineteen years of age.

Interesting differences also were observed between the heights and weights of students in the various colleges and universities. The tallest college men are in the Universities of Toronto, Harvard, Princeton, Yale, Leland Stanford, and California, and the heaviest men in Harvard, Toronto, Leland Stanford, Yale, Cali-

---

[1] Diehl, H. S., "The Heights and Weights of American College Men and College Women," *Human Biology*, vol. 5, Nos. 3 and 4, pp. 445 and 600, September and December, 1933.

fornia, and the University of Texas. Although some of the differences in height and weight among the students of certain institutions are small, University of Toronto men average a full 1½ inches taller than the men of the University of Wisconsin and 2½ inches taller than the men of the College of the City of New York; and the men of Harvard University average almost 10 pounds heavier than the men of the University of Cincinnati and 8 pounds heavier than the men of Cornell (Table 17).

TABLE 17
COMPARATIVE PHYSIQUES OF MEN IN CERTAIN COLLEGES*

College	Height, Inches	College	Weight, Pounds	College	Body Build†
1. Toronto‡	69.88	1. Harvard	148.20	1. College of City of New York	31.04
2. Harvard‡	69.50	2. Toronto	144.51	2. Harvard	30.88
3. Princeton	69.28	3. Stanford	144.36	3. Wisconsin	30.45
4. Yale	69.24	4. Yale	143.52	4. Stanford	30.14
5. Stanford	69.21	5. California	142.58	5. Yale	29.94
6. California	69.05	6. Texas	142.36	6. Minnesota	29.92
7. Texas	69.01	7. Wisconsin	141.94	7. California	29.90
8. Minnesota	68.56	8. Princeton	141.55	8. Texas	29.89
9. Cincinnati	68.55	9. Minnesota	140.66	9. Cornell	29.84
10. Cornell	68.48	10. Cornell	139.93	10. Toronto	29.58
11. Wisconsin	68.25	11. College of City of New York	139.42	11. Cincinnati	29.50
12. College of City of New York	67.02	12. Cincinnati	138.64	12. Princeton	29.49

* Students of seventeen, eighteen, nineteen, and twenty years of age with equal numbers from each age group.
† These indices of body build have been computed from mean heights and weights according to the formula $wt^2ht^2 \times 1,000$. The smaller indices indicate slighter builds.
‡ Figures for Toronto and Harvard students from G. B. Porter, "Freshmen Grow in Stature," *University of Toronto Monthly*, December, 1937.

Among college women similar differences exist. The young women of Leland Stanford and Smith are taller and heavier than women of any of the other colleges studied. In height the women of Leland Stanford exceed those of Cornell and Michigan State Normal College by more than an inch, and the women of Smith and Leland Stanford average 6½ pounds heavier than the women of the North Carolina College for Women and almost 8 pounds heavier than the women of the University of Texas (Table 18).

CHILDREN TALLER AND HEAVIER THAN THEIR PARENTS

From various studies it appears that college students of today are physically superior to those of earlier days. Mosher reported that Vassar students in 1923 were 1½ inches taller than they were 37 years before. MacKinnon and Jackson found that over a period of 30 years University of Minnesota men had increased ¾ inch in height and 4 pounds in weight. University of Toronto

TABLE 18

COMPARATIVE PHYSIQUES OF WOMEN IN CERTAIN COLLEGES*

College	Height, Inches	College	Weight, Pounds	College	Body Build†
1. Stanford	64.37	1. Smith	123.87	1. Cornell	30.68
2. Smith	64.24	2. Stanford	123.70	2 Michigan State Normal	30.14
3. Wisconsin	63.95	3. Cornell	123.15	3. Minnesota	30.14
4. Texas	63.92	4. Minnesota	121.61	4. Smith	30.02
5. North Carolina College for Women	63.68	5. Wisconsin	121.25	5. Stanford	29.88
6. Minnesota	63.52	6. Michigan State Normal	119.97	6. Wisconsin	29.65
7. Cornell	63.36	7. North Carolina College for Women	117.29	7. North Carolina College for Women	28.92
8. Michigan State Normal	63.09	8. Texas	116.02	8. Texas	28.40

* Students of seventeen, eighteen, nineteen, and twenty years of age with equal numbers from each age group.

† These indices of body build have been computed from mean heights and weights. The smaller indices indicate slighter builds.

freshmen increased 1¾ inches in average height and 7½ pounds in average weight from 1921 to 1937. University of Oxford crews increased approximately 14 pounds in weight from 1850 to 1925. Boles reports that a group of Harvard students today average 1¼ inches taller and 8 pounds heavier than their fathers did when they were undergraduates at Harvard. And American soldiers of the Second World War averaged ⅔ inch taller than those of the First World War. Studies such as these, together with the results of feeding experiments with animals, indicate that in all probability the human race is still below the maximum growth and development of which it is biologically capable.

[132]

Underweight

We have seen that underweight in young persons is associated with high mortality, particularly from tuberculosis (Table 16). This may be due either to a greater susceptibility to tuberculosis among underweight people or to the fact that some of these underweight people already have unrecognized tuberculosis. It is, of course, well known that tuberculosis tends to cause loss of weight. Spaulding found no relationship between weight and susceptibility to tuberculosis in children, although there did seem to be some increased susceptibility among the unusually tall children.

Whatever the cause of the relationship, there can be no doubt that underweight is associated with tuberculosis. Hence, it would seem that gain in weight should be encouraged among young underweight persons as a form of insurance against this disease. However, if the weight gain is carried beyond the "ideal" per age and height, the increased risk from degenerative diseases more than offsets the advantage gained from the greater protection against tuberculosis.

Underweight increases the susceptibility to fatigue and nervousness as well as to organic disease. Fortunately, the fad of being thin is on the decline, and many girls and young women are finding that they have more energy and feel better with a little more weight.

Underweight may result from improper eating habits, inadequate food, functional disturbances of the body, or actual disease. If the basic cause is disease, the underweight may be a valuable first symptom. Hence, the only intelligent way to start on a program for gaining weight is to have a thorough physical examination. If the underweight is found to be a dietary problem, there are two general principles to be followed to gain weight: one is to eat more food, particularly of high caloric value; the other to use up less energy.

HOW TO GAIN WEIGHT

Probably 90 per cent of healthy people can gain weight simply by eating more food. At first they doubt this because they consider themselves hearty eaters, but if they keep a record of their diets over a period of several days and determine, by referring to tables such as those given in Appendix B, what their energy intakes amount to, they are amazed to find that they are not consuming enough food to maintain weight.[2]

In order to gain weight the energy (caloric) intake must be raised so that it exceeds the energy expenditure. A moderately active individual of average size uses up about 2,500 calories per day. In order to gain weight a diet of 3,000 to 4,000 calories should be provided. The practical problem is to provide the necessary calories in the most appetizing and digestible form.

Fat yields more energy, weight for weight, than any of the other foods, but carbohydrates are the most easily converted into body fat. Proteins are the least efficient foods for this purpose.

A quart of whole milk a day not only furnishes about 700 calories but supplies most of the requirements for calcium, phosphorus, and vitamin A. Butter, cream, fatty meats, cheese, mayonnaise and boiled salad dressing, cream soups, pies, custards, ice cream, and similar foods have high caloric value. An egg drink once a day between meals is valuable for its mineral and vitamin content, as well as to supply additional calories. Fresh fruit and vegetables stimulate the appetite and contain valuable vitamins and minerals.[3]

In order to gain a pound a week the diet must be increased by approximately 600 calories per day. The support of greater weight, however, requires greater energy expenditure, so for continued gain the diet must be increased still more.

LACK OF APPETITE

Many underweight persons complain of insufficient appetite. In such cases an effort should be made to increase the appetite by the selection of delectable foods, the taking of orange juice between meals, moderate exercise in the fresh air, and occasionally by the use of tonics or insulin.

[2] For energy requirements see p. 115.
[3] For energy values of common foods see Appendix B.

Lack of appetite does not seriously interfere with the nutritional value of food, so a person who is trying to gain in weight should eat more food than is necessary to provide a feeling of satisfaction. The difficulty of a limited capacity may be overcome also by partaking of foods more frequently than three times a day. An extra meal at bedtime is recommended for gaining weight because it increases food intake without impairing the appetite; while lunches in the morning and in the afternoon reduce the amount of food eaten at the regular meals.

More hours of sleep at night and rest periods after lunch and dinner are valuable adjuncts to diet in an effort to gain weight.

Overweight

Fatty tissue in proper amounts is an essential constituent of the human body. It adds not only to comfort and shapeliness, but also protects health and nutrition to a significant degree. Fat in healthy amounts, approximately 10 to 15 per cent of the total body weight, serves a variety of useful purposes. It acts as a reservoir for food to be used in time of need; it serves as padding or shock absorbing material, protecting the various organs against undue shock or vibration; it keeps the individual warm; it is responsible in large measure for the smoothness and elasticity of the skin, as well as for the normal shape and contour of the body, and it conserves protein in the body. People who lack an adequate amount of fat are undernourished if not emaciated, and are susceptible to all the hazards that go with this condition, such as weakness, anemia, loose skin, flabby muscles, and a diminished resistance to disease, particularly tuberculosis.[4]

On the other hand, the records of every life insurance company show conclusively that obesity is a liability to health and that the hazard of excessive weight increases with age and with the degree of overweight. A simple but impressive way of expressing this is the old rule-of-thumb adage "for every inch by which a man's waist measure exceeds his chest measure, subtract two years from his life expectancy."

Public health authorities proclaim obesity to be "the greatest

[4] Millman, Max, *Today's Health,* American Medical Association, March, 1953.

[135]

single health hazard to human life in the nation today." The hazards of obesity have been described as the five D's: disfigurement, discomfort, disability, disease, and death.

The diseases responsible for the high mortality of overweight people are largely metabolic and degenerative—diabetes, heart disease, apoplexy, Bright's disease, and cirrhosis of the liver. The

FIG. 13. ABDOMINAL FAT

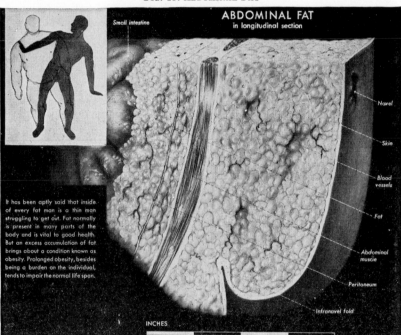

(*Courtesy of Northwestern National Life Insurance Company, Minneapolis, Minn.*)

death rate from diabetes among men who are 25 per cent or more overweight is eight times as high as among men who are of average weight. Overweight seems to be related to these diseases primarily because it interferes with metabolism and throws a greater strain upon the circulatory system. It has been estimated that for each 5 pounds of excess weight the blood vessels are increased by 3 miles. Obese people utilize energy less efficiently and consequently need more food to support the same amount of activity than do thin ones, the basal requirement for an obese

[136]

person being about 50 per cent greater than for a nonfat person of the same weight.

Causes of Obesity

The causes of obesity may be divided into the hereditary, dietary, and glandular groups. Just how heredity influences obesity is not entirely clear. There is a laboratory strain of mice that regularly gets very fat. These mice are neither physically nor sexually active. They get fat by eating excessively. Restriction of food will reduce their fat, but they retain the hereditary urge to eat. In man there are indications that heredity predisposes to obesity. How, we do not know, but there is much to suggest that it is through the nervous control of metabolism and appetite.

The dietary type of obesity merely means that food intake exceeds the energy expenditure of the body. This may be due to habit or to the indulgence of appetite. Psychiatrists report that fat children frequently feel unloved and take comfort in food and fullness. Both dietary and hereditary types are susceptible to control through dietary measures.

In the glandular type of obesity, there is a lowered expenditure of energy because of diminished activity of certain of the glands of internal secretion, usually the thyroid and the pituitary. In such cases fat accumulates even with a normal intake of food. The treatment of this type of obesity is a strictly medical problem.

OBESITY CURES

The "cure" of obesity is one of the richest fields for medical swindlers. The wares which they have to sell, all guaranteed to cure, include elastic belts, corsets, vibrating and exercising machines, reducing foods, bath salts, soaps, creams, and drugs for internal medication.

The wearing of elastic garments may improve the appearance but does not reduce the weight. Active exercise and passive massage increase the expenditure of energy but they also stimulate the appetite. They are effective in the reduction of weight only if accompanied by a control of the diet. Any foods which

[137]

satisfy the appetite and have a low caloric value could properly be called "reducing foods." Those foods, however, which sell at fancy prices and are advertised as of special merit for the reduction of weight should be looked upon with suspicion. Some of these contain laxatives or dangerous drugs, such as thyroid extract or pokeroot. Others, such as most of the reducing breads, have just as high food value as ordinary foods.

Bath salts for reducing weight consist of coloring matter and certain salts, all of which are absolutely worthless for the purpose for which they are recommended. A hot bath, and particularly a hot steam bath, produces temporary loss of weight by sweating. But it is only water that is lost and this is quickly replaced. The various soaps and pastes which are supposed to remove fat consist for the most part of lard, sugar, glycerine, and perfume. There is not the slightest basis for thinking that any of them are of value.

Medicinal preparations advertised for the reduction of weight are either worthless or dangerous. Many contain laxatives which cause a temporary reduction of weight by loss of water. Some contain iodine but this has no effect upon weight except in persons with goiters, and it is dangerous for such persons to take iodine without medical supervision. Many reducing medicines contain dried thyroid extract. This in sufficient quantities increases the rate of metabolism and thus may cause some loss of weight. However, excessive thyroid stimulation is accompanied by nervousness, irritability, and other unpleasant symptoms, and it may produce serious ill effects.

In recent years a drug called "dinitrophenol" has been used both alone and in mixtures with fancy names for the reduction of weight. Its effect upon the body is to increase enormously the rate of metabolism. For this reason it causes a loss of weight but the deaths which have been reported from its use are ample evidence that it is a dangerous drug.

EXERCISE FOR THE REDUCTION OF WEIGHT

Exercise is vastly overrated for the reduction of weight, since under ordinary conditions it is necessary to walk about 36 miles

[138]

to get rid of one pound of fat. Yet, exercise can be a valuable aid in the treatment of obesity, provided it is used with discretion and in conjunction with dietary measures. Discretion is necessary because excessive fat throws a heavy load upon the heart and circulatory system, and it may be dangerous to increase this still more by strenuous exercise. Another disadvantage of exercise is that it increases the appetite and so makes food restriction more difficult. Moderate general exercise, such as walking, and calisthenics which exercise the muscles of the abdomen and back are useful to give a feeling of well-being and to increase the tone of the tissues. It is unwise, however, for the person over forty to carry exercises to the point of exhaustion or shortness of breath.

Weight can be reduced several pounds by sweating, because of the loss of water from the body. This loss, however, is rapidly regained as one takes in fluids to meet the body's needs.

It has been well said that the best exercise for reducing is a rapid movement of the head from right to left when the potatoes and gravy are passed. Another good exercise is to place the hands firmly on the edge of the table and press backward when "seconds" are offered.

WEIGHT LOSS WITHOUT DIETING

Wilder summarizes the measures, other than dieting, advocated for reducing weight as follows:

The wish for something which will permit the glutton to indulge his appetite yet prevent gain in weight without impairing health will probably never be satisfied. The Romans practiced regurgitation; the marble vomitorium in Hadrian's palace is pointed out to every visitor. Brooks, at the Adult Weight Conference, quoted one patient who boasted to him that he was a Roman and did not need to diet. This was a mystery to him, although he said that if he had connected it in his mind with the ruins of Roman banquet halls and Pompeii, he would have known at once what was meant; and later he came to know only too well, for he discovered that many young women have mastered the art of eating their cake and yet not having it. This method of achieving slimness is likely to establish nervous habits. The evil of high colonic flushing practiced by other poorly advised people and the evils attending the chronic use of cathartics are well known.[5]

[5] Wilder, Russel M., "The Treatment of Obesity," *International Clinics*, vol. 4, ser. 43, p. 1, 1933.

[139   ]

THE DIETARY CONTROL OF WEIGHT

There remains the dietary control of food intake as the one safe and effective method of reducing weight. The principle involved is simply that of keeping the energy intake below the energy expenditure of the body. Fat is the body's chief storehouse of excess energy. When more energy is taken in as food than the body can use, some of it, but a relatively small amount, is stored as glycogen (carbohydrate). The rest, whether it be from carbohydrate, fat, or protein in the food, is converted into body fat. The amount of glycogen which the body can store will provide scarcely enough energy to supply the needs of the body for 24 hours, while 1 pound of fat will support moderate activity for almost 2 days. When energy intake is reduced below energy expenditure, the first call is upon the stores of glycogen. But these are soon exhausted, and then the body begins to draw upon the energy which it has stored in the form of fat.

Moderate reduction of weight usually can be accomplished merely by eliminating from the diet foods of high caloric value, such as butter, cream, and other fats and carbohydrates. The quantity of food necessary to satisfy the appetite can be made up by fruits, vegetables, and lean meats.

A reduction of the daily energy (caloric) intake by 600 to 700 calories[6] should result in the loss of about a pound per week. For continued or more rapid loss further restriction of the diet is necessary.

A serious deficiency of many reducing diets is that they do not supply the minimum requirements of the body for protein, minerals, and vitamins. Without these, fatigue, nervousness, digestive disturbances, and an irresistible craving for food develop. On the other hand, patients report that they are not uncomfortable on very restricted diets, if these needs are supplied. Every reducing diet should contain liberal quantities of the vitamins and sufficient minerals and protein to supply requirements (see Appendix B).

[6] The following food portions represent 600 to 700 calories: four slices of bread and four squares of butter; a pork chop and a piece of pie; two pieces of bread with butter and one serving of mashed potatoes with butter or gravy, etc. (see Appendix B).

Another place where a great deal of good can be accomplished . . . is to offset and counteract the silly and asinine claims of people who present, year by year, different reducing diets to women. . . . If there is any one thing we know to be sound, it is that the healthy overweight person must take a diet which is physiologically complete, and which is capable of permitting the body to make physiological repair if he or she succeeds in reducing weight without incurring injury to health. If women could be taught this truth, a great many of them would find that their skins would fit them a good deal better after they have gone down in weight.[7]

In the more difficult cases and in cases of extreme obesity, weight reduction should be preceded by a thorough physical examination. If dietary measures are indicated, the caloric intake necessary to maintain ideal weight should be computed (page 125) and the diet planned so that this amount will not be exceeded. Gradual weight loss is usually preferable to rapid reduction because the subject becomes adjusted to smaller quantities of food and so is more likely to maintain a desirable weight after it has been attained.

If more rapid reduction in weight is desired, there must be a greater limitation of energy foods in the diet. For this purpose diets which supply from 1,000 to 1,500 calories per day have been recommended. Several such diets adequate in proteins, minerals, and vitamins are given in Table 19. Substitutions or additions can be made by referring to the food values given in Appendix B.

A more rapid reduction than was previously thought desirable has recently been shown to be perfectly safe, provided the diet is adequate in protein, minerals, and vitamins. One diet advocated by Strang, McClugage, and Evans[8] supplied approximately 360 calories a day and resulted in weight loss of as much as 4 to 5 pounds a week. Wilder's modification[9] of this diet suggests 500 to 600 calories per day in order that more foods containing vitamin C may be obtained. Vitamins A and D are sup-

---

[7] McCollum, E. V., "Nutrition a Public Health Problem," *Illinois Health Messenger*, vol. 9, p. 92, August 15, 1937.

[8] Strang, J. M., H. B. McClugage, and F. A. Evans, "Further Studies in the Dietary Correction of Obesity," *American Journal of Medical Science*, vol. 179, p. 687, May, 1930.

[9] Wilder, Russel M., "The Treatment of Obesity," *International Clinics*, vol. 4, ser. 43, p. 1, 1933.

TABLE 19

SAMPLE REDUCING DIETS

Breakfast

1 medium grapefruit
1 egg
1 slice toast
½ square butter
1 glass skim milk
Clear tea or coffee

Lunch

Ham omelet (1 egg and 2 tbsp. lean, diced ham)
3 heaping tbsp. squash
Celery and radishes (1 large heart celery; 4 small radishes)
3 tbsp. apple sauce
1 glass skim milk
Clear tea

Dinner

Medium serving chicken
2 tbsp. mashed potato
3 heaping tbsp. beet greens
Cucumber and lettuce salad: 2 leaves lettuce; 12 slices cucumber; 1 slice tomato with lemon or vinegar
1 medium sliced banana
Clear tea ·

1,005 calories

Breakfast

3 medium-sized prunes without sugar
1 thin slice toast
½ square butter
2 thin strips bacon
1 glass skim milk
Clear coffee or tea

Lunch

1 large serving white meat of chicken
½ cup peas
Salad: 2 leaves lettuce; 1 medium-sized tomato
2 asparagus tips—2¾ inches long
½ cup frozen orange juice
1 glass skim milk
Clear coffee or tea

Dinner

1 average serving cold sliced tongue
Salad: 2 lettuce leaves; ⅓ cup shredded cabbage; 1 tbsp. each, pimento and green pepper; mayonnaise
⅔ cup beets
2 stalks celery
1 thin slice graham bread
½ square butter
1 medium-sized peach or ½ canned peach
1 glass skim milk
Clear coffee or tea

1,023 calories

Breakfast

½ glass orange juice
1 thin slice toast
½ square butter
Omelet (1 egg)
1 glass skim milk
Clear coffee

Lunch

Clear broth (fat skimmed off)
2 crackers
Salad: 2 leaves lettuce; ½ cup salmon or tunafish; 2 stalks celery; 2 tbsp. peas; 1 hard-boiled egg
⅔ cup spinach
Fruit cup: ¼ grapefruit; ½ medium-sized orange; ½ banana
½ glass skim milk or buttermilk
Clear tea or coffee

Dinner

1 large serving lean roast beef
⅔ cup cauliflower
⅔ cup string beans
½ cup salad: 1 pkg. lemon Jello; 1 cup grated raw carrots; 4 stalks chopped celery; 2 leaves lettuce
½ cup apple sauce
Clear tea or coffee

1,019 calories

plied in a cod-liver oil concentrate, vitamin B in yeast. Calcium and phosphorus are supplied by giving 2 level teaspoonfuls of dibasic calcium phosphate. Fluids are not restricted.

TABLE 20

BASIC REDUCING DIET*

Breakfast	Lunch	Dinner
1 orange or ½ grapefruit	Clear broth of any kind (fat	Same as lunch, substituting
1 egg, any style but not fried in fat	removed)	various meats, fish, fruits and vegetables
1 slice whole-wheat bread or toast (no butter)†	1 portion† *lean* meat or fish	
1 capsule halibut-liver oil with viosterol	2 portions‡ vegetables from following list	
Coffee or tea in ½ cup of milk (no cream or sugar)	1 portion‡ fruit from following list	
	Coffee or tea with milk as at breakfast	

LIST OF FRUITS AND VEGETABLES ALLOWED

Vegetables		Fruits	
Asparagus	Lettuce	Apples, stewed,	Lemon
Beetroot	Onions	fresh	Melon
Broccoli	Parsnips	Apples, raw	Oranges
Brussel sprouts	Radishes	Apricots	Peaches
Cabbage	Rhubarb	Blackberries	Pears
Carrots	Spinach	Cherries, raw	Pineapple
Cauliflower	Spring onions	Cherries, stewed	Plums
Celery	String beans	Coconut	Plums, stewed
Cucumber	Tomato	Cranberries	Strawberries
Horseradish	Turnip	Gooseberries	
Peas	Watercress	Grapefruit	
Corn		Grapes	

NOTE: Constant use of any one fruit or vegetable should be avoided. Vary articles of diet daily.
List of Meats and Fish Preferred: Beef, veal, lamb, chicken, white fish, haddock, pike, halibut, cod. Fat meats and gravies must be completely avoided.

* Robinowitch, I. M., "Clinical and Laboratory Experiences with High Carbohydrate Low Calorie Diets in the Treatment of Diabetes Mellitus," *New England Journal of Medicine*, vol. 204, p. 687, April 16, 1931. Adapted and utilized for reduction of weight by Dr. B. A. Watson, formerly at Students' Health Service, University of Minnesota.

† Bread is cut 16 slices to the pound. A portion of meat or fish is one-half the size of a slice of bread and of corresponding thickness.

‡ A portion of vegetable or fruit is ⅛ to ½ cup.

A plan of weight reduction which we have been utilizing because of its simplicity provides for an initial rapid loss, followed by more gradual reduction and the maintenance of the desired weight, once it has been attained. The foundation of this plan is a basic diet of approximately 800 calories, adequate in protein, vitamins, and minerals (Table 20).

This diet may be followed from two to four or more weeks unless excessive hunger, fatigue, or weakness develops. The rate at which weight is lost on this diet depends upon the body size and the rate of metabolism, but in general a loss of 3 to 4 pounds per week may be expected.

TABLE 21

EQUIVALENTS FOR BREAD

Substitute for One Slice of Bread	Substitutes for Two Slices of Bread
1 potato (2½ in. diam.)	½ cup of apple sauce
1 banana (medium size)	6 large dates
4 tsp. sugar	¼ cup of hash
1 heaping tbsp. jelly	1 cup of milk
⅔ cup of peas	3 prunes
⅓ cup of lima beans, fresh	3 chocolate drop cookies
¾ cup of cornflakes	1 large muffin
½ cup of oatmeal	½ cup of cream of tomato soup
⅓ cup of rice	⅓ cup of dried apricots
1 egg	1 slice of roast beef, 4 × 4 × ½ in.
2 graham crackers	½ cup of ice cream
½ cup of cooked spaghetti	1 veal chop, medium size, 3 in. thick

After approximately half the desired reduction has been accomplished, the diet may be increased every second day by a slice of bread or its equivalent. A slice of bread provides approximately 80 calories. Some of the equivalents of a slice of bread for the purposes of this diet are given in Table 21. These and others which may be selected from Appendix B increase the variety and improve the palatability of the diet.

PREDICTING WEIGHT LOSS

Reduction of weight by dieting occurs because the body is expending more energy than is provided in the food. This difference is made up by the utilization of body fats. A gram of fat upon oxidation yields 9.3 calories, or a pound of fat about 4,500 calories. Hence, for every pound of weight loss there must be a deficit of 4,500 calories in energy intake in relation to energy expenditure.

On the basis of this knowledge one can estimate weight loss by a simple calculation of the difference between energy expenditure and energy intake. For example, a lawyer or business executive thirty-five years of age, 5 feet 10 inches tall, and weighing 190 pounds without shoes or clothing, decides to reduce by following this diet. His ideal weight, according to standard tables (see Table 14), should be 160 to 165. Since the energy utilized at rest amounts to 11 calories per pound per day (see page 116), his basic requirement is about 1,800 calories per day. Leading a semiactive life increases this by about 40 per cent, or to 2,500 calories. Because of his overweight condition he actually needs considerably more than this, probably 40 to 50 per cent more, or about 3,600 calories, to maintain present weight.

On the basic diet shown in Table 20 he will get about 800 calories per day. Therefore he must utilize his own body fat to supply 2,800 calories. In a week this deficiency totals about 20,000 calories, or the energy contained in 4½ pounds of fat. As the weight is reduced or the diet increased, the loss becomes smaller.

MAINTAINING DESIRABLE WEIGHT

By the time that our hypothetical subject attains normal weight, he should have increased his food intake to about 2,500 calories and on this diet should maintain his weight. Failure to do so means that we have underestimated or overestimated his activity. If he gains on this diet, he should decrease the quantity by one or more slices of bread, or the equivalent, per day. If he loses, he should increase his diet in a similar manner. The regulation of his weight is entirely in his own hands.

By selecting a dietary program with the advice of a physician and following it intelligently and conscientiously, every normal person can reduce weight. Those who fail to do so usually are unwilling to forego the transitory pleasure of indulging the appetite for the greater joy of health, vigor, and longer life in the future. Others are successful in reducing weight but gradually slip back into their old dietary habits. Of 224 employees of the Metropolitan Life Insurance Company who had successfully reduced their weights under the guidance of the Medical Department, the majority had regained weight by the end of the first year, and the group as a whole showed an average gain of over half the amount lost during treatment. By the end of the fifth year the group had regained on the average 10 per cent more weight than they had lost during treatment.

Like "old soaks" who occasionally sober up, some persons engage in alternating periods of dieting and gluttony. This may enable them to preserve their self-respect but probably has little other value. To be of real benefit, weight reduction must be followed by the maintenance of normal weight.

If certain diseases exist, such as actual or suspected tuberculosis, anemia, and certain nervous conditions, dieting should not be undertaken. But for every case in which dieting is undesirable there are scores whose health and efficiency will be benefited by a reduction of weight.

The usual experience of those who get rid of excess weight is that they feel better and have more physical and mental energy than when they were overweight. Persons with high blood pressure, diabetes, and heart disease frequently experience relief of symptoms and improvement of their physical condition when weight is reduced.

Such results are adequate compensation for the inconvenience and effort required to maintain a desirable weight. Better, however, than to reduce weight is to learn in early adult life the importance of preventing obesity. It is easy to lose 2 pounds but difficult to lose 20. Habitual moderation in eating and a reduction of energy foods whenever there is a tendency to exceed one's ideal weight is the best way to avoid the hazard of obesity.

DISCUSSION SUGGESTIONS

1. Discuss the factors which may influence the weight of normal individuals.
2. What is the difference between average weight and best weight? How does this difference change with age?
3. Discuss the relation of weight to mortality. What diseases are most common in persons who are overweight? What ones in persons who are underweight?
4. Discuss the reasons for the physical superiority of college students.
5. Is it probable that there will be any increase in the average height and weight of American men and women? Why?
6. What are the causes and the advantages or disadvantages of underweight?

7. Outline a program and diet for an individual of your age who wishes to gain weight and estimate the rate of gain that can be anticipated.
8. What are the causes and the advantages or disadvantages of obesity?
9. Discuss exercise, baths, and drugs for the reduction of weight.
10. Outline a program and diet for an individual of your age who is 60 pounds overweight and wishes to reduce. Estimate the rate of weight reduction that can be anticipated.
11. What precautions must be taken in the use of reducing diets?

REFERENCES AND READING SUGGESTIONS

1. Diehl, H. S.: "The Heights and Weights of American College Men and College Women," *Human Biology*, vol. 5, pp. 444 and 600, September and December, 1933.
2. Dublin, Louis I., and H. H. Marks: "Mortality among Insured Overweights in Recent Years," Association of Life Insurance Medical Directors of America, New York, 1952.
3. Jollife, Norman: "Reduce and Stay Reduced," Simon and Schuster, Inc., New York, 1952.
4. Mayer, Jean: "The Care of the Disrespective Mice," *Harper's Magazine*, October, 1953.
5. Newburgh, Louis H.: "There Is Only One Way to Get Thin," *Rotarian*, p. 25, November, 1943. Condensed in *The Reader's Digest*, p. 31, November, 1943.
6. Paterson, Donald: "Physique and Intellect," Appleton-Century-Crofts, Inc., New York, 1930.
7. "Are We Growing Bigger?" *Journal of the American Medical Association*, vol. 107, pp. 1054–1055, September 26, 1936.
8. "Overweight and Underweight," Metropolitan Life Insurance Company, New York, 1953.
9. "Fat Can Be Fatal," Northwestern National Life Insurance Company, Minneapolis, 1951.

Chapter VII

DIGESTIVE DISTURBANCES

THE dietitian insists that food be adequate in calories, proteins, vitamins, and minerals; the sanitarian that it be free from disease-producing germs; but the average man merely asks that it be pleasant to the taste, satisfy his appetite, and "agree" with him.

Rare indeed is the man or woman who has not at some time experienced the demoralizing effect of "misery" in the solar plexus. Pain in this region refuses to be ignored; and if it is frequent or constant, attention is almost certain to center upon it. This invariably makes matters worse, for stomachs are retiring, sensitive creatures, with a job to do and an insistence upon doing it in their own way. Pamper them or attempt to regulate them and they become temperamental. Give them too much attention and they become jealous for more.

An evening devoted to the radio is enough to lead one to the conclusion that most, if not all, people of this country suffer from indigestion. Grand-opera stars, crooning cowboys, and news commentators help to sell stomach tablets, yeast, salts, and crystals for "what ails you." Fortunately the average American is not so badly off as the announcers of these programs would have us believe. But it is certain that indigestion would very soon become a universal complaint if people followed the advice of alleged prophets of health with something to sell.

The types of digestive disturbances causing abdominal discomfort are numerous. Sometimes the basis is true organic disease but much more frequently the disturbances are functional rather than organic in nature. In any case, abdominal disturbances merit careful investigation and intelligent treatment.

The good old diagnoses of indigestion and dyspepsia were discarded by physicians along with the frock coat and professional whiskers; yet the public still finds these terms useful to designate various types of abdominal discomfort. When a person says that he has indigestion, he may mean anything from a loss of appetite, bad taste in the mouth, eructations of gas, gaseous distention, cramps, or mild discomfort—to nausea, vomiting, and diarrhea; and the basic trouble may be a serious disease or a mild functional disturbance. Among the organic diseases which produce such symptoms are appendicitis, gallstones, ulcers of the stomach or duodenum, and cancer of the stomach or intestinal tract. All these are serious and demand careful diagnosis and medical or surgical treatment.

Dyspepsia

Dyspepsia or indigestion is a vague, unscientific term used to designate various types of discomfort in the region of the stomach. Dyspepsia may be due to unimportant functional causes, or it may be an early symptom of serious disease.

The late Dr. A. B. Rivers of the Division of Medicine of the Mayo Clinic summarized the results of a survey relative to the occurrence of dyspepsia among a large number of patients who came to the clinic for examination. This analysis shows that about half of the men forty years of age and older who complained of dyspepsia were found to have ulcer of the stomach, gall-bladder disease, or cancer of the gastrointestinal tract or accessory organs. Of women of the same age group, two out of five were found to be suffering from gall-bladder disease, ulcer or cancer of the stomach, or cancer of the pancreas or intestine. Of the men of sixty who came to the clinic because of dyspepsia, 39 per cent were found to have cancer; in men of seventy or older cancer was demonstrable in 58 per cent of the cases. In women,

[149]

also, cancer of the stomach is an important cause of dyspepsia, although its development occurs at a slightly higher age than in men.

Dr. Rivers rightly calls attention to the following fact:

Almost any evening, during the height of the radio programs, it is possible to hear four or five smooth-tongued announcers advising rapid and inexpensive methods of curing gastrointestinal difficulties. Drugstore shelves are filled with attractively displayed means of curing indigestion. The highways are bordered by signs indicating how the passers-by can quickly return to the happy state wherein they can again enjoy their food.

Magazines and newspapers daily carry therapeutic advice regarding gastronomic disturbances for the benefit of their dyspeptic readers.[1]

Only the gullible are taken in by such advertising but there are hundreds of thousands of these who are sacrificing health and even life itself upon this altar of ignorance and commercialism.

Cancer of the Stomach

Cancer of the stomach is responsible for about 25,000 deaths annually in the United States. This represents approximately one-eighth of all cancer deaths. Unfortunately, cancer of the stomach rarely produces definite symptoms early in the disease, at the time that the possibilities of cure would be the greatest. In fact, the early symptoms are usually nothing more than mild "indigestion." Eventually a physician is consulted and a diagnosis made, but all too frequently—and tragically—precious time is wasted trying suggestions of friends or preparations advertised for the cure of indigestion.

Persistent indigestion, any pronounced change in usual bowel habits, or blood in the stool demand a careful examination by a competent physician. Usually nothing serious will be found, but in order to play safe the possibility of cancer should be considered in every person over thirty-five years of age who has any of the symptoms listed above. A good examination is cheap insurance against a serious disease as well as against the mental anguish of worrying unnecessarily about it.

[1] Rivers, A. B., "The Dangers of Treating 'Indigestion' by Advertised Nostrums," *Proceedings of the Staff Meetings of the Mayo Clinic*, vol. 13, p. 87, February 9, 1938.

Ulcers of the Stomach and Duodenum

Ulcers of the stomach and duodenum are a common cause of so-called "chronic dyspepsia." About one person out of ten at some time will have an ulcer. Ulcers usually result from an excessive flow of the stomach's acid-containing digestive juices. It is now

Fig. 14. The Human Stomach

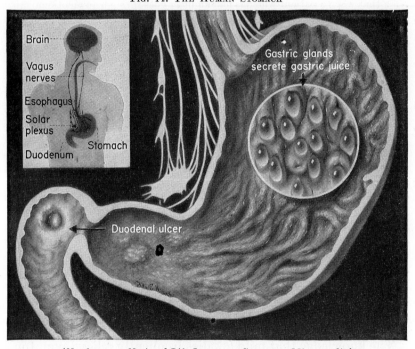

Brain

Vagus nerves

Esophagus

Solar plexus

Stomach

Duodenum

Gastric glands secrete gastric juice

Duodenal ulcer

(*Northwestern National Life Insurance Company, Minneapolis.*)

recognized that nervous tension, worry, and emotional strain, even more than food and drink, stimulate the flow of these juices. The successful treatment of ulcer, therefore, depends upon the elimination of mental tension and turmoil as well as upon medical or surgical measures.

Duodenal ulcers (Fig. 14) rarely, if ever, are cancerous. On the other hand, 20 to 30 per cent of gastric ulcers (ulcers of the stomach) are cancerous. It is imperative, therefore, that the exact

[151]

nature of an ulcer be diagnosed as early as possible to determine what type of treatment is necessary.

Since most ulcers are accompanied by excessive secretions of acids, smooth, nonirritating diets and mild alkalies, such as soda, usually relieve symptoms and facilitate healing. Dr. Walter Alvarez[2] even suggests

. . . that when a patient who has had an ulcer goes through an emotional crisis he should immediately start taking food every hour or two. He shouldn't wait for the expected flare-up or hemorrhage or perforation. The extra feedings are probably most needed between the hours of 10 P.M. and 3 A.M.

Explaining the reasons for this advice, Dr. Alvarez says:

A man of 50 who had always been well discovered one day that the man who for twenty years had been his brother-in-law, his closest friend and his business partner had been falsifying the books in order to steal from him. All that night he lay awake in great mental distress, and next day he had a big gastric hemorrhage. Another man, a physician, after examining a woman's stomach with a roentgenoscope (an x-ray apparatus for viewing the body on a screen), discovered that he had used a current of 60 milliamperes instead of the usual 3 milliamperes. After lying awake all night worrying over the expected burn and resultant damage suit he found himself almost incapacitated by the pain of a bad ulcer. Another man, when a violent strike in his factory distressed him terribly, had a big hemorrhage. A woman who adored her peppery little daughter-in-law one day inadvertently offended her and brought down on her head a storm of abuse which nearly killed her. Next day a long-healed ulcer flared up and perforated. A women who heard that her soldier husband had just been killed at the front promptly had a hemorrhage.

The knowledge that mild alkalies frequently relieve symptoms of gastric distress forms the basis for practically all the indigestion cures offered to a credulous public. The undirected use of such preparations in many cases is perfectly harmless and may give relief, but occasionally an ulcer may rupture or become malignant (cancerous) or the symptoms supposedly due to an ulcer may be the first warning of a beginning cancer. To seek relief of symptoms by self-medication is hazardous.

[2] Alvarez, Walter C., "How to Avoid Flare-up of Peptic Ulcer," *Journal of the American Medical Association*, vol. 125, p. 903, July 29, 1944.

Appendicitis

Appendicitis is an important cause of death in every age group, yet most of the 2,600 annual deaths from appendicitis can be explained by a single word—neglect. The risk increases with each day and hour that a "stomach-ache" of unknown cause persists. Proper attention to abdominal pain, early medical care, and immediate operation, when indicated, are the secrets of preventing deaths from appendicitis.

Appendicitis is an inflammation of the appendix—a small "dead end" of the large intestine—which is located in the lower right part of the abdomen. When an operation is performed within 24 hours of the beginning of the attack less than 1 per cent of the patients die, but the risk is increased to approximately 12 per cent when operation is delayed until the fourth or fifth day. The use of cathartics during an attack of appendicitis greatly increases the risk. A recent study of appendicitis in a large Eastern city showed that, of patients with appendicitis who took no laxatives, 1 in 62 died, of patients who took one laxative, 1 in 19 died; and of patients who took more than one laxative 1 in 9 died.

When the public can be trained to realize that abdominal pain, particularly if accompanied by nausea or vomiting and constipation, may indicate appendicitis, that cathartics may do irreparable harm, and that a physician should be consulted immediately, many lives will be saved each year.

FUNCTIONAL DISORDERS

The most common cause of so-called "indigestion" is a functional disturbance of the digestive tract. That is, all the structures are normal; the trouble is that they do not function or act normally. However, the discomfort produced is real and may be indistinguishable from actual disease; hence, one should not assume that persistent abdominal symptoms are functional, even though vague and indefinite, until the possibility of actual disease has been ruled out. Once the possibility of organic disease has been eliminated, the reason for the functional disturbance may be sought in the character of the food, the habits of eating, or the nervous or emotional state.

ROUGHAGE IN THE DIET

The physical character of food is responsible for symptoms of dyspepsia in many people. Roughage, such as bran, fibrous fruits, and vegetables, is helpful in the correction of some cases of constipation, but the mechanical irritation which roughage produces leads to most distressing symptoms in others. The bowel fills with gas, discomfort increases, and the constipation may become more persistent. What such intestinal tracts need most is rest. This may be accomplished by starvation but these people need nourishment; hence, a soft nourishing diet is desirable. For the average person the use of bran in the diet cannot be recommended.

NERVOUS INDIGESTION

It has long been known that food is most digestible and nutritious if it is appetizing, served under pleasant conditions, and eaten in a happy frame of mind; but only in recent years has physiological research been able to explain the manner in which such factors influence digestion. We now know that the nervous system may affect the digestion in at least two ways: it may stimulate or retard the secretion of digestive juices; and it may increase or decrease the muscular contractions of the intestinal tract. Nervous stimuli are aroused largely by the emotions and reach the digestive tract through the autonomic (involuntary) nervous system.

The smell, taste, sight, and even the thought of appetizing food literally makes the mouth of a hungry person water. Coincident with this increase in the flow of saliva there is an increase in the secretion of the gastric juice and probably of other digestive juices. This is nature's preparation for the digestion of the anticipated food. The more attractive the food and the better its taste, the greater will be the amount of this secretion. Fear, pain, anger, and other strong emotions prevent this psychic secretion and so interfere with digestion if food is taken. Pavlov and others have shown, by placing food directly into the stomach, that some secretion of digestive juices occurs even in the absence of the stimuli of taste, smell, and sight, but for continuing health and normal digestion this psychic secretion is necessary.

AUTOINTOXICATION

Patients in certain anxiety states may vomit food which is practically unchanged from its original condition, although it has been in the stomach for several hours. When such undigested food passes down the intestinal tract, it is acted upon by putrefactive bacteria with the production of toxic substances. These in turn may give rise to symptoms of lassitude, headache, fatigue, and abdominal discomfort. Such a condition is commonly called "autointoxication." Its prevention or correction must be accomplished through the control of nervous and emotional factors and not by the use of cathartics or "intestinal antiseptics."

EMOTIONS AFFECT DIGESTION

The effect of emotions upon the movement of the stomach and intestines has been observed in both man and animals. An ancient Hindu custom required persons suspected of a crime to chew a mouthful of rice and after a time to spit it out upon a fig leaf. Dry rice was taken as proof that the fear of being discovered had prevented the secretion of saliva, and the suspect was adjudged guilty. Fear and apprehension also may produce diarrhea or constipation. And milder degrees of concern or worry over the affairs of everyday life frequently result in spasticity of the musculature of the intestinal tract. This is usually accompanied by gaseous distention and discomfort, frequently described as a sensation of the intestines being "tied up in knots."

Alvarez says of this condition:

It has long been known, even to the layman, that disgust, excitement, fear, anxiety, anger, fatigue, pain or injury will stop or reverse the movements of the digestive tract. A child who has suffered injury or severe fright shortly after a meal will often after several hours return the food quite unchanged. I remember once examining a neurotic young man with a fluoroscope and finding every bit of barium meal, eaten six hours before, still in the stomach. There were no symptoms or signs of organic disease, so I began inquiring and I learned that all that day he had been much upset over a political row in his lodge which, that very evening, was to be fought to a finish. Later, when he was calm, his stomach emptied perfectly.

When, in 1896, Cannon began his classic experiments on animals, he discovered that the slightest uneasiness, discomfort, or anger experienced by the animals would immediately stop all movement in the stomach and bowels. For this reason he had to use elderly female cats, well used to handling and with pleasant dispositions: old tabbies that would lie quietly under the x-ray screen and purr.

That the currents in the digestive tract can be reversed by worry was well shown by a neurotic young woman who one day received a menacing letter from the income tax collector. This so frightened her that, instead of going to see what the trouble was, she took to her bed and vomited day and night for a week. She stopped only when, after learning what had happened to upset her, I went to the Customs House and appeased Uncle Samuel with $3.85; which shows, incidentally, that not all medicine comes out of bottles.

Practically, what can be done to improve matters? How can a patient get back a psychic use and a psychic tone that he or she has lost? Obviously, of course, by resting, by getting sleep, by avoiding worry and annoyance, by cultivating a better technique at meal-time. As Brillat-Savarin has said, "Animals eat, man eats, the man of intellect alone knows how to eat." According to him, no dinner guest should ever be invited again unless, with the coming of each dish to the table, his face would seem to light up and his eyes to shine with anticipation.

It is easy enough to remind patients that "Better still is a dry morsel and quietness therewith than a house full of feasting with strife." The problem for them is how to avoid the strife and worry and care. For many it is impossible. Doubtless all that can be done at times is to postpone the meal until strong emotion has passed, calm has been restored, fatigue has lessened, and hunger has returned. In other words, we should accept Macbeth's advice and let good digestion wait on appetite and health on both.[3]

COLITIS

Axel Munthe, in his "Story of San Michele,"[4] suggests that colitis was invented to serve as a respectable diagnosis when appendicitis began to wane in popularity because surgeons insisted upon operating. People wanted a diagnosis safe from the surgeon's knife and they were given colitis. Whether or not this was the origin of the diagnosis, functional colitis today is a very real

[3] Alvarez, Walter C., "Ways in Which Emotion Can Affect the Digestive Tract," *Journal of the American Medical Association*, vol. 92, p. 1231, April 13, 1929.

[4] Munthe, Axel, "The Story of San Michele," E. P. Dutton & Co., Inc., New York, 1930.

and distressing condition. In many cases it is the end result of attempts to correct by physical means a spastic, irritable bowel, tied up with a sensitive, overwrought nervous system. Bulky diets, cathartics, and enemas are the measures usually employed. What such persons need is a bland, nourishing diet and relaxation. To accomplish this, either a solution of, or an adjustment to, one's emotional problems is necessary.

THE PREVENTION OF NERVOUS INDIGESTION

Many persons tire themselves out by putting too much energy and emotion into trivial tasks. Women in particular must be exhorted to break themselves of the habit of getting all stirred up over little things and of reviewing at length painful or annoying experiences which a more sensible person would promptly forget. Others must be taught to go to bed earlier at night and some must, for a time, retire from leadership or active participation in church, civic or social work. Some can get their grip again if they will only rest in bed on Saturday afternoons and Sundays. Many take their holidays too strenuously; they drive too far in automobiles, they work too hard in their gardens, or they do things that leave them more tired on Monday morning than they were on Saturday night. They must learn the truth of Mosso's statement that all their energy comes from one source, and that when mentally tired it is not wise to exercise so strenuously as to still further take away from the small store of strength.[5]

Eating as an Art. The French are said to eat enthusiastically and the British apologetically; while Americans are famous for their atrocious eating habits.

The health of many people would be improved if they would make an art of eating. This art should include coming to meals with an even temperament and without undue fatigue. If one is tired a rest before dinner should be arranged. The meal should be appetizing, the surroundings attractive, and the dining room quiet. Eating should be slow: the best flavors of foods are lost unless they are thoroughly masticated. Thorough mastication also improves digestion and reduces the quantity of foods desired. Liquids should not be used to carry foods from the mouth to the stomach. The taking of water during meals when there is no food in the mouth is not harmful; ice water, however, particu-

[5] Alvarez, Walter C., "Treatment of Nervous Indigestion," *Journal of the American Medical Association*, vol. 89, p. 440, August 6, 1927.

larly on an empty stomach, diminishes the secretion of the digestive juices. Overeating should be avoided; it is a wise habit for adults to discontinue eating before the appetite is completely satisfied. Pleasant conversation, a leisurely attitude, a bowl of soup at the beginning of the meal would prevent many cases of indigestion. Actually the eating habits of most of us are abominable. We rush through our breakfasts and lunches without taking time to relax or to masticate our food. By dinnertime we are fatigued—so we stimulate ourselves by turning on the radio or going out to eat in some place so noisy that conversation is impossible. Here most of us overeat and make no effort to select food suited to the type of life which we lead.

Constipation

It is reported that the American people spend 50 million dollars a year for cathartics. Actually very few people need cathartics, and many more are harmed than are benefited by them.

Constipation is not a specific disease which can be prevented or cured by any single form of treatment. In fact, an exact definition of constipation is difficult; for a condition of the bowels which one person considers normal, another may interpret as evidence of constipation. There is not even agreement as to the optimum frequency of bowel movements. Some persons in good health regularly have two or three bowel movements per day, while others equally well have only one bowel movement in two or three days. The desire for defecation occurs when a sufficient volume of material from the intestinal tract has reached the rectum. The periodicity with which this occurs depends upon the activity of the musculature of the intestinal tract and upon the quantity of indigestible material in the diet. Most persons in good health have one bowel movement a day, but there is no inexorable rule of nature which makes this necessary. The attempt to regulate the bowels in accordance with one's ideas concerning the frequency with which they should act is the cause of much ill-health and invalidism. In general one's bowels will function best if they are let alone. Many persons who think they are constipated are not constipated at all and develop real difficulties only by their efforts to regulate artificially the activities of the intestinal tract.

CAUSES OF CONSTIPATION

The most frequent causes of constipation are overactivity of the musculature of the intestinal tract, underactivity of this musculature, and disease, usually of an inflammatory nature, within the abdomen. Intelligent treatment of constipation must be based upon the relief of the conditions which produce it; and with such a variety of causes it is obvious that no one method of treatment can be satisfactory. In some conditions a laxative is beneficial; but if the bowel is already overactive, the use of cathartics or irritant diets, although giving temporary relief, will eventually aggravate the condition. If constipation is due to appendicitis, cathartics are certain to increase the seriousness of the condition and may lead to rupture of the appendix.

So, with constipation possibly an illusion or, if it actually exists, only a symptom, the wisdom of obtaining a thorough examination to determine its cause before attempting treatment becomes apparent.

PREVENTING CONSTIPATION

The prevention of constipation should be based upon normal, wholesome management and not upon dietary fads. The following are some simple general rules to accomplish this:

1. Eat a normal, balanced diet. Bulk and roughage are provided by fruits and vegetables. Stewed fruits, particularly prunes, may well be used occasionally to obtain regularity of movement.

2. Make a regular habit of going to the toilet each morning, preferably just after breakfast. This is the time that regularity can be most easily established.

3. Develop the habit of nervous relaxation. Nervous tension, especially at mealtime, is likely to lead to an overactive, spastic intestine.

4. Drink reasonable but not excessive quantities of water. A glass of water after rising in the morning frequently aids in the establishment of regularity of defecation.

5. Take some regular exercise. Walking is frequently adequate, although if there is a tendency to constipation, bending and leg-raising exercises which strengthen the abdominal muscles are helpful. Strenuous exercise is undesirable.

"SPASTIC CONSTIPATION"

In the type of constipation due to an overactive, irritable, spastic bowel, the actual cause may be a rough, irritating diet, the habitual use of cathartics, or actual disease of the intestines, or it may be secondary to emotional or nervous tension or to disease in other parts of the body or abdomen. The usual symptoms which accompany this type of constipation are abdominal pain or tension, gaseous distention of the bowel with belching, tenderness over the colon, and small, mushy, or ball-like stools. In the more advanced and severe cases headaches, fatigue, nervousness, nausea, and vomiting may be present. Effective treatment of this condition requires careful medical supervision and wholehearted cooperation on the part of the patient, and such treatment should be begun before the disease has become chronic. Experimentation with self-medication will only make matters worse and the condition more difficult to correct.

The careful following of a proper regime of treatment usually gives satisfactory results, although improvement may be slow. It is too much to expect that the "bad habits" of years will be corrected in a few days or even a few weeks. Some of the more obstinate cases require a short period of "education" in the hospital in order to get results.

SIMPLE CONSTIPATION

When constipation is due to a sluggishness of the musculature of the intestinal tract, stimulation of the colon is necessary. Cathartics accomplish this by increasing the fluid content of the intestines. A better way is to increase the bulk of indigestible material in the diet. This means more leafy and fibrous vegetables, fruits raw and cooked, and whole-grain cereals. Bran, in the form of cereal, bread, biscuits, or crackers, is useful in some cases but highly irritating in others. In obstinate cases of this type of constipation the diet may be supplemented with agar-agar, or psyllium seed.

Agar-agar (Japanese seaweed) when moist provides a nonirritating indigestible material which gives bulk to the diet. A dessertspoonful with each meal is usually adequate. The granulated form of agar is just as satisfactory as the various commercial preparations and less expensive.

Psyllium seeds, when moist, provide both bulk and lubrication. Two teaspoonfuls at each meal, mixed with any convenient food, are recommended in mild cases.

In the past, mineral oil, or liquid petrolatum, was extensively used to soften the intestinal contents. Recent studies, however, have shown that mineral oil prevents the absorption of vitamin A and may have other deleterious effects. Its use, therefore, is no longer advised.

Acidophilous milk and milk sugar are useful in certain cases to correct constipation and to overcome intestinal putrefaction. Yeast, too, may be helpful in the correction of this type of constipation. The yeast cells cause fermentation of certain foods in the intestinal tract, thereby inducing increased intestinal activity. On the other hand, if fermentation is already occurring, yeast may aggravate the condition.

THE CATHARTIC HABIT

This consideration of constipation would not be complete without reemphasis of the fact that much of the constipation which people attempt to correct is either nonexistent or unimportant and that the attention which is given to it and many of the measures adopted for its relief are much more likely to aggravate the condition than to improve it.

The cathartic habit, developed by many persons in an effort to practice what advertisers call "intestinal hygiene" or "internal cleanliness," is pernicious. Cathartics produce very definite results, and patients who take them are likely to assume that the alleged benefits will follow. If they do not, more of the same treatment is usually resorted to until finally a habit has been established. Even the taking of enemas can become just as truly

[161]

a habit as the taking of drugs. Under certain conditions the temporary use of cathartics is beneficial, but their habitual use is almost certain to result in chronic ill-health.

HALITOSIS

Malodorous breath has been christened "halitosis" by an advertising agency interested in promoting the sale of a mouthwash. Its basis is the Latin word *halitus*, meaning breath or vapor.

Advertisers have educated the public to attribute this unpleasant condition to decayed teeth, to diseases of the mouth, nose, throat, or sinuses, or to the fermentation or putrefaction of food particles between or around the teeth. Any of these conditions may give unpleasant odors to the breath. Recent scientific studies of this condition lead to the conclusion that

. . . essential halitosis is the excretion on the breath of malodorous fats, fatty acids or volatile substances resultant from some fault in the digestion or metabolism of fat. The noxious volatile matter is absorbed from the intestinal tract, is partly excreted in the bile, but in the main is picked up by the circulating blood, which in transversing the lungs parts with the substance which is exhaled on the breath.

Patients suffering from true halitosis are amenable to the therapeutic test of a low fat diet. If a reducing diet, low in fats (40 to 60 Gm. a day), is administered, a prompt disappearance of the halitotic odor occurs.

Mouth washes containing pleasantly odorous materials serve to hide or mask true halitosis as a temporary measure but fail completely to meet the problem, since the source of the fetor is in the intestine and the metabolism.[6]

DISCUSSION SUGGESTIONS

1. Explain the terms dyspepsia and indigestion. Is it safe to treat these conditions with commercially advertised medications which give relief in some cases? Why?
2. What are the early symptoms of cancer of the stomach?
3. Why are the symptoms of gastric ulcer frequently relieved by mild alkalies or by bland diet?
4. Should the diet regularly contain large amounts of bran or other roughage? Why?
5. Explain the relation of the emotions to digestion.

[6] Crohn, Burrill B., and Rudoph Drosd, "Halitosis," *Journal of the American Medical Association*, vol. 117, p. 2244, December 27, 1941.

6. What is meant by autointoxication? Is it proper to treat this condition with "intestinal antiseptics"? Why?
7. Explain what is meant by colitis and the proper means of dealing with the condition.
8. Discuss the statement that most deaths from appendicitis are unnecessary.
9. Discuss the possible influence of eating habits upon health.
10. What are some of the common misconceptions concerning constipation?
11. Outline methods for the prevention and the treatment of constipation.
12. Discuss the cathartic habit.

REFERENCES AND READING SUGGESTIONS

1. Aaron, Harold: "Our Common Ailment—Constipation: Its Cause and Cure," Dodge Publishing Company, New York, 1938.
2. Alvarez, W. C.: "Nervous Indigestion," Paul B. Hoeber, Inc., Medical Department of Harper & Brothers, New York, 1931.
3. ———: "How to Live with Your Ulcer," Wilcox & Follett Co., Chicago, 1951.
4. Cannon, W. B.: "Digestion and Health," George J. McLeod, Ltd., Toronto, 1936.
5. Montague, J. F.: "I Know Just the Thing for That," The John Day Company, Inc., New York, 1934.
6. Wolberg, L. B.: "The Psychology of Eating," Robert M. McBride & Company, New York, 1936.

Chapter VIII

DIETARY DANGERS

DIETARY dangers may result from errors of omission or commission. The hermit in his isolation develops scurvy or pellagra because he lacks fresh vegetables; the infant acquires rickets because parents have been ignorant or negligent about providing cod-liver oil or vitamin D in some other form; the dietary faddist lacks vitality and resistance because of a deficiency of proteins or minerals. On the other hand, the glutton eats his way to the grave; and the cook, the butcher, or the baker may countenance insanitary conditions which lead to contamination of the best of foods.

A knowledge of what goes on behind the scenes in many establishments which are engaged in the production, preparation, and sale of food would cause us to reject many of the foods which we purchase. It is impossible to be certain that all of our foods are safe; but it is not difficult to avoid most of the hazards involved in eating and drinking.

Dietary Fads and Fallacies

The food faddist, with his missionary spirit and his pet prescription of health, is always with us. Each one has a different prescription from that of his predecessors but is just as zealous in his efforts to convert mankind to it. Some of these fads are dispensed in a spirit of charity. Others are well paid for by those seekers after health who have more money than good sense. Of the many types of dietary fads the following are most common:

Vegetarianism. The disciples of this fad usually follow it either because they consider animal foods deleterious to health or because they object to the destruction of animals to supply food for man. This latter reason is purely sentimental; but the former merits consideration.

Professor E. V. McCollum, leading authority on nutrition, has written that "a vegetarian diet, supplemented by fairly liberal amounts of milk, is the most satisfactory type of diet that man can take." But this is not true vegetarianism. In fact, milk, butter, eggs, cheese, and other dairy and animal products are rarely left out of the diets of vegetarians. Hence, most "vegetarians" are not really vegetarians but only abstainers from meat.

Most health fads are based upon a certain amount of truth and in this regard vegetarianism is above the average. We have pointed out that fruits and vegetables are the best source of most of the vitamins and minerals, and that the legumes and the cereal grains are the cheapest energy foods. On the other hand, the body must have a certain amount of protein. This probably could be obtained, as is done by herbivorous animals, from the plant kingdom, but large quantities of food would have to be consumed and even then there would be danger of deficiency. Furthermore, the human digestive tract is not adapted for an exclusively herbivorous diet. For man, animal foods, such as meat, eggs, milk, and dairy products, improve the palatability of the diet and provide the proteins which are most completely and easily utilized by the body.

The Water Fad. This is usually followed on the theory that one should practice "internal bathing" just as one bathes one's hands and face. For this there is no scientific basis whatever. A glass or two of water the first thing in the morning may aid in the maintenance of regular bowel movements. Hot or cool water before breakfast seems to be beneficial to some persons but produces distress in others.

Raw Foods Fad. The advocates of eating foods raw almost exclusively can find some justification in the fact that cooking may reduce the vitamin and mineral content of certain foods. On the other hand, cooking not only improves the flavors of many foods but also makes them more easily digested. Thorough cooking is also an important factor of protection against diseases which are transmitted by foods. Raw foods are exposed to many possibilities of contamination and may carry the causative organisms of such diseases as typhoid fever, amebic dysentery, and hookworm. Meat should always be cooked and fruits and vegetables thoroughly washed before use.

Alkaline Foods. Advertisers of foods and drugs have acquainted the American public with the term "acidosis." They are not specific as to what they mean by it but they assure us that it is a menace to health and that we should guard against it by eating foods or taking drugs which will alkalize the body. Citrous fruits—oranges, lemons, grapefruit—are particularly recommended for the prevention of colds and influenza. Actually there is no evidence that acidosis is related to these conditions, nor that acidosis ever occurs except in certain definite disease conditions.

The Mixing of Foods. It is asserted, too, that the mixing of certain types of foods is deleterious; that acid and alkaline foods, or that proteins and carbohydrates, should not be eaten at the same meal. The alkaline-acid bugaboo should disappear with an understanding that upon oxidation most fruits and vegetables yield both acid and alkaline residue. Nature has combined these foods, so it seems unreasonable for us to attempt to separate them artificially in the diet. In an average, balanced diet the acid- and alkali-producing foods are so well balanced that no thought needs to be given to them.

Dieting. For the obese individual, dieting is a valuable health measure, but dieting by young women of normal weight is neither healthful nor beautiful. Extreme underweight in young persons apparently predisposes to tuberculosis, and the ill-balanced diets frequently adopted are likely to be lacking in essential foods. In their efforts to remain thin many persons form the habit of going without breakfast. This is undesirable; for the body needs food to support the day's activity and it is better to supply this in moderate quantities than it is to overload the stomach once or twice a day and starve it the rest of the time. In many countries it is the custom to eat even more than three meals a day.

Ptomaine Poisoning*

Severe disturbances of the digestive tract accompanied by nausea, vomiting, and diarrhea are usually labeled ptomaine poisoning. The word "ptomaine" implies that there has been decay of protein foods with the formation of poisonous substance. Theoretically this could occur but actually it rarely if ever does. Hence, the term "ptomaine poisoning" is really a misnomer.

The disturbances which go by this name belong to one of several groups: first, they may be due to poisonous substances in the food; second, they may be caused by disease-producing germs consumed with the food; and, third, they may be due to an individual peculiarity or sensitivity which causes an abnormal reaction to certain foods which in themselves are perfectly wholesome.

True Food Poisoning*

In the class of true food poisoning belong mushroom poisoning, milk sickness, shellfish poisoning, botulism, and the occasional poisoning caused by decomposed food.

Mushroom Poisoning. Although very few varieties of mushrooms contain deadly poison, these are responsible for a considerable number of deaths in the United States each year. Unfortunately for the amateur, there is no rule-of-thumb test by which the deadly ones can be identified. The "silver spoon test," the belief that poisonous mushrooms do not grow on wood, and various generalizations concerning appearance are all unreliable. In fact, one of the most deadly mushrooms, the *Amanita phalloides*, is pure white in color and unusually innocent and delectable looking. One way to be safe in the eating of mushrooms is to use only those which have been raised commercially or which can be positively identified. The collection of mushrooms is an interesting study but the tasting of them a hazardous avocation.

Shellfish Poisoning. Within recent years on the west coast a considerable number of persons have been made ill and some

* See also Appendix D.

[167]

deaths have occurred from eating shellfish, particularly mussels and clams. The poisoning seems to be due to certain forms of microscopic aquatic life which these shellfish at times take as food. In the shellfish the poison is most concentrated in the liver. Even the broth made from such shellfish may be poisonous. To avoid this hazard one should forego the use of shellfish gathered from certain areas during the summer months.

Botulism is caused by a deadly poison (toxin) which is secreted by the botulinus germ as it grows in certain foods. The name "botulus" means sausage, to which the first recognized cases of this disease were traced. Since that time botulism has been traced to various animal and vegetable foods. In chickens, turkeys, and ducks it produces a disease known as "limberneck."

The botulinus germ multiplies only in the absence of air, but as it grows it liberates a powerful poison. This is taken into the body with the food, absorbed from the intestinal tract, and carried by the blood to the central nervous system, where it produces paralysis. Nausea and vomiting, the usual symptoms of food poisoning, do not occur because the botulinus toxin causes little or no disturbance of the intestinal tract. Upon the central nervous system, however, it is one of the most potent toxins known, 1/25,000,000 ounce being enough to kill a guinea pig of average size. Dickson reports that a patient died after "nibbling" a portion of a pod of spoiled string bean; that another died after tasting a small spoonful of spoiled corn; and that a third was ill after tasting a pod of a bean which she did not swallow. The botulinus spores resist boiling, but the toxin is destroyed by heating to 175 degrees Fahrenheit for a few minutes. Consequently, botulinus poisoning usually follows the eating of canned foods which are not cooked before serving.

Outbreaks of botulism have been traced to fish, ham, sausage, beef, turkey, chicken, cottage cheese, string beans, corn, berries, peas, spinach, and ripe olives. In Soviet Russia botulism has been caused chiefly by smoked, dried, or salt fish which is used as a food without cooking. A vegetable salad served as a midnight lunch on a farm in North Dakota was responsible for thirteen fatal cases of botulism. A total of sixteen persons partook of a salad consisting of carrots, peas, and cut string beans. Three of the group had been drinking "moonshine" and vomited during or just after the lunch. All the others became ill and died. In this instance, as in numerous others, home-canned string beans were responsible.

Over 400 outbreaks of botulism have been reported in the United States in the past 50 years. These outbreaks have resulted in more than 1,000 cases and over 700 deaths.

Commercially canned foods, because of the greater heat used in the canning process, are much less likely to be a menace than home-canned foods. In fact, for more than ten years no reported outbreaks of botulism have been traced to commercially preserved foods.

The botulinus bacillus is widespread in the soil, particularly of the West and Middle West. It is destroyed or its growth prevented by sufficient heat, acid mediums, and 10 per cent salt brine. In order to guard against the hazard of this poisoning, nonacid foods, such as string beans and corn, should be processed in a pressure cooker with an accurate gauge or thermometer. Such foods that are processed in any other manner must be reboiled for at least 15 minutes before tasting or using. All jars or other containers of canned foods should be discarded when there is any bulging, leaking, abnormal odors, or other sign of spoilage. The spoilage may be so slight as to be undetectable. Hence, continued outbreaks of botulism may be anticipated until there is an end to the serving of home-canned vegetables as salads. Thorough heating is the greatest safeguard against botulism.

Insecticide Danger. The widespread spraying of fruit trees and vegetables with insecticides containing arsenic and lead or DDT has introduced a new hazard in connection with certain foods. An outbreak of "food poisoning" in California a few years ago was traced to the eating of broccoli which had been sprayed with arsenic.

Analyses of cabbage procured from a public market in the southeastern part of the United States showed an arsenic content of from 0.02 to 0.45 grain and of lead from 0.09 to 1.24 grains per pound. From 1 to 2 grains of arsenic may be toxic or even fatal to an adult. It is thus evident that a pound of these particular cabbages contained from one-fourth to one-half of a toxic or fatal dose of this element alone. In addition, the amounts of lead present were by no means small. Similar degrees of contamination were found in certain other foods, such as fresh apples, apple pomace, and cauliflower.

. . . Ingested lead accumulates in the viscera and particularly in the bones and is gradually and continuously released. The continued presence and circulation of small amounts of lead throughout the organism may eventually impair health. The onset of symptoms, such as loss of appetite, malaise, loss of body weight, weakness, fatigue on exertion, anemia, gastrointestinal disturbances, pains in the joints and later paralysis, may be so insidious that chronic poisoning by lead-contaminated foods is not at first suspected.

. . . Some assume that the spray residue is washed away by rains or is blown away by winds, but the evidence available at the present time indicates that this is not the case. Most of the lead arsenate is gradually taken up by the vegetation grown on that soil.

. . . The producer should be compelled to remove spray residues as completely as possible, preferably by the hydrochloric acid rinse procedure, from the surface of apples and other deciduous fruits intended for interstate commerce. He should not use the skins of sprayed fruits in the preparation of cider, vinegar, jelly, stock feed or other products. He should never use lead arsenate or other arsenical sprays on vegetables, such as cabbage, cauliflower, Brussels sprouts, broccoli, spinach, kale, celery and beans, which are consumed in their entirety. As an added precaution, the consumer should always wash thoroughly before using all fruits and vegetables that may have been exposed to metallic sprays. These measures are at best only palliative, and the only satisfactory permanent solution of the problem is the absolute elimination of dangerous substances as sprays. This, of course, would necessitate the perfection of other insecticides, harmless to man and to domestic animals. According to Hanzlik, "This is actually being done experimentally, and it is not too much to hope that practical success will soon be achieved."[1]

Just how extensive or serious this danger is there is no way of knowing. Some manufacturers of infant foods are refusing to accept fruits or vegetables which contain DDT or other insecticides that cannot be removed in processing. Certainly, it is reasonable to take the precaution of thoroughly washing vegetables and of discarding the skins and cores of fruits which have been sprayed. Some states require that all such fruits be washed in an acid solution before being marketed.

[1] Editorial, "Hazards of Contaminated Fruits and Vegetables," *Journal of the American Medical Association*, vol. 109, p. 135, July 10, 1937.

Decomposed Foods. Poisoning from foods in which partial decomposition or decay has occurred is rare in adults but more frequent in infants. Many foods such as buttermilk, cheese, sauerkraut, and vinegar are products of partial decomposition by bacteria, molds, or yeast. When this decomposition affects carbohydrates we call it "fermentation," when it affects proteins, "putrefaction." It is particularly in the bacterial decomposition of proteins that substances which are toxic or irritant to the intestinal tract may be formed. Such changes are most likely to occur in foods not adequately refrigerated[2] during the summer months. These products are of low toxicity and in adults rarely cause symptoms. In infants, however, they may produce severe and serious nausea, vomiting, and diarrhea.

Practically all protein foods are susceptible to such decomposition, but milk and milk products are particularly likely to be involved. The reasons for this are that milk is an ideal medium for the growth of bacteria, that it contains proteins which easily decompose, and that it is used in relatively large quantities in the diets of infants. Pasteurization will destroy disease-producing bacteria that may be in the milk, but it does not kill all the putrefactive bacteria, nor does it have any effect upon the products of their growth which are already in the milk. The receipt of a bottle of ice-cold milk gives one a great sense of security, and justifiably so; but if it were possible to see beyond the pasteurization plant to the insanitary conditions on the farms where some milk is produced, to the manner in which it is handled and transported to market, one might hesitate before using it, particularly for infants. In its raw state such milk is a danger to anyone. Pasteurized, it is safe for adults and relatively safe for children. Infants, however, should have milk which first is just as clean and sanitary as it is possible to make it, then properly pasteurized, refrigerated at all times, and finally boiled before use.

Milk sickness is the common name of an interesting, although at present rare, disease. In the early days many pioneer settlements, particularly in the South and West, suffered severely

[2] Adequate refrigeration means a temperature of 45 degrees or less at all times. A thermometer should be used to determine refrigerator temperatures.

from it and some are said to have been abandoned because of it. Lincoln's mother, Nancy Hanks, died of this disease. Milk sickness in man is always associated with a similar disease, called "trembles," in domestic animals. The human disease is caused by the use of milk from cows which have fed on certain poisonous plants, especially white snakeroot and the rayless goldenrod. As virgin pasture lands have been brought under cultivation, the disease has rapidly declined.

Food Infections*

Most of the cases of so-called "ptomaine poisoning" or "food poisoning" are really food infections; that is, the symptoms are due not to poisoning but to actual infections of the intestinal tract by germs which enter the body with food or drink. Most of these infections are accompanied by nausea, vomiting, diarrhea, and a little fever. In adults they may cause more or less incapacity for several days but are rarely serious. In children, particularly very young children, these are major infections.

This disease, frequently called "summer complaint" of children, although greatly reduced in recent years, remains a prominent cause of death in children under ten. Food and drink are responsible for most of these infections. Hence, adequate care in the selection and preparation of foods and better sanitation in their handling are all that is necessary to eliminate them. If parents will only make use of available information concerning the preparation and care of infant foods, many children's lives can be saved (see diarrhea and enteritis, Tables 3 and 4).

In adults meat is the food most commonly responsible for these infections, and germs belonging to the so-called "salmonella" group are the usual causative organisms. These germs are related to paratyphoid bacilli but are less virulent. Meat and meat products may contain these germs either because they came from infected animals or because they became contaminated in the slaughterhouse. Flies, cats, dogs, mice, rats, and human carriers may serve as sources of such contamination.

The germs from human sources most commonly involved in food

* See also Appendix D.

[172]

infections are staphylococci or streptococci. They may get into the food from hands or from droplets from the nose and mouth.

As a rule food infections occur only when enormous quantities of the germs are consumed. Thorough cooking and boiling destroys them. Consequently, the foods most likely to cause trouble are those in which the germs have had a chance to multiply and which have not been thoroughly cooked just before serving. Hashes, meat salads, custards, and dairy products which have been handled or prepared some hours before use are the types of foods most frequently involved. Hence, it is wise to avoid such foods unless one knows under what conditions of sanitation and refrigeration they have been kept. Foods which have been thoroughly cooked just before serving are the wisest choice in restaurants and hotels. In the home careful selection and handling of foods, adequate refrigeration, and thorough cooking are the best safeguard against food infections.

An outbreak of food poisoning in a large general hospital is a typical example of this type of infection. In this case, 22 per cent of the 390 patients and over 50 per cent of the 610 personnel were affected. The outbreak was confined to those who ate chicken salad. The causative agent was probably introduced by human hands subsequent to the cooking, which had been done the day before serving.[3]

The more serious infections contracted through food and drink include typhoid fever, dysentery, streptococcic infections, and various parasitic diseases, such as trichina and tapeworm infestation. Typhoid and paratyphoid fever in the United States today are disseminated largely by carriers of these germs engaged in the preparation of food. Of 21 cases of typhoid fever recently reported in Los Angeles, 11 were traced to carriers and 10 of these 11 carriers were grandmothers. Milk and milk products are most frequently involved in the spread of these diseases because, if the germs get into milk, they multiply rapidly whenever the milk gets warm. Pasteurization destroys

[3] Lumsden, L. L., C. A. Nau, and F. M. Stead, "A Study of An Outbreak of Food Poisoning in a Hospital in Galveston, Texas," *Public Health Reports*, vol. 58, p. 1497, October 8, 1943.

these germs, so there is no danger of infection from milk that has been properly pasteurized and safeguarded from contamination after pasteurization. Only bottled milk should be used for purposes other than cooking. Other foods which may disseminate these diseases are the same as those responsible for the less severe food infections; that is, foods which favor bacterial growth, tend to be exposed to infection through handling, and are served cold or without thorough cooking. Avoidance of such foods at public eating places will reduce the danger of contracting these diseases.

A serious epidemic recently reported was caused by the streptococcus. It was spread by ham which had been cooked and handled by a woman who was in the pre-eruptive stage of scarlet fever. The result was 24 cases of scarlet fever, 56 cases of septic sore throat, and 22 patients with other symptoms such as diarrhea, vomiting, etc.

Dysentery is a common and serious disease in wartime among both military and civilian populations. It causes prostration with fever, vomiting, and severe and frequently bloody diarrhea. There are two types of dysentery, bacillary and amebic (pages 658 to 660). Either may be contracted by drinking contaminated water, by eating infected foods, or by contact with persons harboring the dysentery organisms.

Although hookworm commonly enters the body through the skin of the feet of persons who walk barefoot upon infected soil, it may be contracted from food. Fresh, uncooked vegetables, such as lettuce, radishes, and celery, which have been grown in contaminated soil are particularly dangerous.

Animal foods are the source of several parasitic infestations of man. Beef may transmit the beef tapeworm; pork, the pork tapeworm and trichina; and fish, the fish tapeworm. Meat inspection gives some protection against the beef and pork tapeworm, but fish and most of the meat which is slaughtered and used locally are not inspected. Furthermore, the inspection of meat does not include an examination for trichina. Concerning this the U.S. Bureau of Animal Industry issued the following warning:

[174]

No method of meat inspection has yet been devised by which the presence or absence of trichina in pork can be determined with certainty, and the government meat inspection does not include inspection for this parasite. All persons are accordingly warned not to eat pork or sausage containing pork, whether it has been officially inspected or not, until after it has been properly cooked. Pork when properly cooked may be eaten without danger of infection. Fresh pork should be cooked until it becomes white and is no longer red in color in all portions of the meat, at the center as well as near the surface. Dry, salt pork, pickled pork, and smoked pork previously salted or pickled, providing the curing is thorough, are practically safe as far as trichinosis is concerned, but as the thoroughness of the curing is not always certain, meat should always be cooked before it is eaten.

At a recent National Conference on Trichinosis it was reported that reliable evidence, based on autopsy findings, indicates that some 25,000,000 persons in the United States are infested with trichinae. Most of these infestations are symptomless, but it is estimated that some 16,000 of about 350,000 who acquire new infestations each year ingest enough of parasites to produce illness.

Public health measures for the prevention of this disease depend upon the cooking of all garbage that is fed to hogs and upon refrigeration at below freezing temperatures of all pork and pork products from garbage-fed hogs. Within the home or in public eating establishments additional protection can be assured by thorough cooking of all pork and pork products before eating (see also page 755).

The cysts of the tapeworm which occur in beef, fish, and pork are likewise readily destroyed by heat. Smoking and drying will not destroy these parasites. In certain sections of Europe, where raw fish is considered a delicacy, the fish tapeworm is very prevalent. In this country cases have developed as a result of eating or tasting uncooked or partially cooked fish. Beef or pork is rarely eaten raw, but "rare" beef may contain living parasites. The avoidance of uncooked or inadequately cooked fish and meat is insurance against these infections.

Milk—A Potentially Dangerous Food

Of all foods in the dietary of man milk is the most nearly perfect. Unfortunately, however, milk is an ideal food not only for man but for many of his microscopic enemies as well. It is difficult to obtain, transport, and deliver in a sanitary condition and is the only animal food extensively used by man in a raw state. Disease-producing germs may get into milk either from a diseased animal or from human beings who have contact with the milk.

The diseases of animal origin which one may get through milk are tuberculosis, undulant (Malta) fever (also called brucellosis), foot-and-mouth disease, and intestinal ailments resulting in diarrheal conditions, especially in children. In addition milk may be contaminated with disease-producing germs by persons who handle milk or milk products. A few germs accidentally introduced into the milk at the time of milking may develop into many millions by the time the milk is consumed. The diseases of human origin most commonly spread by milk are typhoid fever, septic sore throat, scarlet fever, and diphtheria. In the twenty years from 1908 to 1927, 429 milk-borne outbreaks of typhoid fever with a total of approximately 15,000 cases were reported in the United States.

Epidemics of scarlet fever traceable to raw milk are reported every year. One that occurred in Oswego, New York, involved 300 cases of scarlet fever and was traced to raw milk from a single cow. Fortunately the disease-producing germs found in milk are easily killed by heating the milk to a temperature which does not change its value as a food. This process of heating, called "pasteurization," is the health measure which makes it possible to produce and distribute milk on a large scale and still have it a safe food.

The usual method of pasteurization is to hold the milk at a temperature of 142 to 145 degrees Fahrenheit for at least 30 minutes and then cool it rapidly. Another approved method is to heat it to 160 degrees Fahrenheit for 15 seconds.

Important as pasteurization is, it is not all that is desirable in a milk supply. In addition milk should come from healthy cows, be collected in a clean, sanitary manner, kept in sterile containers at low temperatures, and transported as rapidly as possible to the pasteurization plant. Clean, high-grade, pasteurized milk from healthy cows is an objective toward which every community should work. Of all these safeguards, however, pasteurization is much the most important. At the present time approximately 90 per cent of the milk used in American cities of 10,000 population and over is pasteurized, but all too many smaller communities are still exposed to the hazard of raw milk. Milk products, such as butter, cream, and cheese, also should be pasteurized because they, too, may transmit disease.

Raw Milk

Raw milk is claimed by some of its advocates to have greater nutritional value than pasteurized milk. There is, however, no real evidence that pasteurized milk is inferior to raw milk as a food, even for infants. A study by the U.S. Public Health Service compares the rates of growth and the illnesses of 1,875 children who received heated milk with the growth and illnesses of 1,762 children who were fed predominantly on raw milk.[4] Both groups received in addition to the milk the average American child's diet. The conclusions of this study are that children who are fed pasteurized milk or other heated milk thrive as well as children who are fed raw milk and contract certain communicable diseases less frequently.

Pasteurization decreases somewhat the vitamin C content of milk, but since milk is not a dependable source of vitamin C this is of no importance. A milk diet should always be supplemented with orange juice or some other good source of vitamin C.

The individual's part in safeguarding himself and his family against the hazards connected with nature's best food is to use only milk products which are properly pasteurized and to demand milk which is clean and wholesome even before pasteurization. For infants the very best quality of milk, preferably certified, should be obtained and then boiled.

Care of Milk in the Home

If pasteurized milk cannot be obtained, the milk used in the home should be subjected to heat treatment which will destroy

[4] Frank, L. C., F. A. Clark, W. H. Haskell, M. M. Miller, F. J. Moss, and R. C. Thomas, "Do Children Who Drink Raw Milk Thrive Better Than Children Who Drink Heated Milk?" *U.S. Public Health Reports*, vol. 49, p. 1951, September 23, 1932.

any disease-producing organisms that may be present in the milk.

Directions for Home Pasteurization of Milk

Small pasteurization equipment is now available for home use. These pasteurizers are of the 30-minute holding type and many are equipped with an automatic timing device which relieves the housewife of the necessity of constantly watching the milk during the pasteurization process.

For home pasteurization of milk without special equipment the U.S. Department of Agriculture gives the following instructions:

Fill the lower part of a double boiler with enough water to reach the bottom of the top part of the boiler. Bring water to a vigorous boil. Pour milk in top part of boiler. Place cover over double boiler and heat until the milk reaches 165° F. With experience one can estimate the time needed and use a thermometer only for final temperature check. When milk reaches 165° F place the top part of the double boiler containing the milk immediately in a dishpan of cold water and cool to 60° F or less.

For more rapid modification of this method place the milk in a sauce pan or kettle of suitable size for the quantity of milk desired. Put pan containing the milk over direct heat, stirring continuously with a metal spoon to prevent formation of undesirable scum. Keep an accurate dairy thermometer in the milk and watch the temperature carefully. As soon as the milk reaches 165° F place the pan of milk in a larger pan of cold water, stirring occasionally as milk cools. When the temperature drops to under 150° F cover and stir less often. Cool to 60° F or less.

Other practical suggestions for the care of milk and cream in the home, made by the Minnesota Department of Health, are as follows:

Milk may become unfit for human food, especially for babies, by improper care in the home. Improper care usually consists of failing to keep the milk cold, in allowing it to freeze, in failing to clean the top of the bottle, in pouring it into unclean or unsterilized utensils, and in exposing it unnecessarily in uncovered dishes to dust, flies, and odors. Milk cannot be properly kept without ice or mechanical refrigeration except in cold weather.

The milk should be kept in the original bottle and not poured into a pail or pitcher for storage. It should not be poured back into the bottle after it has been exposed in another vessel. Keep the milk bottle covered with the cap or with a clean, inverted tumbler.

Sanitary Food Handling

Health departments the country over are making rapid strides in safeguarding the basic sources of food and drink from contamination with the germs of communicable diseases. But several important questions can still be asked concerning the delivery of these to the ultimate consumer; namely, are the food handlers themselves free of communicable diseases, are they cleanly in their personal habits, are the methods which they employ in the serving of foods sanitary?

A few cities require that all food handlers who are working in public eating places be given physical examinations before employment. Theoretically, this would seem to offer the public a considerable degree of protection, particularly since we know that some individuals are chronic carriers of the germs of such diseases as typhoid fever, dysentery, and diphtheria. Actually, however, the number of these carriers is so few and an adequate examination for the detection of carriers so expensive and so impractical to administer that food-handler examinations are rarely considered feasible as a general public health measure.

In spite of this, individual families employing domestic servants to handle foods, live in the home, and be closely associated with members of the family, would do well to insist upon physical examinations before employment to insure freedom from active tuberculosis if for no other reason. A few years ago a Vienna physician wrote feelingly on this subject because three of his four children became ill with tuberculosis and one died as the result of infection from a nursemaid who had been with the family for many years and had had a mild cough which she and the family had considered as caused by "chronic bronchitis."

More important and more practical as a general health measure than the physical examination of food handlers is the insistence on personal cleanliness, which means, primarily, frequent and thorough washings of the hands and adequate medical supervision of acute illnesses among employees. A cook could well be a typhoid carrier all of her life without ever infecting anyone if she always washed her hands thoroughly after use of the

[179]

toilet and before handling foods. On the other hand, a person who had had a physical examination last week might develop a mild diphtheritic sore throat this week and, if she continued on the job, might spread the infection to others. The employees of food-handling establishments should not continue on the job when they are ill and should be certified as noninfected by a physician before returning to work.

Eating utensils which are inadequately sterilized before use also may serve as the means of transmission of infection. During the influenza epidemic of 1918, an epidemiologic study of some 66,000 troops showed that there was an influenza rate of 51 per thousand troops among those whose mess kits were mechanically washed and sterilized, as compared to a rate of 252 per thousand among troops who washed their own mess gear in common tubs of warm water. Another study of influenza among 252,000 inmates of public institutions showed an attack rate of one-third as great in those institutions which used machine washing of dishes as in the institutions which employed hand washing.

Many public eating establishments neither thoroughly clean nor sterilize cups, glasses, and silverware after they have been used. Drinking glasses in saloons and roadhouses repeatedly have been found to contain tens of thousands or even hundreds of thousands of germs per glass, many of them capable of producing disease. The soda clerk in the drugstore rarely washes glasses and frequently dips them in filthy water which is veritably alive with bacteria. One investigator reported that the rinse water used for glasses had a bacterial count slightly in excess of that usually found in sewage. Common drinking cups have long since been outlawed but in many establishments which serve food and drink they are still with us in actuality. Public health ordinances which require reasonable sanitary precautions in the handling of food and drink should be insisted upon—and then enforced. In Wheeling, West Virginia, the Health Department publishes in the newspapers laboratory reports of the number of bacteria found upon drinking glasses, forks, and spoons in the various eating establishments of the city. The New York City Department of Health recently held up the permit renewals of 286 restaurants until they installed satisfactory facilities for washing utensils in hot water. Adequate facilities for the employees to wash their hands and insistence that they be utilized are required by some health departments. A similar requirement should be set up and enforced in every community.

The Health Department of Washington, D.C., has set up regulations concerning the washing of eating and drinking utensils used in restaurants and hotels and gives the following advice to the general public:

DISINFECTION FOR THE FAMILY EATING UTENSILS

Use not only as an emergency measure when there is sickness in the family or during an epidemic, but regularly for the continuous (day to day) prevention of disease distribution through eating utensils.

GENERAL INSTRUCTIONS

A. Remove adhering food particles, especially grease, from used dishes.

B. Wash glasses first, next silverware, then dishes, and finally pots and pans. Place on draining rack and air dry.

C. The following methods are for the average family of four, allowing about 10 utensils per person. For a larger family renew the solution or use a proportionately larger quantity. Use either of the following suggested methods:

Combined Cleanser and Chlorine Solution. To 1½ gallons of hot water add washing soda or other *inorganic* washing powder or cleanser (not common soap as that destroys the germicidal properties of the chlorine disinfectant). Then add the chlorine powder to make a 220 p.p.m. (parts per million) solution as directed on the container.

Separate Cleanser and Chlorine Solution. By this method use an oblong dish pan divided in the center by a partition into two compartments. In one wash with a hot inorganic cleanser solution and in the other disinfect by immersion of the utensils for three to five minutes in a hot chlorine solution made so as to have 100 p.p.m.

NOTE: Chlorine disinfectant powder is sold at drug stores and by hotel and dairy supply houses under various trade names.

DIRECTIONS FOR MAKING A STOCK SOLUTION OF CHLORINE (SODIUM HYPOCHLORITE)

1. Place one pound of chlorinated lime (bleaching powder) and one pound of sodium carbonate (washing soda) in a large bottle.

2. Add one gallon of water and shake vigorously. Let stand for 24 hours.

3. Syphon or pour off clear liquid (stock solution) into a clean bottle and keep tightly corked.

[181]

4. To make a disinfectant solution of 200 parts per million of available chlorine use in the proportion of one ounce of this stock solution to one gallon of water.[5]

Food Sensitivity

"One man's food is another man's poison" is one way of saying that some persons develop peculiar reactions to foods which for others are perfectly wholesome. Such reactions are called "food idiosyncrasies," "sensitivities," or "allergies." A variety of symptoms may result from these conditions but most common among these are hives, certain eczemas, transient swellings of various parts of the body, "sick headaches" (migraine), dyspepsia, nausea, vomiting, diarrhea, bronchial asthma, and nasal congestion and discharge. These symptoms, of course, may be due to other causes as well as to allergy.

Allergic reactions are very selective, so much so that a person may react to one of the proteins of milk or eggs and not to others. Still, symptoms of hypersensitiveness frequently are precipitated or aggravated by nonspecific physical, chemical, or mechanical irritants or physiological disturbances. For example, persons with indigestion as a result of food sensitivity usually are worse after cathartics, roughage, or other irritating substances in the diet, and a nose which is stuffy because of spinach, eggs, or chocolate in the diet or feathers in the pillow or a dog or cat about the house may be kept in a condition of chronic irritation by smoke, dust, sprays, or "nose drops."

The foods to which one may become sensitive include practically the entire diet, although spinach, lettuce, strawberries, sea foods, chocolate, and eggs are the most common offenders.

The cause and the exact mechanism of the development of these sensitivities are still largely a mystery. Heredity is an important factor but not the only one involved.

First-born children in all families and youngest children in large families are reported by Dr. S. M. Feinberg to show the greatest frequency of allergic diseases. This he believes may be

[5] Riis, Roper W., "Many a Germ twixt Cup and Lip," *Survey Graphic*, New York, December, 1937. See also Cumming, J. G., and N. E. Yongue, "Eating Utensil Sanitation," *American Journal of Public Health*, vol. 26, p. 237, March, 1936.

due to the type of nutrition. First-born children and youngest children in large families usually receive special care and are frequently overfed. He regards overfeeding in childhood of significance in producing allergic diseases.

Some physicians believe that these sensitivities are purely of nervous origin. This is an extreme point of view, although there is a nervous element in many of these cases. There are even persons who make semi-invalids of themselves by imagining that they are sensitive to one food after another.

The diagnosis of the allergic or sensitive state and the determination of the foods or other substances involved is a piece of medical detective work sometimes very difficult to solve. Skin tests with extracts of the suspected foods and the adoption of diets from which certain foods are eliminated are some of the special procedures which supplement a careful history of the conditions under which the attacks occur.

DISCUSSION SUGGESTIONS

1. What are some of the more common dietary fads? What fallacies underlie these?
2. Why is the term "ptomaine poisoning" a misnomer?
3. What conditions are justifiably considered as true food poisonings, food infections, and food toxemias?
4. How can the mushroom collector avoid mushroom poisoning?
5. Explain what is meant by botulism, how this disease affects its victims, and how it can be prevented.
6. Discuss the possible hazard from insecticides used as sprays on fruits and vegetables.
7. What is the cause of "milk sickness"?
8. What are the more serious bacterial infections which one may get from foods? What types of food are most likely to transmit such infections?
9. What parasitic infestations may one get from meat? Which of these is the most common? How may these be prevented?
10. Why is milk a potentially dangerous food? What diseases are most commonly transmitted through milk? How may this be prevented?
11. What are the advantages and disadvantages of raw milk?
12. How should milk be cared for in the home?
13. What provisions are there in your community to insure the sanitation of foods and to prevent their contamination by food handlers? What recommendations would you make for improving these?

[183]

14. Why is it desirable that domestic servants be given physical examinations before employment?
15. Explain what is meant by food allergy, the symptoms for which it may be responsible, and the usual methods of prevention.

REFERENCES AND READING SUGGESTIONS

1. Alvarez, W. C.: "How to Live with Your Allergy," Wilcox & Follett Co., Chicago, 1951.
2. Andrews, John: "Methods of Sanitizing Eating and Drinking Utensils," *U.S. Public Health Reports*, vol. 59, p. 1103, August 25, 1944.
3. Frank, L. C.: "What Everyone Should Know about Milk," *U.S. Public Health Service Bulletin*, Washington, D.C., 1934.
4. Goldsborough, L. S.: "Must Our Pork Remain Unsafe?" *Reader's Digest*, p. 27, March, 1950.
5. Lane, Edward A.: "Food Poisoning," *Today's Health*, vol. 30, p. 28, June, 1952.
6. Spencer, Steven M.: "Food Poisoning Can Get You, Too," *The Saturday Evening Post*, p. 25, January 5, 1952.
7. Riis, R. W.: "They Guard Our Food and Drugs," *Reader's Digest*, June, 1952.
8. Roueché, Berton: "Family Reunion," (Botulism) *The New Yorker*, January 3, 1953.
9. Samuels, Florence E.: "The Allergic Patient and His World," Charles C Thomas, Publisher, Springfield, Ill., 1953.
10. Tanner, F. W., and L. P. Tanner: "Food-borne Infections and Intoxications," Garrard Press, Champaign, Ill., 1954.

Chapter IX

STIMULANTS AND NARCOTICS

THE good fellowship, sociability, and pleasant stimulation associated with the use of tea, coffee, tobacco, and alcohol make difficult an unprejudiced consideration of their influence upon health. The fanatic, on the one hand, depicts them as insidious poisons which undermine character as well as health. Commercial interests, on the other, portray their use by superb physical specimens of young manhood and womanhood, implying in some instances and actually stating in others that their use is beneficial to health and essential to the full enjoyment of life. The truth lies somewhere between these extremes.

To place under one heading substances so vastly different in chemical composition and in physiological effects is somewhat like putting a Maltese kitten and a Bengal tiger in the same category. Our justification for doing so is that they have certain important characteristics in common. For example, all of them depend for their effects on a druglike action, and all are more or less habit-forming.

Tea, Coffee, and Cocoa

Widespread use of tea, coffee, and cocoa by peoples in many different parts of the world is curious and unexplained. Coffee originated in Arabia, tea in China, and cocoa in Brazil and Central America. Unless one is accustomed to them, they are not pleasant to the taste and they produce relatively little drug effect, nothing like the habit-forming cocaine, opium, and alcohol. There is a Chinese legend that tea leaves were first eaten by a Buddhist ascetic who noted their stimulating effect and used them to aid him to stay awake for nine years contemplating Buddha.

For our purposes tea and coffee may be considered together because the important constituent of both is caffeine. Although tea leaves contain more than twice as much caffeine as coffee beans, an ordinary cup of either contains approximately a grain and one-half of caffeine, the dosage commonly used when caffeine is prescribed for medicinal purposes.

Cocoa contains a drug called "theobromine," which is similar to caffeine both in chemical structure and in physiological effects except that it is less stimulating to the brain. Tea and coffee have no food value, and the food value of cocoa without milk or sugar is negligible.

The effects of various amounts of caffeine on the body have been extensively and carefully studied. Consequently, it is now well established that the amount of caffeine in two cups of coffee or tea ordinarily increases the volume and the rate of blood flow, the rate and depth of respiration, and the heat production of the body by 10 to 20 per cent.

The effects upon digestion are not so definite or so uniform. Some workers report a slowing of digestion, others an acceleration, and still others that it has no effect upon digestion at all. Hawk, of the University of Chicago, found no evidence in a hundred normal young men of permanent interference with digestive function from taking two to six cups of coffee daily; although at times about half of the cases reported indigestion, gas formation, diarrhea, or constipation, which seemed to be related to the drinking of coffee.

One of the most definite effects of caffeine is to increase the output of the urine. Experimentally it has been shown that the caffeine in five cups of coffee or tea increases the secretion of urine by 400 to 500 per cent or more. Whether the continued stimulation of the kidneys by caffeine causes any damage is debatable. Hawk thinks that it may, although most physicians believe that the kidneys become so accustomed to caffeine that they are not injured by it even when it is taken over a long period of time.

The most common cause for restricting the use of tea or coffee is the stimulating effects of caffeine on the nervous system. Ordinarily these effects are said to be a "heightening of the intellectual faculties and an increased capacity for physical and mental work"; but occasionally insomnia, nervousness, and headaches result from even the moderate use of tea or coffee. Lashley found that after an injection of caffeine rats were much more active in a circular treadmill than normally, but that their performance in the maze was less accurate and their ability to learn apparently retarded. Most of the studies on man seem to indicate that small doses of caffeine increase motor and mental efficiency and activity, although Hawk reports that in his studies two to six cups of coffee per day interfered with sleep and produced nervousness, inability to concentrate, and in some cases headache and dizziness.

Such disagreement concerning the immediate effects of caffeine makes it small wonder that there is considerable difference of opinion as to whether the habitual use of caffeine beverages is beneficial, harmful, or indifferent. Continuous use undoubtedly results in the development of some tolerance but this disappears rather promptly when caffeine is discontinued.

Coffee drinking by children is uniformly condemned by medical opinion. Yet the American Child Health Association reports that 39 per cent of 35,000 fifth-grade children in 86 cities of the United States had some tea and coffee every day, and 15 per cent had two or more cups. Among the foreign-born population the consumption of these beverages by children was still higher. The effects of caffeine on children have not been shown to be different from that on adults, but any drug stimulation of children, normally so highly active, is clearly undesirable. Furthermore, the use of tea and coffee by children tends to crowd milk, with its essential food elements, out of the diet.

Medical opinion, though by no means unanimous, is that the

habitual use of caffeine beverages in moderate amounts, even if long continued, is not injurious to normal adults. On the other hand, excessive quantities probably are bad for anyone; and people who are particularly susceptible to caffeine or are afflicted with nervousness or certain other diseases undoubtedly do better to forego tea and coffee entirely.

Benzedrine, a more powerful stimulant than caffeine, should be used only when ordered by a physician (see page 233).

Tobacco

In 1773 Samuel Johnson wrote, "Smoking has gone out." But if it ever did, it was well rekindled, for a hundred and eighty years later over 5 billion dollars are spent each year for tobacco in this country alone.

Tobacco seems to have been one of America's contributions to civilization. The mound builder smoked his pipe; and the cliff dwellers of Arizona and New Mexico smoked cigarettes rolled in the husks of corn. The early explorers learned its use from the Indians and called it tobacco because of the Y-shaped pipe, *tobocos*, in which it was smoked. Later the Portuguese named it *nicotiana* because Johannes I. Nicotius, French ambassador to Portugal, introduced the plant into that country.

THE "VERTUES OF TOBACCO"

European physicians at first believed that tobacco had great medicinal properties, and for a time it could be obtained only from a pharmacy on a physician's prescription. A Dr. Everard of London in 1659 wrote a book entitled: "Panacea; or the Universal Medicine, being a Discovery of the Wonderful Vertues of Tobacco Taken in a Pipe, with its Operation and Use both in Physick and Chyrurgery." Among the "vertues" which he ascribed to tobacco were: to cure deafness, a drop of the juice in each ear; to cure headaches, a green tobacco leaf on the head; for redness of the face, apply the juice or the ointment of the tobacco leaf; for a toothache, tie a tobacco leaf over the aching region; for a cough, boil the leaves and shake the sirup on the stomach; for stomach pain, and to take away the "crudities of the stomachs of young and old," "apply hot tobacco leaves over the region of the belly and reheat whenever they get cool." This is an impressive list of "vertues" but the end is not yet, for he goes on to recommend tobacco in the form of ointments, concoctions, powders or leaves for burns, wounds, cancers, sciatica, diseases of the liver, of the spleen, of the womb, worms, colic, warts, corns, nettles, and mad-dog bites, etc. Smoking, on the other hand, was not so highly thought of by this seventeenth-century physician, who says that

. . . young men must take great care how they suck this smoke for the custom and too much of it brings a grave out-of-order and makes them hot so that they lose their good temper and are beyond the bounds of health. Tobacco causes vomit and is an enemy of the stomach. Is it not a filthy thing and utterly to be detested that man, who is a more prudent creature, should be ensnared by the wanton enticement of this smoke of tobacco? To be deprived of his stomach? To be consumed by wasting his radical moisture? To be tormented with fever, to be vexed with many other infirmities? Are not these grave rewards for taking his pleasure? I think with Galen that it were better if any man have brains in his head to die a thousand times, than to lead such a life.

TOBACCO—A CURSE OR A BLESSING?

Oscar Wilde lauds the cigarette as "the perfect type of the perfect pleasure. It is exquisite and it leaves one unsatisfied. What more can you want?" Dumas, on the other hand, "is firmly convinced that tobacco saps the brain as surely as alcohol."

Thackeray writes that "the cigar has been one of the greatest creature comforts of my life—a kind companion, a gentle stimulus, and an amiable anodyne, a cementer of friendships," while the acrimonious Swinburne says: "James the First was a knave, a tyrant, a fool, a liar, a coward; but I love him, because he slit the throat of blackguard Raleigh, who invented this filthy smoking."

Oliver Wendell Holmes, physician and author, wrote in his younger years: "I must not smoke so persistently; I must turn over a new leaf—a tobacco leaf—and have a cigar after each cigar." Later in life: "I think tobacco often does a great deal of harm to the health. I myself gave it up many years ago. I think

[189]

self-narcotization is a rather ignoble substitute for undisturbed self."

Scientists, too, differ on this subject. Charles Darwin says: "Nothing soothes me more after a hard day's work than a cigarette," while Luther Burbank asserts that "men who smoke one cigar a day cannot be trusted with some of my most delicate work. Cigarettes are even more damaging than cigars."[1]

Thus the controversy goes on, while the consumption of tobacco increases at an unbelievable rate. A generation ago smoking was more or less of an occasion; today the smart cigarette, the plutocratic cigar, and the complacent pipe are everywhere. From 1910 to 1952 the consumption of cigarettes in this country increased from approximately 10 billion to approximately 500 billion annually. This increase paralleled the development of new techniques in advertising: including the press, radio, motion pictures, television, skywriters, billboards, exhibits, sampling, etc. In 1952 our national expenditure for tobacco was 5 billion dollars, as compared with an expenditure of about 20 billion dollars for clothing, 4 billion dollars for all public education, 2 billion for private education and research, and about 5 billion for medical and hospital care.

It is difficult for most smokers to explain just why they enjoy smoking. Sociability, custom, and nervous habit are undoubtedly factors. But the failure of efforts to promote denicotinized tobacco, even by government edict, indicates that the seductive qualities of tobacco are dependent upon the drug effect of its chief chemical constituent, nicotine.

NICOTINE—A POWERFUL DRUG

Nicotine is a colorless, oily compound which in concentrated form is one of the most powerful poisons known. A drop applied to the tongue of the guinea pig or the shaven skin of a rabbit is sufficient to cause death. Less than one-fiftieth of a drop injected into the vein of a man causes a slowing of the heart rate, a rise in blood pressure, and a decrease in the temperature of the skin.

[1] Hamilton, A. E., "This Smoking World," Appleton-Century-Crofts, Inc., New York, 1927.

One cigar contains enough nicotine to kill two adults if injected into the circulatory system. The death of a child was reported recently from swallowing snuff. The Census Bureau reported 288 fatal cases of nicotine poisoning in the United States for the years 1930–1934 inclusive.

The amount of nicotine absorbed from tobacco varies with tobaccos and with the method of use. When tobacco is powdered and used as snuff, the proportion of nicotine absorbed is higher than with either chewing or smoking. Chewing, in turn, results in greater absorption than smoking. And there is more absorption from the smoking of tobacco in a pipe than in a cigar and more from a cigar than from a cigarette. There is evidence also that the smoke of damp tobacco contains more nicotine than that of the same tobacco thoroughly dried. For this reason it is claimed that smokers who chew the ends of their cigars absorb more nicotine than those who use a holder.

"STRONG" TOBACCOS

Tobacco itself varies greatly in nicotine content. Havana tobacco contains approximately 1.5 per cent of nicotine; Maryland tobacco, 2.0 per cent; Virginia tobacco, 6.0 per cent; Kentucky tobacco, 8.0 per cent. Contrary to general belief, there is no relation between the so-called "strength" of a tobacco and its nicotine content. "Strength" depends primarily upon the presence of aromatic substances which are formed during the fermentation of tobacco before drying.

THE EFFECTS OF TOBACCO

The effects of tobacco upon the body vary from those which are so slight that it is impossible to measure them, to acute poisoning. The latter is accompanied by symptoms of faintness, dizziness, cold clammy skin, rapid pulse, weakness, and sometimes nausea, vomiting, and diarrhea. These symptoms occur most frequently in persons unaccustomed to the use of tobacco, but habitual smokers at times experience similar effects. These effects are of short duration and probably have little if any influence upon the general health.

Of greater interest and importance is the effect of tobacco in nontoxic quantities over long periods of time. On this question there is much positive opinion but relatively few scientific data. In some cases smoking seems to soothe the nerves and calm the spirits. In others it gives rise to headaches, giddiness, insomnia, and nervous irritability. Serious visual damage may result from the excessive use of tobacco.

The advertising claims that certain cigarettes are less irritating than others is an obvious admission that all are irritating to the membranes which line the nose, throat, and respiratory passages. Not infrequently smoking is the cause of a persistent, irritating, and even debilitating cough.

EFFECTS UPON THE CIRCULATORY SYSTEM

Upon the heart and circulatory system the effects of tobacco occasionally are dramatic, producing pain in the region of the heart, irregularities of the heartbeat, and possibly even heart failure. Distinguished physicians even suggest that in certain individuals tobacco may be a factor in the development of angina pectoris and high blood pressure.

Investigators at the Mayo Foundation discovered that the smoking of two standard cigarettes resulted in an increase in metabolic rate and consistent changes in the tracings of the electrical impulses generated by the heart. The subjects were habitual smokers and inhaled during smoking.

Another group at the Mayo Clinic report that their studies show a definite relationship between coronary heart disease and heavy cigarette smoking and that heavy cigarette smokers develop coronary disease at a relatively young age.

In addition to these rather unusual effects of tobacco on the circulatory system there have been many observations which show that smoking quite regularly causes first a slowing and then an increase in the pulse rate and a rise in blood pressure. These effects occur in habitual as well as in occasional smokers.

Analyzing the evidence available on this subject the editor of the *Journal of the American Medical Association* concluded that the use of tobacco "even in moderate quantities seems to lower the efficiency of the heart under strain."

Drs. Wright and Moffat of New York have reported that the smoking of a single cigarette causes a marked drop in the temperature of the fingers and toes. In a hundred cases the average drop was 5.3 degrees Fahrenheit, and the greatest drop 15.5 degrees Fahrenheit. Coincident with the drop in temperature a slowing or stopping of the blood flow in the capillaries frequently occurred. Some of the most severe toxic symptoms and greatest temperature changes occurred in individuals who were experienced and heavy smokers. They also found that practically identical effects are produced by various standard brands, by denicotinized, and by mentholated cigarettes.

This decrease in the temperature of the fingers and toes following smoking is probably due to the same physiological mechanism that is responsible for the relationship between smoking and Buerger's disease. In this disease gangrene of a limb occurs as a result of the blood supply being cut off, first by spasm of the arteries and then by the formation of a clot, or thrombus, within the vessels. In a large series of patients with this disease it was found that 80 per cent were sensitive to tobacco, as compared to 36 per cent of smokers without Buerger's disease and to 16 per cent of nonsmokers. Naturally, then, physicians advise against the use of tobacco by patients with this disease. In other types of diseases of the blood vessels experiments indicate that smoking may exaggerate symptoms rather than cause them.

EFFECTS UPON DIGESTION

A cigar, a cigarette, or a pipe after a meal may aid digestion or may give rise to indigestion, gaseous distention, spastic constipation, and occasionally even chronic colitis.

EFFECTS UPON THE RESPIRATORY SYSTEM

Tuberculosis frequently has been attributed to smoking, but there is no evidence to justify this. Tobacco smoke, however, does contain substances which are irritant to the mucous membranes of the respiratory tract, and excessive smoking invariably increases cough and asthma. Smoker's throat, smoker's cough, smoker's larynx, and smoker's bronchitis have become common medical terms. It has been reported that pulmonary complications after abdominal operations are six times as frequent in persons who smoke ten or more cigarettes a day as in nonsmokers.

The most serious effect, however, that investigators are coming to believe smoking has upon the respiratory tract is its possible role as a contributory factor in the development of cancer of the lung. A recent report by the British Medical Research Council states that the risk of dying of cancer of the lung increases with the amount smoked. "Among men 45 to 64 years of age" they state that "the death rate in non-smokers is negligible, while in the heavier smoking groups it is estimated to reach three to five deaths per 1000." "The risk," they add, "is appreciably less for pipe smokers than for cigarette smokers."

A recently published preliminary report of an extensive study by the American Cancer Society concludes that "men with a history of regular cigarette smoking have a considerably higher death rate than men who have never smoked or men who have smoked only cigars or pipes." Their data indicate also that the higher death rates among smokers as compared to nonsmokers are due largely to cancer of the lung and to coronary artery disease.[1a]

Studies such as this—and there are a number of them—are strongly suggestive, though not conclusive, evidence of a causative relationship between cigarette smoking and cancer of the lung; other studies may change the picture. Until they do, this possible relationship cannot be ignored.

EFFECTS UPON LONGEVITY

From a study of the life histories of 6,813 men, of whom 2,094 were nonusers of tobacco, 2,814 moderate smokers, and 1,905 heavy smokers, Professor Raymond Pearl of Johns Hopkins University concluded that smoking is unquestionably associated

[1a] Hammond, E. C., and D. Horn, "Smoking and Death Rates," *Journal of the American Medical Association*, Aug. 7, 1954.

with a definite impairment of longevity and that the degree of this impairment is proportional to the amount of tobacco habitually used (Table 22). Heavy smokers experience the greatest average reduction in longevity, but even moderate smoking shows a measurable and significant impairment of longevity.

TABLE 22
TOBACCO SMOKING AND LENGTH OF LIFE[*]

The number of survivors at 5-year intervals starting at the age of thirty of (a) 100,000 white males who were nonusers of tobacco; (b) 100,000 who were moderate smokers but did not chew tobacco or take snuff; and (c) 100,000 who were heavy smokers but did not chew or take snuff.

Age	Nonusers	Moderate	Heavy	Age	Nonusers	Moderate	Heavy
30	100,000	100,000	100,000	65	57,018	52,082	38,328
35	95,883	95,804	90,943	70	45,919	41,431	30,393
40	91,546	90,883	81,191	75	33,767	30,455	22,338
45	86,730	85,129	71,665	80	21,737	19,945	14,498
50	81,160	78,436	62,699	85	11,597	10,987	7,865
55	74,538	70,712	54,277	90	4,573	4,686	3,392
60	66,564	61,911	46,226	95	1,320	1,366	938

* Pearl, Raymond, "The Search for Longevity," *Scientific Monthly*, vol. 46, pp. 462–483, May, 1938.

FATIGUE AND SMOKING

Smoking is said to result in some temporary stimulation and relief of fatigue, due, it seems, to a stimulation of the adrenal glands by nicotine. This effect, however, is of short duration and is usually followed by even greater fatigue than that which is relieved. Many persons report that they are more fatigued at the end of the day when they are smoking heavily than when they smoke occasionally or not at all.

From a study of six patients whose main symptom was fatigue, Segal concluded that cigarette smoking can be the cause of fatigue and that in some people fatigue can be relieved by stopping smoking.

TOBACCO AND MENTAL EFFICIENCY

There is no agreement concerning the effects of tobacco upon mental efficiency. William Dean Howells says: "If one hath

[195]

been poring long over a book or has toiled with a pen, it quick-eneth the brain and dispels the clouds that overset the mind." Likewise, Dunlap, director of the Psychological Laboratory at Johns Hopkins University, reports that they

> . . . found evidence of improvement due to smoking in complicated opera-tions comparable to the mental requirements of driving an automobile or an airplane. In various investigations we have found that after smoking the person works more steadily, that is, with less spurts or slack. We have not investi-gated the effects of smoking over long periods of time such as months, nor has anyone else. We cannot say that smoking is beneficial or harmful; as regards the alleged immediate detrimental effects, we can say that it is not proved.[2]

On the other hand, Professor O'Shea of the University of Wisconsin concluded from a carefully conducted experiment on "Tobacco and Mental Efficiency" that, while individuals vary in their reactions to tobacco, the usual effect of smoking is to slow down and disturb the intellectual processes. Likewise, Bush of the University of Vermont, who tested the effects of smoking on fifteen college students, found losses in the fields of imagery, perception, and association, with an estimated 10 per cent de-crease in mental efficiency. Earp of Antioch College found that the scholarship of student smokers was lower than that of non-smokers, and that scholarship was lowest among smokers who inhaled. It is evident from such reports that conclusive evidence is not yet available as to the effect of tobacco upon creative mental activity.

SMOKING BY WOMEN

Since the emancipation of women has been extended to the use of tobacco, the question is frequently raised as to the prob-able effect of smoking upon women and through them upon their children and upon succeeding generations. As to its effect upon women themselves there is no reason to be more alarmed than there is concerning its effect upon men. As to its effect upon an unborn child there is more question.

[2] Quoted by Hamilton, A. E., "This Smoking World," Appleton-Century-Crofts, Inc., New York, 1927.

Nicotine administered to a pregnant animal has been shown to be harmful to the offspring. Doctor Clinton H. Thieness of the University of Southern California, after most careful experimentation, reports that the second generation of female rats treated with toxic doses of nicotine experiences only one-third as many periods of sexual activity as normal rats. This effect is not observed in the first generation but appears in the second and in subsequent generations. This same careful investigator reports that the animals treated with nicotine give birth to as many offspring as the normal rats used as controls, but only one-half as many of the offspring of mothers who have been treated with nicotine live to the age of weaning. This may be due to lowered vitality at birth, to the nicotine in the breast milk, or to less good care on the part of the mothers because of the depressing effect of the nicotine which they receive. In considering the possible application of the experiments to smoking by women, one must realize that these animals were given doses of nicotine large enough to cause convulsions every day from infancy to adult life.

Smoking by a pregnant woman produces an increase in pulse rate of the unborn child; and 4 ounces of breast milk from mothers who smoke six to eight cigarettes per day has been found to contain enough nicotine to kill a frog. A sufficient quantity of this certainly would affect the infant. As to the practical importance of this observation we have no information. It is perfectly conceivable that a package of cigarettes a day might be injurious to the unborn babe or the nursing infant, while three or four cigarettes might be no more injurious than a cup of coffee.

SMOKING BY CHILDREN

It has long been agreed, even by the tobacco interests themselves, that the use of tobacco by growing boys and girls is unhealthful and dangerous. Japan has a national law prohibiting the use of tobacco by boys and girls under legal age. Nicotine and tobacco have been reported by some investigators to cause retardation of the growth of animals; but other investigators have failed to confirm these results. Physicians have reported the stunting of the physical and mental growth of children working in tobacco factories, but these observations have never been satisfactorily controlled.

SHOULD ONE SMOKE?

In spite of all the careful studies and observations of the effects of tobacco upon man and animals we are still unable to give a final answer as to the ultimate effects of moderate smoking upon health. There is abundant evidence that the excessive use of tobacco is deleterious and that individual susceptibility to tobacco varies enormously. Instances have been reported in which irregular heart action lasting for days or weeks followed moderate smoking. Furthermore, except for some possible nervous relaxation there is no known beneficial effect which tobacco exerts upon the body. On the other hand, as Hamilton says in his book, "This Smoking World":

> Who knows but that even the physiological damage which is sometimes done by unenlightened excess of the use of tobacco may be compensated, in the end, by the vast amount of spiritual ice-breaking and the sparks of friendship kindled by that curious instrument of human intercourse which has found a place in the vestpocket of mankind?

The decision to smoke or not to smoke should be made, but probably never will be, by weighing the pleasure which it gives, on the one hand, against the cost and possible risk involved, on the other. If the decision is to smoke, smoking should be in moderation. Mark Twain, J. P. Morgan, and hosts of others smoked excessively to the end of long and useful lives, but the average man or woman is undoubtedly better off to smoke moderately or not at all.

What constitutes moderation is also an individual matter. Susceptibility to tobacco varies immensely and so does the susceptibility of the same individual under different conditions. The effect of a cigar leisurely smoked after dinner may be quite different from its effect if smoked when one is tired, hungry, and nervous. In general, if one has a chronic cough or is nervous and easily fatigued when smoking heavily, the only intelligent procedure is to reduce or, for a time at least, discontinue the use of tobacco. Many persons break themselves of the habit and feel the better for it.[3]

To those who wish to smoke with the least danger of impairing health and vitality, Dr. James J. Waring gives the following suggestions:[4] (1) Do not smoke until past the age of twenty-one years. (2) Use cigarettes, not more than five daily. (3) Do not inhale or blow smoke through the nose. (4) Smoke only immediately after meals. (5) At least once a year stop smoking for a month or more. (6) Have a health examination periodically.

Alcohol

Alcohol is a seductive mistress whose virtues and vices it is difficult to weigh impartially. Some years ago we decided that, having put an end to war, we would likewise be rid of the demon rum. This done, we promptly began to resent our own interference with "legitimate" business, "legitimate" thirst, and individual liberty. The saloon with its swinging doors was gone, but the mysterious and enticing speakeasy took its place. People began to boast of their bootleggers, and an enormous illicit business in rum and crime grew up. Then came the depression, and we were assured that if we would repeal prohibition gangdom would disappear and prosperity and happiness return. So we voted back our liquor and we are still hoping that it will wash away our troubles.

THE EFFECTS OF ALCOHOL

Alcohol is a poison to living tissue. In reasonably concentrated solutions it will destroy plant, bacterial, and animal life. This is a serious indictment of something that we use as a beverage. But we might answer that other ingredients of our diet, such as salt, iodine, and even water itself, are deadly poisons if taken in sufficient quantities. The difference is that, whereas these substances in proper amounts are essential to life and rarely if ever are used

[3] McElvoy, J. P., "Are You a Man or a Smokestack?" *The Reader's Digest*, p. 102, August, 1944.

[4] Waring, James J., "Hygiene for the Smoker," *Hygeia*, vol. 3, p. 320, June, 1925.

to excess, alcohol supplies no nutritional need and is frequently taken in toxic quantities.

Even small amounts of alcohol produce definite and measurable effects upon the body. The chief of these is the depressant action upon the nervous system. Alcohol is generally thought to be a stimulant, but, except for the small amount of energy produced in its oxidation, this is entirely erroneous. The feeling of exhilaration is the result of the depressant action on the higher brain centers, the ones which control restraint. With inhibition and restraint removed a feeling of exhilaration results if the effect of the alcohol is supplemented by the stimulation of companionship or activity. In the absence of such stimulation the narcotic effect of depression and sleepiness may be the only one observed. Larger quantities of alcohol paralyze one nerve center after another and eventually lead to unconsciousness. This last stage is identical with that obtained in ether anesthesia; in fact ether is a very volatile and active derivative of alcohol.

Through Cassio, Shakespeare said, "O God! that men should put an enemy in their mouths to steal away their brains; that we should, with joy, pleasure, revel, and applause, transform ourselves into beasts."[5]

Nervous control and motor coordination are definitely reduced by alcohol. Grim evidence of this is the large number of automobile accidents which occur to drivers who have been drinking. Moderate amounts of alcohol interfere with attention, concentration, memory, judgment, and reason. The learning process in men and animals is adversely affected. Speed of performance is slowed and errors increase.

An analysis of the deaths from poisoning in the state of Massachusetts over a 10-year period showed that in 4,505 cases death was directly related to the ingestion of alcohol. If the fatal accidents and suicides that occur during intoxication are included the figure is higher.

A committee of the British Medical Association on the "Relation of Alcohol to Road Accidents" stated that such moderate quantities of alcohol as three

[5] *Othello,* Act II, Scene III.

ounces of whisky diminish attention and control and reduce the rapidity and accuracy of coordination of movements of the eyes, hands and legs. These effects are more likely to lead to an accident, the greater the speed. The reaction time is increased from 0.1 to 0.4 second by alcohol, and in addition drivers unconsciously accelerate their speed. Tests made on twenty subjects by means of a motor driving apparatus showed that 2⅔ ounces of whisky increased the rate of driving 6 per cent and driving errors 13 per cent.

American data suggest that a third or a fourth of fatal road accidents are attributable to the action of alcohol on the drivers. A new method of investigation is now being tried—determination of the alcohol content of the blood or urine. It has been shown that from 40 to 63 per cent of persons having one part per thousand of alcohol in their blood are under its influence. The conclusion is that the only safe course for the automobile driver is total abstinence, which should be practiced several hours before driving as well as during it, owing to the slowness with which alcohol disappears from the blood.[6]

After-dinner drinks may be perfectly harmless if no important activities are undertaken at such times, whereas the drink taken before driving a car, running machinery, or performing any task that demands accurate decisions or mental acuity might be dangerous. The drinker should observe the following rule: For every two drinks, he should wait three hours before undertaking important activities.[7]

Among the physiological effects of alcohol is a dilation of the blood vessels resulting in a flushing of the skin and a sensation of warmth. This is usually accompanied by a slight fall of blood pressure and an increase in pulse rate. Larger doses depress the heart action and cause an increase in blood pressure. There is some evidence also that the continued use of alcohol may lead to a deposit of fat in the heart muscle with a consequent loss of its reserve power.

ALCOHOL AND PHYSICAL EFFICIENCY

Observations on soldiers indicate that those not supplied with alcoholic drinks are able to march farther and are in better con-

[6] "Alcohol and Automobile Accidents," *Journal of the American Medical Association,* vol. 108, p. 984, March, 1937.

[7] "The Amount of Alcohol That Can Be Tolerated," *Journal of the American Medical Association,* vol. 153, p. 1414, December 12, 1953.

dition at the end of the day than those to whom it has been given. Concerning its use a leading athletic coach of the country says:

Liquor and athletics just don't go together. There isn't a responsible coach in the country who tolerates drinking when men are in training. I've seen promising athletes fade out of the picture because they got to drinking between training seasons. Even "pro" athletes have to fight shy of liquor if they want to stay at the top. Every once in a while you read about some "pro" who has gone down the skids because of drink. For every chance that a fellow who starts drinking in college can come through all right, there are too many chances that he will come to grief.[8]

SOCIAL AND ECONOMIC EFFECTS OF ALCOHOL

No consideration of the effects of alcohol upon health is complete without brief mention of the moral, social, and economic aspects of the problem. The saloon in which the workingman squanders his weekly pay is an important contributing factor to the poverty, the malnutrition, and the illness of his family which result therefrom. Various studies have shown that illness, death, and delinquency rates among children in such homes are many times higher than among children whose parents provide them with decent, wholesome living conditions. The young man whose vision of the sordid nature of prostitution is dulled by alcohol all too frequently discovers to his sorrow that he has contracted syphilis or gonorrhea, and many a girl takes her first step on the road to sex delinquency when under the influence of liquor.

Still more important than these effects of alcohol upon physical health are its effects upon mental health. Rare indeed is the child who can grow up with a normal wholesome attitude toward life in a home in which one or both parents are intemperate drinkers. The drunken father bullies his children and inspires in them both fear and disgust. Alcohol always has had a disorganizing influence upon the family and is responsible for more family conflicts and broken homes than any other single cause. Probably every reader knows personally of promising young men whose careers have been wrecked and whose homes broken because of drink. In the past drinking, at least to excess, was confined

[8] From *Allied Youth*, p. 4, October 28, 1936.

largely to men. What the end results of the modern competition of women in this regard will be only time will tell.

ALCOHOL ADDICTION

Alcohol is definitely a habit-forming drug. Some persons are able to take small amounts at irregular intervals over a period of years and then stop taking it without difficulty. Others find that one drink leads to another with increasing frequency until addiction becomes firmly established. The mental processes, the craving, and the depravity of alcoholics are very like those of drug addicts. In fact, Charles Jackson's portrayal of a drunkard's mind and soul in "The Lost Weekend"[9] is reminiscent of De Quincy's "Confessions of an English Opium Eater."

There is frequently a relationship between alcoholism and barbiturate or opium addiction. The first step is the use of barbiturates to alleviate the "hangover" from alcohol. The next step is an increase in dosage and dependence upon the barbiturates. Addiction may stop here or it may be transferred to stronger narcotics, such as veronal, opium, or morphine.

RESISTANCE TO DISEASE

It has long been an impression of physicians that pneumonia is particularly common and serious among heavy drinkers. This observation finds support in laboratory experiments which show that rabbits are rendered more susceptible to pneumococcus and streptococcus infections by hypodermic injections of alcohol or ether.

DISEASES CAUSED BY ALCOHOL

Concerning alcoholism the distinguished Sir William Osler wrote that when a large amount of alcohol is taken the effect is chiefly upon the nervous system and is manifested by muscular incoordination, mental disturbance, and narcosis. The face is flushed, the pulse full, the respiration slow and deep. Unconsciousness is present but rarely so deep that the patient cannot be aroused. Muscular twitching may occur but rarely convulsions.

[9] Jackson, Charles, "The Lost Weekend," Rinehart & Company, Inc., New York, 1944.

[203]

Dr. Osler cites the following as the chief effects of the continued use of considerable quantities of alcohol:

Nervousness, as evidenced by unsteadiness of the muscles, tremors of the hands and tongue. The mental processes may be dull, particularly in the early morning hours. Irritability of temper, forgetfulness, and a change in the moral character gradually come on. The judgment is seriously impaired, the mind enfeebled, and in the final stages dementia may supervene. Epilepsy and neuritis may result from chronic drinking.

Stomach symptoms, commonly described as "catarrh," are frequent. The appetite is usually impaired and the bowels constipated. The toper has a furred tongue, heavy breath, and in the morning a sensation of sinking at the stomach until he has had his drink.

Cirrhosis of the Liver. Alcohol produces definite changes in the liver, leading ultimately to a form of hardening or cirrhosis. There are cases in which comparatively moderate drinking for a few years has been followed by cirrhosis; on the other hand, the livers of persons who have been steady drinkers for 30 or 40 years may show only a moderate grade of cirrhosis. For years before cirrhosis develops, heavy drinkers may present an enlarged and tender liver, with at times swelling of the spleen.

The *kidneys, heart,* and *arteries* also may show definite degenerative changes from alcoholism.

Delirium tremens is a type of psychosis, or insanity, resulting from the long-continued action of alcohol on the brain. A spree by an habitual drinker is likely to bring on an attack. At the outset of the attack the patient is restless and depressed and sleeps badly, symptoms which cause him to take alcohol more freely. After a day or two the characteristic delirium sets in. The patient talks constantly and incoherently; he is incessantly in motion and desires to go and attend to some imaginary business. Hallucinations of sight and hearing develop. He sees objects in the room, such as rats, mice, or snakes, and fancies that they are crawling over his body. The terror inspired by these imaginary objects is great and has given the popular name "horrors" to the disease. Approximately twenty-five thousand persons per year

[204]

are being admitted to state psychopathic hospitals with diagnoses of acute or chronic alcoholic psychoses. Many more are cared for in general hospitals and by private physicians. About 10 per cent of these patients die during an acute attack. The others recover, but recurrence is almost the rule if drinking is continued.

DOES ALCOHOL WEAKEN THE RACE?

The effect of alcohol upon the race has been the subject of both speculation and experimentation. Speculation concludes that, since children of drunkards are frequently weaklings and defectives, the use of alcohol is deleterious to the racial stock. That this may be true cannot be denied. On the other hand, children of intemperate parents usually grow up under such conditions of inadequate care, faulty nutrition, and unhealthy environment that they would be handicapped, no matter what their natural endowment.

Several carefully controlled studies have investigated the effects of alcohol upon successive generations of laboratory animals. Summarizing these studies Dr. Pearl says:

Experiments by various workers on such different forms of life as guinea pigs, fowls, rats, mice, rabbits, frogs, and insects, agree in showing a beneficial effect of alcohol on the race. This beneficial effect appears to be produced chiefly as the result of a remarkably sharp and precise selective action of this agent upon germ cells in developing embryos, killing off the weak and defective, and leaving the strong and sound to survive and perpetuate the race.[10]

In accord with this is Stockard's[11] suggestion that the action of alcohol in eliminating unfit individuals may have benefited the races of Europe. All dominant races have used alcohol, and it is possible that this, through the elimination of some of the weaker and less desirable germ cells, has contributed to the preservation of a biologically superior stock. Stockard considers it unlikely that human beings have injured or eliminated their normally resistant germ cells with alcohol.

[10] Pearl, Raymond, "Alcohol and Longevity," p. 227, Alfred A. Knopf, Inc., New York, 1926.

[11] Stockard, C. R., "Alcohol, a Factor in Eliminating Racial Degeneracy," *American Journal of Medical Sciences*, vol. 82, part 2, p. 469, April, 1924.

ALCOHOL AND THE LENGTH OF LIFE

The combined experience of 43 American life insurance companies over a period of 25 years shows that the death rate among "very moderate drinkers" is 18 per cent higher than the rate among insured lives generally, 50 per cent higher among those who had a history of past intemperance, and 86 per cent higher among steady but so-called "moderate drinkers." The "very moderate drinkers" used two glasses of beer or one glass of whisky daily and the steady "moderate drinker" more than two glasses of beer or one glass of whisky daily but were accepted as temperate and standard risks. The Northwestern Mutual Life Insurance Company reported a similar mortality experience among its policyholders. Neither of these studies gives rates for persons who only occasionally use alcohol and then in moderation.

Dr. Pearl[12] concluded, from data which he collected firsthand on a group of 2,000 persons, that heavy drinking definitely shortens life, but that moderate drinking is not necessarily associated with an increased mortality rate.

THE MEDICINAL VALUE OF ALCOHOL

There is not a single disease in the treatment of which alcoholic beverages have been shown to be of definite value. Even in the treatment of snake bite it not only is worthless but is more likely to be harmful than beneficial.

A summary of the opinions of a group of prominent physicians concerning the therapeutic uses of alcohol is presented in the following quotation from Dr. Haven Emerson's book "Alcohol and Man":

As a solvent of various medicaments alcohol performs a useful, perhaps indispensable function, and the pharmacist requires it to compound many of our widely used therapeutic preparations. The therapeutic part played by alcohol in these preparations is very limited. As a therapeutic agent, alcoholic beverages have a place in rendering more comfortable and peaceful the disturbances of chronic disease and old age. Sometimes it is useful to increase

[12] Pearl, Raymond, "Alcohol and the Duration of Life," *American Mercury*, vol. 1, p. 213, February, 1924.

appetite. Beyond this there are very few conditions needing alcohol and alcoholic beverages in their treatment. Much of the use of alcohol and alcoholic beverages of the past no longer exists for better therapeutic measures have replaced them. It seems a fact that in both private and hospital practice the utilization of alcohol and alcoholic beverages by the better trained physicians has decreased greatly and is continuing to decrease.

ALCOHOL AND VENEREAL DISEASE

One who acts as a health adviser to young people again and again hears the story that illicit sexual relations were engaged in and venereal disease contracted while under the influence of alcohol. The director of the Student Health Service of one of our large universities reported that practically every student who contracts venereal disease does so while under the influence of alcohol.

Alcohol paralyzes the inhibitions and is an excitant to sexual excess. The prostitute, the seducer, and others connected with the traffic are all familiar with the effectiveness of alcohol in this regard; and if the hesitant prospect is not already under the influence of alcohol, it is obligingly provided.

Alcohol also aggravates existing venereal infection, impedes the progress of cure, and reactivates quiescent infections. Knowing this, the physician prohibits alcohol, even in small amounts, to patients under treatment.

THE PROS AND CONS OF ALCOHOL

As a medical and health problem, alcoholism is exceedingly widespread and serious. One study reports that there are 3,700,-000 "excessive drinkers" in this country, that is, persons who drink too much for their own good. Of these some three-quarters of a million are problem drinkers, people for whom drinking has become a serious illness. This is exclusive of the many millions of "social drinkers" who can "take it or leave it alone." About 60 per cent of the problem drinkers are mentally ill to start with; that is, with them drinking is a symptom of the illness rather than a cause. For the other 40 per cent the trouble starts with drinking; some with social drinking, others with compensatory, occupational, or situational drinking.

When all the facts are assembled, most of the entries concerning alcohol are on the debit side of the ledger. It shortens life, produces certain specific diseases, lowers physical and mental efficiency, weakens judgment, and destroys discretion. But, you say, these are the results of excessive amounts of alcohol—the results of intemperance. What about its occasional use in moderation? On this point we have less definite information. It may be entirely harmless. Certainly there is no specific evidence that it is deleterious. But can its use be kept occasional and moderate?

In this connection the action taken by the Royal Academy of Medicine of Belgium is of significance. This took the form of the following motion, which was unanimously adopted for transmission to the minister of public health:

> In conformity with its previous utterances in the matter of the necessity for a vigorous fight against alcoholism, the Academie royale de medicine disapproves categorically of any restoration of the legal right to the consumption of spirituous beverages in public places. The Academie regrets that from time to time attempts are made to exact from parliament repeal of legislation which possesses a high moral significance and the effects of which have been salutary. The Academie hopes that in future the concept that, of all the duties incumbent on the state, the most imperious is that of protecting the race against the forces of moral degradation and physical deterioration, will cease to be contested.[13]

On the other side of the ledger we find that alcoholic beverages add delectability to a dinner, stimulate the appetite, engender conviviality, and afford release from care. A good wine adds materially to the pleasure of those who truly appreciate it. To them it is sacrilegious to debase it by intemperate use.

Of alcoholic drinks, light wines are the usual choice of the connoisseur and are least likely to be injurious. Their alcoholic content varies from 7 to 10 per cent, but there is little likelihood of using them to excess. Beer contains less alcohol but tends to be fattening and is more likely to be used in increasing amounts. The distilled liquors, such as whisky, brandy, and gin, have high alcoholic content and are responsible for most of the occasional drunkenness and habitual intemperance.

[13] *Journal of the American Medical Association*, vol. 109, No. 16, p. 222, July, 1937.

A PERSONAL DECISION

At some time in life everyone is confronted with the question: What shall be my attitude toward liquor and what course shall I follow? It has been well said that "the most important thing about liquor is that it shall be unimportant." Let us be unemotional about it, acquaint ourselves with the available facts, decide how much real pleasure it holds, count the cost, estimate the hazards, and make an intelligent decision. Above all, let us not be coerced into the use of alcohol by the advertising of the liquor interests which suggests that to use it is the only socially acceptable course to follow.

On most college campuses a few years ago it was decidedly the "smart" thing to drink. Today this is much less true and most students consider drunkenness something to be ashamed of. Some persons who drink to excess do so because they are miserable and hope to escape the realities of life; others because they are trying to compensate for feelings of inferiority by demonstrating that they can "drink with the best of them"; others because they wish to be good fellows and believe that one drink after another is the way to do so; and still others—and most habitual drunkards belong in this group—because of an inherent weakness of character. None of these reasons for excessive drinking is consistent with good mental health.

Many do not care for alcoholic beverages; others for economic, social, or personal reasons decide to forego them. Still others are unable to keep the use of alcohol within the bounds of moderation. To all of these the only sound advice is to avoid it entirely.

If, on the other hand, the moderate use of alcohol adds materially to one's pleasure or happiness; if its use can be a pleasant occasion instead of a controlling habit; if "one can sip the cup but not drain it"; if it can be kept one's servant instead of becoming one's master; then it may be used with little if any danger to health; then it may be worth the cost; and then and only then can it justifiably have a place in one's life.

Narcotics

Literally narcotics are drugs which produce sleep. These include opium, morphine, and their derivatives, and the bar-

[209]

biturates. Practical usage, however, includes as narcotics other habit-forming drugs, such as cocaine and cannabis (marijuana).

Few if any drugs are more valuable than those which relieve pain and produce sleep. The first medication given to a wounded soldier on the battlefield is an injection of morphine. This eases his pain and relieves his anxiety. It frequently saves lives by preventing shock, by helping to control hemorrhage, or by giving needed rest when life's flame is almost out.

In 1680 the famous physician Sydenham wrote, "Among the remedies which has pleased Almighty God, to give man to relieve his suffering, none is so universal and so effectatious as opium." A similar appraisal would be valid today. Yet opium and its derivative morphine are responsible for most of the drug addiction in the world today. Other important habit-forming drugs are heroin, cocaine, marijuana, and the barbiturates. Alcohol is also narcotic (sleep-producing) and habit-forming but it is considered in a separate category.

NARCOTIC ADDICTION

Opium addiction, in the form of opium smoking, has been known for centuries in the Orient. Prior to the Second World War strong efforts were made through international agreements to control the production and the distribution of opium. However, in the Orient, opium and heroin are used as an instrument of warfare. They are forced upon the people in one manner or another until they become addicted to them. From then on they are degraded victims of their conquerors, who controlled the supply of the drugs which have become indispensable to them.

In this country the seriousness of opium addiction was not recognized until early in the present century. As late as 1909, 118,000 pounds of opium were legally imported and distributed for smoking purposes in the United States. In this same year, however, the United States promoted the First International Opium Commission which met in Shanghai. Since that time the United States has led the world in its efforts both to control the use of narcotics at home and to secure the adoption of international agreements to limit the manufacture and sale of narcotics to strictly medicinal purposes.

In 1914 Congress passed the Harrison Narcotic Act. Under this law all dispensaries of opium, morphine, cocaine, and their derivatives are required to be licensed and registered, to keep an accurate and permanent record of all drugs received and disposed of, and to dispense these drugs only for medicinal or scientific purposes. This law is intended to prevent the improper use of these drugs. To a great extent it does this, but there has always been an illicit trade or "black market" in these drugs. Some are smuggled into the country; others are produced and sold illegally. Although the prices charged are unbelievably high, the craving of the unfortunate addict causes him or her to pay any price or sacrifice anything to obtain these drugs.

The number of narcotic addicts is not known. When the Harrison Narcotic Act was passed it was estimated that there were 150,000 to 200,000 narcotic addicts, mostly women, in this country. According to a recent estimate the addicts in this country now number about 48,000, mostly men—approximately 1 addict per 3,000 population. The reduction has been largely due to the vigorous enforcement of the Harrison Narcotic Act and to the provision of federal facilities for the treatment of addicts.

It is estimated that one-third of addicts acquire the habit before the age of twenty and two-thirds before the age of thirty years. Physicians are very cautious in the administration of narcotics, with the result that less than 5 per cent of addicts develop the habit as the result of proper medicinal use. The other 95 per cent acquire the habit from associates or "peddlers."

Opium. Opium is derived from the juice of unripe seed capsules of the poppy plant, *Papaver somniferum*, a native of Asia Minor. The dried juice forms a brown gummy mass which is used for smoking; powdered, it becomes the drug opium. From opium are extracted by chemical processes morphine, codeine, papaverine, and several other drugs. Of these by far the most important is morphine. Morphine in small doses deadens pain and produces sleep. For these purposes it is invaluable, yet, even when used medicinally, the dangerous habit-forming properties

[211]

of the drug must never be forgotten. Investigators are constantly attempting to find or produce a drug which will have the beneficial effects of morphine without its addictive possibilities. Closely related to morphine chemically is codeine. Codeine has much less narcotic action than morphine and little addictive possibilities. Heroin, on the other hand, which is also closely related to morphine and derived from it, is the most dangerous addictive drug known. When first produced, it was thought to be less habit-forming than morphine, but experience indicated a very different situation. It is estimated that 75 per cent of the addicts use heroin. The dangers of this drug caused the Federal Government several years ago to forbid both its manufacture and its sale in this country.

Cocaine. Cocaine is obtained from the leaves of the coca tree, native to Peru and Bolivia. For many years the Indians of these countries have chewed the leaves of these trees for stimulation and to decrease fatigue. The alkaloid cocaine is obtained from these leaves.

Medicinally, the most important action of cocaine is its ability to block nerve conduction by local application. For this reason it is used as a local anesthetic for certain operative procedures. For most purposes cocaine has been replaced by substitutes, such as procaine or Novocain, which are less toxic and non-habit-forming. The toxic effects of cocaine are so unpleasant that there are few pure cocaine addicts in the United States.

Addiction to cocaine is based not upon its anesthetic effects but upon the stimulation of the central nervous system which it causes. The first effects are garrulity, restlessness, and excitement. The sense of fatigue is diminished and the addict greatly overestimates his muscular and mental capacity. Hallucinations and ideas of persecution, mental deterioration, digestive disorders, emaciation, and sleeplessness are common. Most addicts take the drug by injection although many inhale a cocaine powder that is commonly called "snow."

Marijuana. Marijuana, or hashish, is obtained from the flowering top of Indian hemp, *Cannabis indica*, a plant which grows wild in many parts of the world, including the United

States. Hemp is used commercially for the manufacture of twine, rope, bags, and clothing. The drug cannabis has no medicinal value but is habitually used for its psychic effect by millions of people in all parts of the world. It is either smoked as "reefer" cigarettes, chewed, or drunk. In this country most addicts are maladjusted adolescents.

The effects of this drug are almost entirely on the central nervous system. It produces a dreamy state of partial consciousness in which the subject's ideas are disconnected and uncontrollable. The subject may have a feeling of well-being, exaltation, and excitement; or he may sink into a depression or panic state. Delirium may ensue. Violent acts have been committed under the influence of this drug. Its continued use results in mental deterioration.

Barbiturates. The barbiturates, which are sold under various trade names such as Luminal, Amytal, Seconal, Nembutal, etc., are habit-forming for some persons. Taking these drugs because of sleeplessness and nervousness, subjects may become dependent upon them somewhat as they become dependent upon alcohol or the opiates. Self-medication with these drugs is therefore inadvisable. Approximately two-thirds of the states have passed laws preventing the sale of barbiturates except on a physician's prescription.

CAUSE OF ADDICTION

Narcotic addicts as a group are emotionally immature childlike persons, who never have made a proper adaptation to the problems of living. They experiment with the use of these drugs for adventure, for the pleasant sensation supposed to ensue, for the relief of fatigue, or for escape from reality. Most normal individuals find the results disappointing and unpleasant, but a few weaker ones have taken their first steps toward addiction. Little do they realize how the first few steps take them on a downward path from which there is no turning back.

Once addiction is established the victim is no longer his own master. These powerful drugs give rise to an abnormal craving which will not be denied and which can be satisfied only by more of the drug. No matter what the cost in money, reputation, or professional advancement the drug addict must have his customary doses of narcotics. If the supply is interrupted, the addict becomes virtually insane and will sink to poverty or crime to satisfy his craving. Withdrawal causes such severe suffering that few addicts have the moral courage and strength to discontinue the habit. Over 50 per cent of the inmates of corrective institutions in New York City are drug addicts and 90 per cent of that number are young people. Every young drug addict is a potential criminal.

PREVENTION OF ADDICTION

Law enforcement and education are the two most effective measures for the prevention of drug addiction. Confirmed addicts need hospital treatment. The U.S. Public Health Service provides this treatment in special hospitals for narcotic addicts. To be admitted, the individual patient must make application to the Surgeon General of the U.S. Public Health Service.

Efficient enforcement of the narcotic laws and apprehension of those engaged in the illicit traffic of narcotic drugs will eliminate the availability of the drug to both confirmed and potential addicts. Public appreciation of the seriousness of the problem is necessary for such law enforcement and control.

Education of boys and girls concerning the illicit traffic in drugs and the dangers of addiction will prevent many of them from taking that first ill-considered step toward addiction. This, combined with the development of wholesome social interest and activities, will eliminate the clubs and dens of narcotic users and marijuana smokers.

DISCUSSION SUGGESTIONS

1. Discuss the physiological effects of caffeine. Is there evidence that its habitual use is harmful?
2. What is the drug contained in tobacco and what effect does this have upon animals?
3. Upon what does the "strength" of tobacco depend? Is strength an indication as to the nicotine content of tobacco?
4. Discuss the more important physiological effects of smoking. What real evidence is there that smoking is deleterious?

5. Is there any evidence that smoking by a mother may be harmful to her offspring?
6. If one decides to smoke, what precautions should be observed?
7. Discuss the more important physiological effects of alcohol.
8. What is the relation of the use of alcohol to automobile accidents? To resistance to disease? To physical efficiency?
9. Discuss the social and economic effects of alcohol and their relation to health.
10. What is the relation of the use of alcohol to the length of life? What diseases may be caused by alcohol?
11. Discuss the medicinal value of alcohol.
12. What, if any, justification is there for the use of alcoholic beverages?
13. Discuss the reasons you think that most people have for drinking.
14. What is the effect of the various narcotic drugs upon the nervous system?
15. Explain the relations between crime and narcotic addiction.
16. Would you as an employer give a position to a person who used narcotic drugs of any kind? Why?
17. How can narcotic addiction be controlled?

REFERENCES AND READING SUGGESTIONS

TEA AND COFFEE

1. Hawk, P. B.: "A Study of the Physiological and Psychological Reactions of the Human Organism to Coffee Drinking," *American Journal of Physiology*, vol. 90, p. 380, 1929.
2. Hollingsworth, H. L.: "The Influence of Caffeine Alkaloid on the Quality and Amount of Sleep," *American Journal of Psychology*, vol. 23, p. 89, 1912.
3. ———: "The Influence of Caffeine on Mental and Motor Efficiency," *Archives of Psychology*, No. 22, April, 1912.
4. ———: "The Influence of Caffeine on the Speed and Quality of Performance in Typewriting," *Psychological Reviews*, vol. 19, p. 66, 1912.
5. Lashley, K. S.: "The Effects of Strychnine and Caffein upon the Rate of Learning," *Psychobiology*, vol. 1, p. 141, 1917.

TOBACCO

1. Brean, H.: "How to Stop Smoking," Vanguard Press, Inc., New York, 1951.
2. Earp, J. Rosslyn: "The Student Who Smokes," The Antioch Press, Yellow Springs, Ohio, 1925.
3. Hamilton, A. E.: "This Smoking World," Appleton-Century-Crofts, Inc., New York, 1927.
4. Narr, Ray: "Cancer by the Carton," *Reader's Digest*, December, 1952.
5. Riis, Roger William: "How Harmful Are Cigarettes?" *Reader's Digest*, January, 1950.

6. Wood, Frank L.: "What You Should Know about Tobacco," Zondervan Publishing Company, Grand Rapids, Mich., 1944.

ALCOHOL

1. Bacon, Selden: "The Facts about Alcoholism," *U.S. News & World Reports*, October 2, 1953.
2. Hagaard, H. W., and E. M. Jellinek: "Alcohol Explored," Doubleday & Company, Inc., New York, 1942.
3. Jellinek, E. M., and Mark Keller: "Alcoholism in the United States of America, 1940–1948," *Quarterly Journal of Studies of Alcohol*, New Haven, Conn., 1952.
4. Lovell, Harold: "Hope and Help for the Alcoholic," Doubleday & Company, Inc., New York, 1951.
5. "What You Should Know about Alcoholism," U. S. Public Health Service, Washington, D.C.
6. Yahraes, Herbert: "Alcoholism is a Sickness," 5th ed., Public Affairs Pamphlets, New York, 1948.
8. Lay Supplements issued by *Journal of Studies on Alcohol*, New Haven, Conn.
   a. The Problems of Alcohol.
   b. Production and Properties of Alcoholic Beverages.
   c. Alcohol and Industrial Efficiency.
   d. Facts on Delirium Tremens.
   e. Alcohol, Heredity, and Germ Damage.
   f. Alcoholic Beverages, Health, and Length of Life.
   g. What Happens to Alcohol in the Body.
   h. Alcoholic Beverages as a Food and Their Relation to Nutrition.
   i. Facts on Cirrhosis of the Liver.
   j. How Alcoholic Beverages Affect the Body.
   k. How Alcoholic Beverages Affect Behavior.
   l. Alcohol and Crime.
   m. Government and the Alcohol Problem.
   n. Moderate and Excessive Users of Alcoholic Beverages.

NARCOTICS

1. Chester, Francis: "Shot Full; The Autobiography of a Drug Addict," Methuen & Co., Ltd., London, 1938.
2. "Conferences on Drug Addiction among Adolescents," The Blakiston Company, New York, 1953.
3. Howe, Hubert S.: "Narcotics and Youth," Brook Foundation, West Orange, N. J.
4. Steven, Alden: "Make Dope Legal," *Harper's Magazine*, November, 1952.

5. Taylor, Norman: "Flight from Reality: The Marvelous History of Hashish, Marihuana, Opium and Opiates, Peyote, the Coca Leaf, Alcohol, Tobacco, Coffee and Other Drugs and Stimulants," Duell, Sloan & Pearce, Inc., New York, 1949.
6. Walton, R. P.: "Marihuana; America's New Drug Problem," J. B. Lippincott Company, Philadelphia, 1938.
7. Williams, H. S.: "Drug Addicts Are Human Beings (the Story of Our Billion Dollar Drug Racket, How We Created It and How We Can Wipe It Out,)" McGraw-Hill Book Company, Inc., New York, 1938.
8. "What You Should Know about Drug Addiction," U. S. Public Health Service, Washington, 1952.

Chapter X

EXERCISE—FATIGUE—REST

THE advice for keeping fit most frequently given by physicians and laymen alike is plenty of sleep, an adequate but not excessive diet, and regular, moderate exercise and recreation. There are people who are healthy with little or no exercise, but the vast majority of us feel better, sleep better, and get more fun out of life if we take regular exercise and enjoy some recreational sport.

Every generation of man until the present depended largely upon physical activity for its livelihood. But modern life has changed this. Urbanization, mechanical transportation, innumerable laborsaving devices, and specialization in human endeavor have made it possible to live with a minimum of physical activity. Will this undermine health and eventually result in physical deterioration of the race?

A minimum of exercise is necessary for healthy living. If that minimum of exercise is not performed, muscles lose strength and flexibility to the point where they will be predisposed to orthopedic difficulties. One of our most common orthopedic difficulties—backache—is frequently caused by such lack of exercise. If strength of trunk muscles and flexibility of back and leg muscles drop below a certain level, backache frequently results.

Proponents of exercise point to the physical perfection of the ancient Greeks, to the great endurance of primitive peoples, to the exuberant health of physically active youth, and to the an-

[218]

cient adage "a sound mind in a sound body." According to some "physical culturists," exercise and diet will prevent everything from neurasthenia to cancer, from baldness to flat feet.

Others feel that we have been uncritical and have gone too far in our enthusiasm for physical exercise. They point out that the animals that live longest are those which take the least exercise. The indolent tortoise has been known to live 200 to 300 years, and the elephant, which lumbers lazily about, frequently attains 150 to 200 years. On the other hand, the more physically active animals have relatively short spans of life, the dog living only 10 to 15 years, the hare 7 to 8, and the mouse 3 to 4.

The Effects of Exercise upon the Body

The most obvious effect of regular exercise on the body is an increase in muscular development. Soft, flabby muscles become hard and firm. This improves personal appearance, increases strength and endurance, and enables one to enjoy physical activities.

More directly related to health, however, are the effects of exercise upon the general metabolic processes of the body. The rate and the force of the heartbeat are increased, breathing becomes deeper and more rapid, and heat production and perspiration are increased.

The energy to support exercise is derived from the oxidation (burning) of food substances, largely carbohydrates and fats. This results in an improved appetite and increased elimination, and in children a stimulation of growth.

One occasionally hears the term "athletic heart" but even physicians do not know exactly what it means. In fact, recent investigations of the subject have led to the conclusion that there is no such thing as athletic heart.

The heart is a muscular pump which, like other muscles, tends to enlarge as a result of strenuous work. The hearts of very active animals like the squirrel and rabbit are relatively larger in proportion to body size than the hearts of less active animals. On the other hand, this enlargement is merely muscular development and is in no sense an evidence of damage.

[219]

This muscular pump of ours performs enough work every 24 hours to lift a weight of 10 to 15 tons to a height of 5 to 6 feet; and it keeps this up day after day, year after year. Furthermore, on many occasions it is suddenly called upon to increase enormously the amount of work which it is doing. Hence, it is of vital importance to keep the heart in as good condition as possible at all times. Moderate exercise will aid in this and so is beneficial rather than detrimental.

Studies of the effect of exercise upon the human heart have been made in connection with the National Games in Vienna, the Olympic Games in Amsterdam, and the Marathon races in Boston. All sorts of tests were used in these examinations but in each instance the conclusion was that amateur athletics, even as strenuous as the Olympic games, have no deleterious effect upon the normal heart. The Vienna studies suggested, however, that some types of professional athletics, such as rowing, long-distance swimming, and bicycle riding, may be followed by evidence of heart damage.

EXERCISE TO REDUCE WEIGHT

Exercise increases the combustion of carbohydrates and fats and so is frequently advocated for the reduction of weight. In principle this is reasonable, but the difficulty arises from the fact that exercise also stimulates the appetite and so leads to an increased consumption of food. To be effective in the reduction of weight, exercise must be combined with dietary control. Exercise alone is futile.

EXERCISE AND LENGTH OF LIFE

Some years ago Dr. Pearl[1] reported that an analysis of the mortality statistics of Englishmen, the most comprehensive and accurate in existence, shows a direct and positive relationship between the expenditure of physical energy as indicated by occupation and the age at death. This means that, after deducting deaths from accidents and from hazards peculiar to the various

[1] Pearl, Raymond, "Studies in Human Biology," The Williams & Wilkins Company, Baltimore, 1924.

occupations, a high death rate tends to be associated with those occupations which involve hard physical labor. This relationship prevails whether the labor is performed chiefly indoors or outdoors.

Another very different approach to this problem was made by Dr. Pearl[2] under the controlled conditions of his laboratory when he observed the relation of the length of life of a species of flies to their activity. From this study he concluded that the more rapid the rate of energy expenditure the shorter the duration of life. In other words, the length of life varies inversely with the rate of living.

The early deaths of certain prominent college athletes have led to a rather general impression that participation in intercollegiate athletics tends to shorten life. The implications of this are of such importance that an extensive study of the question was made some years ago under the direction of Dr. Louis I. Dublin.[3] This study comprised a computation of the death rates, twenty or more years after graduation, of 5,000 college athletes and 5,000 nonathletes.

The first analysis showed a 3 per cent lower death rate among the athletes than among the preferred risk of life insurance policy-holders. Next a comparison was made among the athletes in the different sports. This gave rather surprising results, for the highest death rate was among the athletes who had won letters in baseball; next came those who had won letters in crew; next in track; and at the bottom of the list was football. And still below the football players were those who had won letters in two or more sports. On first thought this might suggest that the more strenuous the sport or the more extensive the participation the greater the benefit to health. Actually, it probably indicates nothing more than that it requires a better physique to win a letter in football or in two or more sports than in baseball, crew, or track.

The slightly lower death rate among athletes than among the

---

[2] Pearl, Raymond, "The Rate of Living," Alfred A. Knopf, Inc., New York, 1928.
[3] Dublin, Louis I., "Longevity of College Athletes," *Harper's Magazine*, vol. 159, p. 229, July, 1928.

accepted risks for life insurance suggested that possibly athletic participation was beneficial rather than detrimental. On the other hand, it is known that college graduates as a group are unusually good insurance risks. This led to a second study in which the death rate for the 5,000 athletes was compared to the rate for 5,000 of their classmates who did not participate in athletics. Between these groups no differences of any significance appeared.

An interesting supplement to this study was a computation by Dr. Dublin of the death rate for those students, athletes and non-athletes, who had attained scholastic distinction as indicated by election to honorary scholastic societies. Queerly enough, this group had a death rate lower than either the athletes or non-athletes. In other words, if one desires a long life it may be better to "make" Phi Beta Kappa than to win a letter in college sports.

PHYSICAL FITNESS[4]

Fitness is a state of mind and body in which the tissues have power and efficiency. A program of physical fitness includes the teaching of good personal hygiene. This in turn means enough sleep, proper nutrition, controlled exercise and rest periods, mental hygiene and recreation. The person who is fit has a great deal of what sport writers call "bounce." His mind and body are resilient and elastic. He recovers promptly from minor bruises to his tissues or his personality.

The great victories which were won in the Second World War by American troops all over the world were not won by men who were physical weaklings. The American soldier proved himself to be a competent fighter. He represented a selection of the best physical specimens of our nation, developed to fighting efficiency by the training program of our armed forces.

On the other hand, there are evidences of physical deficiencies in our population which are capable of prevention and in many instances of correction. Many of the 4,000,000 men who were rejected for military service during the Second World War could have been made physically fit had the advantages which medical

[4] Adapted in part from "Health and Physical Fitness," by Morris Fishbein, *Hygeia*, p. 815, November, 1946.

science and physical education have to offer been made available to them. Many were pampered and soft and in need of physical conditioning. It is folly for a nation as wealthy and efficient as ours to fail in its utilization of what medical science has to offer for developing a nation that is physically fit.

Improvement of physical fitness must begin even before birth, with proper prenatal care. It must continue through infancy with an immunization program that will prevent many of the infectious diseases of childhood and their crippling complications. It must go on through nursery and kindergarten, where sound habits of nutrition begin to be established. It must carry through grade school, high school, and college, where sound instruction in health habits and physical activities, including competitive sports, should be integrated in the curriculum. Finally, when the boy or girl has left school, there must be continuing participation in healthful living, sports, and recreational pastimes to maintain the physical fitness that the schools have established.

Recent studies[5] show that school children of certain areas in our country are much less fit muscularly than their counterparts in certain European countries. While 57 per cent of our children failed to pass a battery of six simple muscle tests, only 9 per cent of the Europeans failed. The progressive mechanization of our country has all but eliminated spontaneous physical activity in our children. It is necessary to make a conscious effort to replace this lack.

PHYSICAL FITNESS AND NATIONAL EMERGENCIES

Whether or not physical exercise is essential to good health or longevity in normal times, there can be no question as to the importance of physical fitness in times of war or preparation for war. A national emergency places upon every citizen, and particularly upon men and women of college age, a deep personal obligation both to themselves and to their country in the matter of health and physical fitness.

[5] Kraus, Hans, and Ruth Hirschland: "Muscular Fitness and Orthopedic Disability," *New York State Journal of Medicine*, January 15, 1954; and "Health and Muscular Fitness," *Journal of the American Association for Health, Physical Education and Recreation*, December, 1953.

Recognizing this, many colleges and universities are providing special programs and facilities to assist their students to meet this obligation. Physical examinations, tests of physical fitness and of knowledge concerning the essentials of personal and group hygiene are offered. On the basis of these findings personal advice is given, facilities for the correction of physical defects are made available, and individualized programs of physical activity and instruction are provided. It is the moral responsibility of every physically qualified student to avail himself of this opportunity to make himself physically fit for the service which he may be called upon to render in the defense of his country.

A RATIONAL RECREATION PROGRAM

Whether or not exercise improves the health or adds to the length of life, it is common experience that a certain amount of regular exercise contributes to a feeling of well-being. Furthermore, exercise which involves play and recreation, and relieves nervous tension and mental fatigue in so doing, is not only pleasant but beneficial.

How much and what kind of exercise one should take merit careful consideration. The growing child and the normal young man and young woman thrill with the exhilaration of strenuous sports. They fatigue to the point of exhaustion but recover promptly with a period of rest. But not so with those of middle age and beyond. For them moderation is of vital importance, especially if they have been inactive for a long time. Higher levels of physical activity can be maintained by regular exercise.

Just how much exercise a person of a given age can safely take it is impossible to say. Individual variability is too great to permit of generalization. A game of tennis may be perfectly safe for one person of forty but folly for another. The safe limit for exercise depends upon the condition of the heart, the condition of the muscles, the type of exercise, and the regularity with which it is taken. Two general suggestions, however, will serve as sound advice for anyone. The first is to determine periodically the condition of the heart and general health by careful, thorough physical examinations, administered by a physician. The other is to keep the exercise below the point of physical exhaustion. A sense of pleasant relaxation or moderate fatigue after exercise is desirable, but exercise to the point of extreme fatigue may do serious damage and is likely to be more deleterious than no exercise at all.

Proper balance of rest and exercise is required. Heavy exercise occasionally or even once a week may be more detrimental than helpful. Heavy eating, smoking, and drinking between exercise occasions "add insult to injury."

The type of exercise to be preferred depends upon one's physical condition. Young people can safely enjoy vigorous competitive sports such as tennis, handball, and squash, but most older persons do better to limit themselves to less strenuous activities. Walking, golf, swimming, sailing, skating, and horseback riding are among the sports that one can enjoy and safely participate in throughout life. To be of greatest benefit, physical activities should involve recreation as well as exercise and take one out of doors into the fresh air and sunshine. Regularity is important if one is to get the most enjoyment and benefit out of exercise.

Setting-up Exercises. In the modern physical education program formal exercise drills have been largely replaced by recreational sports. There are times, however, when it is difficult or impossible to get even an outdoor walk. For such occasions the "daily dozen" is offered (see posture exercises on page 226).[6] Setting-up exercises have been discredited mainly because they have been "given so atrociously." If well given and well directed, they are an important supplement to sports and often the only practical substitute.

POSTURE[7]

Good posture is an asset to any man or woman, boy or girl. It improves personal appearance; suggests poise, self-confidence, health. Many an applicant for a position makes an unfavorable first impression because of poor posture.

[6] See also Tunney, Gene, "It's More Fun to Be Fit," *The Reader's Digest*, vol. 40, p. 17, February, 1942.

[7] Note report on your own posture, Appendix C.

The importance of posture to health has been grossly exaggerated, but after all the chaff has been blown away there still remains a distinct relationship between the two. Stooped shoulders and exaggerated spinal curvatures throw extra strain upon the muscles of the legs and back. A protruding abdomen permits sagging of the abdominal organs, which in turn interferes with function. All of this predisposes to fatigue, and fatigue in turn predisposes to poor posture; thus, a vicious cycle is set up.

The makers of kidney pills have succeeded in associating backache and kidney disease in the minds of most people. In reality true kidney disease is rather rare, and when it does occur it is almost never accompanied by backache. On the other hand, backache, which is common, is usually due to poor posture or flat feet or both. Relief is obtained not by taking kidney pills but by correcting the cause of the trouble.

Poor posture may be due to heredity, to habit, to fatigue, to poor development and use of the muscles of the back, abdomen, and legs, or to a combination of these factors. For the improvement of posture, exercise is a basic requirement if trunk-muscle weakness and poor flexibility of back and hamstring muscles are involved. Rest, until muscular fitness is restored and emotional balance attained, is important. Correction of poor habits, proper seating and sleeping facilities are essentials.

Whatever the cause of poor posture, the chances of correcting it are greatest in childhood and decrease progressively with age. The habits of children are still in a formative stage; their ligaments and muscles are still adaptable and their bones not completely calcified.

POSTURE EXERCISES

Posture exercises should be prescribed on an individual basis after proper evaluation of the person's needs. This includes muscle tests and structural evaluation. In general, however, exercises which are useful to improve posture are those which tend to strengthen the muscles of the back and abdomen. Some simple exercises to accomplish this are as follows:[8]

[8] Quoted with permission from "Standing Up to Life," Metropolitan Life Insurance Company, New York.

1. *Lying on the Back; Hands Back of Neck.* Take a deep breath and raise chest high; keep chest up and exhale by pulling abdomen in hard.

2. *Same Position; Knees Bent, Feet Pulled Up.* Pull abdomen in hard and then relax part way; also done standing with hands clasped on top of head.

3. *Sitting in a Chair; Trunk Bending Forward.* Incline trunk forward from the hips, keeping spine straight. This is the position which should be taken when bending forward to write or to do any other kind of desk work. The absence of the lowered chest and rounded back and shoulders of the incorrect position is striking. This exercise may be done standing.

4. *Standing; Abdominal Retraction.* Stand with the heels four inches away from the wall, but with the hips, shoulders, and head touching the wall; flatten the lower part of the back against the wall by pulling in the abdominal muscles. This causes a downward rolling motion in the lower part of the back and flattens the lumbar curve. Holding this position, come away from the wall with the weight well forward on the balls of the feet. This suggests the correct standing position, but it should be held in a graceful, flexible manner.

5. *Standing; Leg Raising.* Stand with hands on hips, back flat and chin in; raise leg forward without bending the knee; lower it; repeat with other leg. This exercise teaches how to hold the back flat while balancing the body and doing a leg exercise.

6. *Carrying the Head Forward, Clasp Hands behind the Head.* Force the head back against their pressure, keeping chin in. This strengthens the muscles of the back of the neck.

7. *Spinal Curvatures.* "Stand tall," holding the back straight, rise on the toes with the arms extending forward and up, stretching the arms and the body.

8. *Distended Abdomen.* This condition may be successfully prevented and largely overcome by doing Exercises 2 and 4.

PAINFUL ARCHES

Our lowly, misused, misshapen feet are at last coming into their own. A doctor in eastern Canada and imitators in various parts of this country have been "curing" all sorts of human ills merely by twisting the foot—and "pulling the leg." Sufferers flocked to this little Canadian village from all over the country; and many came away benefited. But they were helped, not by the foot twisting, but by their faith in the quackery and by a better fitting pair of shoes than they had before.

As a matter of fact, painful feet are responsible for an enormous amount of backache, headache, fatigue, nervous irritability, and other related disturbances. The prevalence of arch trouble is suggested by the enormous number of so-called "corrective" shoes on the market. Some of these are beneficial, but a shoe salesman is hardly a dependable health adviser.

That the problem is not merely one of shoes or of exercise is shown by the following quotations from the Metropolitan Life Insurance Company's pamphlet on this subject:

CORRECT POSITION OF FEET IN STANDING

Most foot troubles come from an improper use of the feet in standing and walking—sometimes an incorrect posture is taken because of the pressure of an uncomfortable shoe, sometimes because of carelessness or ignorance.

In standing, point the feet straight to the front and place them from two to four inches apart. Support the weight on the outside of the feet. Frequently remind yourself of this correct position while standing by "gripping the floor" with all the toes. This exercise lifts the long arch and places the whole foot in a correct position. Standing for a long time in this position is less tiring than when the feet are turned out or the ankles are allowed to bend in.

FAULTY SHOES CAUSE FOOT MISERY

Shoes should be so made that the inner edge of the sole is straight. When the inner edge of the sole curves toward the middle of the toes, it crowds the toes and forces the great toe into an unnatural position. Shoes should be long enough and wide enough for the toes to lie straight and slightly separated. They should be roomy over the toes, and fit snugly around the heel and over the instep.

Take plenty of time when buying shoes. Try on both shoes of a pair. Shoes may seem to be comfortable when you stand with your weight distributed upon both feet, but when you throw all the weight upon one foot, the shoe may feel quite different, and you may find it not at all comfortable.

Some women say they must wear high heels to be comfortable. Yet high heels are undoubtedly the cause of many sore feet, aching backs and touchy tempers. They are frequently the cause of the falling of the front arch, painful callouses, contracted toes and corns.

High heels tend to tilt the body forward unnecessarily in standing and walking. When that is done, the body must use muscular effort to hold itself upright. In doing so, the spine may be curved unnaturally and the abdominal organs thrown out of place.

Some persons may be able to wear high heels all their lives without injury or discomfort. Others may go for many years apparently unharmed. But usually a time comes, during or after middle life, when both feet and body rebel against unnatural treatment, and ailments of many kinds develop.

If a woman persistently wears high heels, the muscles at the back of her leg will grow short from lack of use. Then, if she tries to come down suddenly to sensible heels or to tennis shoes, she will feel a tremendous strain upon the heel cord. In such cases, relief may be had by going back to the higher heels and coming down gradually to the lower.

ARCH TROUBLES AND THEIR CAUSES

The most common foot ailment is that known as "fallen arch," "flat-foot" or "weakfoot." It is the flattening of the long arch that extends from the heel to the great toe. One of the first symptoms is a pain under the arch and up the back of the leg. There is a change also in the print made by the wet foot. The normal footprint is narrow in the middle and wide at the heel and at the toes. The flat foot leaves a footprint that is almost the same width through its entire length.

Some persons are born with flat feet, and apparently suffer no distress from them, unless called upon to do an unusual amount of foot work. Persons whose feet become flat, however, feel various pains and aches, become extremely tired after a little walking or standing, and their ankles tend to bend in.

As implied earlier, one of the causes of flatfoot or fallen arch is toeing out. Another is improper shoes; another, lack of exercise for the foot muscles.

A very painful condition of the foot is the flattening of the anterior or metatarsal arch, which extends across the ball of the foot from the base of the great toe to the base of the little toe. At this point, specialists say, 90 per cent of the foot troubles of women are to be found.

The first warning of an unnatural condition of this arch is pain in the three outer toes and directly under the ball of the foot. Another sign is a painful callous in the middle of the ball of the foot. Such a callous shows that there is irritation in this particular spot, resulting from the arch having dropped.

This trouble is frequently due to a sole that bends down under the ball of the foot and bends up at the sides. This allows the short front arch to drop. The pain may be relieved to some extent by changing to shoes with soles that are flat. A spot of thin padding, about the circumference of a half-dollar, under the ball of the foot, placed slightly back of the center of the arch; or a band of rubber webbing or adhesive plaster bound around the foot, back of the arch, may give relief.

A doctor with special experience in treating feet is needed for foot troubles. It is not wise to buy various arches and supports or special shoes without the advice of a doctor or an orthopedic specialist.

The feet, including the toes, are made for walking. With the growing use of the automobile, and with elevators to take the place of stairs, men and women are walking less and less, thereby frequently causing the foot muscles to become flabby and various foot troubles to develop. Walking in com-

[229]

fortable, well-fitted shoes is one of the best ways to keep the feet healthy. For curing foot troubles, special exercises are often prescribed by the physician.

EXERCISES TO STRENGTHEN THE FEET

Exercise 1. *Outward Roll.* Remove shoes and stockings. Stand with weight on both feet; feet about 6 inches apart. Roll the feet outward twelve to thirty times, so that the weight of the body is supported on the outer edge of the feet. Lift the inner parts of the feet clear of the floor at each roll.

Exercise 2. *Rising on Toes, Barefoot.* Stand with feet parallel, 6 to 8 inches apart. Rise on the ball of the foot, twisting heels inward and trying to grasp the floor with the toes.

Exercise 3. *Lifting Arch, Barefoot.* Stand with feet parallel. From the abnormal position with the feet relaxed and the ankles bending in, tighten up to a straight leg, straight ankle position. This will lift the arch from the floor, and hold it in the normal position. It may not be easy at first to do this exercise without lifting the inner edge of the foot, but the exercise is so helpful that the ability to do it is worth considerable effort.

Exercise 4. *Walking on Toes, Barefoot.* Not so easy, but wonderful for strengthening the toes. Walk on tiptoe until you find you must drop back on the whole foot.

Exercise 5. *Flexing Toes, Barefoot.* Flex the toes, then "fan out," extend, and relax them.

Exercise 6. *Ankle Bending, Barefoot.* Sit on a chair, resting your legs on another chair of the same height; your knees stiff; feet and toes stretched out in slightly pigeon-toed position. Then count four, at the same time bending the ankles and bringing the toes toward you as much as possible. You will feel a noticeable pulling of the calf muscles.

NOTE: These exercises should be begun gradually so as to avoid excessive fatigue of the muscles involved. When possible, they should be performed morning and evening. Do one exercise three or four times, then go on to the next until all have been done. Then repeat the whole series.

Fatigue

Fatigue is familiar to all mankind. In moderate degrees it brings pleasant relaxation and serves as nature's best sleeping potion. On the other hand "The man who said 'the harder the toil the sweeter the rest' was never profoundly tired."[9]

The sensation of fatigue is really a sensation of pain, produced by the action of certain toxic products upon the nerve centers of the brain. These toxins may be produced in the muscles as a by-product of the oxidation of food substances to supply energy for

[9] John Muir.

the support of physical activity; they may be the toxins from a general or a localized infection in the body; or they may be absorbed from the digestive or respiratory tracts. But whatever their source, they enter the blood stream and are circulated throughout the body, modifying activities and producing sensations far removed from their point of origin.

Muscular fatigue from physical activity is first recognized as a sensation of moderate discomfort, but if the activity is continued this gradually develops into true pain, which eventually becomes so excruciating that the continuation of the activity is impossible. In fact, fatigue may well be considered a protective mechanism, for pain causes cessation of muscular activity before the muscles are completely exhausted. Evidence of this is the fact that electrical stimulation will cause a muscle to contract after the limit of voluntary contraction has been reached.

War correspondents commented repeatedly upon the fatigue of the men in combat zones. One of them described this fatigue as follows:

In the morning you start out tired, and by the end of the day a deadly fatigue sets in. You can see it in a man, for fatigue is a poison just like a noxious drug. His yellow face, bad breath, rivulets of sweat, glazed eyes— these are only some of the physical symptoms of fatigue, and from them come other more disastrous effects.

As hours and days pass you fall more and more often. When you have got a load on your back, that sometimes means broken limbs, and it always means further accumulation of fatigue. Your resistance to cold becomes less, your digestive organs work badly, your nerves become even more frayed. You lose weight, sleep, confidence. Every day more and more men go under.[10]

ACUTE AND CHRONIC FATIGUE

Acute fatigue is the inevitable result of severe physical or emotional activity. The condition of health and of physical training influences the susceptibility to fatigue and the rate of recovery. Children fatigue more easily than adults but also recuperate more quickly. Extreme fatigue is never beneficial and may be deleterious, particularly to older persons.

[10] Mathews, H. L., "Road of Mud, Fatigue and Glory," *The New York Times Magazine,* December 26, 1943.

[231]

Various acute infections, such as influenza, tonsillitis, and colds, cause fatigue very similar to that produced by physical activity. Recovery from this fatigue is usually prompt after the termination of the infection.

Chronic fatigue is a different story. It lowers vitality day after day, week after week. Rest gives temporary, but only temporary, relief, and life hardly seems worth the effort. Such fatigue is evidence of ill-health.

It is common knowledge that tuberculosis may cause chronic fatigue; but so also may sinus infection, diabetes, heart disease, and a host of other diseases. In alcoholics and drug addicts fatigue is a prominent symptom; in some persons the use of tobacco causes chronic fatigue. A diet which is inadequate in proteins, vitamins, or certain minerals results in fatigue even though its energy content is sufficient. Eyestrain, constipation, indigestion, painful feet, poor posture, disturbances of certain glands of internal secretion, and nervous instability and emotional strain are among the other common causes of chronic fatigue.

THE EFFECTS OF FATIGUE

The most striking effects of fatigue are upon the nervous system, where it produces irritability, nervousness, restlessness and insomnia. Trifles become disturbing. Enthusiasm is gone; attention distracted; judgment warped. The whole world looks drab. The most amiable disposition is ruined by it. Child specialists tell us that many behavior problems in children are due to nothing more or less than fatigue.

There is considerable evidence that fatigue lowers resistance to disease. And it very definitely interferes with recovery from infections. The death rate from influenza is highest among those who refuse to "give up," and the patient with tuberculosis who tries to build up his health by physical exercise, even in the out-of-doors, is throwing away his chance for recovery.

RELIEF OF FATIGUE

For the relief of fatigue one thinks first of rest. And rest, physical and mental, is important; but unfortunately even for fatigue there is no panacea.

Fatigue is a symptom which will disappear only when the basic trouble is corrected. Therefore, the starting point for relief of chronic fatigue should be a determination of its cause. If this happens to be diabetes or sinus infection or faulty nutrition, medical science has a very definite solution to offer. If painful arches are at the bottom of the trouble, proper shoes and exercises will give results. If one's job is monotonous, physical and mental efficiency will be improved by making a change in jobs for part of the day. If worry or nervous tension is the inciting cause, a game of bridge, an engrossing book, a good play, or a game of golf is the best treatment.

The drugs which are used for the relief of fatigue may be divided into two groups: those which depress sensation and so lessen the feeling of fatigue, and those which stimulate the higher nervous centers to carry on in spite of fatigue. The former group is made up primarily of alcohol and the narcotics, such as morphine and cocaine and their derivatives. Alcohol may cause a temporary diminution in the sense of fatigue, but this is followed by even greater fatigue and depression than existed before. Morphine and cocaine depress sensibilities but are dangerous habit-forming drugs which should never be used except under the direction of a physician. The federal narcotic agents tell us that it is common practice for narcotic peddlers to employ accomplices who offer these drugs to their boy and girl associates to "give them a lift" from the fatigue of the day's work so that they can enjoy the evening's fun. The narcotic peddler gets his "pound of flesh" by draining the very lifeblood out of those who become addicts.

Caffeine has long been used as a stimulant to offset fatigue, and, except for the nervousness and insomnia which it causes in some persons, no known ill effect results from its use. The same cannot be said for the so-called "pep pills"—benzedrine sulphate tablets—which are coming into use by students, particularly when studying for examinations. These tablets are more powerful stimulants than caffeine but they make some persons so nervous and jittery that they are unable to sleep or do concentrated work for several days. A few serious toxic results have been reported from their use.

[233]

Clearly, the attempt to obtain relief from fatigue by drugs, either depressant or stimulating, is unsound. Fatigue is nature's warning that rest is needed. To silence this warning signal or to whip one's body along in spite of it can only lead to catastrophe.

Rest

Facilities for exercise abound on every hand. Nearly every community has its gymnasium and its playground. Great national organizations, educational institutions, and even governments support athletic programs. Many industries and some department stores operate rest and relaxation rooms for their employees. But who ever heard of providing a place for rest and relaxation for the general public? The very suggestion seems fantastic. Yet how many weary, footsore people are crowded into the business districts of our cities every day? People for whom a few moments of relaxation would give life a different hue. People who need rest, not exercise.

Industries, studying the work records of employees throughout the day, find that efficiency declines toward the latter part of the morning, improves after lunch, and then declines again more rapidly in the afternoon. They find also that accidents are most frequent during the periods of accumulating fatigue; and that 15-minute rest periods in midmorning and midafternoon result in increased efficiency which more than compensates for the time "wasted."

Many individuals have made similar discoveries concerning their own well-being. One of the most famous surgeons in the world long made it an inviolate rule to have a 15- or 20-minute rest each day after lunch. No matter where he was or how pressed for time, he slipped away for a brief doze and returned refreshed. This practice of relaxation undoubtedly was an important factor in the maintenance of his health and vitality through many years of a strenuous and useful life.

The habit of relaxation is worth cultivating. A few minutes on a davenport or comfortable chair with the eyes closed, the mind at rest, and every muscle relaxed will do much to conserve physical and nervous energy. At first complete relaxation probably can be attained for only a few minutes at a time but this should be increased to at least 10 or 15 minutes once or twice a day.

The time may come when we shall have rest clubs as well as athletic clubs; but not yet. We are still too much inclined to boast of the small amount of rest on which we can get along. We still cling to the mad desire to get everything done in a day. To entice the average American to rest in the daytime one must camouflage the rest with mysterious measures such as light treatments, massage, or sun bathing. Possibly when as a nation we have grown up, we shall learn, as many of the old-world countries have learned, to take life more leisurely, to get a little more out of life as we go along, with a friendly chat and a cup of tea to break the tension of the day.

Sleep

From birth until death the body is never completely at rest. Energy expenditure goes on even during sleep. On the other hand, sleep is the nearest one ever comes to absolute rest. It is the time when the body's stores of vital energy are replenished. This respite from activity is essential to life. The longest that anyone has been known to live without sleep is not quite ten days. Laboratory animals deprived of sleep die of exhaustion.

Scientists have not yet agreed concerning the physiological mechanism which produces this condition in which we spend about a third of our lives. One of the most widely quoted theories is that sleep is due to a decrease in the blood supply to the brain. Another theory is that the accumulation of waste products in the blood produces fatigue of the brain cells so that activity ceases and sleep results. Still another theory suggests a special sleep-producing toxin.

The existence of such theories is evidence that the exact mechanism of sleep is not well understood. It is agreed, however, that during sleep certain definite physiological changes occur. Pulse rate and blood pressure are decreased; respirations are slower and deeper; and glandular secretions diminish. Consciousness is lost but the subconscious portion of the brain continues its activity. Evidence of this is found in the answers to questions which may be given during sleep, without the sleeper's regaining consciousness, and the ability of many people to awaken at specified hours when they wish to do so.

The intensity of sleep varies throughout the night, being deepest during the second and third hours and then becoming progressively lighter until waking. Noises, excitement, worry, and dreams affect the restfulness and diminish the benefits of sleep.

It is familiar knowledge that most deaths occur during the early morning hours. This is the time when vital processes, as indicated by temperature, metabolism, blood pressure, and heart action, reach a low point. Hence, it is easily intelligible that the spark of life should succumb to exhausting diseases at this time. But it does not explain the frequency of apoplexy and sudden death from heart disease in persons who retired apparently in good health. Similar attacks occur during waking hours as the result of unusual stress, strain, or effort, which throws an extra burden upon brittle arteries or a weakened heart.

Why these accidents should occur during sleep when the blood pressure is lowered and the work of the heart reduced has long been a puzzling question. The explanation of some of these cases may be contained in the observations of MacWilliam of the University of Aberdeen. Dreams, as is well known, are of very short duration; a long, complicated dream transpires in a matter of a few seconds. During some of these brief dreams there is intense emotional excitement during which the pulse rate increases, the heartbeat becomes more forceful, and the blood pressure rises. In one case MacWilliam reports that the pulse increased from 70 to 90 beats per minute and the blood pressure from 130 to over 200 millimeters. This means an intense strain suddenly thrown upon the heart and blood vessels—a strain under which a weakened heart or blood vessel may give way.

For years it had generally been supposed that restful sleep was quiet and relatively motionless. "Sleeping like a log" implied a perfect night. Ingenious scientists, however, who devised instruments and cameras to record and photograph every movement of the sleeper, tell us that a sleeper rarely remains in one position

THE
HUMAN
BODY

THE HUMAN BODY

An accurate knowledge of the architecture of the human body is of great importance to students in hygiene, nursing, and physiology. The anatomical plates on the following pages have been specially prepared and included in this text to provide a ready reference source not only of the various structures of the body, but also of their relationships to one another.

The various body systems are shown in the natural color of healthy tissues, and special attention has been paid to labeling the structures and organs that are usually discussed in college-level courses. It is suggested that frequent reference to this section will prove invaluable in helping the student visualize more clearly the body as a functional organism. To facilitate their use, certain illustrations have been placed on facing pages for easier comparison, and the same general body outlines have been used throughout. Furthermore, all structures are shown in proportionate size to afford a clearer understanding of their size and the space they occupy in the body.

These illustrations were prepared by Robert J. Demarest, Medical Illustrator, in consultation with a number of medical authorities.

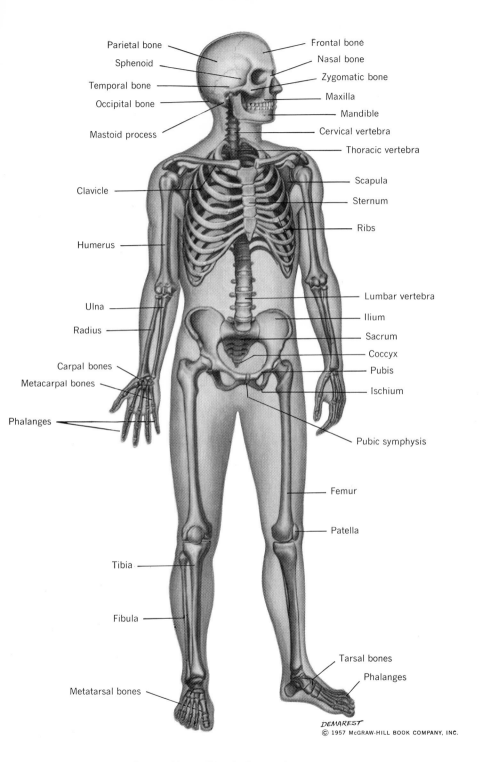

Parietal bone

Sphenoid

Temporal bone

Occipital bone

Mastoid process

Clavicle

Humerus

Ulna

Radius

Carpal bones

Metacarpal bones

Phalanges

Tibia

Fibula

Metatarsal bones

Frontal bone

Nasal bone

Zygomatic bone

Maxilla

Mandible

Cervical vertebra

Thoracic vertebra

Scapula

Sternum

Ribs

Lumbar vertebra

Ilium

Sacrum

Coccyx

Pubis

Ischium

Pubic symphysis

Femur

Patella

Tarsal bones

Phalanges

DEMAREST

© 1957 McGRAW-HILL BOOK COMPANY, INC.

PLATE A   SKELETAL SYSTEM (anterior view)

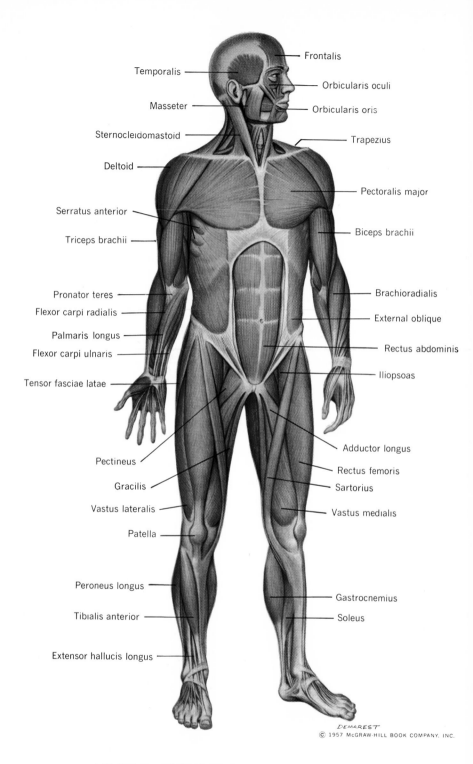

Frontalis

Temporalis

Orbicularis oculi

Masseter

Orbicularis oris

Sternocleidomastoid

Trapezius

Deltoid

Pectoralis major

Serratus anterior

Biceps brachii

Triceps brachii

Pronator teres

Brachioradialis

Flexor carpi radialis

External oblique

Palmaris longus

Rectus abdominis

Flexor carpi ulnaris

Iliopsoas

Tensor fasciae latae

Adductor longus

Pectineus

Rectus femoris

Gracilis

Sartorius

Vastus lateralis

Vastus medialis

Patella

Peroneus longus

Gastrocnemius

Tibialis anterior

Soleus

Extensor hallucis longus

DEMAREST
© 1957 McGRAW-HILL BOOK COMPANY, INC.

PLATE B   MUSCULAR SYSTEM (anterior view)

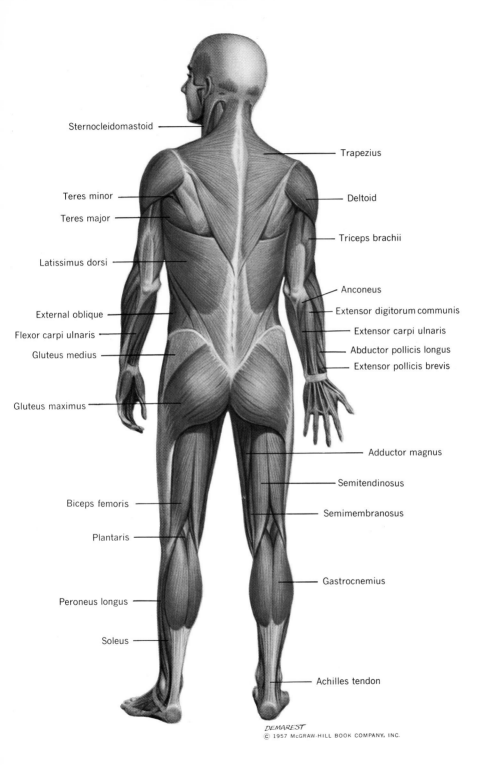

Sternocleidomastoid

Trapezius

Teres minor

Deltoid

Teres major

Triceps brachii

Latissimus dorsi

Anconeus

Extensor digitorum communis

External oblique

Extensor carpi ulnaris

Flexor carpi ulnaris

Abductor pollicis longus

Gluteus medius

Extensor pollicis brevis

Gluteus maximus

Adductor magnus

Semitendinosus

Biceps femoris

Semimembranosus

Plantaris

Gastrocnemius

Peroneus longus

Soleus

Achilles tendon

PLATE C   MUSCULAR SYSTEM (posterior view)

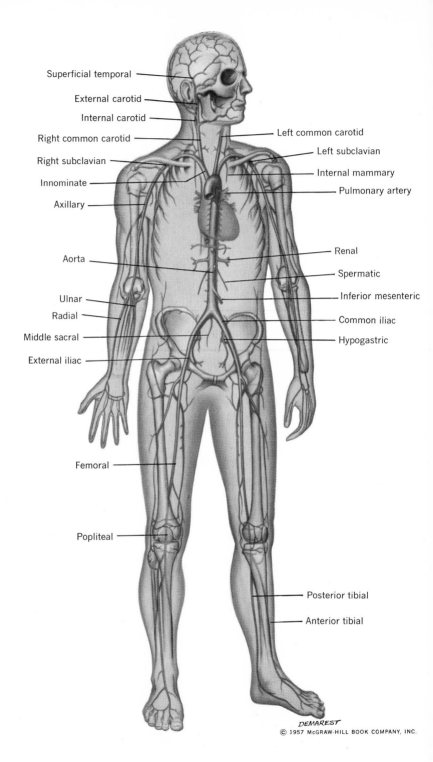

Superficial temporal

External carotid

Internal carotid

Right common carotid

Right subclavian

Innominate

Axillary

Aorta

Ulnar

Radial

Middle sacral

External iliac

Femoral

Popliteal

Left common carotid

Left subclavian

Internal mammary

Pulmonary artery

Renal

Spermatic

Inferior mesenteric

Common iliac

Hypogastric

Posterior tibial

Anterior tibial

DEMAREST
© 1957 McGRAW-HILL BOOK COMPANY, INC.

PLATE D ARTERIAL SYSTEM

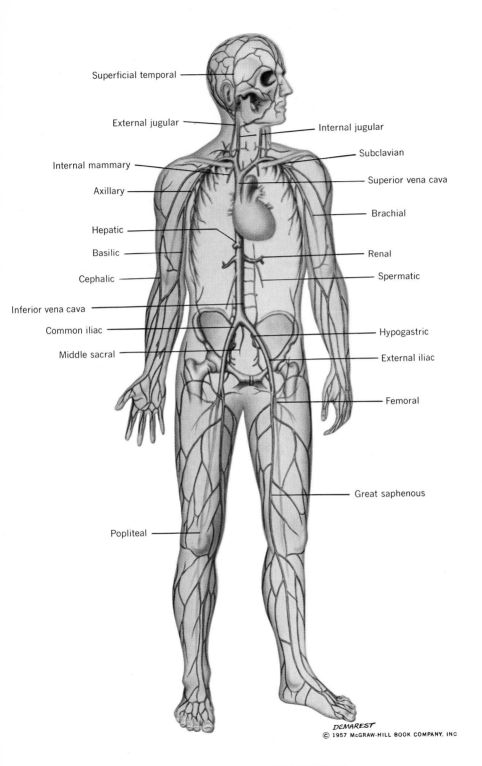

Superficial temporal

External jugular

Internal jugular

Subclavian

Internal mammary

Superior vena cava

Axillary

Brachial

Hepatic

Basilic

Renal

Cephalic

Spermatic

Inferior vena cava

Common iliac

Hypogastric

Middle sacral

External iliac

Femoral

Great saphenous

Popliteal

DEMAREST
© 1957 McGRAW-HILL BOOK COMPANY, INC

PLATE E   VENOUS SYSTEM

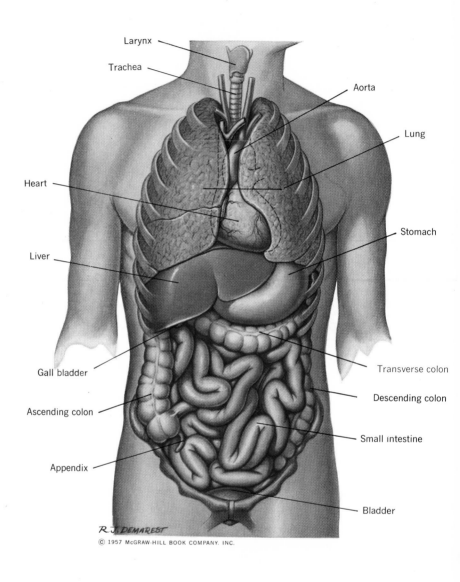

Larynx

Trachea

Aorta

Lung

Heart

Stomach

Liver

Gall bladder

Transverse colon

Descending colon

Ascending colon

Small intestine

Appendix

Bladder

R. J. DEMAREST

PLATE F   VISCERA

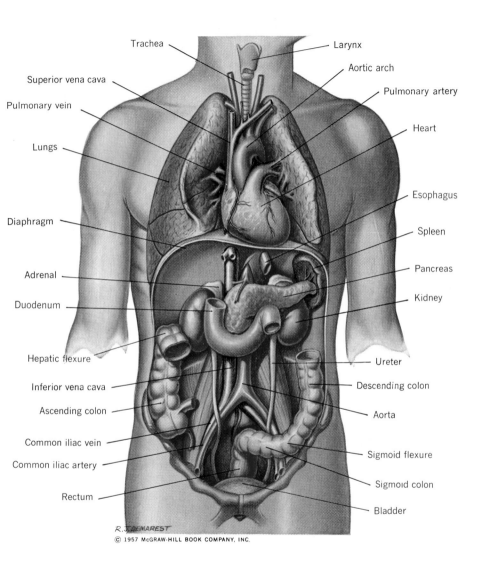

Trachea

Larynx

Superior vena cava

Aortic arch

Pulmonary artery

Pulmonary vein

Heart

Lungs

Esophagus

Diaphragm

Spleen

Adrenal

Pancreas

Duodenum

Kidney

Hepatic flexure

Ureter

Inferior vena cava

Descending colon

Ascending colon

Aorta

Common iliac vein

Sigmoid flexure

Common iliac artery

Sigmoid colon

Rectum

Bladder

R. J. DEMAREST

PLATE G   VISCERA (deep structures)

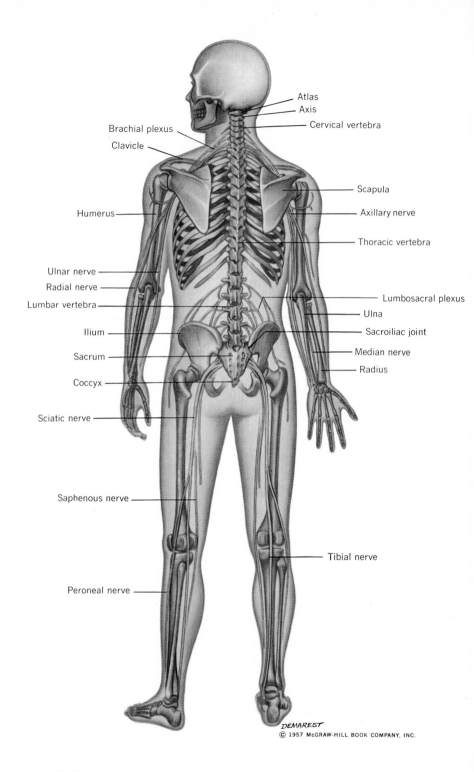

Atlas
Axis
Cervical vertebra
Brachial plexus
Clavicle
Scapula
Humerus
Axillary nerve
Thoracic vertebra
Ulnar nerve
Radial nerve
Lumbar vertebra
Lumbosacral plexus
Ulna
Ilium
Sacroiliac joint
Sacrum
Median nerve
Coccyx
Radius
Sciatic nerve
Saphenous nerve
Tibial nerve
Peroneal nerve

DEMAREST
© 1957 McGRAW-HILL BOOK COMPANY, INC.

PLATE H   SKELETAL SYSTEM (posterior view showing spinal nerves)

INDEX

ABOUT THE ARTIST

ROBERT J. DEMAREST's medical illustrations have appeared in many texts and medical journals as well as in several popular weekly magazines. Such a variety of uses clearly indicates the appeal of the life-like medical illustrations this young artist does. Trained at the Art Students' League and the School for Medical Illustrators, Demarest on graduation was honored as the recipient of the Saunders' Fellowship in Medical Art at the University of Pennsylvania. Mr. Demarest is currently associated with the College of Physicians and Surgeons, Columbia University.

for more than 10 to 15 minutes at a time. He shifts his arms and legs; he tosses and rolls at intervals all night.

The general effects of loss of sleep are fatigue, poor general health, irritability, nervousness, inability to concentrate, and lowered perseverance of effort. Accuracy, memory (particularly), and speed are adversely affected.

The hours of sleep necessary to relieve fatigue and restore physical and nervous energy vary with many factors, such as age, the degree of fatigue, the state of general health, and nervous and emotional control. The infant under one month of age sleeps from 21 to 23 hours a day. The child of six to eight years requires approximately 12 hours of sleep. The boy or girl from thirteen to fifteen requires from 9 to 10 hours. For the average person of middle age the normal requirement is approximately 8 hours. With the approach of old age the sleep requirement again increases.

INSOMNIA

The inability to sleep is not a disease itself and is rarely due to disease. Its beginning is usually traceable to nervousness, worry, or pain. Caffeine interferes with the sleep of some people but has no appreciable effect upon others. Moderate fatigue induces sleep but excessive fatigue results in restlessness and insomnia.

Most people who have difficulty in sleeping become obsessed with the fear that they will be unable to sleep. This leads to emotional disturbances which make sleep and rest still more difficult.

For the prevention of insomnia physical exercise sufficient to produce moderate fatigue is usually helpful. A leisurely walk in the fresh air may be all that is necessary. A warm bath, not a hot one, and a glass of warm milk at bedtime aid in relaxation and hence are useful to induce sleep. The various milk drinks which advertisers claim are aids to sleep probably have no more value than milk alone, but people like to be fooled.

Until recently sleep-producing drugs were little used except to control pain, but their consumption in this country has been increasing at an enormous rate. For this purpose the barbiturates, sold under fancy names and at fancy prices, are most widely employed. Used occasionally and upon the advice of a physician, these are distinctly useful drugs. They bring welcome sleep to many distraught persons. But the regularity with which they are taken and the reliance placed upon them by an increasing number of persons are cause for concern. Stimulation throughout the day with tobacco, coffee, and alcohol, and sleep at night with the aid of drugs can lead only to disaster.

Furthermore, some of the widely used sedatives contain a drug, called "amidopyrin" or "pyramidon," which destroys the white blood corpuscles of certain people. As a result of this, resistance to infection is so lowered that a common cold may result in sudden death. During a recent three-year period 1,300 deaths in the United States were attributed to the use of pain-relieving or sedative medicinal preparations containing these drugs. Only a small proportion of people are thus affected by it, but there is no way of knowing to whom it will be toxic; hence, the only safe course to follow is to avoid all medications which contain it. This obviously can be done only by refusing to use medicinal preparations with trade names unless the ingredients are known.

DISCUSSION SUGGESTIONS

1. Discuss the adage "a sound mind in a sound body."
2. Explain the physiological effects of exercise. Is there evidence that regular, strenuous physical exercise will improve health and prolong life?
3. Discuss the term "athletic heart."
4. Outline what you think would be a rational exercise program for an attorney forty-five years of age.
5. Do setting-up exercises have any value? If so, what?
6. Why is good posture an asset? How may posture be improved?
7. Discuss the psychological, anatomical, and physiological aspects of poor posture.
8. What is the proper position of the feet in standing and walking?
9. Discuss the causes, the effects, and the prevention of painful feet.
10. What are the causes and the effects of fatigue? Are these all undesirable?
11. Discuss the various methods which are used for the relief of fatigue.
12. Explain the value of rest periods during the day in industry.
13. What physiological changes occur during sleep?
14. What are the usual causes and the best methods of preventing insomnia?

REFERENCES AND READING SUGGESTIONS

1. Bartley, S. H., and E. Chute: "Fatigue and Impairment in Man," McGraw-Hill Book Company, Inc., New York, 1947.

2. Cureton, Thomas: "Physical Fitness Work Book," The C. V. Mosby Company, St. Louis, 1947.
3. Jacobson, E.: "You Must Relax," McGraw-Hill Book Company, Inc., New York, 1934.
4. ———: "You Can Sleep Well," McGraw-Hill Book Company, Inc., New York, 1938.
5. Kraus, Hans: "Therapeutic Exercises," Charles C Thomas, Publisher, Springfield, Ill., 1949.
6. Martin, Rudley: "How to Care for Your Feet," *Hygeia*, vol. 25, p. 845, November, 1947.
7. Read, Dudley B.: "Keep Fit and Like It," McGraw-Hill Book Company, Inc., New York, 1939.
8. Steinhaus, A. H., and others: "How to Keep Fit," Consolidated Book Publishers, Chicago, 1943.
9. "Posture from the Ground Up," Metropolitan Life Insurance Company, New York.
10. "Sleep," Metropolitan Life Insurance Company, New York.
11. Maisel, A. J.: "Why Do We Get So Tired—And What Can We Do about It?" *Today's Health*, September, 1954, and *The Reader's Digest*, September, 1954.

Chapter XI

SUNLIGHT AND FRESH AIR

YEAR after year the awakening of life, the unfolding of nature under the vitalizing energy of the sun's rays, presents convincing evidence that the sun exerts a powerful influence upon living things. Observing this, primitive people from the equator to the poles have worshiped the sun and have erected temples to the Sun God. Some of these ancient temples included terraces for sun bathing.

There was then, and there still is, much of mystery and magic concerning the beneficial effects of sunlight. This has made possible its exploitation by uncritical and unscrupulous charlatans and has been the basis of much fanaticism in connection with its use.

What Is Light?

To you and to me light is that which enables us to see, but to the physicist light consists of waves of electromagnetic energy which travel through space at the rate of 186,000 miles per second. It requires about eight minutes for light to travel from the sun to the earth, 92,900,000 miles. The astronomer uses the speed of light to measure distance, his unit, the light-year, being the distance that light travels in a year, about six million million miles. The most distant stars which can be seen with the unaided eye, the Andromeda nebula, are 800,000 light-years away.

In the rainbow one sees the effect of passing sunlight through drops of water. The scientist achieves this same effect, that is, the sorting out of light-waves according to their length, by the use of a prism. This throws the long light-waves in one direction and the short waves in the other, with waves of intermediate length being serially arranged between the two extremes. By so doing he finds that only about 13 per cent of the electromagnetic waves in sunlight are visible to the human eye. The longest of the visible rays we see as red, the shortest as violet, with blue, green, yellow, and orange between. About 80 per cent of the electromagnetic waves in sunlight are longer than the visible red rays. These rays are called "infrared" and produce heat. They have considerable penetrating power, as one may sense inside a window on a sub-zero day. The remaining 7 per cent of the waves in sunlight are shorter than the visible violet and are called "ultraviolet" rays.

The proportion of these various waves in sunlight is always the same, but the relative amounts of them that reach the earth vary enormously with the season of the year and the condition of the atmosphere. They are at their maximum when the sun is directly overhead and the atmosphere perfectly clear. Smoke, dust, and fog impede the passage of all these rays but most seriously reduce the ultraviolet, which has the least penetrating power. Even window glass filters out most of the ultraviolet in sunlight. During the winter months, when the sun's rays are most oblique, the ultraviolet rays which reach the earth are frequently reduced to 10 per cent of the amount which reach the same localities during the summer.

ULTRAVIOLET LIGHT

The light rays which have the greatest known effect upon health belong to the ultraviolet group. In order to be effective these rays must penetrate the superficial layers of the skin of animals or the leaves of plants. For maximum effect, direct and unobstructed exposure is necessary. Still, there is sufficient deflection of these rays by various objects or by particles in the air so that some ultraviolet reaches points which receive no direct sunlight.

[241]

The stimulating effect of direct sunlight may be observed in the difference between the growth of flowers and shrubs on the shady and on the sunny side of a house. That this difference is due largely to ultraviolet light can be demonstrated experimentally. In a study conducted by the Massachusetts Agricultural College, at the end of 38 days radishes which had been exposed to ultraviolet light were 69 per cent heavier and head lettuce 76 per cent heavier than radishes and lettuce from the same batch of seeds and raised under identical conditions except that the plants did not receive any direct ultraviolet irradiation. In another experiment a dozen hens under ordinary conditions laid 124 eggs in 16 weeks, while a second dozen hens from the same broods which were exposed to ultraviolet light for 10 minutes each day laid 479 eggs in the same space of time. Such observations have led to the equipping of chicken houses with artificial light to provide ultraviolet rays or with window glass such as quartz or Vitaglass, which permits the passage of the ultraviolet rays of sunlight.

The effect of ultraviolet light upon the health of mankind is due largely to its influence upon the utilization of calcium and phosphorus. This influence is exerted indirectly through the formation of vitamin D, which is produced by the action of ultraviolet light upon certain sterols (oils) in the skin. Other effects of ultraviolet light upon the body are a small increase of certain types of white blood corpuscles, a temporary reduction of blood pressure, and a slight increase in the pulse and respiratory rates.

Ultraviolet rays destroy bacterial life, most bacteria being killed by 2 hours of exposure to sunlight in the middle of the day. On the other hand, the idea that exposure of the body to light will destroy bacteria within the body is without foundation, for ultraviolet rays do not penetrate as much as $\frac{1}{25}$ inch into the normal skin.

INFRARED RAYS

The red and infrared rays produce heat when they come in contact with objects which absorb them. Dark clothing is said to look hot and light clothing cool, and so they are, for dark colors absorb these rays while light colors refract them. Infrared rays coming in contact with the body produce heat, and heat relieves pain, brings relaxation, and stimulates blood flow.

LIGHT AND HEALTH

Although the importance of sunlight to health is beyond question, the enthusiastic advocates of light treatments and sun bathing make claims for it far beyond any possible justification. A booklet circulated to physicians lists ninety-four diseases which are supposed to be benefited by ultraviolet irradiation of the body. In this list we even find such conditions as appendicitis, acidity of the stomach, fractures, obesity, and tonsillitis. This booklet was written by a physician but was prepared for and circulated by a company which sells sun lamps. Such exorbitant claims interfere with the better understanding and the intelligent use of light in the field of medicine.

Actually there is only one disease which is definitely due to insufficient sunlight, and that is rickets. Infants uniformly develop this disease unless they are exposed to ultraviolet radiation or are supplied with vitamin D in some other way. It is not necessary, however, to expose the entire body to ultraviolet light in order to obtain the beneficial effect from it, for it has been shown that generalized rickets can be cured by exposing only a small portion of the skin to the light.

Certain other diseases, although not due to a lack of sunlight, are favorably influenced by properly administered light treatments. Noteworthy among these are certain skin diseases, such as acne and psoriasis; tetany; and tuberculosis of bones, glands, peritoneum, and intestines. In other forms of tuberculosis the use of ultraviolet light may be detrimental. Sunlight aids in the healing of wounds on the surface of the body and in some cases seems to have a beneficial effect upon the appetite, digestion, hemoglobin formation, and general well-being of individuals who are below par as a result of severe illness or protracted ill-health. It is well known that children with rickets are unusually susceptible to colds, bronchitis, pneumonia, measles, whooping cough, and

[243]

tuberculosis; hence, ultraviolet light has been widely advocated for the prevention of these conditions. Carefully controlled studies, however, have failed to establish its value in this regard.

THE DANGERS OF SUNLIGHT

The irritating effects of sunlight upon the skin are a universal experience each spring or summer. Moderate exposure produces a sensation of warmth and relaxation followed by a slight flushing of the skin, while prolonged exposure results in irritability and sleeplessness and inflammation of the skin with blistering and destruction of tissue. Absorption of toxic products from such areas may result in severe generalized reactions. Patients may have headache, vomiting, fever, nausea, and general malaise from an overdose of sunshine without any blistering or even redness of the skin.

The tanning which follows exposure to sunlight is nature's effort to protect the body from the irritating effects of the sun's rays. Chronic irritation is known to be one of the causes of cancer. The skin is as susceptible as any other part of the body to such irritation. Skin cancer occurs most frequently on the exposed parts of the body, and among persons who work outdoors or who tan themselves excessively.

A curious susceptibility to light occasionally shows in the development of hives or skin rashes from even a brief exposure to ultraviolet rays. Still more unusual and puzzling are the individuals who develop multiple cancers of the skin as a result of exposure to light. These persons, usually children, get along satisfactorily as long as they are kept in the dark, but exposure to light causes the appearance of brown, pigmented areas, much like freckles, which gradually develop into multiple skin cancers. In medical terminology this is "xeroderma pigmentosa."

Another ill effect of excessive tanning is the drying and wrinkling effect of the sun's rays upon the skin. Those who wish to avoid looking old before their time should not attempt to bake themselves to an Indian brown each summer. If they do, they must expect wrinkles, like those of the Indians, in middle or later life.

[244]

SUNSTROKE, HEAT PROSTRATION, AND HEAT CRAMPS[1]

Normal persons differ greatly in the ability to withstand heat, the very old, the very young, the obese, and those with systemic disease being most easily affected by it. Alcoholics and persons who have once had sunstroke are particularly susceptible to its effects and require especial protection against it. Excessive exposure to heat may give rise to heat prostration, heatstroke, or heat cramps.

Heat prostration, or heat exhaustion, is a condition in which collapse and depression of the nervous system predominate. Extreme weakness, dizziness, pallor, and perspiration are the common symptoms. Consciousness is not lost. The temperature is normal or nearly normal. The onset usually occurs during the exposure to heat but may be delayed for several hours. Ordinarily recovery is rapid and complete.

Heatstroke, or sunstroke, is a much more serious condition. The onset may be sudden, with delirium, stupor, and instantaneous death, or it may be more gradual with mental excitement or depression, dryness of the mouth and skin, dizziness, and headache. The temperature becomes very high—frequently 107 to 110 degrees. The skin is intensely hot and usually dry but may be moist.

Heat cramps, also called "stoker's cramps," are painful muscular spasms, particularly of the abdominal muscles and of the extremities. They may, however, be so generalized as to simulate epilepsy. They are due to excessive sweating from hard labor in furnace rooms, foundries, metal mines, etc. The patient is usually pale, nauseated, dizzy, and depressed. His temperature is normal and his pulse is rapid but strong.

The immediate treatment of all heat-induced disturbances demands removal of the patient to the coolest place available, rest in the recumbent posture, and the supplying of salt and water. The patient should be urged to quench his thirst with

---

[1] The following consideration of this subject has been largely quoted or adapted from Dr. Bernard Fantus, "Therapy of Disturbances Due to Heat," *Journal of the American Medical Association*, vol. 103, p. 990, September 29, 1934.

water containing a level teaspoonful of salt to a quart. Milk, orangeade, and lemonade should be given every 2 hours and a physician called. In extreme heat exhaustion, stimulation with coffee or aromatic spirits of ammonia, 15 drops in water, may be beneficial. In heat stroke rapid cooling of the body is imperative. This may be accomplished by removing most of the clothing and sprinkling the patient with a sprinkling can or watering hose, while maintaining a constant current of air by fanning.

Preventive treatment is identical for the various disturbances due to excessive heat. It must embrace (1) increasing heat elimination, (2) lessening heat production, and (3) minimizing exposure to heat, while (4) maintaining the heat regulating center in optimum functional condition.

When the human body must maintain its normal temperature in spite of an external heat near to or even above that of the system, its chief defense is the evaporation of sweat. Therefore the production of sweat should be favored. This requires the ingestion of an abundance of water, maybe from twelve to fifteen glasses a day. The frequent taking of small quantities is better than large drinks at long intervals. This is especially true when the circulation is enfeebled. Carbonated drinks are preferable because they leave the stomach more rapidly, as the stomach does not absorb water. Profuse sweating robs the body of large amounts of salt. Therefore salt should be taken in unusual amounts, four to five teaspoonfuls daily, with the food or the drink. A level teaspoonful to a quart of water or 1 gram tablet with each tumblerful is the best concentration. This becomes less necessary after acclimatization has occurred, which in part consists of the ability to secrete extremely dilute sweat. The liberal use of fruit juices is particularly important.

When sweat production is not free enough, the skin—most especially the head and hair—should be kept wet with cold water, and frequent cool baths may be required.

Sweat cools a person only when it evaporates. The sweat that runs off "in streams" is lost as far as heat regulation is concerned. Sweat evaporation must therefore be favored by loose, light, thin, non-constricting clothing or practically no clothing at all and by exposure to air currents produced by fans or between open shaded windows.

Heat production should be minimized by reducing muscular exertion as much as possible when the heat is intense. The midday siesta is a hygienic necessity in hot climates. Work should be done in the cooler part of the day. Work that must be done during very hot weather should be carried on in short periods alternating with rest.

Food should be light and highly digestible, moderate in amount and largely consisting of carbohydrate, with avoidance of fats because of their high caloric value and of protein because of the large amount of heat freed during its assimilation. Juicy fruits should be especially favored.

Exposure to the direct rays of the sun should be avoided, for the visible and the ultraviolet rays are the most dangerous, especially when they impinge directly on the head. Should such exposure be unavoidable, tropical helmets should be worn. Forced marching in heat and sunshine should be done in open formation so as to prevent heat and humidity stagnation, and it necessitates frequent halts in the shade. During a halt one should, if possible, avoid resting directly on the ground, for the air just above the sunned ground is hottest.

The heat regulating mechanism should be protected against intoxication by liquor and other narcotics, as well as by coffee, tea, or tobacco, for all these have an unfavorable effect on it and, in the last analysis, on the heat regulating center upon which devolves the business of maintaining the normal body temperature.[2]

SUN BATHING

Sun bathing has enthusiastic devotees, who tell of health being restored and vitality preserved by the simple and pleasant expedient of regularly exposing the body to the rays of the sun. The true sun worshiper, undaunted by the winter's cold, finds for himself a protected spot where he may carry on his rituals uninterrupted the year around. He labels as amateurs the multitudes who cover the beaches during the summer months but lose their enthusiasm under the blasts of the autumn winds.

Sun bathing *in moderation* is doubtless beneficial to most persons. Its chief physiological effects have been enumerated, but in addition there is a stimulating effect of ultraviolet light upon the skin and a general physical and nervous relaxation, with psychic as well as physical benefits therefrom. Of its psychic effects Stuart Chase says:

Interminable, drowsy conversations were always in progress. We talked of law, science, government, women, crime, sports, history, races—without passion, with a detached philosophy which held, I am convinced, an authentic wisdom. The sun nourishes that wisdom, that all-pervading power. Beating down upon us it ironed out the taut impetuosity, the nervous, hasty judgments, the bile and the bitterness of men who walk the streets of cities in their clothes. Unclothed and in our right minds we lay, at peace with the

[2] Fantus, *loc. cit.*

world, detached and lazy, like the gods upon Olympus, speculating upon the foibles of humanity, not caring greatly where the race was going or why.[3]

An English physician reports that:

. . . none are brighter in their spirit than those who are sun-worshipers in the most literal sense, and not only are they more vigorous, more alert, gayer in spirit, but there is a stimulating effect upon the mentality of patients receiving insolation. The effect of sun treatment upon the nude recumbent patients at Alton and Hayling Island was to raise their mental activity on the average of 10 per cent above that of the ordinary child. If all school children had the benefit of at least one or two months of insolation annually there is no doubt that it would have a profound effect upon their education generally and the improvement of both their bodies and their minds.[4]

Woodruff,[5] on the other hand, suggests that excessive sunlight is a cause of backwardness in the tropics and recommends that examinations for promotion in the army not be held there because of the universal loss of memory experienced.

Nudism. The growth of nudist cults has been attracting attention in various parts of the world. Advocated as a health measure, it is in reality only an exaggerated form of sun and air bathing. Since, however, as much benefit may be obtained by exposing a portion of the body to the sun's rays as by complete exposure, it would seem that the nudists could well adopt practices which would be less sensational and more aesthetic.

ARTIFICIAL SUNLIGHT

In recent years the American market has been flooded with devices for providing "sunlight" indoors. The better of these give off a considerable proportion of ultraviolet radiation. Others give off no ultraviolet rays whatsoever. Light treatments prescribed by a competent physician are of real value in a limited number of conditions; but their excessive and indiscriminate use by all sorts of pseudomedical practitioners is blatant quackery and tends to discredit them entirely.

[3] Chase, Stuart, "Confessions of a Sun-worshiper," *The Nation*, vol. 178, p. 762, June 26, 1929.

[4] Gaubain, H., "Effects of Sun, Sea, and Open Air in Health and in Disease," *Practitioner*, vol. 118, p. 137, March, 1927.

[5] Woodruff, C. E., "The Effect of Tropical Light on White Men," Medical Art Agency, New York, 1905.

Fresh Air

Everyone knows that fresh air is important to health. Yet most of the ideas as to what is meant by fresh air and why it is important are erroneous.

One can live for weeks without food, for days without water, but only a few minutes without air. Air is drawn into and expelled from the lungs about eighteen times a minute. The blood takes up oxygen from this air and discharges carbon dioxide, also called "carbonic acid gas," into it. This has long been known and upon it most of the impressions concerning the relation of air to health have been built. On the other hand, the physical conditions of the air with which the body is continuously surrounded have been largely ignored. Extremely hot or cold air has been known to influence comfort, health, and even life itself, but not until recently have these physical conditions of the air been carefully studied. Now they are conceded to be of the greatest importance in ventilation and in air conditioning.

THE COMPOSITION OF AIR

The air consists of a mixture of gases which surround the earth. Of these nitrogen makes up 78 per cent; oxygen, 21 per cent; carbon dioxide, 0.04 per cent; and argon and various other rare gases, a little less than 1 per cent. Altitude makes some difference in the amount of oxygen in the air, but analyses have shown that at similar altitudes air from many parts of the world is surprisingly uniform in composition. The breathing of air reduces the oxygen and increases the carbon dioxide content by approximately 5 per cent.

OXYGEN AND CARBON DIOXIDE OF NO PRACTICAL IMPORTANCE IN VENTILATION

An old method of testing the condition of the air in a room was to light a candle and observe how it burned. If the flame was dim, this was said to be evidence that ventilation was bad and that the oxygen was being depleted. Scientifically this conclusion is valid, but practically the test has no value, because even under conditions of very poor ventilation the oxygen is never reduced to a degree which would be indicated by this test.

The tragedy of the Black Hole of Calcutta, in which all but 23 of 146 prisoners perished overnight in a room 18 by 14 by 10 feet, is usually attributed to suffocation. The two small windows on one side of the room, however, were adequate to supply all the oxygen necessary. Consequently, it has been concluded that the deaths were caused, not by a lack of oxygen or an excess of carbon dioxide, but by the physical condition of the air, that is, the high temperature, the high humidity, and the accumulation of noxious vapors.

Our bodies have become adjusted to functioning best in an atmosphere containing about 21 per cent of oxygen. On the other hand, the actual amount of oxygen in the air may vary considerably without producing any ill effects. At high altitudes, such as Pike's Peak, the air contains only about two-thirds as much oxygen as at sea level. Newcomers to these altitudes experience increases in the rate of the pulse beat and of respiration, but no harm results. And after a time even these effects disappear, for the body becomes adjusted, in part by an increase in the number of red blood corpuscles, to the lower oxygen concentration.

Nitrogen, which constitutes about 78 per cent of the air, is an inactive gas with no effect upon the body. Carbon dioxide also is essentially a nonpoisonous gas. Charged waters and sparkling wines contain it in concentrated form, yet they cause no ill effects. Outdoor air normally contains about 4 parts in 10,000, but the atmosphere in the crowded sections of cities may contain about five times this much. It is now recognized that a concentration of 3 per cent in the air we breathe, that is, 300 parts in 10,000, produces no unpleasant symptoms; and that although 5 per cent, 500 parts in 10,000, causes an increase in the rate of respiration, it is not really toxic. The carbon dioxide content of the air of homes and office buildings rarely exceeds two-tenths of 1 per cent, 20 parts per 10,000. To have any noticeable effects upon the body it would have to be fifty to one hundred times as great as this. Hence, we need have no concern about the oxygen and carbon dioxide content of the air of the buildings in which we live and work.

AIR PRESSURE

The human body adjusts to moderate changes in atmospheric pressure without difficulty, but marked increases or decreases in atmospheric pressure may seriously affect health. Conditions of increased pressure are found chiefly in mines or tunnels. Men can work under these increased atmospheric pressures provided they accustom themselves gradually to the change. The greater pressure causes an increase in the amount of oxygen and nitrogen dissolved in the blood. This produces no ill effects so long as one remains in the high-pressure atmosphere, but it may have serious consequences if one passes quickly to an atmosphere of low pressure. With the reduction in atmospheric pressure the excess gases dissolved in the blood are released. The oxygen causes no difficulty because it is immediately taken up by the tissues; but if the reduction in pressure is sudden, the nitrogen, which is not utilized by the body and which takes some time to pass through the membranes separating the blood vessels from the air sacs of the lungs, tends to form bubbles in the blood stream, just as the carbon dioxide in a bottle of ginger ale forms bubbles when the cap is removed. These bubbles are carried along in the blood stream and tend to plug some of the tiny blood vessels. This causes a disease commonly called "the bends," or caisson disease, the usual symptoms of which are nose bleed, abdominal pain, nausea, vomiting, dizziness, paralysis, and unconsciousness. Prevention of caisson disease depends upon gradual decompression.

Low atmospheric pressures are having practical health importance with the perfection of airplanes to fly at high altitudes. The difficulties are due to the diminished amount of oxygen available in the rarefied atmosphere. The first noticeable signs of oxygen deficiency are impairment of mental concentration, disturbance of muscular coordination, accelerated pulse and respiration. These have been observed at altitudes of 8,000 to 12,000 feet, an elevation frequently used in transcontinental flying. More severe degrees of oxygen deficiency produce faulty judgment, symptoms typical of alcoholic intoxication, hilarity or pugnacity, and instability; and muscular effort causes great fatigue and may injure the heart.[6] Greater degrees of oxygen-want cause unconsciousness and eventual death. To prevent these conditions, aeronautical engineers have perfected sealed cabins for planes which fly at high altitudes, with oxygen introduced from tanks in order to maintain the desired concentration. Combat pilots and crews have oxygen supplied to them from tanks by means of tubes and inhalation masks.

THE BODY MUST BE COOLED

The greater importance of the physical over the chemical properties of air is apparent from an experiment in which subjects were placed in sealed glass chambers, the air conditions of which could be regulated and recorded. When distress was reported by the subjects in the chambers, the temperature was about 85 degrees Fahrenheit and the humidity high. Analysis of the air showed some increase of carbon dioxide and a slight reduction of oxygen. This, however, was not responsible for the discomfort, for the breathing of fresh air from a tube leading to the outside gave no relief, and persons on the outside experienced no discomfort from breathing the air of the chamber from a tube. But relief did occur when the temperature was lowered, the humidity decreased, and the air set in motion.

Heat is constantly being produced by the body, and unless this is promptly eliminated the body temperature will rise, discomfort will ensue, and in time life will be destroyed. The chief methods for getting rid of body heat are by direct transference to the surrounding air and by evaporation. When the temperature of the air is lower than the temperature of the body, heat loss is largely by direct transference; but when the temperature of the air is higher than the temperature of the body, evaporation becomes the more important method of the heat loss. Both these mechanisms are influenced by the humidity and motion of the air.

[6] Barach, A. L., "Pilot Error and Oxygen Want," *Journal of the American Medical Association,* vol. 108, p. 1868, May 20, 1937.

HUMIDITY OF THE AIR

We used to feel sorry for people who lived in damp houses but now we are told that colds, coughs, and other illnesses may be reduced by maintaining a proper humidity of the air in our homes and offices. This may be correct, but as yet we have no evidence that humidification of air reduces illness. It does add materially to comfort at certain temperatures; but of more than this we cannot at present be certain.

Humidity of the air is expressed in terms of the percentage of moisture in the air to the total amount of moisture which the air could hold at that temperature. A humidity of 100 per cent means that the air is saturated. Experiments have shown that greatest comfort is experienced at a temperature of 68 degrees Fahrenheit with a humidity between 40 and 50 per cent. To maintain this humidity, moisture must be added to the air of buildings during the winter and withdrawn during most of the summer.

The apparent paradox that a humid day in the summer is oppressively hot and a damp day in the winter bitterly cold is due to the fact that at high temperatures humidity decreases heat loss by reducing evaporation; and at low temperatures it increases heat loss by facilitating the direct transfer of heat from the body to the air.

MOTION OF THE AIR

Air which immediately surrounds the body soon becomes warm and moist; hence, motion of the air increases heat loss both by evaporation and by direct heat transfer. Some circulation of the indoor air is desirable, but drafts are uncomfortable and give rise to vasomotor disturbances which predispose to colds and other respiratory infections.

"BAD AIR"

All too frequently one is forced to experience the unpleasant effects of bad, or so-called "vitiated," air. Physical discomfort, headache, and restlessness or lassitude result from even a short

[253]

period in a hot, stuffy, malodorous room. Prolonged exposure to such conditions may cause loss of appetite, nausea, dizziness, digestive disturbances, and general ill-health. These effects, however, are due not to a reduction of oxygen or an increase of carbon dioxide but to improper temperature and humidity and unpleasant odors.

THE VALUE OF OUTDOOR AIR

The air has long been thought to be associated in some mysterious way with health and disease. The ancient Romans observed the prevalence of a disease characterized by chills and fever in regions that were low and damp and named this disease "malaria"—bad air. Science has explained away the mystery of this association but rendered it none the less real by showing that malaria is caused not by the inhalation of swamp air but by the bite of a mosquito.

During the great plague of London in the seventeenth century and the epidemic of cholera in New Orleans a hundred years ago, citizens were required to keep bonfires burning in the streets in order that the air might be sterilized. A survivor of the New Orleans epidemic left the following note in his diary:

> The cholera has been raging with unabated fury for fourteen days. It seems as if the city were destined to be emptied of its inhabitants. During this time a thick, dark, sultry atmosphere filled our city. Everyone complained of a difficulty in breathing, which he never before experienced. The heavens were stagnant as the mantled pool of death. There were no breezes. At the close of the fourteenth day, about eight o'clock in the evening a smart storm, something like a tornado, came from the northwest, accompanied by heavy peals of thunder and terrific lightning. The deadly air was displaced immediately, by that which was new, fresh, salubrious, and life-giving. The next morning shone forth all bright and beautiful. The plague was stayed. In the opinion of all the medical gentlemen who were on the spot, that change of weather terminated the epidemic.[7]

The modern campaigns for fresh outdoor air in the interest of health have been based largely upon the remarkable recovery of Dr. Edward Livingston Trudeau from tuberculosis in the Adiron-

[7] Saxon, Lyle, "Fabulous New Orleans," Appleton-Century-Crofts, Inc., New York, 1928.

dacks and the establishment by him of the world famous sanatorium for outdoor treatment of this disease at Saranac Lake, New York. Most of Dr. Trudeau's patients improved, as he had done, under his treatment of fresh air, rest, and nourishing food. But he gradually changed his conception of the relative importance of these measures. Dr. Lawrason Brown, late chief of the medical service of the Trudeau Sanatorium, said:

> This brings up the problem of the treatment by exposure to fresh air. I question whether the too long prolonged exposure of weakened, or, indeed, of any patient to chilly or cold air may not defeat the very purpose at which we aim, the stimulation of the patient. I am sure that in the future this part of the treatment will be revised as much as the diet has been changed in the last twenty-five years.[8]

A few years ago pneumonia patients were treated in cold rooms or sleeping porches. Today such treatment would be considered criminal, for it was shown during the First World War that the death rate from pneumonia was four times as great among the patients who were treated in cold wards as among those who were treated at normal room temperatures. Minor respiratory infections, such as common colds and bronchitis, also respond better to treatment in temperatures of 68 degrees Fahrenheit than in cold air.

Outside air is usually very moist in summer and very dry in winter. The capacity of air to hold moisture is just about one-fifth as great at 20 as at 70 degrees Fahrenheit. Consequently, when outside air at 20 degrees Fahrenheit and with a 50 per cent humidity is brought into a building and heated, the capacity of this air to hold water is so increased that the relative humidity drops to 10 per cent. Consequently, the suggestion so frequently heard that the humidity indoors during the winter months may be increased by opening the windows is erroneous.

Air with a 10 to 20 per cent humidity is extremely dry and absorbs moisture from every possible source. Evaporation from the skin is so rapid in it that one feels chilly at temperatures of 68

[8] Brown, Lawrason, "Changes in Sanatorium Procedure," *Journal of the Outdoor Life,* vol. 31, p. 251, July, 1934.

to 70 degrees, while at the same temperature with a relative humidity of 40 to 50 per cent one would be comfortable.

POLLUTION OF AIR

The outside air in most urban communities instead of being pure is grossly polluted by smoke, dust, and gases. In Chicago actual measurements show that every month more than 50 tons of dust and dirt are deposited for each square mile in the downtown district; in New York, about 100 tons; in Cleveland, 120 tons; and in parts of St. Louis almost 200 tons. During the winter much of this comes from the incomplete combustion of coal; in the summer from dust blown into the air from streets, playgrounds, parking lots, or distant farms. In addition to this solid material, such air contains large amounts of ammonia, chlorine, carbon monoxide, sulfur dioxide, and other gases.

An idea of the condition of the air in our cities may be obtained by approaching them by airplane on a clear day when there is little wind. Long before the city itself is visible a brownish-purple haze of dust and smoke comes into view. In many cities this is so great that it shuts out much of the ultraviolet light of the sun's rays. In this instance, distance fails to lend enchantment to the view, for these clouds of dust and smoke are rarely visible to the inhabitants of the city who are surrounded by them.

Over the past several years heavy industrial pollution of the air combined with fog, frequently called *smog*, has caused a great deal of respiratory distress and illness and considerable numbers of deaths in several localities. Sixty-three persons died when smog settled over the Meuse Valley of France in 1930. In the village of Donora, Pennsylvania, 20 persons died when smog settled over that area in 1948. In London during the heavy fogs of December 1952 the number of deaths reported was so high that a special study of the situation was made, the conclusion of which was that approximately 4,000 of these deaths were brought about by fog.[9]

Such pollution of the air, whether from industries, apartment houses, or private residence, is unnecessary and disgraceful and

[9] *American Journal of Public Health*, June, 1953.

can be eliminated if the public would become sufficiently interested to follow the example of cities like Pittsburgh and do something about it.

Even in rural areas the outside air practically always contains some contamination. During certain seasons of the year dust storms fill the atmosphere with dirt for hundreds or even thousands of miles. The protective mechanisms of the body filter out much of this dust in the air which we breathe, so that man may live in a dusty atmosphere for a considerable period of time without demonstrable harm. On the other hand, the inhalation of dust is unpleasant, and certain industrial dusts, such as silica and asbestos, are particularly harmful. In recent years the industries in which these dusts are involved have made great strides in protecting workers from this special dust hazard.

At certain seasons of the year the atmosphere in both city and country also contains pollens of plants and trees. By these, the 5 per cent of the population that is susceptible is made miserable with hay fever or asthma. Such sufferers have long since discovered that they can secure relief by moving during the pollinating seasons to regions where the pollens to which they are sensitive do not exist.

AIR-BORNE INFECTION

More than three-quarters of the illnesses in temperate climates the world over are caused by diseases in which the usual portal of entry of the causative germs is the nose and mouth. Nationwide periodic surveys from 1928 to 1931 showed that influenza and pneumonia caused more days in bed than any other disease. Colds and bronchitis ranked second, tuberculosis third. The diseases spread through the nose and mouth caused a total of 218 days in bed for every 100 persons, as against 167 days in bed from all other causes combined.

The germs of these diseases leave their hosts in expired air or in nose and throat discharges and reach their new victims through the air or through hands, food, drinking glasses, or inanimate objects. Transmission of infection through the air may take one of two forms. The more obvious is so-called "droplet infection,"

[257]

in which the germs are carried on droplets of moisture expelled from the nose and mouth. These are rapidly removed from the air by gravity. The second form is called "air-borne infection" and refers to dried residues of infected droplets or droplet nuclei which are so small that they can remain alive suspended in air for periods which may permit their wide dissemination.

Research studies have demonstrated that living bacteria may be carried by air currents from room to room and from place to place in a large building and that it is possible to destroy most of these bacteria by passing the air through large tubes in which it is exposed to ultraviolet light.

Summarizing the present status of scientific knowledge of air-borne infection, Dr. Stuart Mudd of the University of Pennsylvania writes, "Air of enclosed places is the principal vehicle for the dissemination of respiratory diseases. The rationale for rendering air safe for human occupancy has been laid down in the laboratory and in suitably controlled human environments. The means are ultraviolet radiation, dust suppressive measures, and the use of germicidal vapors of hypochlorous acid and of propylene and triethylene glycol."[10]

A few years ago there was a great deal of promotion of ultraviolet light to reduce the disease-producing germs in the air. Currently various machines which throw glycols into the air are being advertised for the same purpose. Under experimental conditions both methods are effective, but neither has yet been shown to reduce respiratory infections under the conditions under which we live and work. Just what the eventual practical application of all this will be it is impossible as yet to know.

VENTILATION

The purpose of ventilation is to provide indoors the atmospheric conditions which are most comfortable and healthful. Fresh-air enthusiasts maintain that this can best be accomplished by the introduction of outdoor air. Children are told that in order to obtain a perfect health rating they must sleep with

[10] Mudd, Stuart, "Current Progress in Sterilization of Air," *American Journal of Public Health*, vol. 34, p. 578, June, 1944.

their windows wide open, no matter what the outside temperature. Up until the last few years this was accepted as sound advice, but scientific studies of ventilation have changed many of our ideas on this subject and have provided us with a more intelligent basis upon which to proceed.

It is now established that the essential purpose of ventilation is to provide indoors the atmospheric conditions of temperature, movement, and humidity which will effectively remove heat from the body surface without objectionable drafts. In practice this means a room temperature of 68 to 70 degrees Fahrenheit, a relative humidity of 40 to 50 per cent, and moderate air movement. Ventilation also should provide sufficient air exchange to avoid the accumulation of unpleasant odors.

The ventilation of sleeping quarters should be regulated in accordance with outside atmospheric conditions, keeping in mind the fact that drafts are undesirable and that sleep is most restful in an atmosphere which is cool, rather than warm or cold.

AIR CONDITIONING

The conditioning of air is an attempt to provide those conditions of purity, temperature, motion, and humidity in which individuals are most comfortable and can function most efficiently. Air is first filtered and washed so that smoke, dust, gases, and even pollens are removed. Eventually it may also be sterilized.

Hay fever and asthma sufferers, if their symptoms are due to pollens, are usually comfortable in air which has been purified in this manner. Furthermore, many hay fever sufferers can tolerate small amounts of pollen without symptoms and so can be relatively comfortable during the hay fever season by spending their sleeping and working hours in air from which all pollen has been filtered.

The temperature of conditioned air averages 68 to 70 degrees Fahrenheit and the humidity 40 to 50 per cent. For maximum comfort temperature and humidity need to be adjusted in relation to the outside temperature, both being somewhat higher in summer and lower in winter.

Many types of air conditioning are now being offered for sale.

[259]

Some are effective, others worthless. In new office buildings installations for air conditioning are rapidly being included in standard specifications. The units for individual rooms are less satisfactory, although some of these materially improve the condition of the atmosphere. For the home of moderate size the simplest and in general the most satisfactory method of air conditioning is to combine this with a warm-air heating system. With such a system the air can be filtered, warmed, and moistened in the winter and filtered, cooled, and dried in the summer.

Progress in air conditioning is so rapid that the not too distant future may find most homes, schools, and office buildings provided with conditioned air. Then hay fever will be a rare affliction, the nuisance of dust in the home will disappear, and the discomfort of underheated, overheated, and improperly humidified rooms will be a thing of the past.

We shall then look back upon the open window age when the fresh air faddists reigned supreme as we now look back on the age when food and drink were not conditioned and when flies swarmed about the rooms we occupied.[11]

DISCUSSION SUGGESTIONS

1. What is light? Explain what is meant by the visible spectrum; by infrared rays; by ultraviolet light.
2. Explain the more important effects of ultraviolet light upon health.
3. Of what use is infrared radiation in medicine?
4. What are the symptoms of heat prostration? Of heat stroke? Of heat cramps?
5. How may these be prevented and how should each be treated?
6. What are the values of sun bathing?
7. What do you understand by fresh air?
8. What physiological processes does the air influence?
9. Discuss the effects of changes in the atmospheric pressure of the air upon the body.
10. What physical factors of the air are most important to health and comfort?
11. What do you understand by "bad air"?
12. Explain the ill effects which pollution of the air may have upon health.
13. What conditions of the atmosphere should conditioning of the air provide? Are these conditions important to health? If so, in what way?

[11] Myers, J. A., "Why Condition the Air?" *Hygeia*, vol. 13, p. 22, January, 1935.

REFERENCES AND READING SUGGESTIONS

1. Clark, J. H.: "Lighting in Relation to Health," The Williams & Wilkins Company, Baltimore, 1931.
2. Kovacs, Richard: "Nature, M. D. Healing Forces of Heat, Water, Light, Electricity, and Exercise," Appleton-Century-Crofts, Inc., New York, 1934.
3. Luckeish, M.: "Artificial Sunlight," D. Van Nostrand Company, Inc., New York, 1930.
4. Macfie, Ronald: "Sunshine and Health," Henry Holt and Company, Inc., New York, 1927.
5. Mayer, Edgar: "The Curative Value of Light," Appleton-Century-Crofts, Inc., New York, 1932.
6. Myers, J. A.: "Why Condition the Air?" *Hygeia*, vol. 13, p. 22, January, 1935.
7. National Tuberculosis Association: "Air and Sunshine," New York, 1932.
8. Winslow, C.-E. A.: "Fresh Air and Ventilation," E. P. Dutton & Co., Inc., New York, 1926.
9. ——— and L. P. Herrington: "Temperature and Human Life," Princeton University Press, Princeton, N. J., 1951.

Chapter XII

SPECIFIC DISEASE PREVENTION

THE time may come when communicable diseases will be so completely eradicated that they no longer will constitute a hazard of any consequence. This has been attained with certain ones. Against certain others, control measures unfortunately have not been so successful. In some instances great reductions in the prevalence of these diseases have been made, but the hazards of infection are still with us. To these diseases conditions of modern life make more or less exposure inevitable. Hence, it becomes of importance to maintain individual resistance at the highest possible level.

Resistance to Disease

We frequently speak of increasing individual resistance by exercise, fresh air, good food, and rest. All these measures are important for the maintenance of health but they do not afford protection against communicable diseases. An athlete in the best of health is just as susceptible to measles, smallpox, or scarlet fever as is his friend who leads a sedentary life.

Resistance to communicable diseases depends upon the possession by the body of specific protective substances, the so-called "antibodies," which destroy infections or counteract their poisonous products. The body may procure these protective substances either by manufacturing them itself or by obtaining them from some other person or some animal which has produced them.

The human or animal body produces antibodies when stimulated to do so by the presence of disease-producing microorganisms or their poisonous products. Practically, this may occur as a result of infection with the microorganisms of a disease or by vaccination; that is, by introducing into the body some of the dead or greatly weakened microorganisms or minute amounts of their poisonous products. The immunity or resistance thus developed is spoken of as an "active immunity" because the body produces its own protective substances. Such immunity is relatively slow in developing but tends to last a considerable period of time. In some instances this may be a few months, in others a few years, in still others a lifetime. For example, a lifelong active immunity usually follows attacks of smallpox or typhoid fever; while the active immunity following vaccination against smallpox lasts only 5 to 10 years and against typhoid fever approximately 3 years.

The other type of specific resistance or immunity is obtained by injecting into the body some of these protective substances which have been produced by a person who has had the disease or by an animal into which the germs or their poisonous products have been injected. In either instance the protective substances are found in the blood. If taken from some other person, the liquid part of the blood, with or without the corpuscles, may be injected directly; or the constituent of blood, gamma globulin, which contains the antibodies may be extracted, preserved, and used as needed. If from animals, the protective substances are removed from the blood, concentrated, and standardized before injection. The resistance or immunity thus obtained is present immediately after the injection but lasts a relatively short time, at most a few months. The degree of protection or resistance depends upon the quantity of protective substances injected. This so-called "passive immunity" is given when there is need for immediate protection, as when one is actually ill with a disease or when infants, who are particularly susceptible, have been exposed to a disease against which such protective substances are available.

Misconceptions Concerning Immunizations

Much misinformation and misunderstanding prevail concerning artificial immunization. Practically everyone has heard that there are vaccinations or inoculations against certain diseases, but whether these are safe and of established value is not generally known. Furthermore, there is, in addition to honest doubt and questioning, a certain amount of definite, organized propaganda against immunization procedures.

Some of the enemies of immunization are merely misinformed, misguided cranks. Others use it as an argument for securing adherents to some particular form of treatment or disease prevention. Even some of the latter, in their ignorance, are perfectly sincere in their opposition; but it is difficult to believe in the sincerity of practitioners of some of the so-called "healing cults" who during an epidemic of smallpox seek vaccination for themselves while advising their patients to avoid it.

The question most frequently raised concerning artificial immunization is whether it may not be deleterious to inject these dead or weakened germs or their products into the body; particularly is this true when several vaccinations are suggested. This is a natural and perfectly proper question, but the answer is obvious if one considers that when one contracts these diseases and recovery occurs, it is practically always complete, even though enormous quantities of the infection have permeated the body. In vaccinations the quantities introduced into the body are definitely known and are far below the amounts which will cause damage. Such injections do not produce so great or so prolonged an immunity as usually follows an attack of the disease, but neither do they carry the hazard of prolonged illness, serious complications, and even death itself that accompanies natural infection.

It is difficult for physicians, and impossible for the public, to keep accurately informed concerning the value of all of the immunizations which are proposed. Manufacturers in this field

[264]

are constantly offering and advocating new preparations. Some of these are of merit, but for others there is no excuse whatsoever. Among the vaccinations of greatest practical value in this country are the following:

Smallpox Vaccination*

A person living today cannot possibly realize what smallpox meant before the days of vaccination. Smallpox was just as inevitable then as measles is today. In fact, it was considered a children's disease, just as chicken pox, whooping cough, and measles are considered children's diseases today; for hardly anyone ever reached adult life without having had it. It has been estimated that 60 million people in Europe died of smallpox during the eighteenth century. A French physician in 1754 wrote that "Every tenth death was due to smallpox and one-fourth of mankind was either killed by it or crippled or disfigured for life."

Smallpox has been present in India, China, and Egypt for thousands of years, but it did not become prevalent in Europe until about the sixteenth century. Charles IX and Louis XIV in France carried scars of the disease and Louis XV died of it. George Washington contracted smallpox in the West Indies. Queen Mary of England died of smallpox in 1694 at the age of thirty-three. More than a century later the historian Macaulay wrote the following description of the epidemic in which she had died:

That disease, over which science has since achieved a succession of glorious and beneficient victories, was then the most terrible of all the ministers of death. The havoc of the plague had been far more rapid; but plague had visited our shores only once or twice within living memory; and the smallpox was always present, filling the churchyards with corpses, tormenting with constant fears all whom it had not yet stricken, leaving on those whose lives it spared the hideous traces of its power, turning the babe into a changeling at which the mother shuddered, making the eyes and cheeks of the betrothed maiden objects of horror to the lover.

Toward the end of the year 1694, this pestilence was more than usually severe. At length the infection spread to the palace and reached the young and blooming Queen. She received the intimation of her danger with true

* See also Appendix D.

greatness of soul. She gave orders that every lady of her bedchamber, every maid of honor, nay, every menial servant who had not had the smallpox, should instantly leave Kensington House. She locked herself up during a short time in her closet, burned some papers, arranged others, then calmly awaited her fate.[1]

Smallpox was introduced into Mexico by the Spaniards very soon after the discovery of America. Within a short period 3½ million persons were said to have died of the disease in Mexico alone. Rapidly the disease spread to the North American Indians, and it has been estimated that half of them died of it in a short time.

Smallpox is a disease which varies enormously in severity. In prevaccination days it was always severe, being fatal to between 20 to 30 per cent of its victims. But just prior to the beginning of the twentieth century a very mild form of smallpox appeared in Florida and spread very rapidly over the whole of the United States. Since then this mild, nonfatal type of the disease has predominated to such an extent that people have become careless about maintaining immunity to it. This is unfortunate, for whenever a sufficient proportion of the population becomes susceptible an epidemic of smallpox is possible. Whether this is mild or severe depends upon which type of infection happens to be introduced.

In the winter of 1924–1925 such a calamity occurred. People had become negligent about vaccination and when the malignant type of smallpox was brought into this country several serious epidemics occurred. In Minneapolis alone during December and January of that year there were approximately 1,000 cases of smallpox with 300 deaths. During this winter 17 cities of 100,000 population or more reported deaths from smallpox and some of these, notably Detroit, Toledo, and Camden, had very high rates.

As a result of these outbreaks people became alarmed and rushed to be vaccinated. Evidence of repeated carelessness in this regard was reappearing in 1936, when 7,813 cases of smallpox were reported in the United States, more than in any country of the civilized world except India. In the winter of 1952–1953

[1] Macaulay, Lord, "The History of England," edited by C. H. Firth, vol. 5, p. 2468, Macmillan & Company, Ltd., London, 1914.

approximately 5,000 persons died from smallpox in Calcutta's worst epidemic in 50 years. In this country, on the other hand, only 21 cases of smallpox were reported in 1952 for the entire United States, a new low record.

The greatest mass vaccination campaign ever undertaken was conducted in New York City in the winter of 1947. In less than one month more than 6,500,000 persons were vaccinated, over 5,000,000 of these within two weeks after the mayor of the city appealed for universal vaccination. The reason for this appeal was the occurrence of several cases of malignant smallpox.

FIG. 15. SMALLPOX IN RELATION TO VACCINATION, UNITED STATES, 1919–1929

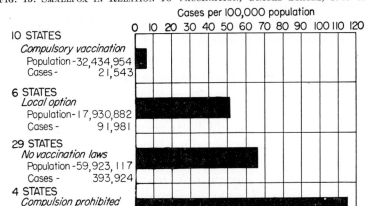

This campaign limited the outbreak to 12 cases and 2 deaths. This is a remarkable accomplishment, particularly as compared to what happened in 1901 when the city had less than half its present population and 1,859 cases and 410 deaths occurred before a similar epidemic was brought under control.

The occurrence of smallpox is in no way influenced by climate, soil, age, or occupation. It affects alike the rich and the poor, the clean and the dirty. It spreads wherever the contagion finds susceptible people. The one and only method of controlling it is to raise individual resistance by means of vaccination.

Vaccination as we know it today was developed by Edward Jenner in England in 1796. Prior to this many persons were

[267]

immunized by *inoculation* of material which was taken from a smallpox sore and rubbed into a slight abrasion of the skin. This practice had been in vogue for centuries in India and China. Mild cases of smallpox actually developed in persons thus inoculated. It is said that an English physician was granted a life annuity of 10,000 pounds per year for performing this service for Catherine the Great of Russia.

Vaccination, although still confused in the minds of some with inoculation of smallpox material, is an entirely different procedure. The vaccine is obtained not from patients with smallpox but from healthy calves which have been inoculated with cowpox, or from laboratory cultures of cowpox virus on chick-embryo culture medium. In the preparation of this vaccine the most careful surgical technique is used, after which the vaccine is tested for purity and then accurately standardized.

The technique of vaccination is to introduce a very small amount of vaccine into the skin—usually of the arm. In a few days the skin becomes red and swollen and one typical cowpox lesion develops. This should be protected from dirt, kept dry, and not touched. Shields should not be worn. Usually no bandage is necessary.

There is no longer any possible question concerning the efficacy of vaccination for the prevention of smallpox. In many countries of the world and in certain states of this country vaccination against smallpox is compulsory. In such countries and states smallpox is practically unknown. But where vaccination depends upon individual initiative, smallpox finds a fertile field.

Complications of vaccination are occasionally reported, but they occur very, very rarely; possibly once in 100,000 vaccinations. Certainly the risk is infinitesimal in comparison with the protection conferred by vaccination. The dangers of vaccination claimed by the antivaccinationists are practically all fallacious or of such antiquity that they do not apply to modern vaccination.

The duration of the immunity as a result of vaccination is variable. For 5 to 7 years the protection is of a high grade, after which the immunity gradually decreases until it is completely lost 5 to 10 years later. The first vaccination should be performed before a child reaches his first birthday. This gives a high-grade immunity, which should never be allowed to disappear completely. The second vaccination may well be done at the time of beginning school and subsequent vaccinations at intervals of 5 to 10 years and whenever one has been exposed to smallpox. By following this program, resistance will be kept at such a level that subsequent vaccinations will cause no inconvenience and yet immunity to smallpox will be maintained. It is disgraceful today for any intelligent person to contract smallpox.

Diphtheria Immunization*

In 1952 approximately 5,000 persons, mostly children, in the United States got diphtheria and some 250 of them died. This represents about one seventy-fifth of the death rate which prevailed in 1900. No more striking illustration of this reduction can be given than that the number of American boys who died in 1944 on European battlefields was smaller than the number of American children who died from diphtheria in 1900, when the population of the country was only 76,000,000.² Although this is one of medical science's most brilliant achievements, the results are still not satisfactory when children still are dying needlessly from this disease.

If reasonable use were made of available scientific knowledge, diphtheria would soon become as rare as cholera and yellow fever. We have a test which determines who are susceptible; we have an immunizing agent which gives prolonged immunity; we have an effective antitoxin for treatment of the susceptible persons who develop the disease. Nothing more could be desired. But it remains for the public to utilize this service which physicians are prepared to render.

Diphtheria is caused by a bacillus which sets up an infection in the throat and gives off a toxin (poison) which is absorbed into the blood stream and carried throughout the body. This affects primarily the nervous system, causing paralysis, and the heart muscle, causing heart failure. If one is to recover from diphtheria,

* See also Appendix D.
² *Bulletin of American Association for the Advancement of Science*, September, 1944.

[269]

this toxin must be neutralized by antitoxin which the body produces or which is injected for treatment.

Diphtheria germs are disseminated in the nose and throat discharges of patients and carriers and are spread by droplets of moisture in the air or by hands, drinking glasses, and other objects which can retain and transmit infection. Fortunately, these germs have a distinctive appearance under the microscope so

Fig. 16. Trend in Diphtheria Deaths in New York City

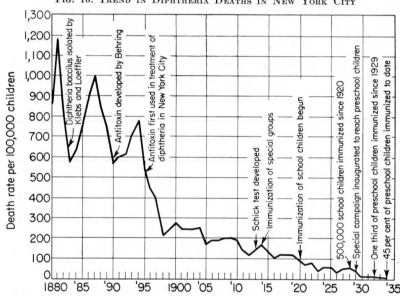

Crude annual death rates for diphtheria per 100,000 children under 10 years of age, 1880–1934. (*L. I. Dublin and A. J. Lotka, Twenty-five Years of Health Progress, Metropolitan Life Insurance Company, New York, 1937.*)

that it is possible by means of nose and throat cultures to identify individuals who have these germs in the nose or throat.

The most important of the measures for the prevention of diphtheria is the active immunization (vaccination) of children. This is accomplished by the injection of a minute but definite amount of modified diphtheria toxin (poison). This material is called toxoid. Toxoid has been used in millions of cases and found effective and entirely harmless. Most deaths from diphtheria occur among children under five years of age; hence, at the age of six months every healthy child should be immunized against

[270]

diphtheria. At this age the need for protection is most urgent and the procedure is perfectly safe.

The Schick test, which is a dependable test of immunity against diphtheria, consists of the injection into the skin of the forearm of a very small but definitely measured amount of diphtheria toxin. If redness results, it is called a positive test and indicates that the individual is susceptible to diphtheria. No redness in two days indicates immunity. With infants and young children this test is rarely used, because so many of them are susceptible that it is better to immunize them all than to attempt to pick out the few who might be naturally immune. Among older children and adults, however, the proportion of immune individuals is greater. Hence, this test gives information of distinct value.

Diphtheria antitoxin, which is prepared from the blood serum of a horse treated with diphtheria toxin, contains protective substances which neutralize the diphtheria toxin, and so is useful for treatment or temporary protection. Before the use of antitoxin, which was developed about the beginning of the present century, approximately one person out of every three who got diphtheria died. With antitoxin available there would be practically no deaths if the antitoxin were administered at the very onset of the disease and in sufficient dosage.

With toxoid to give prolonged protection there should be less need of antitoxin for treatment; but as long as immunization depends upon individual initiative, we shall need antitoxin to try to save those who are the unfortunate victims of their own or their parents' negligence. Even antitoxin will not save them all. Some will come too late or will not come at all and so will be additional sacrifices upon the altar of ignorance, prejudice, and procrastination.

Scarlet Fever Prevention*

Scarlet fever is another disease for which we have a skin test for immunity, an immunizing agent to give prolonged protection, and a serum containing protective substances (antitoxin) for

* See also Appendix D.

treatment. The materials used for these purposes act in the same manner as in diphtheria but are somewhat less effective.

The cause of scarlet fever is a streptococcus, very similar to the ones which cause tonsillitis, septic sore throat, rheumatic fever, and erysipelas. These germs enter the body through the nose or mouth and set up an infection on the tonsils and in the pharynx. This stage of scarlet fever is indistinguishable from tonsillitis. However, as the scarlet fever microorganisms grow in the throat, they give off a toxin which is absorbed into the blood stream and carried throughout the body. This toxin is responsible for the characteristic red rash from which scarlet fever gets its name and

FIG. 17. SCARLET FEVER DEATHS BY AGE GROUPS

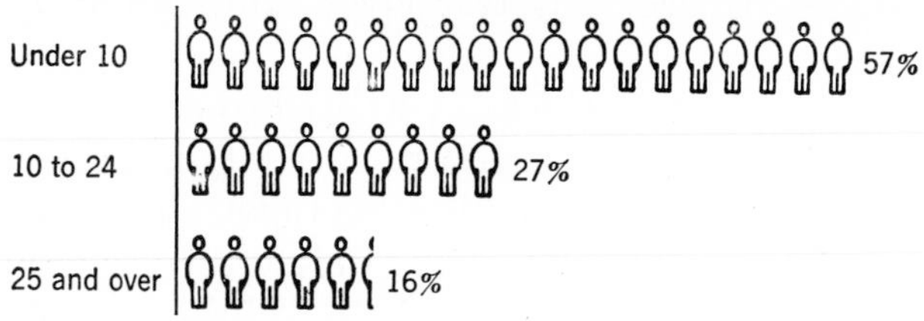

Under 10 .... 57%

10 to 24 .... 27%

25 and over 16%

Age distribution of total deaths from scarlet fever in Minnesota. (*Minnesota State Department of Health.*)

for the nephritis which may occur during scarlet fever. The complications of sinus, ear, and mastoid infections are due to the extension of infection from the pharynx to these regions.

In mild cases of scarlet fever, sometimes called "scarlatina," the rash may be so slight as to be hardly noticeable. Although many of these patients are hardly sick at all, they should be isolated just like other cases because they serve as sources of infection, and persons who get the disease from them may have severe attacks.

The scarlet fever germs are contained in the nose, throat, and ear discharges of patients, mild cases, which are frequently unrecognized, and carriers. The old idea that the skin which peels off during convalescence is the source of infection is erroneous, except in so far as this skin has been contaminated by discharges from the nose, throat, or ears. Transmission of the infection from person to person is by contact with patients or carriers, or by

[272]

means of droplets of moisture expelled from their noses or mouths, or through milk or other inanimate objects, such as drinking glasses, towels, and doorknobs, which harbor the germs.

The Dick test is used to determine whether one is immune or susceptible to scarlet fever. Persons who develop a slight redness of the skin at the site of the test are susceptible to scarlet fever, and those who show no redness are probably immune. It is of distinct practical value to have this information in regard to children and physicians, nurses, and others who are likely to be exposed to scarlet fever.

The material used as a vaccine to stimulate the development of a prolonged immunity consists of scarlet fever toxin. A series of five injections is used, the amount contained in the first injection being smallest, with subsequent injections somewhat larger. The reason that relatively little is known of scarlet fever immunization is that physicians and public health officials have not urged it as they have urged immunization against smallpox and diphtheria. For this there are several reasons. One is that, although scarlet fever is much more prevalent than diphtheria, it has been relatively mild in recent years. A second is that it is always difficult to secure the widespread acceptance of an immunization procedure which requires as many as five visits to a physician. A third is that the unpleasant, although not serious, reactions which occasionally follow the injections give rise to some opposition.

These are practical considerations which have caused public health workers to hesitate to promote immunization against scarlet fever. Furthermore, the effectiveness of the sulfonamides, penicillin, and other antibiotics in the treatment of scarlet fever reduces the need for immunization.

Antityphoid Vaccination*

In civil life typhoid fever has been almost wiped out by the sanitation of water, milk, and food supplies. In the Army and Navy, however, sanitary measures have been supplemented by the use of typhoid vaccine. This vaccine consists of dead typhoid

* See also Appendix D.

germs, a definite number of which are introduced into the body in order to stimulate the development of resistance to the disease.

The efficacy of typhoid vaccination in increasing resistance to this disease is beyond question. But the hazard of typhoid fever has been so greatly reduced that few people in civil life consider it necessary to keep up individual resistance by means of vaccination. This is a reasonable course to follow when the sanitary status of one's water, food, and milk supply is known. On the

Fig. 18. Death Rates from Typhoid and Paratyphoid Fever in the United States since 1900

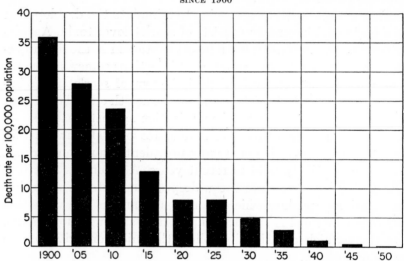

other hand, when one is traveling about, particularly in foreign countries, typhoid vaccination is cheap insurance against a very serious disease.

Whooping Cough Vaccine*

Whooping cough, which in 1950 caused the death of 1,168 American children, almost as many as diphtheria, measles, and scarlet fever combined, is the most distressing as well as one of the most serious of the diseases of infancy. It is caused by a known germ which is present in the secretions from the nose and throat (see Figs. 19 and 20).

* See also Appendix D.

[274]

The early symptoms, and in some cases the only symptoms, are those of a common cold. Hence, infants can be protected against infection only if they are safeguarded against exposure to colds or acute respiratory infections. Although vaccination against whooping cough was tried for some years with questionable success, a new vaccine is giving more encouraging results. Many of the vaccinated children are completely protected and the majority of those who do contract whooping cough after vaccination have it in a much milder form than unvaccinated children. This immunization seems to offer new hope of protecting our children against one of the most dread diseases of infancy.

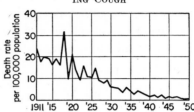

FIG. 19. TREND IN DEATHS FROM WHOOPING COUGH

Rates per 100,000 persons 1 to 14 years of age. (*Data from U.S. Office of Vital Statistics.*)

FIG. 20. WHOOPING COUGH DEATHS BY AGE GROUPS

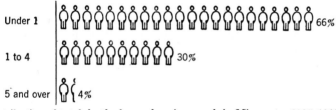

Under 1   66%

1 to 4   30%

5 and over   4%

Age distribution of total deaths from whooping cough in Minnesota, 1927–1946. (*Data from Minnesota State Department of Health.*)

Whooping cough is most serious during infancy, so this vaccine should be given during the first year of life. A mixture of whooping cough vaccine and diphtheria toxoid is giving good results. Since whooping cough in older children and young adults is less serious, immunization is not advised for these age groups.

Immunization Against Measles*

Measles, although frequently considered trivial, is a serious disease in infancy. In fact, the possibility of death from measles

* See also Appendix D.

[275]

is seventeen times as great if contracted by a child under one year of age as by a child of six. This difference points the way toward which efforts to combat measles may be directed. Complete prevention of a disease which, even in its early stages, is so highly communicable is impossible unless a specific immunizing agent against it can be developed. But postponement of the disease until school age when it is relatively without danger should be attempted and in many cases can be achieved (see Fig. 21).

FIG. 21. MEASLES DEATHS BY AGE GROUPS

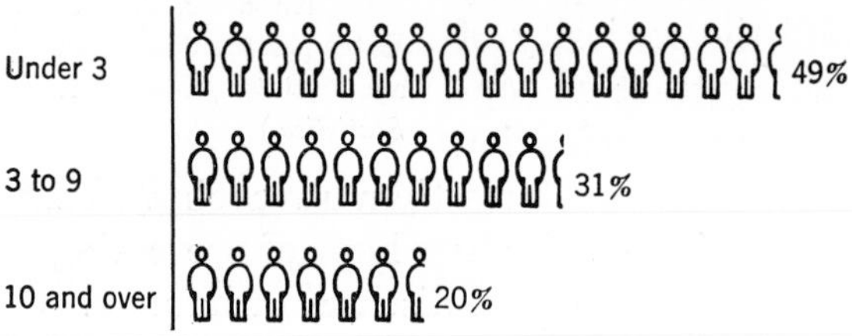

Age distribution of total deaths from measles in Minnesota, 1927–1946. (*Data from Minnesota State Department of Health.*)

The cause of measles is a virus, a tiny germ spread by discharges from the nose and throat. Early symptoms resemble an ordinary cold. It is in this stage that measles is most highly contagious. Hence, measures for the protection of infants against acute respiratory infections in general will also reduce their exposure to measles.

In addition to such general procedures there is available a specific preventive measure which can be utilized by physicians for the protection of children known to have been exposed to measles. This is the injection of gamma globulin, placental extract, or whole blood. Blood from one of the parents may be used for this purpose. The principle involved is to give the infant some of the protective substances which have been present in the blood of persons who have recovered from measles. If such injections are given within 5 days after exposure, the disease is usually prevented; if given from the fifth to the eighth day, a mild form of measles may develop, but complications are rare.

[276]

Injections given after the eighth day following exposure usually have little or no effect upon the course of the disease. The protection from such injections is temporary but usually long enough to safeguard a child during a current epidemic. The following year the child will again be susceptible, unless he had a mild form of the disease. Each year that an attack of measles can be postponed means a material reduction in the danger to the child.

Tetanus Toxoid and Antitoxin*

Tetanus is the scientific name for the disease commonly called "lockjaw." The widespread belief that tetanus is most likely to develop in wounds contracted by stepping on a rusty nail has a scientific basis. The normal habitat of tetanus germs is the intestinal tract of horses and other herbivorous animals. Hence, these germs are likely to occur wherever there are excreta from these animals. Barnyards, highways, fields, and gardens in which manure is used as a fertilizer are practically certain to abound with highly resistant forms of this organism.

Protection against tetanus is obtained by the injection of tetanus toxoid, which gives prolonged immunity against the disease. After being shown to be both effective and harmless, this toxoid was administered to all persons in the United States Army and Navy during the Second World War. The result was that only 4 cases of tetanus developed among more than 10,000,000 men in our armed forces, and only 2 of these were the result of battle casualties.

It is now recommended that tetanus toxoid be given to all children in infancy. This will provide prolonged protection, but "booster doses" should be given whenever an injury occurs that might be contaminated with tetanus organisms.

Tetanus antitoxin, which like diphtheria antitoxin is prepared from horses, gives a passive protection against tetanus toxin. This is useful for the prevention of the disease in persons who receive deep wounds in areas where tetanus organisms are likely to be present and who have not been immunized with tetanus toxoid.

* See also Appendix D.

[277]

Immunization against Poliomyelitis*

Poliomyelitis, or "infantile paralysis," as it is commonly called, is an acute communicable disease which is characterized by symptoms of a generalized infection and by the destruction of groups of motor cells in the central nervous system, with resultant paralysis. It is caused by a living virus which, at least in certain stages of its development, is small enough to pass through the pores of a porcelain filter. This germ enters the body through the nose or mouth and is disseminated in the nose, throat, and intestinal discharges of patients, mild unrecognized cases, and carriers.

The hazard of death or crippling from this disease is small in comparison to the hazard from accidents, but its effects are at times so tragic that parents tend to become panicky whenever poliomyelitis is reported in the community.

The majority of cases occur in children under five years of age and during the months of July, August, and September. Transmission is most probably by close contact with patients or carriers or through articles recently contaminated by them. It is possible that intestinal discharges may play a role in the spread of this disease. Drying does not kill the virus and it has been demonstrated in the dust of the sickroom.

Studies of the blood serum of the adult population in different parts of the country show that 50 to 80 per cent contains antibodies against the virus of poliomyelitis. This indicates that most persons at some time or other have been infected with this virus and that paralysis is the exception rather than the rule.

The most important single point in a program for the prevention of poliomyelitis is the early diagnosis of the cases and the recognition of the disease in the many mild cases in which paralysis does not develop. Unfortunately there are no early symptoms or signs which are diagnostic of this disease. Most patients have a sore throat, fever, headache, and constipation or diarrhea with or without vomiting. Irritableness, drowsiness, and a desire to be let alone are common. These symptoms are rather typical but

* See also Appendix D.

TABLE 23

IMMUNIZATIONS OF PUBLIC HEALTH IMPORTANCE IN THIS COUNTRY

Disease	Immunizing Material	Immunity Produced		Recommended	
		Type	Dependable Duration	For Whom	When
Smallpox	Cowpox virus	Active	5 to 10 years	All normal persons	1st—3 to 9 months of age. 2d—entrance to school Later—every 5 or 6 years and during epidemics
Diphtheria	1. Toxoid	Active	5 to 10 years	All normal children and susceptible adults especially exposed	1st—3 to 6 months of age. 2d—entrance to school and at 5 year intervals to age 15 For susceptible adults such as nurses and physicians
	2. Antitoxin	Passive	2 to 3 months	Infants and young children	If not immunized and closely exposed to disease
Typhoid and paratyphoid fever	Dead germs	Active	2 to 3 years	Susceptibles	Exposed to disease or traveling in foreign countries
Whooping cough	Dead germs	Active	Several years	Infants, children	4 months of age
Measles	Immune blood serum, gamma globulin, or placental extract	Passive	Few weeks	Infants	When exposed to disease
Tetanus	1. Toxoid	Active	Probably 5 to 10 years	Children Adults	In infancy When likely to be exposed
	2. Antitoxin	Passive	Few weeks	Children Adults	After injuries likely to be contaminated, if toxoid has not been administered
Rabies	Attenuated virus	Active	Undetermined	Anyone	When exposed to saliva of suspected animal
Combined immunization	Diphtheria and tetanus toxoid and whooping cough vaccine	Active	5 to 10 years	Infants	3 months of age Repeat at school age without whooping cough vaccine
Poliomyelitis	Dead or attenuated virus	Active	Not yet known	Infants and other susceptibles	Infancy or later if susceptible

they occur also in other diseases and may be absent in definite cases of poliomyelitis.

Fortunately research workers have recently developed laboratory tests which make the identification of poliomyelitis virus and of antibodies against poliomyelitis relatively simple and rapid. When generally applied these tests should provide information which will be of great value in dealing with outbreaks of this disease.

The removal of tonsils and adenoids greatly increases the chances of having the bulbar type of the disease if one gets "polio." There is also some evidence that vaccinations or immunizations against diseases such as smallpox, diphtheria, etc., if given during an epidemic of poliomyelitis may increase the likelihood of getting this disease.

During every epidemic of poliomyelitis many children develop paralysis and horrible deformities because of improper treatment or no treatment during the febrile and postfebrile stages of the disease. Active treatment, utilizing hot packs during the acute stage, with early movement to prevent disuse atrophy and deformities, is the principle of the treatment which was recommended by Sister Elizabeth Kenny and is now widely utilized throughout this country.

The respirator, the so-called "mechanical lung" or "iron lung" which has received so much publicity, is useful only to keep alive certain patients, some of whose respiratory muscles have been paralyzed, until other muscles can take over the function of respiration. If they are unable to do this, the patient can never live outside the respirator.

When the blood of most adults was found to contain antibodies against the poliomyelitis virus, efforts were made to use such blood and blood serum to prevent and treat the disease. The results, however, were uniformly discouraging until gamma globulin, which contains the antibodies of the blood in concentrated form, became available. Studies of this product seem to indicate that it gives partial protection against poliomyelitis for a few weeks' time.

Of much greater possibilities are the several vaccines against this disease which are currently under study. One of these consists of killed poliomyelitis virus, the others of live virus which has been weakened or attenuated in one of several ways. In experiments with animals and with small groups of children all of these vaccines show real promise; and the one vaccine which has been tried in a large nationwide study has proved more than 80 per cent effective in preventing paralytic poliomyelitis. The duration of the protection provided by this vaccine, which consists of dead virus, has not yet been determined; but it now appears certain that this vaccine or one of the others under study will provide us with a safe and effective means of preventing this dread disease.

Other Immunizations

Numerous other vaccines and serums are produced. Cold vaccines and BCG vaccine against tuberculosis are considered elsewhere. Acne vaccines are of value in about one-third of the cases.

Certain other serums and vaccines, such as those against yellow fever, cholera, Rocky Mountain spotted fever, anthrax, and botulism, are of definite scientific value but are of little general use in this country because of the infrequency of the diseases against which they give protection. Vaccines for yellow fever, plague, cholera, and typhus are given to all members of the military services who are sent to parts of the world where these diseases are prevalent.

Artificial immunization has been one of the most valuable preventive measures contributed by science. We can now be protected by vaccination or other injections against many dread diseases and we are hopeful that the future may provide us with completely effective vaccines against such diseases as influenza, tuberculosis, pneumonia, the common cold, and poliomyelitis; and that the people will utilize the protective measures which science has made available to them.

DISCUSSION SUGGESTIONS

1. What basis is there for the statement that civilization increases the prevalence of communicable diseases?

[281]

2. Does physical fitness provide protection against communicable diseases? Explain why.
3. Define active immunity. How may its development be stimulated? For what practical purposes is artificial active immunization useful?
4. Define passive immunity. How is it produced? Of what practical value is it in the prevention or treatment of disease?
5. Outline the history of smallpox in the United States. What are the possibilities of epidemics in the future?
6. What is smallpox vaccination? Explain the preparation of smallpox vaccine.
7. How does modern vaccination differ from the old-time practice of inoculation?
8. At what ages and at what intervals would you recommend smallpox vaccination? Why?
9. What is the cause of diphtheria and how is it transmitted?
10. Explain what diphtheria toxin is. What is it used for?
11. What is diphtheria antitoxin? What is it used for?
12. What is the Schick test? What is its significance? Would you expect to find a larger proportion of persons of a given age reacting positively to this test in urban or in rural communities? Why?
13. Discuss the prevention of diphtheria in the individual; in the community.
14. What is the cause of scarlet fever? To what other diseases is it closely related? How is it transmitted?
15. What is the Dick test? What is its significance?
16. Discuss the prevention of scarlet fever in the individual; in the community.
17. Of what does typhoid vaccine consist? What is its value?
18. How is tetanus contracted? How may it be prevented?
19. What reason is there for thinking that infection with the virus of poliomyelitis is widespread and that paralysis is the exception rather than the rule?
20. What is the seasonal prevalence of poliomyelitis? What are the early suggestive symptoms?
21. Discuss the importance of and immunization against whooping cough and measles.
22. Discuss the present status of our efforts to prevent poliomyelitis.
23. Against what diseases other than the foregoing have effective immunizing agents been developed?
24. Outline a program to secure the more widespread utilization of scientifically established immunizing procedures.
25. Check your own immunization record, Appendix C.

REFERENCES AND READING SUGGESTIONS

1. Anderson, Gaylord, and Margaret Arnstein: "Communicable Disease Control," 3d ed., The Macmillan Company, 1953.

2. Blakeslee, Alton L.: "Polio Can Be Conquered," Public Affairs Pamphlet, New York.
3. Delano, Jane A.: "American Red Cross Textbook on Home Hygiene and Care of the Sick," New York, Blakiston Division, McGraw-Hill Book Company, Inc., 1947.
4. DeKruif, Paul: "Microbe Hunters," Harcourt, Brace and Company, Inc., New York, 1926.
5. Park, W. H., and A. W. Williams: "Who's Who among the Microbes," Appleton-Century-Crofts, Inc., New York, 1929.
6. Smith, Geddes: "Plague On Us," Commonwealth Fund, Division of Publications, New York, 1943.
7. Stern, B. J.: "Should We Be Vaccinated?" Harper & Brothers, New York, 1927.
8. Thomas, Ruth: "The Why and How of Immunization," *Hygeia*, vol. 25, p. 626, August, 1947.
9. Winslow, C.-E. A.: "The Conquest of Epidemic Disease," Princeton University Press, Princeton, N.J., 1942.

Text-Films

The following McGraw-Hill Text-Film on Health Education is recommended for use with this chapter of the text, as well as with Chapters II and XIII.

The Body Fights Bacteria (17 min sd MP). The film describes the counterbalances to human disease: (1) the body's own defenses, (2) artificial immunization, (3) drugs. Animated drawings, live photography, and action photomicrography are employed in the discussion.

Silent follow-up filmstrip based on material contained in the motion picture offers opportunity for review, testing, and further discussion.

Chapter XIII

COLDS AND INFLUENZA

THE cold is the commonest of all human ills. A survey by the American Institute of Public Opinion found that for the week ending November 15 colds were reported in one-third of American homes, with an estimated total of 18 million persons affected. A corresponding survey for the week ending October 11 showed one-fourth of all families reported colds, with an estimated 13 million individuals affected. Few persons go through a winter without at least one cold; and the average frequency is two to three attacks per person per year. About one-fourth of the population has three or more colds and about the same proportion less than two colds annually.

The loss of time due to colds is enormous. Industry reports that employees lose on the average 1 to 3 days annually on account of this disease. Children of school age lose about 2 days a year from colds, with the children in the lower grades suffering more attacks and more serious colds than those in the higher grades. A survey by the New York State Department of Health showed that 57 per cent of patients who sought medical service from physicians outside the big cities did so because of colds or tonsillitis. The American Cold Foundation estimates the cost of colds in this country as 400 million dollars per year.

Colds themselves are never fatal and rarely serious. Their great danger lies in their complications, of which pneumonia, ear and sinus infections, and mastoid disease are the most common.

The "common cold" is not a clear-cut disease entity like diphtheria, smallpox, or scarlet fever but covers various disorders of the nose, throat, and even the lower respiratory tract. If one wishes to appear more scientific, one may speak of coryza, rhinitis, pharyngitis, laryngitis, or bronchitis. But even this will not clarify the situation, for a cold may be a rhinitis today, a pharyngitis tomorrow, and a laryngitis and bronchitis the following day. And coryza usually is present in the early stages of a cold but it also occurs in hay fever, influenza, measles, etc. If it ever becomes possible to differentiate colds according to the germs or physical agents which produce them, then our terminology may be more exact. But until that time the term "common cold" will continue to indicate various disorders of the nose, throat, and chest, characterized primarily by nasal discharge, soreness or dryness of the throat, and cough.

Colds occur in every land from the poles to the equator, although in tropical and semitropical climates they are less severe and less frequently followed by complications than in colder regions. Head colds reach the high point for the year in October and November but are prevalent all through the winter months. Sore throat and influenzal infections also begin in the fall but reach their high point in March.

The Cause of Colds

Colds, as the name suggests, were long thought to be related to atmospheric conditions, but recently attention has been centered upon specific microorganisms which have been described as their cause. There is, however, abundant evidence that general factors as well as specific microorganisms play a part in the production of colds. Of the direct and the contributory causes of colds the ones of greatest importance are as follows:

A Filtrable Virus. A microorganism so tiny that it will pass through the pores of a porcelain filter and cannot be seen even with ordinary microscopes is at present being accorded greatest consideration as the cause of colds. Kruse, in Germany, suggested the existence of such a virus in 1914 when he introduced the filtered nasal discharge of a patient with an acute cold into the nasal cavities of thirty-six members of his bacteriology class. Fifteen, or 42 per cent, of these students developed typical head colds, while no colds developed in twenty-nine uninoculated members of the class. Investigators in this country obtained similar results and concluded that common colds, at least of a certain type, are infectious and that a causative filtrable virus occurs in the nasal secretions of persons with colds. This virus can be transmitted from person to person but is not highly infectious. Under certain conditions it will stay alive a long time; under other conditions it dies quickly. It seems probable that this virus is responsible for most epidemics of colds.

The usual symptoms of this "virus cold" in human subjects are stuffiness of the nose, sneezing, sore throat, and headache. No fever occurs during the course of the attack, the duration of which is approximately one week. This mild course, however, occurs only if the subjects are carefully isolated from all possible contacts with other persons. Otherwise, the acute process is usually followed by secondary infections with other microorganisms which happen to be present in the nose and throat. These secondary infections persist 2 or 3 weeks, are accompanied by a thick, yellow discharge, and may involve the sinuses, ears, and lower respiratory tract.

Bacteria. Several different bacteria, much larger than viruses, have been reported by competent bacteriologists to produce typical colds. Most of these bacterial colds seem to begin with a severe sore throat, with coryza appearing later as the infection extends upward into the nasal passages.

Although a distinction is usually made between influenza and the common cold, either may give rise to nasal symptoms. In fact, Doull and Bahlke state that, in an epidemic of influenza among the resident nurses of Johns Hopkins Hospital, 51 per cent of the patients exhibited coryza as a "first day" symptom.

The Transmission of Colds. The cold virus is found in abundance in the nose and throat during the early stages of a cold but disappears in three to four days. Consequently, a patient is very infectious just as he is coming down with a cold but ceases to be a menace in a few days. Most communicable colds enter the body through the respiratory tract, although investigators report several cases of acute colds in which the mode of transmission seems to have been by means of food.

The rapidity with which acute colds may spread through a community is illustrated by the observations of Heinbecker that practically 100 per cent of the natives of certain Eskimo villages developed acute respiratory infections with sneezing, coughing, and spitting within 72 hours after the arrival of his exploring party.

Allergic Colds. One of the baffling maladies of man is the condition or group of conditions known as "allergy" or "hypersensitiveness." Persons in an allergic state react in an abnormal manner to substances which of themselves are essentially harmless. It has been estimated that 10 to 20 per cent of persons exhibit some type of hypersensitiveness. Just why this develops we do not know. Heredity is a predisposing factor but does not completely explain the condition.

The substances to which people may become sensitive are legion, but most common among these are pollens of plants and trees; emanations from animals such as dogs, cats, rabbits, and horses; substances such as feathers, wool, lint, and face powder; eggs, milk, meat, chocolate, strawberries, melon, spinach, lettuce, and various other foods.

Varied also are the symptoms which allergic conditions may produce. The portion of the body most frequently affected is the nasal mucous membrane, in which the reaction causes swelling, congestion, and watery discharge. During the summer these symptoms are called "hay fever." In the lower respiratory tract, allergic reactions produce asthma; in the skin, hives and certain types of eczema.

The substances which give rise to these reactions usually are inhaled with the air or ingested with the food. When inhaled they are most likely to affect the respiratory tract, although they may be absorbed and produce symptoms, such as hives, in other parts of the body. Foods may cause nasal symptoms, asthma, hives, headaches, or other allergic manifestations.

[287]

Between the common cold and allergic reactions of the nasal mucous membrane there is great similarity. In fact, a "rose cold" is the same condition which later in the summer is called hay fever. Some people suffer from such symptoms periodically or continuously throughout the year, and usually think that the trouble is a cold or sinus infection. Relief sought along those lines, however, can lead only to disappointment.

After an allergic condition of the nasal mucous membrane has continued for a long period of time, particularly if medicated oils or similar preparations are dropped, sprayed, or otherwise introduced into the nose, secondary infections are likely to develop. In such cases treatment of the infection is unsatisfactory unless the fundamental allergic condition is recognized and corrected. An allergic state is a contributory factor of sufficient importance in chronic or recurrent colds and chronic sinus infection to be considered in every case.

Climatic Factors. It is difficult to determine accurately the influence of the weather upon the development of colds. It has long been common knowledge that colds are most frequent during the winter months and that colds frequently develop following exposure to drafts or chilling of the body. On the other hand, arctic explorers tell us that members of their parties and Eskimos with whom they come in contact go all winter long without colds even though exposed to extreme and rapid changes of temperature. They pass suddenly from temperatures of 80 to 90 degrees in the igloos to 30 or 40 degrees below zero on the outside. They may fall into the water and have their clothes become solid ice on them or be soaked to the skin with perspiration and shiver to keep warm. But still they do not take cold. On the other hand, contact with the outside world through trading vessels or through visits to trading posts is almost certain to start an epidemic of colds.

In this country there is apparently a distinct and definite relationship between the occurrence of colds and the temperature. The Metropolitan Life Insurance Company finds that colds among their employees tend to increase whenever there is a distinct drop in outside temperature. The Johns Hopkins investigators found that during the winter months the attack rate of colds rises when the temperature falls below its ordinary level. On the other hand, the daily range of temperature, the humidity, the rainfall, the wind velocity, the percentage of sunshine, and the atmospheric pressure apparently have no relationship to the occurrence of colds.

The general belief that one can avoid colds by moving to a different section of the country finds little support in several studies conducted by the U.S. Public Health Service. Careful records were kept of the occurrence of colds in certain student and family groups in different parts of the country. The students were from Harvard University, Mount Holyoke College, Johns Hopkins University, Georgetown University, Tulane University, University of Chicago, Ohio State University, University of Utah, University of Arizona, and University of California. The attack rates in these student groups were remarkably uniform, showing no consistent relation to latitude, longitude, or climate. The occurrence of epidemics in the several groups in widely different localities showed a striking time correspondence. Whether the students used sleeping porches, well-ventilated bedrooms, or poorly ventilated bedrooms for sleeping purposes did not materially affect their susceptibility.

Physical Factors. Anything which produces irritation of the membranes of the nose and throat may produce symptoms of nasal congestion and discharge, commonly described as a cold. Usually these symptoms are of short duration unless the injury to the mucous membrane has opened the way to bacterial infection. In such a case the infection may be severe and prolonged.

Many things irritate the mucous membranes of the nose. When the autumn wind fills the atmosphere with dust, colds increase. Tobacco smoke is an irritation to the membranes of the nose and throat of certain people in whom smoking may be a factor in keeping up a low-grade irritation. The irritating gases in storage battery shops, garages, chemical plants, etc., produce congestion of the nose, and overheated air, such as occurs in most American homes during the winter, predisposes to colds.

Drafts. Exposure to drafts and chilling of portions of the

[289]

body frequently result in congestion of the nose which may develop into a typical acute cold. Just why this should occur is not entirely clear. In some cases the congestion and discharge disappear with the restoration of uniform temperature. In others, this nonspecific reaction is followed by bacterial infection which becomes a typical cold and runs the usual course of two to three weeks.

Other Factors in the Production of Colds. Spiesman of the University of Illinois reported studies which show that persons who have frequent colds almost all experience a much greater and more prolonged reduction in the temperature of the nasal mucous membrane upon a chilling of the skin than do individuals who are not susceptible to colds. This is probably due to a disturbance in the control of blood flow to the skin and mucous membranes. The cause of this disturbance is not known but those conducting the study believe that the susceptibility to colds is reduced by cold baths and a diet high in fresh fruits and vegetables and low in wheat products and carbohydrates.

Other nonspecific factors which in many cases seem to be related to colds are fatigue, constipation, overeating, malnutrition, nervousness, and poor ventilation. The importance of most of these factors is difficult to measure, but it is logical to assume that persons who are in good physical condition will be less affected by the factors which predispose to colds than those whose physical condition is below par.

The Prevention of Colds

Many measures, specific and general, are advocated and advertised for the prevention of colds. If these measures were really effective, like vaccination for smallpox or vitamin D for rickets, there could be no doubt concerning their value; but they are not. This much is agreed to by all. The question is: Have they any merit at all? Do they measurably reduce the frequency or the severity of colds? These are difficult questions but we can at least review the available information on the subject.

Avoidance of Exposure. In the communicable type of cold, exposure to infection, direct or indirect, is the method of spread.

Hence, avoidance of exposure to persons with colds is a rational preventive measure. Unfortunately, under the conditions of modern life the avoidance of exposure to colds is an impossibility. We can, however, minimize the degree of exposure and materially reduce the danger of infection by the practice of such simple hygienic measures as thorough washing of the hands before meals and after contact with objects likely to contain infective material; keeping the hands away from the nose and mouth; avoidance of direct exposure to persons with colds, particularly during the first three days of the disease, and the use of individual drinking glasses even within the family. A different colored drinking cup or glass for each member of the family is a simple way to reduce the probability that every cold will become a family affair.

Hardening Processes and Sleeping Porches. Cold baths, outdoor exercises, the use of sleeping porches, and similar measures are advocated for the prevention of colds on the theory that they will make the skin and mucous membranes less sensitive to temperature changes. A controlled study, however, in which medical and public health students of Johns Hopkins University served as subjects, indicated that outdoor exercise had no influence on the frequency of colds and that the only effect of sleeping with wide-open windows was that a larger percentage of colds were accompanied by cough.

It may be healthful for a person accustomed to it and in the prime of physical condition to sleep in zero or near-zero temperatures; but for persons who lead a relatively inactive life and spend most of their time indoors, moderation is the wiser course to pursue. The most refreshing nights of the year are in the spring and fall, when with wide-open windows the temperature of the sleeping room is between 50 and 60 degrees. To maintain similar conditions throughout the rest of the year would be ideal. In summer this is difficult to accomplish, but in winter temperature can be controlled by regulating the amount of outside air.

Vaccines. Cold vaccines—not cold "serums" as they are frequently called; there is no serum for colds—consist of killed bacteria or bacterial extracts. The common vaccines contain various mixtures of the bacteria most commonly found in the nose and throat of persons with colds. The theory upon which vaccines are usually advocated is that they stimulate the development of an immunity against colds. However, since colds themselves produce little or no immunity, it is hardly reasonable to assume that injection of the killed germs, even if they cause colds, will do so. Rather it seems that when vaccines are of benefit it is because they temporarily desensitize the person to certain bacteria to which he happens to be sensitive or allergic. This is analogous to the injection of pollens for the prevention of hay fever.

Vaccines for the prevention of colds were extensively used some years ago, but carefully controlled studies fail to show much if any value from their use. Several of these studies were carried out at the University of Minnesota. Two widely used vaccines were studied; one given by injection, the other put up in capsules and taken by mouth. Only individuals who reported that they usually had four or more colds per year were included in the study. For the purposes of the study four groups, *A*, *B*, *C*, and *D*, were set up, to which the subjects were assigned in order. The individuals in group *A* were given the recommended series of injections of the hypodermic vaccine; those in group *B* were given injections of sterile water according to the same directions; group *C* received supplies of the oral vaccine, which they took throughout the winter according to instructions; and group *D* received capsules of similar appearance and with the same instructions, but these capsules contained only milk sugar. Careful records were kept of the number of colds experienced by each subject during the period of the study. Groups *B* and *D* were the "control" groups, so essential in scientific studies. The individuals in them thought that they were receiving vaccine and the physicians who recorded the colds contracted had no information as to the group to which any individual belonged. Over the 2-year period group *A* contained 272 individuals; group *B*, 276; group *C*, 370; and group *D*, 378.

These studies showed that the individuals in the control groups *B* and *D*, who received no vaccine whatever, reported 63 and 68 per cent fewer colds, respectively, during the period of the study than these same individuals reported that they had had during the previous winter. This is very significant since these individuals received nothing of any value for the prevention of colds. It shows how easily and how unjustifiably enthusiastic one may become concerning any procedure or preparation, no matter how worthless, for the prevention of colds if skillful advertising or well-meaning but uncritical friends recommend it. Most advertisers of vitamin concentrates, alkalization, nose drops, and gargles do not claim that their products will reduce the frequency of colds by more than 60 to 70 per cent.

The individuals who received the hypodermic vaccine reported 73 per cent less colds during the study than they reported they had had during the previous winter and an average of 1.6 colds per person per year during the study as compared to 2.1 colds for the control group. This difference occurred both years of the study and so doubtless is significant. It is questionable, however, in view of the large number of injections required, whether this difference has any practical value. That is, how many people would wish to undergo the expense and inconvenience of all these vaccinations in order to reduce by 25 per cent the number of colds which they will probably have during the year?

Oral vaccines, administered in either capsules or tablet form, are extensively promoted and widely used for the prevention of colds. The Minnesota studies, however, as well as the studies of other investigators, indicate that they are of even less value than the injected vaccine. This is the only conclusion possible, since the group which received the vaccine reported an average of 1.8 colds per person as compared to 1.7 colds for the control group.

The most recent study at the University of Minnesota was an evaluation of a vaccine which is sprayed into the nose. Some encouraging results have been reported for this type of vaccine, but in the student groups tested, the results were entirely negative.

Another type of vaccine occasionally used for the prevention of chronic or recurrent colds is called an "autogenous" vaccine. This, too, consists of dead bacteria but, instead of a heterogeneous mixture, the bacteria in it are obtained from the nose and throat of the patient himself. These inoculations are usually given weekly throughout the fall, winter, and spring months. While not uniformly successful, such vaccines are more likely to be of benefit than those that are prepared without regard to the particular individual for whom they will be used.

From these and other careful studies we must conclude that there is no satisfactory evidence that cold vaccines are of value when used routinely in large groups of individuals. For this reason their indiscriminate use is clearly unjustified.

Ultraviolet Light. A few years ago the exposure of the body to ultraviolet light during the winter months was widely advocated for the prevention of colds. The logic for this was that colds are more frequent during the season of the year when the ultraviolet rays in the atmosphere are at a minimum.

Some of the early investigators of this subject reported encouraging results, but the Johns Hopkins University workers failed to find any significant reduction in the number of colds which occurred in a group of medical students who received regular ultraviolet irradiation during the winter months as compared with a group who received no such treatment.

Vitamins are much advertised for the prevention of colds, especially vitamin A, as found in cod-liver oil, halibut-liver oil, and carotene, and vitamin D, as found in cod-liver oil and viosterol. Advertisers would have us believe that if we get enough of these and other vitamins in tablets, oils, specially treated foods, cough syrups, or even cough drops, the common cold will be a thing of the past. But let us examine the facts of the situation.

Vitamin A deficiency (see Chapter IV) in animals unquestionably increases susceptibility to respiratory infections. On the other hand, since this vitamin is found in the average diet, is not destroyed by heat, is stored by the body, and is necessary in only minute amounts in order to prevent symptoms of deficiency, it clearly does not follow that its addition to the average diet will increase resistance to respiratory infections. Barenberg and Lewis supplemented the diets of one-half of the children in an institution in New York with vitamin A but found no lower incidence of colds among these children than among those who received no vitamin supplement. More recently Shibley and Spies administered vitamin A in the form of halibut-liver oil over a period of 56 weeks to a group of approximately 100 students of Western Reserve University. Careful records were kept of the frequence of colds in this group as compared with the frequence in a group of 100 other students on ordinary diets. At the end of the year they reported that neither the frequence nor the severity of colds was affected by the addition of this vitamin to the diet. There was, however, some suggestive evidence that the duration of colds during the winter months was two or three days shorter among the group that had received the vitamin A supplement.

Vitamin D, in the form of viosterol, is occasionally suggested for the prevention of colds, probably because rachitic children are unusually susceptible to respiratory infections. But here again the results of actual studies show that children who are given viosterol throughout the winter have just as many colds as children who do not receive it. The addition of vitamin D to the diet, particularly of children, during the winter months is very desirable. Its value lies not in any specific effect that it has in the prevention or cure of colds, but in its influence upon general nutrition and upon the development of the bones and teeth.

Cod-liver oil, which contains both vitamin A and vitamin D, has been reported to reduce the frequency of colds in children. On the other hand, Hess, Barenburg, and Lewis found that the daily administration of cod-liver oil had no influence upon the susceptibility of a group of infants to respiratory infections.

Vitamins B, C, D, and E are sometimes thought to be related to infection because animals on diets in which these vitamins are lacking exhibit unusual susceptibility to infection. Such animals, however, are always in a greatly weakened condition; hence, their increased susceptibility cannot be accepted as evidence that the addition of extra quantities of these vitamins to an adequate diet will prevent infections.

A controlled study, similar to that with cold vaccines, was carried on at the University of Minnesota to determine the value of vitamins for the prevention of colds. One group was given large doses of vitamin C alone and another group large doses of multiple vitamin capsules (A, B₁, B₂, C, D). The control group took capsules that were indistinguishable from the vitamin capsules but contained no vitamins. The results of this study, which was carried on throughout a year, gave no indication that large doses either of vitamin C or of the multiple vitamins had any important effect on the number or the severity of infections of the upper respiratory tract.

To summarize, one can only conclude that specific evidence is not available to prove that the addition of vitamins to the average diet increases resistance to colds.

Nose and Throat Operations. Abnormal conditions of the nose and throat, such as adenoids, diseased tonsils, and nasal obstruction, are important factors in increasing susceptibility to colds. Hence, benefit may be expected from operative procedures when they are clearly indicated and properly performed. On the other hand, indiscriminate operating upon the nose and throat does more harm than good (see Chapter XIV).

Ventilation. Overheating is the aspect of ventilation which is most clearly related to the prevalence of colds. A temperature of 68 to 70 degrees with a 40 to 50 per cent humidity seems to be optimum for comfort and health. Humidity alone has not been shown to be of importance, but an adequate amount of moisture in the air enables one to be comfortable at lower temperatures than would otherwise be possible.

Habits of Living. Hygienic living, with particular reference to diet and to the avoidance of fatigue, overeating, and constipation, improves general health and so should reduce susceptibility to, at least, certain types of colds.

Nasal Hygiene. Nasal sprays, nose drops, gargles, and antiseptics are extensively advertised during the winter months for the prevention of colds. Beautiful girls and important-looking men are pictured gargling their throats or dropping mysterious medications into their noses. Millions of dollars' worth of such preparations are sold, in spite of the fact that there is no evidence whatsoever that the use of any medicinal preparation, oil, or antiseptic is of any value for the prevention of colds. Some mouthwashes, gargles, and antiseptics may destroy germs but none of them acts instantaneously nor are they effective in the weak solutions which could be tolerated by the membranes of the nose and throat. Furthermore, only a very small proportion of the mucous membrane of the nose and throat can possibly be reached by sprays and gargles (page 311). Nor can one be certain that the use of these preparations is harmless, for they tend to paralyze the cilia of the nose whose function is to get rid of bacteria or other foreign matter, and most of them contain substances which may keep up a low-grade chronic irritation.

Diet for Prevention of Colds. The dietary measures most frequently recommended for the prevention of colds include a high protein diet, a low protein diet, and large quantities of citrus fruits, the last presumably to produce alkalization. Appealing though such theories may sound, none of them is based upon scientific evidence or established fact.

The Treatment of Colds

There is no subject upon which one gets so much free and worthless advice as the treatment of colds. It is not necessary to look for it. It is impossible to avoid it. Most of this comes from advertisers who are making greatly exaggerated or entirely unjustified claims for some medicinal preparation. But friends and neighbors are always willing to suggest their pet remedies.

It is frequently said that if you treat a cold you can cure it in fourteen days and that if you do nothing about it you will be well in two weeks. And a favorite prescription is a couple of dozen soft linen handkerchiefs and ten days in bed. Skepticism as to the value of most treatment of the common cold is amply justified.

The types of treatment which we shall consider are those of established or accepted value and those which, even though worthless, are extensively used. No treatment known is a specific cure for the common cold. It is possible, however, to minimize the physiological disturbances which the cold produces and thus decrease the severity of symptoms and the probability of complications.

Specifically, the measures which seem of greatest value in the

[297]

treatment of colds are those which control or reduce the severity of the reaction of the nasal mucous membranes. In both the infectious and noninfectious types of colds congestion and swelling of these membranes occur, usually accompanied by a watery discharge. This reaction apparently lowers their resistance to infection by any germs which happen to be present. Thus, control of the reaction tends not only to relieve these symptoms but to shorten the duration by decreasing the probability of secondary infection. Certain general measures, such as rest, are of value because by conserving energy they aid the body to build up resistance.

Sweating Out a Cold. Exercise is a method of treatment for the common cold utilized by many people. They describe it as "sweating out" a cold. What they actually experience is relief of nasal stuffiness and discharge as a result of the exercise. This occurs because, with an increase in the flow of blood to the muscles and skin, nasal congestion is diminished. Such relief, of course, is only temporary, but occasionally it seems to prevent further progress of the cold. Usually, however, symptoms recur when the body gets chilled, and the cold becomes more severe than before.

Hot Baths. A hot bath is a favorite early treatment for colds. These baths may consist of hot water, hot air, or steam—a Turkish bath. In each case the blood vessels of the skin are dilated and the blood flow through them is increased, with a concurrent reduction of nasal congestion. If hot baths are followed by rest in bed with sufficient covers to prevent cooling, the effect is prolonged and the possibility of its being of more than temporary benefit is increased.

Physiotherapy. Massage of various types with or without other forms of physiotherapy increases blood flow through the muscles and skin and gives relief of about the same degree and the same value as exercise or hot baths.

Strict Bed Rest. "Go to bed when you have a cold and stay there until you are well" is good advice for the treatment of colds. Its value lies in protecting others from exposure, in increasing general resistance, and in keeping the body warm. Unfortunately, like most good advice, this is rarely followed. People just will not stay in bed unless they feel ill.

In treating the colds of students at the University of Minnesota, no effort is made to have them stay in bed unless their colds are accompanied by fever, general aching, or other symptoms which indicate that the infection is rather severe. If such symptoms exist, there can be no doubt about the importance of bed rest, not only to hasten recovery but to reduce the probability of pneumonia or other serious complications.

Water for Colds. Large quantities of liquids have long been considered a valuable aid in the treatment of colds. These may be taken in the form of water, lemonade, orange juice, or any other drink. The purpose is to increase excretion, thereby presumably aiding in the elimination of the toxic products produced by the infection. Whether this really occurs no one knows, so we must conclude that the practice is based upon assumption rather than scientific evidence of its value. In fact, the preliminary report of a study on this subject suggests that persons with acute colds get along just as well when they let thirst determine the fluid intake as when they attempt to force or to restrict fluids.

When colds are accompanied by fever, there is an increase in the fluids lost by evaporation. These need to be replaced but nature takes care of this by increasing the thirst.

Catharsis for Colds. Cathartics of various kinds have long been used as a home remedy for colds and are included in many of the cold medicines advertised to the public. The reason for their use has been the assumption that catharsis aids in the elimination of the infection. Logically, there is no reason to think that this could occur, but, like sheep, most people continue to do what others have done. A few years ago two controlled studies of this common practice were made, both of which concluded that cathartics are of no value in the treatment of the common cold.

Antiseptic Gargles. Gargles of many kinds are advertised for the treatment of colds. Their claims are based upon alleged antiseptic properties. Under conditions of sufficient concentration and adequate time some of them probably will destroy bacteria.

But in the weak concentrations in which they are used and in the short space of time that they are retained in the throat they are not antiseptic. Furthermore, gargles reach only a small portion of the mucous membrane of the throat. Consequently, for practical purposes their antiseptic properties are negligible.

The Application of Heat. Hot irrigations or hot gargles, on the other hand, are widely used by physicians for the treatment of throat infections. Their purpose is to apply heat to inflamed tissues, a principle employed in the treatment of infections generally. The solution commonly used for this purpose is ordinary table salt in the proportion of half a teaspoon of salt to a glass of water. The solution should be as warm as can be comfortably tolerated. Gargling should be as long and as frequent as is convenient.

Counterirritation. Hot or cold compresses, mustard plasters, or medicated ointments applied to the outside of the throat or chest are widely utilized in the treatment of colds. Some of them probably increase somewhat the blood flow to the skin, but they have never been shown to be of value for the treatment of colds.

The Medicinal Treatment of Colds. More drugs are sold for the treatment of colds than for any other condition. Some are prescribed by physicians, but the great majority are sold through radio, newspaper, or billboard advertising.

Certain of these preparations are supposed to alkalize, others to acidify, the system. Some stimulate secretions; others suppress them. There is no reason, logic, or scientific evidence to support the claims which are made for most of them.

The cold medication of greatest age is the old-fashioned Dover's powder. This was first proposed by Thomas Dover in the latter part of the seventeenth century for the treatment of gout. Originally it contained powdered opium, powdered ipecac, and potassium chlorate and was administered with a half pint of grog. Some time later the potassium chlorate and the grog were omitted and the powder of opium and ipecac came to be used for colds. This was probably because the preparation had obtained a reputation as a sweating powder and sweating was supposed to be beneficial.

[300]

A Critical Study of Cold Medications. Several years ago a series of studies was instituted by the Health Service of the University of Minnesota to determine the value of various forms of treatment of the common cold. These studies were specifically planned to avoid prejudice for or against any particular medication. To accomplish this the following procedure was adopted. Physicians wrote prescriptions for "cold medication." These prescriptions were filled by a pharmacist who used in sequence the various medications being studied at the time. Neither physician nor patient knew what medication had been given. After 48 hours of treatment the patients reported the results on cards prepared for this purpose. Upon the basis of these reports the effectiveness of the medication in each case was estimated. Finally, the pharmacist's record was obtained and the results tabulated according to the various medications which were used.

At the outset of the study some of the tablets and capsules contained only milk sugar. These were included so that those making the study might know what proportion of patients would recover without treatment in the 48-hour period for which results were reported. In other words, the group who received sugar tablets, thinking that they contained medication, served as a control group for the rest of the study. The importance of having this control was clearly shown by the results, for approximately 35 per cent of the students who got sugar tablets reported improvement or cure of their acute colds within 48 hours. Some of these experienced such prompt and remarkable improvement that they were moved to comment that these tablets were the most effective treatment that they had ever tried for their colds. The fact that such a large percentage of persons with colds recover spontaneously within a few days is the reason that it is possible to sell almost any preparation for the treatment of colds, provided it is supported by an effective advertising program.

The medications studied in this manner included practically every medicinal preparation which there was any reason to think might be beneficial. The results may be grouped into several classifications: (1) those of greatest value, (2) those of moderate value, (3) those of little or no value.

[301]

The medications of greatest value, according to this study, were all derivatives of opium. This is particularly interesting in view of statements by De Quincey and other writers on opium that addicts, while using opium, are free from colds. It also explains why the use of Dover's powder has continued these many years. In fact, the study showed that the value of Dover's powder is due entirely to the opium which it contains and that its action is not dependent upon sweating.

Some opium derivatives, although effective for the treatment of colds, are clearly undesirable for general use, either because of the danger of habituation to them or because of the considerable proportion of persons who experience unpleasant symptoms following their use. In this study several opium derivatives which carry no practical danger of habituation were tried in different combinations, proportions, and dosages. Finally, a preparation consisting of equal parts of codeine and papaverine was selected as most valuable for this purpose. Of 1,500 students who were given this preparation for the treatment of acute head colds, between 70 and 75 per cent reported definite improvement or complete relief within 24 to 48 hours. While taking this medication these students were up and about attending classes. Had they remained in bed while using it, it is possible that even better results might have been obtained. The earlier in the course of the cold this is used, the better the results. The most effective way to use it is to have it available to take at the very onset of coryza. This preparation, commonly called copavin, is available through physicians, who should decide when and in what dosage it should be used.

The medications which according to this study might be considered to be of moderate value for the treatment of colds are codeine alone, papaverine alone, powdered opium, Dover's powder, quinine, and aspirin. The proportions of individuals who reported benefit after the use of these preparations ranged from 57 per cent for powdered opium down to 48 per cent for aspirin.

Other medications gave results little if any better than those reported for the sugar tablets. These included a calcium-iodine preparation, an aspirin-phenacetin-caffeine combination, atropine sulphate, soda, and a 1 per cent ephedrine solution dropped into the nose. The aspirin-phenacetin-caffeine combination is widely sold under various trade names for the treatment of colds and headaches. Atropine sulphate, or belladonna from which atropine is derived, is the important constituent of the widely used "coryza and rhinitis tablets." According to these studies, although atropine frequently produces temporary dryness of the nose and mouth, its effect is of short duration and apparently has little if any influence upon the progress of the cold.

Ephedrine constricts blood vessels. Hence, when solutions containing ephedrine sulphate are dropped into a congested, stuffy nose, they usually give relief. For this reason, ephedrine is included in most of the preparations which are used as sprays and nose drops. Unfortunately this relief from ephedrine is of short duration—so short, in fact, that the proportion of students who reported lasting benefit was no greater than the proportion who thought they were benefited by a sugar capsule.

Commercially advertised preparations for the treatment of colds are legion. Radio and television have given vendors of alleged cold remedies a new medium through which to reach the public and they are making the most of it.

Two of the nationally advertised and most widely sold of these cold remedies were included in this study. These were taken out of their original containers and dispensed in such a manner that patients did not know what they were receiving. The directions, however, were those contained on the original package. One of these is taken by mouth, a so-called "internal medication." The other is dropped into the nose. The results reported after the use of the internal medication were a little, but very little, better than those reported after the sugar tablets. The results with the nose drops were even worse. In fact, the percentage of students who reported benefit after their use was a little less than the percentage who thought they were benefited by sugar tablets. There is even some evidence that the use of medicated oils in the nose during the acute stage of colds, although giving temporary relief, tends to aggravate the irritation of the inflamed mucous membrane. Yet people spend millions of dollars each year for these and other worthless preparations.

From these studies the following conclusions can be drawn:
1. Medications that give most relief are all derivatives of opium.
2. A preparation consisting of equal parts of codeine and papaverine is of greatest benefit.
3. Aspirin, soda, and quinine are of little or no value.
4. Advertised cold remedies give essentially the same results as are obtained with sugar tablets.
5. Use of medicated oils in the nose during the acute stage of colds tends to aggravate irritation of the inflamed mucous membrane.

Sulfonamides and Antibiotics for Colds. These "wonder drugs" are valuable in so many infections that it is natural that they should be tried on colds, particularly since they are of definite value in certain complications of colds. Well-controlled studies, however, have failed to show them to be of any benefit in acute colds. And there are certain objections and even dangers to their use in minor respiratory infections.

Antihistamines for Colds. Recently drugs known as the antihistamines have been extensively advertised for the prevention and treatment of colds. These preparations usually relieve allergic symptoms. Critical studies, however, have failed to show them of any value in real colds.

The Commercial Aspect of Colds. The sale of preparations for the prevention and treatment of colds has become big business, so big in fact that *Fortune Magazine*[1] devoted a major article to it some years ago. Concerning this business *Fortune* says:

> The least of the cold soother's worries is his formula. What goes into his pills or syrups or salves is distinctly a secondary consideration. How to sell his concoction is what chiefly worries the aspiring manufacturer of cold remedies. He is in a business where competitors are many and scruples are few.

Such information should serve as a warning in regard to the claims made by newspaper, billboards, and radio advertisers; but the customer needs also to beware of the cold remedies which the prescribing druggist recommends.

[1] "The Cold Business," *Fortune Magazine*, vol. 6, p. 26, October, 1932.

Several years ago an investigator, feeling that he was coming down with a cold, visited seven different drug stores in Chicago and asked for remedies for his cold. With one exception, he obtained in each drug store three items. The bill for the three items averaged $2. None of these remedies duplicated others. Some were entirely useless; some might have given temporary symptomatic relief; others were prescriptions which were apparently pet hobbies of the druggists "consulted." The seventh druggist suggested that the investigator return to his home, go to bed and call a physician; adding, that the undertaker across the street was exceedingly busy during this particular period.[2]

Influenza

"Influenza" and "grippe" are terms used to designate acute infections of the respiratory tract in which constitutional symp-

Fig. 22. Trend in Deaths from Influenza

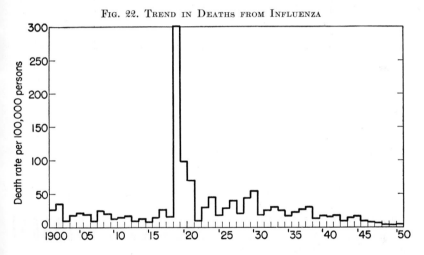

toms are more pronounced than in the common cold. Although coryza frequently accompanies influenza and grippe, the latter conditions are characterized more particularly by headache, sudden onset, backache, fever, chills, prostration, sore throat, and cough. The fatality rate from influenza is low, most patients recovering in 3 to 4 days, but cough and weakness may persist for some time.

[2] "Norwich Capitalizes on Colds," *Journal of the American Medical Association*, vol. 116, p. 56, January 4, 1941.

Fig. 23. Influenza Deaths by Color, Sex, and Age

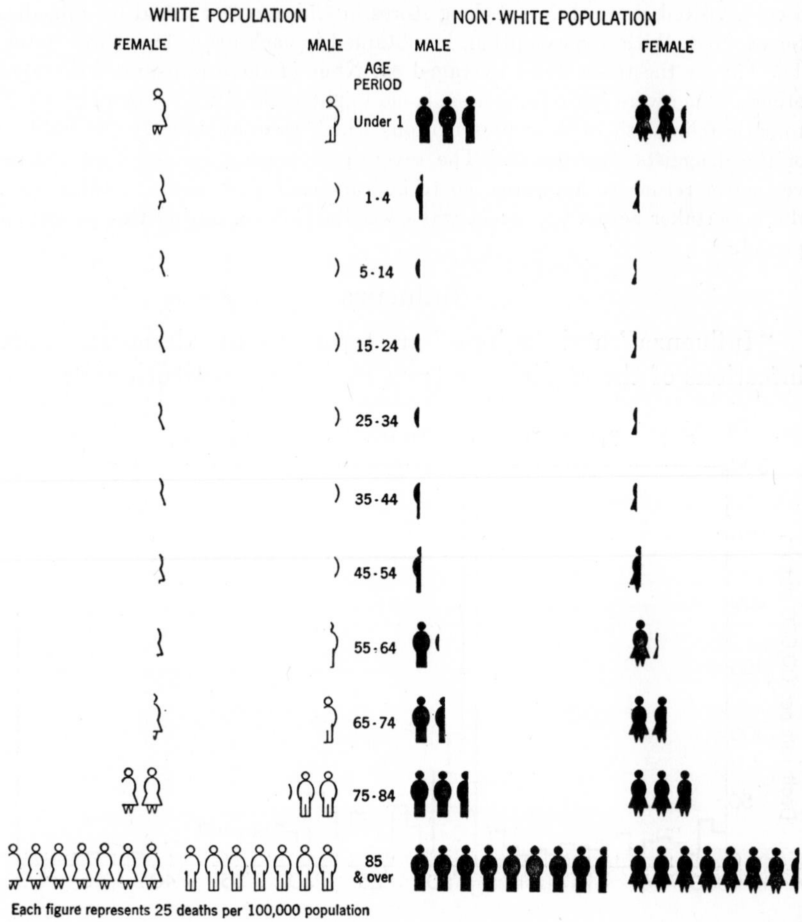

Each figure represents 25 deaths per 100,000 population

Averages of annual death rates per 100,000 persons by color, sex, and age. Ages one to seventy-four years. (*Data from U.S. Office of Vital Statistics.*)

Just what is the relationship or the difference between grippe and influenza is not clear. The symptoms and physical findings are similar. In general, however, the term "grippe" is usually used to designate the relatively mild infections which occur with greater or less frequency almost every winter, while the term "influenza" is used for the more severe infections which occasionally occur in epidemic form.

[306]

Influenza is an acute infectious disease. At different times various germs have been considered its cause. Andrewes, Laidlaw, and Smith in England[3] and Francis in this country[4] have proved the cause to be a filtrable virus. These workers, using filtered nasal secretions from patients with influenza, have succeeded in infecting ferrets, mice, and human volunteers. This is very important. But of even more immediate practical value is the vaccine which Francis has developed for the prevention of influenza. This vaccine was widely used during the war. In general it seems to reduce the occurrence of influenza among vaccinated persons to about one-third the rate among the unvaccinated. Unfortunately, the general usefulness of this vaccine is limited by the appearance of new strains of the virus against which the vaccine is ineffective.

Lacking a completely effective preventive vaccine, we must also utilize general measures to combat this disease. The virus of influenza is highly infective and is transmitted from person to person by means of discharges from the nose and mouth. Measures to reduce contact with infected persons should be observed, although they are not completely effective.

The great danger from influenza is not the disease itself but the pneumonia which so frequently complicates it. This may develop in spite of all precautions, but it is most frequent among persons who remain up and about while ill. Consequently, the most valuable advice which can be given to patients with influenza is "go to bed when you have any fever and remain there until thoroughly recovered." Other measures are helpful but should be prescribed by a physician in accordance with the needs of the individual patient.

DISCUSSION SUGGESTIONS

1. What is meant by the common cold? Explain its importance.
2. What are the causes of colds?
3. Discuss the relation of climate to colds.

[3] Andrewes, C. H., P. P. Laidlaw, and W. Smith, "The Susceptibility of Mice to the Viruses of Human and Swine Influenza," *The Lancet*, vol. 11, p. 859, October 20, 1934.
[4] Francis, Thomas, Jr., "Epidemiological Studies in Influenza," *American Journal of Public Health*, vol. 27, p. 211, March, 1937.

4. What is the possible importance of chilling and of drafts to colds?
5. Does sleeping with wide-open windows influence favorably or unfavorably the occurrence of colds?
6. Discuss the value of vaccines for the prevention of colds.
7. What evidence is there that vitamins are of value for the prevention or treatment of colds?
8. Discuss the use of nose drops and antiseptic gargles for the prevention and treatment of colds.
9. Why are hot baths useful for the treatment of colds?
10. Discuss the studies outlined concerning the medicinal treatment of colds.
11. What is meant by a "control" in such studies? Why is this necessary?
12. Discuss the present status of scientific knowledge concerning the cause, the method of spread, and the prevention of influenza.

REFERENCES AND READING SUGGESTIONS

1. Diehl, Harold S.: "Medicinal Treatment of the Common Cold," *Journal of the American Medical Association*, vol. 101, p. 2042, December 23, 1933.
2. ———, A. B. Baker, and D. W. Cowan: "Cold Vaccines: An Evaluation Based on a Controlled Study," *Journal of the American Medical Association*, vol. 111, p. 1168, September 24, 1938.
3. ———: "Cold Vaccines: A Further Evaluation," *Journal of the American Medical Association*, vol. 115, p. 115, August 24, 1940.
4. ———: "Vitamins for the Prevention of Colds," *Journal of the American Medical Association*, vol. 120, p. 1268, December 19, 1942.
5. ——— and D. W. Cowan: "Intranasal Vaccine for the Prevention of Colds," *Annals of Otology, Rhinology and Laryngology*, vol. 53, p. 286, June, 1944.
6. Dingle, J. H.: "Common Virus Infections of the Respiratory Tract," *Journal of the American Medical Association*, vol. 136, p. 1084, 1948.
7. Editors of *Fortune Magazine:* "Our Common Enemy, Colds," Robert M. McBride & Company, New York, 1934.
8. Francis, Thomas, Jr.: "Epidemiological Studies in Influenza," *American Journal of Public Health*, vol. 27, pp. 211–225, March, 1937.
9. ———, J. E. Salk, and W. N. Brace: "The Protective Effect of Vaccination against Influenza B," *Journal of the American Medical Association*, vol. 131, p. 275, 1948.
10. "Status Report on Antihistaminic Agents in the Prophylaxis and Treatment of the Common Cold" (Council Report); "Antihistaminics for Colds" (Editorial), *Journal of the American Medical Association*, vol. 142, pp. 566, 570, February 25, 1950.
11. Stuart-Harris, C. H., "Influenza and Other Virus Infections of the Respiratory Tract," The Williams & Wilkins Company, Baltimore, 1953.

Chapter XIV

CARE OF THE NOSE, THROAT, AND EARS

MOST of the acute infections to which man is heir are contracted through the nose and throat. Common colds, influenza, tonsillitis, pneumonia, scarlet fever, diphtheria, infantile paralysis, and so on, through a long list of diseases, find their way into the body through this portal. Measures which reduce the infective material which gains access to the nose and mouth, such as frequent washing of the hands and keeping them away from the face, the use of individual drinking glasses, and the avoidance of exposure to persons with these diseases, are all worth while. There is, however, little or nothing of value in the way of local preventive measures to suggest. In fact, the best advice that can be given to most persons concerning the care of the nose and throat is briefly expressed by: "Whatever you do do, don't."

The alleged value of gargles, nasal douches, jellies, sprays, or drops, the so-called "control by nasal hygiene," is based on nothing more than advertising propaganda. Furthermore, the regular use of such preparations without medical advice is pernicious. These preparations usually give temporary relief of nasal stuffiness but they also interfere with the normal protective mechanism of the nasal mucous membranes and in time may cause sufficient irritation to give rise to a chronic catarrhal condition. When this occurs, the medication still gives temporary relief, so the natural inclination is to use it more frequently.

[309]

There is a possibility also that over a period of time there may be enough absorption of these substances to be deleterious. Sniffers of cocaine or of snuff soon learn that absorption from the mucous membrane of the nose is prompt and efficient. In like manner, other substances are absorbed and in some cases the effects might well be cumulative and toxic.

Obstruction to Breathing

The most frequent cause of obstruction to breathing is the common cold, a condition of such importance that we have devoted a special chapter to its consideration. Uncomplicated colds rarely last more than a week or two, but the sinus infections which may complicate them are frequently protracted. The other common causes of chronic nasal obstruction are adenoids in children, and allergic conditions, nasal polyps, and abnormalities of the nasal septum in older persons. Lasting relief can be expected only by eliminating the cause of the obstruction, whatever this may be. Self-medication merely aggravates the trouble.

Adenoids. The dull, pinched, stupid expression of the mouth-breathing child cries for relief. Susceptibility to colds and ear infections, impaired hearing, and a deformed upper jaw are among the other results of chronic mouth-breathing by children. The usual cause of this is adenoids, an overgrowth of tonsillike tissue located in the upper part of the pharynx behind the nose. Fortunately this can be relieved by a simple surgical procedure.

Abnormalities of the Nasal Septum. The septum is the partition between the two sides of the nose. It is composed in part of cartilage and in part of bone. Theoretically the septum should be straight but it rarely is. In fact, a perfectly straight septum is just as rare as an artistically perfect nose. Although most deformities of the septum are of little or no consequence, they occasionally are of sufficient seriousness to interfere with breathing. This not only is annoying but also predisposes to colds and sinus infection. In such cases an operative procedure to straighten the septum is indicated.

Sinus Infection. The term "sinus infection" is now used almost as loosely as "nasal catarrh" was in the past; many persons

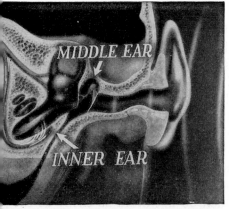

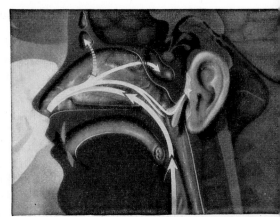

icate, complex mechanism of the human ear.

The health of nose, throat, and ears is closely related.

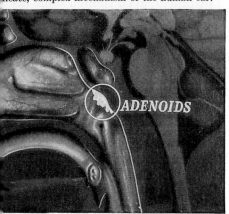

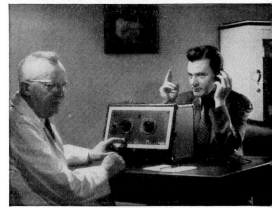

Adenoids and tonsils are thought to be protective organs. They should be removed only when infected.

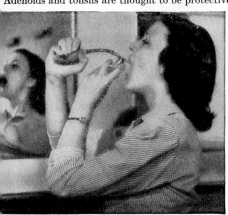

prescribed remedies are *not* recommended.

The audiometer detects the slightest degree of hearing loss.

(From The Nose, Throat, and Ears, a McGraw-Hill Text-Film)

who because of some nasal stuffiness think they have sinus infection do not have it at all. On the other hand, sinus infection is of such frequency and seriousness that it merits careful diagnosis and treatment.

The sinuses are cavities in the bones of the face which are connected by small openings with the nasal cavity and are lined with mucous membrane which is continuous with the mucous membrane of the nose. It is probable that when an acute cold has existed for several days without much improvement, the inflammation has extended to the membranes lining the sinuses, especially to the lower sinuses, which do not drain so easily as the upper group. In the majority of instances, even though some inflammation has extended to the sinuses, the condition will heal promptly as the individual's resistance increases and the natural forces of repair improve under the general measures advisable in these conditions.

The actual cause of sinus disease is infection from the nose, but predisposing factors are violent blowing of the nose—the nose should be blown gently with both nostrils open—a hypersensitive allergic nasal mucous membrane, diving, swimming with the nose in the water, possibly damp climates, and the promiscuous use of sprays, oils, and antiseptics in the nose during acute colds.

Acute sinus infections often clear up without treatment or with the application of such simple measures as heat, steam inhalations, rest, and improved nasal drainage. Occasionally, however, the infection is so severe or drainage so inadequate that pus accumulates in the sinus. This, also, may clear up promptly or it may develop into a subacute or chronic condition. In acute sinus infection local symptoms of nasal discharge, pain, and headache, as well as general symptoms of fever, fatigue, general aching, and cough, are the rule. In chronic sinus disease, on the other hand, the local symptoms may be entirely absent. Occasionally infection from a sinus may be carried by the blood to other parts of the body, such as the joints, kidneys, heart, or brain. A condition potentially so serious calls for adequate medical supervision and treatment.

FIG. 24

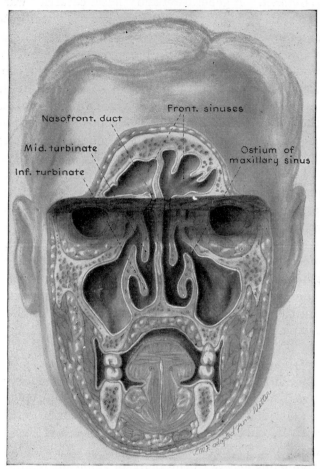

Coronal section of head (semischematic) to show relations and communications of paranasal sinuses. The nasofrontal duct and the ostium of the maxillary sinus connect the frontal sinuses and the maxillary sinuses respectively with the nasal cavity. (*From L. R. Boies, "Fundamentals of Otolaryngology," W. B. Saunders Company, Philadelphia, 1949.*)

Nasal Catarrh. A generation ago "nasal catarrh" was a common complaint. Today it probably is just as prevalent but known by other names. In the seventeenth century nasal discharge was thought to come from the brain. Later it was believed to represent the elimination of poisonous materials from the blood stream, and internal medications were advertised for its cure. Now we know that this condition is due to sinus infection or some other chronic irritation of the mucous membrane and that, to be successful, treatment and prevention must be based upon a determination of the cause.

Nasal Polyps. Chronic sinus infection usually is accompanied by a mucopurulent nasal discharge. This keeps up an irritation of the nasal mucous membrane which, if the membrane is hypersensitive, may eventually result in the formation of grapelike growths called "polyps." In other words, when polyps develop, sinus infection is superimposed upon an allergic condition. The obstruction to breathing in such cases can be relieved by removing the polyps, but unless the allergic condition and then the sinus infection are also corrected the recurrence of the polyps may be expected.

Hay Fever

The sneezing, sniffling, and nose blowing commonly called "hay fever" occur with greater or lesser frequency the year round. In fact, hay fever and related allergic conditions, such as asthma, hives, and certain eczemas, headaches, and digestive disturbances, occur whenever the substance to which an individual is sensitive gains access to the body in sufficient quantities.

Why some people react in this strange manner to substances entirely harmless to others is one of the unsolved mysteries of medical science. This is not because the condition has not been investigated. On the contrary, scientists have devoted a great deal of study to it and have made some progress toward its solution. We know, for example, that heredity is one of the factors in its development; that an individual may become sensitive to a wide variety of substances; that a healthy person can be rendered sensitive for a short period of time by injecting the blood of someone else who is sensitive; that it is usually possible to identify the substances which cause trouble; and that a tolerance to an offending substance may be built up by injecting it first in very minute and then in gradually increasing doses.

The symptoms considered typical of hay fever may be produced by pollens of plants, grasses, or trees, by the dander or hair of animals, by lint, feathers, foods, and many other substances. The pollens, however, are the only substances of this sort which are definitely seasonal. Most cases of spring hay fever are due to grass pollens, although even before the grasses begin to pollinate there are some cases, usually considered spring colds, which are due to the pollens of trees. The pollens of most of the flowering plants are relatively large and heavy and are carried from one plant to another by bees or other insects; hence, they are rarely responsible for hay fever. On the other hand, the pollens of grasses, trees, and many other plants are wind-borne and spell misery to hundreds of thousands of persons each year. Such pollen grains may be carried enormous distances and to great heights by air currents. Lindbergh found a few at a height of 12,000 feet, and they frequently settle out of the upper air hundreds of miles away from their natural habitat and many months after the plants or trees from which they come have ceased pollinating. These pollens, however, do not give rise to hay fever, for symptoms occur only when the concentration of pollen in the air is high. During the pollinating season it is not uncommon to find 1,500 to 2,000 grains of a particular pollen to a cubic yard of air.

An accurate diagnosis of the pollen or pollens responsible for hay fever can be made by placing a minute amount of the pollen on a slight scratch of the skin. Swelling and redness indicate sensitivity to that particular pollen. If, in addition to this evidence of sensitivity, the plant is actually pollinating during the period when symptoms occur, one can be reasonably certain that this is at least one of the pollens causing trouble. It is unusual, however, for a person to be sensitive to one and only one pollen. Hence, in order that diagnosis may be complete, tests must be made with pollens from all the plants which are pollinating during the period of symptoms in the region in which the patient lives.

The most common causes of spring hay fever, frequently called "spring colds" or "rose colds," are the pollens of trees and grasses; while the pollens of ragweed, wormwood, Russian thistle, and pigweed are responsible for most of the fall hay fever. Goldenrod, long thought to be the cause of fall hay fever, has been exonerated. It and other flowering plants have been suspected in connection with hay fever because they happen to flower at the time that weeds with inconspicuous flowers are pollinating.

After the cause of hay fever has been determined, the simplest way to prevent it is to live, at least during the hay fever season, in a region in which the pollens to which one is sensitive do not exist. Another way to reduce exposure to pollen is to spend most of the day during the hay fever season in filtered air. This gives relief in many cases.

For the unfortunate hay fever victims who cannot move away during the hay fever season and whose homes and places of work are not air-conditioned, there is still considerable hope of obtaining relief, for it is usually possible so to increase one's tolerance that one will be free from symptoms or at least reasonably comfortable even though exposed to high concentrations of pollen. This is accomplished by giving a series of injections of the pollens to which one is sensitive. In order to be effective this treatment must be based upon an accurate diagnosis of the causes of the hay fever and the inclusion in the treatment material of all the pollens which are responsible for symptoms. Failure to do these two things has been the reason for many of the unsatisfactory results from this type of preventive treatment of hay fever in the past.

Temporary relief in hay fever and other allergic conditions can frequently be obtained by the use of a group of drugs called antihistamines.

The Tonsils

With so many tonsils being removed one naturally wonders what the tonsils are for. Actually there is no certain evidence of their purpose, although it is generally thought that they have some sort of protective function, ineffective though this seems to be in most cases.

It is probable that the protective function of the tonsil is exercised in this manner. With exposure in early life to the usual infections which find entrance to the body through the nose and throat, the tonsils and adenoids tend to become infected before the deeper portions of the respiratory tract. The products of this infection when absorbed tend to vaccinate the individual against further infection. Since, however, it is impossible to produce a prolonged immunity against the bacteria which cause ordinary nose and throat infections, this is only a temporary protection. With repeated infections changes may occur in the structure of the tonsils and adenoids which make them more or less constant sites of infection and a menace to general health.

In childhood tonsils and adenoids are naturally large but both decrease in size during later life. There are three definite reasons why the removal of the tonsils and adenoids is advisable: (1) repeated attacks of acute tonsillitis or quinsy; (2) enlargement of tonsils and adenoids to the point of causing obstruction to the nose or the eustachian tube; (3) reasonable suspicion that the tonsils are serving as a focus of infection. In the event of a serious disease condition in which other possible foci of infection have been eliminated, it is sometimes advisable to sacrifice the tonsils even though the local condition does not offer adequate proof of tonsil infection.

If tonsils are to be removed, it is well to remember that recent studies indicate that removal of tonsils and adenoids at the beginning of a poliomyelitis season increases the danger of contracting the disease, especially of the bulbar type.

The end results of tonsillectomy in children were analyzed by Dr. Kaiser[1] of Rochester, New York, in a study in which he compared the health of 2,200 tonsillectomized school children over a period of 10 years with the health of a corresponding number of children of similar ages who had been advised to have their tonsils removed but for various reasons had failed to do so. From this study he concludes: (1) that tonsillectomy materially reduces the occurrence of sore throats; (2) that tonsillectomized children are less susceptible to scarlet fever and diphtheria; (3)

[1] Kaiser, A. D., "Results of Tonsillectomy," *Journal of the American Medical Association*, vol. 95, p. 837, September 20, 1930.

that acute head colds and middle ear infections are reduced over a 3-year period by tonsillectomy but are essentially uninfluenced over a 10-year period; (4) that enlargement of the lymph glands of the neck is less frequent among tonsillectomized children; (5) that infections of the lower respiratory tract, such as laryngitis, bronchitis, and pneumonia, occur more frequently among children who have had their tonsils removed; (6) that first attacks of rheumatic fever occur 30 per cent less frequently in tonsillectomized children, but recurrent attacks are not reduced at all; (7) that incomplete tonsillectomies do not offer the same protection against the usual throat complaints and infections as complete removal of tonsils; and (8) that the hazards of tonsillectomy must be considered in deciding upon the operation.

From these data it is clear that miraculous results cannot be expected from removal of the tonsils; but that when definite indications for tonsillectomy exist, sufficient improvement may be expected to amply justify the operation. Kaiser concludes from his studies that "there is substantial evidence that in about 20 per cent of the children the tonsils are either hypertrophied or diseased and therefore have an unfavorable influence on the physical development of the child. Such tonsils should be removed."[2]

Tonsillectomy is not a dangerous procedure if adequate precautions are taken to safeguard against accident. Undoubtedly many tonsils have been needlessly removed in the past and more will be sacrificed in the future. On the other hand, the indications for the removal of tonsils and adenoids are being more accurately defined and medical opinion on the subject of tonsillectomy is becoming more and more conservative.

The Conservation of Hearing

Helen Keller, deaf, dumb, and blind, is credited with saying that she would value above all other senses the sense of hearing, that instrument of intercourse with others without which the sound of the human voice is lost and one becomes engulfed in an

---

[2] Kaiser, A. D., "Significance of the Tonsils in the Development of the Child," *Journal of the American Medical Association,* vol. 115, p. 1156, Oct. 5, 1940.

indescribable loneliness. In the following paragraphs E. F. Benson vividly describes his sensations during a brief period of absolute stillness:

I had sat down on the topmost bluff of these cliffs, having tethered my donkey down below. . . . No breeze of any sort was stirring, but the air, pure, hot, invigorating, was absolutely still. At that moment I suddenly felt as if something was dreadfully wrong, though I did not at once guess what it was. Then came the thought, the identification of what was wrong: it seemed as if the world was dead; then came the reason for it: it was because there was no sound. For a moment I listened in order to verify this—listened with poised breath and immovable limbs. Yes, I was right: there was no sound of anything at all; for once the ears were deprived of the delicate orchestra that goes up, a hymn of praise, day and night from the earth. It was like a dreadful nightmare.

I first tried coughing, to see if it would be companionable, but that did not do; I coughed, and then silence resumed its reign. I lit a cigarette. I moved, rustled, even got up and walked a little, kicking the pebbles that lay about in the sand. But that was no use, and I perceived where the defect was. I knew I was alive, and could make sounds, but what I wanted was some evidence that something else was alive. But there was none.

I cannot describe the horror of this. Momentary as was the sensation, it was of a quality, a depth of surcharged panic, which comes to us only in nightmares. I was alone, I was not within touch, in this utter stillness, of any other consciousness, and surely this must be hell, the outer darkness of absolute loneliness, which not even the glorious golden orb swung centre-high in the blue could ever so faintly penetrate. Indeed, it and this iridescent panorama at my feet only added some secret bitter irony to the outer darkness. All the light, the colour, the heat, which one had so loved was there still, but life was arrested, and there was nobody.

Then quite suddenly and unexpectedly the farcical happened, for from some hundred yards away down below the steep cliff up which I had climbed came a long discordant bray from my donkey, who perhaps felt lonely, too. But I have never heard a sound which was to the spirit so overpoweringly sweet. I heard that, and gave a long breath, and shouted. "Thank you very much" for the whole glory of the noon, which silence had blackened, was instantly restored.[3]

In such silence the deaf live day after day, year after year. It is small wonder that they become depressed, seclusive, irritable, and dependent.

[3] Benson, E. F., "A Reaping," Tauchnitz, Leipzig, 1909.

It has been estimated that there are in the United States at least 3 million people with sufficient impairment of hearing to merit attention. Many of these, even with progressive deafness, are unaware of the condition. In fact, impairment of hearing is frequently unrecognized and not even given serious consideration until 25 to 50 per cent of the hearing has been lost.

Causes of Deafness

Certain types of deafness are determined before birth. Some of these appear in early life, others with advancing years. Most

Fig. 25

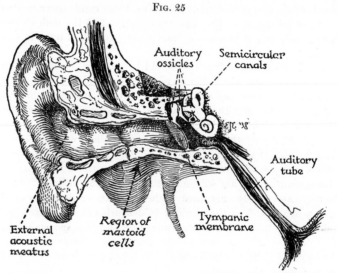

Section of external, middle, and internal ear (semichematic) to show relationships.

deafness, however, is due to inflammatory conditions of the middle ear, to obstruction of the auditory (eustachian) tube, to interference with nasal breathing, to foci of infection in sinuses, tonsils, teeth, gall bladder, or other organs of the body, to the toxins of scarlet fever, diphtheria, or syphilis, to accumulations of wax in the external ear canal, or to certain nutritional, glandular, or general diseases.

Inflammatory conditions of the middle ear are produced by infections which reach the middle ear from the throat by way of the eustachian tube. In children the eustachian tube is straighter and larger than in adults; hence, infection can traverse its course most easily in childhood. An acute infection of the middle ear, even though the eardrum is ruptured or opened, usually produces little or no impairment of hearing, but recurrent or chronic infections are almost certain to result in a greater or lesser degree of deafness.

The complications of "abscessed ears" can in a large measure be avoided if the condition is given the attention it deserves. Unfortunately in the past earache and abscessed ears have been considered as incidental to childhood, like measles or chicken pox. Profuse discharge from an ear attracts attention, but once it has started "drying up" the ear is often forgotten and the infection smolders on until a chronic condition is reached or the infection suddenly flares up to the extent that an operation on the mastoid may become necessary. It is nothing short of criminal to allow an ear to discharge over a long period of time when proper treatment will clear it up. Hearing lost in this manner can never be restored.

The prevention of ear infections depends primarily upon the prevention and treatment of nose and throat infections and general diseases, upon the removal of diseased tonsils and adenoids, and upon care in the blowing of the nose—the nose should be blown gently with both sides open. Deafness from scarlet fever and diphtheria is preventable, for we have a safe and effective immunization against diphtheria and antibiotics are effective in the treatment of scarlet fever. Syphilis, even if acquired, need never develop to the stage at which it affects hearing. Adenoids and tonsils can be removed when indicated, obstruction to breathing relieved, foci of infection eliminated, and general health improved.

In recent years dramatic progress in dealing with middle ear infections has been made possible by the development of the sulfonamide and antibiotic drugs. These are so effective in curing most middle ear infections that operations on the mastoid and even on the eardrum have become rarities. Evidence of this is the one mastoid operation performed in the University of Minnesota hospital in 1950 as compared to 100 such operations in 1936.

[321]

Important also are symptomless infections of the middle ear in children. When unrecognized, these may result in permanent impairment of hearing. The main factor in the development of this condition is a nasopharyngeal infection complicated by eustachian tube obstruction. One method of treating the nasopharynx is to employ small doses of radium. This treatment is simple and without any ill effects.

Wax, which is always present in the external ear canal in small quantities, occasionally accumulates and hardens so that it covers the eardrum and interferes with hearing. When this occurs, it should be removed by a physician. The unskilled use of instruments in the ear may result in injury and infection.

Swimming and diving, in the opinion of most otologists, are not dangerous to the ears in individuals with intact eardrums provided certain precautions are taken. Diving feet first so that water forcibly enters the nose, improper exhaling with the head submerged, and vigorous blowing of the nose after emerging from the water may allow water to get into the sinuses or eustachian tubes and may so irritate the nasal passages that an inflammation of the membranes lining these spaces results. Whenever one has even a semblance of a cold, one should refrain from diving and should keep the head out of water in swimming. Persons who have repeated ear infections or damaged eardrums or have had mastoid operations should use special precautions to prevent water from reaching the middle ear.

What Remains for the Deaf

Life for a deaf person is difficult at best, but if the handicap is recognized early and faced intelligently much can be done to minimize its seriousness. Proficiency in lip reading enables many deaf persons to lead a normal or a relatively normal life, but in order to attain proficiency the study of lip reading needs to be started early. Teachers of handicapped children report that it is far more difficult to teach the deaf than the blind, and that whereas the blind are usually happy the deaf tend to be despondent. To delay preparation for and adjustment to this handicap is tragic.

Improvements in electrical hearing aids are making it possible for the partially deaf to keep their contact with the world. The type of instrument best adapted to each particular case should be advised by an otologist and its use started before the hearing is too seriously impaired. It is the height of folly to waste time and money upon commercially advertised hearing aids or methods for the relief of deafness. Earphone radios, which, like the telephone, transmit sound waves through the bones of the skull to the nerves of hearing, have brought many pleasant and happy hours to the deafened.

Life for the partially deaf could be made much easier if their friends when speaking to them would first attract their attention and then speak distinctly and slowly rather than loudly. Shouting is annoying, irritating, and difficult to understand.

For the one who is hard of hearing Dr. Gordon Berry lays down the following nine commandments:

1. Thou shalt frankly confess thy deafness to thyself and before thy fellowmen. Let there be no deceit nor false pride.

2. Thou shalt not covet thy neighbor's hearing but shall rejoice that thou livest in an age when thy handicap can be made so small.

3. Early and again shalt thou consult thy otologist and accept every scientific aid he can render.

4. Eschew the quack and his devices. Easy and broad is the way to his door and many there be that find it.

5. Thou shalt join and work for a League for the Hard of Hearing where thou wilt receive encouragement and stimulation for thyself and wilt find happiness in serving thy brother. Thus wilt thou march forward with the Federation army that is alleviating deafness throughout the world.

6. So love thy neighbor that thou do everything in thy power to help him when he would have speech with thee. To this end:

7. Thou shalt study lip-reading, in season and out of season.

8. Thou shalt secure and use the best ear-phone thou canst discover.

9. Triumphantly shalt thou rise above thine infirmity; and so conduct thy life that the world hath need of thee.[4]

DISCUSSION SUGGESTIONS

1. Name the more important diseases whose portal of entrance to the body is through the nose and mouth.

[4] Berry, Gordon, "The Psychology of Progressive Deafness," *Journal of the American Medical Association*, vol. 101, p. 1602, November 18, 1933.

2. Discuss the value of antiseptic mouth washes, sprays, and gargles in the prevention of these diseases.

3. Discuss the more important causes and effects of nasal obstruction.

4. What are adenoids? What is the typical appearance of a child with chronically enlarged adenoids?

5. What are the paranasal sinuses? Why is sinus infection a frequent complication of the common cold?

6. Is special treatment always necessary for sinus infections? Why?

7. What is the possible relationship between sinus infection and acute nephritis or rheumatism?

8. What is the condition commonly called "nasal catarrh"? Should this condition be treated with "catarrhal" jellies or sprays? Why?

9. What are nasal polyps? What causes them?

10. What is the basic cause of hay fever and what are the more common substances which produce it?

11. Discuss the specificity of hay fever and the means of preventing it.

12. What are the usual indications for removal of the tonsils?

13. What are the more important effects of tonsillectomy upon health as indicated by a study of 2,200 tonsillectomized children over a period of 10 years?

14. List in order of importance the major causes of deafness.

15. Discuss Dr. Gordon Berry's "nine commandments for the hard of hearing."

16. Note reports of your hearing test and of examination of your nose and throat, Appendix C.

REFERENCES AND READING SUGGESTIONS

1. Davis, Hallowell: "Hearing and Deafness," Murray Hill Books, Inc., New York, 1949.

2. Furstenberg, A. C.: "So You Think It's Sinusitis," *Hygeia*, vol. 25, p. 758, October, 1947.

3. Holden, Harold M.: "Noses," The World Publishing Company, Cleveland, 1950.

4. Kaiser, Albert D.: "Children's Tonsils In or Out," J. B. Lippincott Company, Philadelphia, 1932.

5. Phillips, W. C., and W. G. Rowell: "Your Hearing," The World Publishing Co., Cleveland, 1943.

6. Taylor, H. M.: "Sinusitis and Swimming: Further Observation of Etiological Factors, with Especial Emphasis on Man's Lack of Adaptation to Aquatic Habits," *Journal of the American Medical Association*, vol. 85, p. 7, July 4, 1925.

Text-Films

The following McGraw-Hill Text-Film on Health Education is recommended for use with Chapter XIV of this text.

The Nose, Throat, and Ears (11 min sd MP).   Animated drawings in this motion picture describe the structure and functions of the ears, nose, and throat; it also clarifies the recommended procedures for their care.

Silent follow-up filmstrip based on material contained in the motion picture offers opportunity for review, testing, and further discussion.

Chapter XV

THE CONSERVATION OF VISION

THE eye has been called the "mirror of the soul," for it twinkles with good nature, sparkles with joy, softens with compassion, hardens with adversity, and clouds with despair. In the Orient there is a superstition that the "evil eye" is indicative of a malevolent personality, and in the early days in our own country the appearance of the eye was considered important evidence in trials for witchcraft. But the eye also reflects the state of physical health, its clear, normal luster giving way to the dull, gaunt look of illness, fatigue, or intoxication.

Good vision is essential for success in most occupations and for the enjoyment of the beautiful and interesting things of life. Uncivilized man was dependent upon acuity of vision for his subsistence and even for life itself, and we receive most of our education through our eyes, by means of observation, printed words, and pictures.

The eye is an extremely efficient instrument, functioning almost continuously to provide clear vision for close work in school, office, or shop. In so doing it acts with surprising rapidity, performing upwards of a thousand movements in 5 minutes of reading. It has been estimated that one-fourth of the daily energy expenditure of persons in sedentary occupations is utilized for the purpose of seeing.

Physiologically the eye is a mechanism, much like a camera, which brings the rays of light to focus upon light-sensitive nerve endings in the retina. These, in turn, transmit a stimulus to the brain, where the visual image is perceived. In the lowest types of seeing animals the eye consists merely of a few pigmented cells, sensitive to light, at or near the surface of the body, and connected with some simple nerve structure. In the higher forms of life these structures become more complex and connected with the brain. In addition to these more highly developed eyes, insects and worms retain some of the simple, supernumerary eyes. Most spiders, for example, have eight such eyes, and some worms four or more.

The simplest type of eye can perceive only light, but as one proceeds up the biological scale the visual apparatus becomes more complex and begins to perceive size, shape, distance, and color. Since acute vision is an asset in the struggle for existence, the animals with the most efficient eyes tend to rise in the biological scale.

The shape, structure, and location of the eyes are greatly influenced by the mode of life. Animals that live in the water or are most active at dusk have eyes that admit much light, and some even have a reflecting apparatus within the eye. The eyes of vertebrates are usually located in the head, but starfish have a so-called "eye" at the tip of each of their five rays; clams have rudimentary eyes at the tip of the siphon, which is located at the back of the body; some worms have eyes in their gills; while earthworms have light-sensitive cells over the surface of the body.

Helmholtz, the noted physicist who invented the ophthalmoscope, which enables a physician to examine the interior of the eyeball, is credited with saying that he would have returned to an instrument maker a piece of apparatus as imperfect as the human eye. Truly the eye is far from perfect, but the process of evolution has provided us with a visual instrument which adapts itself amazingly well to the changing demands made upon it.

Until recently, biologically speaking, man lived out of doors and used his eyes chiefly for distance vision. Some change of focus was necessary, but the demands made upon the visual apparatus were but a fraction of what they have been since he changed his mode of living. Several million years of reading the printed page may bring about a better adaptation of these outdoor eyes to the manner in which we now live.

The Cause and Prevention of Blindness

One of the greatest calamities that can befall one is blindness. The occasional genius, such as Milton or Helen Keller, can rise above this calamity, but most persons are crushed by it. It has been estimated that there are 100,000 blind persons in the United States and that in at least 50 per cent of these cases the blindness was due to causes which could have been prevented. Of these causes, the most important are injuries, infections, poisons, and degenerative diseases.

Eye Injuries. Injuries constitute an important cause of blindness in this country. Some of these can hardly be called preventable, but the vast majority could be avoided with reasonable precaution. Children can be taught that they should not use sharp instruments and that certain toys and games are hazardous; industry can safeguard the vision of employees; and individuals can learn to take necessary precautions.

Most industrial eye injuries occur in such occupations as machine operating, chipping, grinding and polishing, mining and quarrying, riveting, welding and cutting, glassmaking, sandblasting, and woodworking operations. In these and other occupations in which fragments of metal, wood, or stone may be thrown about, goggles or masks should be worn. The Chicago Division of the American Steel and Wire Company reports that eye injuries resulting in total loss of vision were reduced from 1 per 643 employees in the period from 1910 to 1915 to 1 per 2,700 employees in 1927 to 1933, and that the reduction in partial loss of vision was from 1 per 750 employees in 1910 to 1915 to 1 per 9,450 employees in 1927 to 1933. This reduction was the result of the use of goggles and the adoption of other protective devices. Injuries on the farm and in many other areas could likewise be greatly reduced by reasonable care and the use of protective goggles.

[328]

First Aid in Eye Injuries. Cleanliness is of the greatest importance in the care of eye injuries. A slight scratch on the surface of the eye may become so seriously infected that the eyesight is lost. The tissues of the eye are extremely delicate. For this reason expert medical attention should be secured whenever there is an injury to the eye.

A Cinder in the Eye. Dust, cinders, and other small particles of foreign material frequently lodge on the surface of the eyeball.

FIG. 26

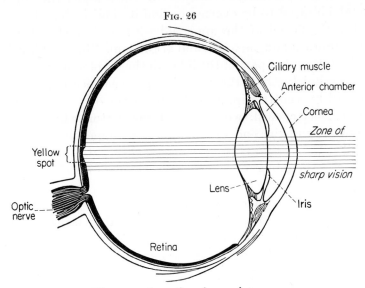

Diagrammatic section of normal eye.

The irritation thus produced results in a flood of tears which usually washes the offending particle away. Occasionally, however, such particles become lodged under a lid and for this or some other reason refuse to be dislodged. In such cases closing both eyes for a few moments without moving the eyeball leads to the accumulation of tears so that with the opening of the eyes the particle may be flushed out. Rubbing of the eyes irritates the tissues and embeds the particle.

If it is not dislodged in this manner, some additional simple measures may be tried with safety; but in so doing the greatest

[329]

of cleanliness must be observed. The tissues of the eye have already been injured and dirty fingers or a dirty handkerchief may result in serious infections of the lids and even the eyeball itself. The first measure to try is to put a few drops of saturated boric acid solution or a drop of castor oil into the eye. If this does not dislodge the foreign body, the assistance of a friend whose hands have been thoroughly scrubbed with soap and water may be secured. If the particle is on the surface of the eyeball or under the lower lid, it usually is easily seen. If it is under the upper lid, the lid will need to be everted to find it. This is done by taking hold of the lashes of the upper lid with the eye closed, pulling gently upward and outward, and at the same time pushing downward on the upper part of the lid with the tip of a finger, a match, or a toothpick. Once the particle has been located, it may be removed by gently wiping with the corner of a clean handkerchief or, better still, with some sterile cotton which has been wound around the end of a match and dipped into boric acid solution. If these measures are not successful, the assistance of a physician should be obtained. Dirty handkerchiefs or hard instruments such as toothpicks, knife blades, and finger nails should never be employed for this purpose.

Cosmetics Dangerous to Eyes. Among the cosmetics offered for the enhancement of beauty are dyes for eyebrows and eyelashes. Some of these contain chemicals which are injurious to the delicate structure of the eye; hence, their use is distinctly hazardous.

Eye Infections. Mild infections of the eye, called conjunctivitis, which may accompany colds, usually clear up with simple treatments. The more severe infections, on the other hand, require medical attention. These may be acute and self-limited or they may be due to serious disease, such as trachoma or gonorrheal ophthalmia, which, if not properly treated, will result in blindness. All infections of the eye are communicable by means of hands, towels, etc., and care is necessary if infection is to be avoided. (See pages 650 and 753.)

An inflamed, granular condition of the margins of the eyelids and the development of sties are frequently associated with eyestrain and with general ill-health. For such conditions a complete physical examination and a careful refraction are more important than local treatments.

Poisons Affect the Vision. Among the poisons which may produce partial or complete loss of vision are tobacco, wood alcohol, and quinine.

Many persons use tobacco for years without any apparent effect upon visual acuity, but others are definitely harmed by it. The eyes tire easily, visual acuity becomes progressively diminished, color vision is lost, and use of the eyes causes severe headache. Such symptoms occur most commonly in pipe smokers, particularly if both tobacco and alcohol are used in excess. If tobacco and alcohol are discontinued completely, the symptoms usually disappear rapidly and vision returns to normal. Such loss of vision occurs most commonly in men who smoke half a dozen or more cigars a day or several ounces of pipe tobacco a week.

Bootleg liquor sometimes contains poisonous wood alcohol and has been reported as the cause of considerable blindness. This usually follows the drinking of even small quantities of the beverage, although an occasional man can drink it over a long period of time without any apparent ill effects.

Quinine probably has caused more blindness than any other one drug. Ringing of the ears, headache, partial deafness, and dizziness are the common toxic symptoms produced by quinine. Less frequent but more serious is loss of vision, which may be partial and temporary or absolute for days, weeks, or life. A knowledge of the possibility of serious harm from the use of this drug should make people less willing to consume it, without medical advice, in various patent medicines for the treatment of colds, fever, and malaria.

Cataracts. Various changes which impair vision may occur in the eye during the later decades of life but most common of these is a cloudiness of the crystalline lens or its capsule, called "cataract." Occasionally this is due to injury or disease but the most common type is the senile cataract, the cause of which is not understood. In the past a cataract was considered a hopeless sentence to blindness for the rest of one's life, but now useful vision can be restored in 97 per cent of patients by means of a simple but delicate operation.

Glaucoma is a serious eye disease which is responsible for one-third of all blindness after forty years of age. Mechanically this is due to an increased pressure within the eyeball. This much we know, but since the basic cause for the increased pressure is not understood we do not have the key to its prevention. However, if glaucoma is recognized early and proper treatment instituted, its progress frequently can be arrested. The early symptoms are headache, pain in the eyes, halos surrounding lights, and rapid loss of vision. Although these symptoms may be due to other causes, their presence makes a careful examination by a competent physician imperative.

Eyewashes

Advertisements for eyewashes with fancy names suggest that these preparations should be used regularly if one desires bright, sparkling, healthy eyes. Eye specialists, on the other hand, never recommend such practices. Dust and dirt are constantly settling on the eyeball but nature removes them by maintaining a constant flow of tears which are gently carried over the eyeball by blinking of the lids. If there is unusual exposure to dust, smoke, or other irritating substances, a few drops of a saturated boric acid solution frequently are soothing.

Common Visual Defects

The common visual defects are nearsightedness, farsightedness, and astigmatism. These rarely lead to blindness but are responsible for an enormous amount of discomfort and inefficiency. Except for the farsightedness of advancing age, these conditions are due to developmental abnormalities in the shape of the eyeball. It has been suggested that race and heredity as well as other factors play a part in their causation, but relatively little is really known concerning their actual cause.

In taking a picture with one of the better cameras one first makes the necessary adjustments of focus, so that the objects which one wishes to photograph are clearly reproduced on the focusing ground glass. In a somewhat similar manner a picture of whatever is in front of the eye is thrown upon the retina. The retina lines the back of the eyeball and contains the nerve endings of vision. If the rays of light from the object at which one is

FIG. 27

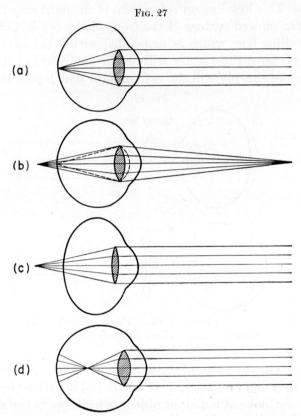

(a)

(b)

(c)

(d)

The focusing of light rays on the retina in normal and in abnormal eyes. (*a*) Normal eye, rays focusing on retina. (*b*) Normal eye, adapted for near vision by accommodation bringing rays to focus on retina. (*c*) Farsighted eye. (*d*) Nearsighted eye.

looking are brought to focus upon the center of this retina, at which the vision is most acute, a clear visual picture is obtained. If not, the image is blurred and indistinct (Figs. 27, 28).

The mechanism of vision requires, first, that rays of light be reflected from an object to the eye. On a dark night we are unable to see objects about us because insufficient light rays are reflected from them, but we can see the new moon which out beyond the earth is reflecting the light from the sun.

After reaching the eye these rays of light must be bent, or refracted, so that they will come to focus upon the proper part of the retina. This bending, or refraction, of the light rays is done in part by the curved surface of the front of the eye but chiefly by the crystalline lens which is suspended within the eyeball. The thicker this lens, the greater will be the curvature of its surface and the more sharply will the rays of light which pass through it

FIG. 28

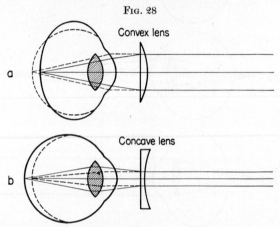

Correction of visual defects by lenses. (*a*) Convex lenses bring the point of focus forward toward the retina in farsighted eyes. (*b*) Concave lenses throw the point of focus farther back toward the retina in nearsighted eyes.

be focused. The thickness of the lens is controlled by a ring of tiny muscles, the ciliary muscles, which surround it within the eyeball.

When one looks at a distant object, a near one in the same line of vision is indistinct. Now, if one focuses upon the nearer object, the distant one is not seen so well. This is because a clear image is obtained only of the object which is brought to focus upon the most sensitive portion of the retina. The other becomes indistinct as it goes out of focus. This shifting of focus is accomplished by a change in the thickness of the lens. In a perfect eye the rays of light from a distant object come to focus upon the retina when the eye is at rest, that is, when the ciliary muscles are inactive and the lens is thin.

Farsightedness (*Hyperopia*). In this condition the eyeball is too short for good close vision. This is a universal condition at birth but usually disappears before there is much use of the eyes for near vision. If it persists, the rays of light with the eye at rest come to focus not on the retina but behind it. Blurring of vision results. This is unsatisfactory, so the ciliary muscles correct the difficulty by contracting and making the lens thicker, thereby bringing the point of focus forward until it is on the retina. This gives clear vision but requires excessive work on the part of these muscles. For short periods of time this gives rise to no difficulties but if it continues muscular fatigue is inevitable. This in turn causes headache, pain in the eyes, nervousness, and general fatigue. This type of visual defect is the one which causes the most severe symptoms of eyestrain.

Important though farsightedness is as a cause of eyestrain, it is rarely discovered by the ordinary vision test, because during the test clear vision is secured by excessive use of the ciliary muscles. Hence, if a child brings a report from school that his vision test shows 20/20 in each eye this should not be accepted as conclusive evidence that his vision is satisfactory. If symptoms of eyestrain are present, a further examination is indicated.

The Use of Drops for Eye Examinations. Much misunderstanding and misinformation exist concerning the use of "drops" for the examination of the eyes. The drops contain a drug, such as atropine or homatropine, which temporarily paralyzes the ciliary muscles. Unless this is done, the activity of these muscles in persons under about forty years of age makes the accurate measurement of certain visual defects impossible. Everyone who needs glasses should have a thorough eye examination, and for a young person this implies the use of drops.

Squints and Cross-eyedness. Sometimes the degree of farsightedness in one eye of a child may be greater than in the other, or one eye may be farsighted and the other normal or relatively normal. When this occurs and both eyes are used, the one eye is under a much greater strain than the other. Since reasonably good vision can be obtained with the use of only one eye, in time the overworked eye ceases to function, first when it gets tired and then continuously. The child does not know that he is using only one eye and for a time no change is noticeable. Eventually, however, the muscles which turn the farsighted eye toward the object of vision seem to realize that, since the eye is not being used, their work is unnecessary, so they too stop working and the condition which we call "cross-eyedness" develops. At first this appears only when the child is tired but eventually it becomes constant. After the unused eye has been fixed in one position for some time, the muscles on the one side of the eyeball become shortened, and those on the other side stretched. This muscular change, however, is the end result and not the cause of cross-eyedness.

The prevention or treatment of cross-eyedness clearly must be based upon a thorough eye examination with all muscles, overacting and underacting alike, put at rest. On the basis of such an examination glasses can be prescribed which will tend to equalize the work of the two eyes and so prevent further progress of the condition. To be successful, however, this needs to be done in early childhood, just as soon as squinting is observed. If the disuse of the one eye has become an established habit, it may be necessary to cover the other eye temporarily in order to put this one back to work.

Farsightedness of Adults (Presbyopia). The crystalline lens of a young child is very elastic and the ability to focus the vision upon near objects correspondingly great. With increasing age the lens loses its elasticity and the power of accommodation is correspondingly reduced. At thirty years of age the power of accommodation is only one-half as great as at ten years of age and at forty-five only one-half as great as at thirty. At the approximate age of forty-five the near point for comfortable vision reaches about 12 inches, the distance ordinarily used for reading. After this age most persons need glasses in order to read with comfort; and since the condition tends to be progressive, the glasses need to be changed every 1 to 3 years.

Nearsightedness. Nearsightedness, or myopia, occurs when the eyeball is longer than it should be. For this reason with the eye at rest the point of focus of distant objects falls in front of the retina and indistinct vision results. The use of the ciliary muscles to make the lens thicker would only move the point of focus farther forward and so make matters worse. Hence, the only way for a nearsighted person to obtain clear vision, without glasses, is to bring the object close to the eye. The glasses prescribed for myopia throw the point of focus backward toward the retina, thereby increasing the acuity of vision.

Although nearsightedness tends to run in families and is more common in some races than in others, its actual cause is unknown. It frequently appears in childhood and progresses somewhat until about the age of twenty-one. Hence, it sometimes has been suggested that nearsightedness may be due to schoolwork. On the other hand, it seems that the condition is just as frequent and develops just as rapidly in children who are out of school as in those who are in school.

Nearsightedness occasionally becomes progressive and if not arrested may lead to serious impairment of vision. Some such cases are associated with malnutrition, focal infections, or general ill-health. Thus the boy or girl with progressive nearsightedness should be placed under the care of a competent oculist and a general physician.

Astigmatism. Astigmatism is a type of visual defect due to an irregularity in the curvature of the portions of the eyeball through which the light rays enter, that is, the cornea and the lens. If either of these surfaces is flatter than normal, there is less bending of the rays of light, with the result that the point of focus is thrown backward. On the other hand, if the curvature is greater than normal, the point of focus is farther forward. In addition to these possibilities some eyes are flat in one direction and excessively curved in the other, and the abnormal curvatures which we call "astigmatism" may be associated with either nearsightedness or farsightedness. Such visual defects frequently cause severe eyestrain. To obtain relief a careful eye examination and accurately prescribed and fitted glasses are essential.

Night Vision

The human eye is able to make certain adjustments to improve vision in dim light. First, and most obvious, it can constrict the iris, thereby causing enlargement of the aperture and admitting more light. We see this as an increase in the size of the pupil. In bright light the iris expands and the pupil becomes smaller. The eye makes these adjustments reflexly.

Second, and even more important, the eye uses a different portion of the retina for night vision. The central posterior area, which is called the "fovea," or yellow spot (Fig. 26), and which provides the clearest vision in the daytime, is blind at night; the nerve endings in the area surrounding the fovea are more sensitive to dim light. For this reason one's vision is best at night if one does not look directly at the object one wishes to see.

Third, chemical changes occur in the cells of the retina which make them more sensitive to light. This change takes time and is spoken of as adapting the eyes to the dark. Adaptation is rapid at first but is not completed for half an hour. Pilots who are night fliers are carefully instructed in how to develop and utilize their night vision. Their life depends upon this as well as upon their planes and their ability to fly them.

Vitamin A deficiency causes night blindness but there is no evidence that the addition of vitamin A to an adequate general diet improves night vision.

Eye Exercises

Exercise of the eye muscles is a valuable adjunct in the treatment of certain cases of muscular imbalance in the eyes, especially in cross-eyed children. When used together with correction of refractive errors by lenses and with muscle surgery, better results may be obtained than without such training. It is not a substitute for other accepted means of treatment.

In addition, certain systems of eye exercises have become popular in which promises are held out of improved vision without the necessity for wearing glasses. There has been no proof that any form of exercise will actually change the refractive index of an eye. The refractive index has been shown to be a mechanical problem which is dependent on the size and shape of the eyeball. The same may be said in regard to the development of color sense, where none exists, by any method of training.

Eye Specialists

There are several groups of individuals who, with more or less justification, consider themselves eye specialists. It is important to be able to distinguish among these and to understand the service which each is qualified to render.

The *oculist* or *ophthalmologist* is a graduate physician who first had a basic training and practical experience in general medicine and surgery and then specialized in diseases of the eye. He realizes that eyestrain or visual defects are frequently associated with and may be the first recognizable sign of disease, either in the eye itself or in some other part of the body, and he considers all such possibilities when making an eye examination. Furthermore, physicians are the only persons permitted to treat disease or to use the drugs which are so necessary for complete eye examinations of young persons. If, after a careful examination, glasses are deemed necessary, the oculist writes a prescription for them which is taken to an optician to be filled.

Opticians are craftsmen, skilled in the grinding of lenses and the making and fitting of glasses according to prescriptions. If eyestrain is to be relieved, lenses must be accurately ground and glasses carefully fitted. It is essential also that frames and nose-pieces be kept in proper adjustment. In some cases of astigmatism even a slight displacement of a lens from its proper position will cause discomfort.

Optometrists are licensed to make visual tests and to prescribe glasses. They are not trained to treat diseases, but graduates of approved schools of optometry are trained to make proper references to physicians. Some optometrists do not limit themselves to the examination of eyes but engage in the selling of glasses or are associated with some store which does so.

Most of the glasses worn in this country are prescribed and sold by optometrists. Many optometrists render valuable services as competent, conscientious, and ethical practitioners. Others are primarily businessmen engaged in the selling of glasses for profit. Fortunately the proportion of ethical optometrists has been increasing rapidly over the past 15 years. These are repu-

[339]

table practitioners and truly merit the title of professional men. Theirs are not the names one sees blatantly advertised.

A word of sound advice for anyone who has or who thinks he has eyestrain is to investigate thoroughly before consulting those who advertise "Eyes examined free." Such establishments are business, not welfare, institutions. They examine eyes free but they make their profit by selling glasses. Hence, those who may need glasses should be careful about whom they consult.

Then there are the "eye specialists" who travel about proclaiming some "newly discovered method" for correcting defective vision without the use of glasses. They usually start with a free lecture but collect the money later. It is amazing how many credulous people pay these fakers for a course of lectures, a book of instructions, or some other equally worthless commodity. As soon as fees begin to dwindle, such specialists hear a call to spread the gospel elsewhere.

Illumination

Although poor lighting is an important factor in the development of fatigue and eyestrain, there is no satisfactory evidence, the advertising of electric light companies notwithstanding, that poor illumination is a cause of defective vision. Our eyes were developed for use out of doors where the intensity of light, even on a cloudy day, is many times as great as in a well-lighted room indoors. Direct sunlight in the middle of the day gives an illumination of approximately 10,000 foot-candles.[1]

The essentials of good lighting are that the light be adequate, uniform, and steady and that glare and shadows be avoided. Under no circumstances should the source of light be in the line of vision. For reading and close work the whole room should be well lighted with additional light centered upon the work. A well-lighted room is bright and cheerful, a poorly lighted one gloomy and depressing. Good lighting improves the spirits, increases efficiency and productivity, and decreases accidents.

In rooms where no close work is done, 1 to 3 foot-candles of

---

[1] A foot-candle is the amount of light at a distance of 1 foot from the flame of a candle of ordinary size, that is, approximately 1 inch in diameter.

illumination are sufficient; classrooms, libraries, and desks should have at least 10 to 15 foot-candles of illumination on top of the desk; and for finer work, such as drawing or sewing, 20 to 100 foot-candles of illumination should be provided. An unshaded, 75-watt gas-filled argon and nitrogen bulb will provide 9 foot-

TABLE 24

ILLUMINATION FROM VARIOUS SIZES OF MAZDA BULBS

Strength of Bulb, Watts	Degree of Illumination,* Perpendicular to Ray of Light at Distance of		
	3 Feet	6 Feet	12 Feet
25	2.2	0.6	0.1
40	3.8	1.0	0.2
60	6.6	1.7	0.4
75	9.2	2.3	0.6
100	13.5	3.3	0.8

* These values are approximate only and then for an unshaded light.

candles of illumination at a distance of 3 feet, 2 foot-candles at a distance of 6 feet, and about ½ foot-candle at a distance of 12 feet.

The colors of the walls and ceiling of a room have a distinct influence upon the amount of light necessary to give adequate illumination. Light colors reflect the light; dark colors absorb it. The illumination at any point in a room is received in part directly from the source of illumination and in part from light which is reflected from the walls and ceiling. The type of shade or reflector over a light makes a great difference in the illumination obtained from it. In fact, many of the most decorative shades render lights practically useless for illumination. The degree of illumination available can be accurately measured by means of an instrument called a "lightmeter." This contains a photoelectric cell which indicates on a dial the intensity of light in terms of foot-candles. In the planning of office buildings, schools, factories, and even homes the advice of an illuminating engineer should be obtained. And in the selection of a lamp to be used for reading or close work, the stamp of approval of the

Illuminating Engineering Society (I.E.S.) gives assurance that the lamp is properly designed to give good illumination.

Glare

Bright light which strikes the eye directly from an unshaded source or is reflected from objects such as glossy paper, polished furniture, clean white snow, or the hood of an automobile causes contraction of the iris with resultant unequal stimulation of the retina. This is commonly described as "glare" and is responsible for a considerable amount of unnecessary eyestrain.

Sunglasses of various sizes, shapes, and hues have become synonymous with sports and vacations from Florida to Alaska and from seashores to mountaintops. As a result they are worn much more extensively than any real need for them would justify. Our eyes possess the capacity to adjust themselves to varying degrees of light intensity. It is a mistake therefore to make a habit of wearing sunglasses whenever one is in bright light. On the other hand, there are situations in which the light is so brilliant or accompanied by so much glare that one is more comfortable if some of this light, particularly the ultraviolet light, is filtered out by special glasses. As a general rule, such glasses should not be worn indoors and should be put on out of doors only when the light is particularly bright. Many kinds of sunglasses are offered for sale and probably most of them are reasonably satisfactory. One should be certain, however, that such glasses do not contain irregular curvatures or flaws that will contribute to eyestrain. For persons whose eyes are particularly sensitive to light, a little tinting in the glasses they regularly wear may provide some comfort.

Color Blindness

When light strikes an object some of the rays are absorbed, some are reflected. The reflected rays which reach the cornea give rise to the sensation of color. If an object reflects all the light rays, it is said to be white. If it absorbs all the light rays, it is said to be black. Objects which we perceive as red, blue, etc., reflect the rays of light of the wave lengths which, when they stimulate the nerve endings, give rise to the sensations of these particular colors.

Color blindness is a condition in which the nerve endings are not sensitive to all the colors. This defect is hereditary. Approximately one man out of 25 and one woman out of 200 have some degree of color blindness. A male will be color-blind if he inherits the defect from either of his parents; while the female will show the defect only if she inherits it from both parents. For this reason women may transmit the defect to their sons without themselves showing it.

Complete color blindness is very rare. These persons see all objects without color; that is, as the blacks, grays, and whites of an ordinary photograph. The most common form of color blindness is the inability to distinguish red from green. This is a distinct handicap in many activities. Traffic lights can usually be distinguished because of their brilliance. The color-blind driver also learns that the top light in the semaphore means "stop" and the bottom light means "go."

It is important for a person to know whether he is color-blind and if so, the extent of his defect. This can be determined by various tests. Such tests should be included in every college entrance physical examination.

Care of the Eyes and Prevention of Eyestrain

Eyes will stand considerable abuse; but if one expects efficient service from them day after day and year after year, they must be given reasonable care. When used for close work, the eyes should be rested at frequent intervals by looking at a blank wall or at some distant object. During illness and convalescence they are susceptible to fatigue and so should be used sparingly. They need protection during infectious diseases, particularly measles.

Reading in bed frequently produces eyestrain because the book, magazine, or paper is not held in a proper position, and lighting is inadequate and poorly placed. Likewise, reading with an unsteady light or on a moving train is fatiguing and likely to cause severe eyestrain. Adequate, steady, and properly located illumination is essential for comfort in the use of the eyes.

Goggles are useful to protect the eyes from dust and wind and are the most important single measure for the prevention of eye injuries in numerous occupations. Tinted lenses reduce the irritation from the glare of the sun in summer and the reflected light from the snow in winter.

When symptoms of eyestrain or of defective vision occur, the eyes should be examined by a competent oculist. However, not everyone with symptoms of eyestrain needs glasses. It is important also to realize that the condition of the eye and the general health are closely related. Defective vision may be due to a specific disease or may be aggravated by poor general health, and eyestrain may give rise to symptoms in remote parts of the body. Finally, when the eye is involved, the best service is none too good, for the possibility of preventing progressive loss of vision and eventual blindness may depend upon the early recognition and proper treatment of glaucoma, trachoma, progressive myopia, or certain general diseases or toxic conditions.

DISCUSSION SUGGESTIONS

1. Enumerate the more important causes of blindness.
2. In what industries are eye injuries most common and what measures are useful in reducing them?
3. How would you proceed to remove a cinder from the eye and what special precautions would you take?
4. What are the usual contributory causes of "granulated" margins of the eyelids?
5. What is conjunctivitis and how is it usually contracted?
6. What are the poisons which most commonly affect vision?
7. What is a cataract? Can it be successfully treated? If so, how?
8. What is glaucoma?
9. Through what structures in the eyeball do the rays of light pass? What is the retina; of what does it consist; and how is it connected with the brain?
10. How is change of focus in the eye accomplished?
11. Define and explain the mechanism of hyperopia.
12. Define and explain the mechanism of myopia.
13. Define and explain the mechanism of astigmatism.
14. Define and explain the mechanism of presbyopia.
15. What type of eye defect is most likely to cause symptoms of eyestrain? Why?

16. Explain the development and the prevention of cross-eyedness.
17. What is the difference between an oculist, an ophthalmologist, an optician, and an optometrist?
18. Explain the reason for the use of drugs in an examination of the eyes.
19. Define a "foot-candle." Approximately how much light should be provided on the top of a desk for studying?
20. Enumerate the more important measures for the prevention of eyestrain.
21. Note reports of your examinations and of changes in vision which occur during your college course, Appendix C.

REFERENCES AND READING SUGGESTIONS

1. Lancaster, Walter B., and Franklin M. Foote, "The Battle against Blindness," *Journal of the American Medical Association*, vol. 145, p. 26, January 6, 1951.
2. Luckeish, M.: "Seeing and Human Welfare," The Williams & Wilkins Company, Baltimore, 1934.
3. Merrill, H. G., and L. W. Oaks: "Your Vision and How to Keep It," 2d ed., G. P. Putnam's Sons (Knickerbocker Press), New York, 1931.
4. Tinker, M. A.: "Illumination and the Hygiene of Reading," *Journal of Educational Psychology*, vol. 25, p. 699, 1934.
5. Bulletins of the National Association for the Prevention of Blindness, New York.
6. Conservation of Vision Pamphlets, American Medical Association, Chicago.

Chapter XVI

SOUND TEETH

THE relationship of the teeth to general health and efficiency was appreciated in a general way long before vitamins or focal infections had been heard of. Toothaches used to be as inevitable as colds; and slave buyers and horse traders inspected the teeth of their prospective purchases before buying. Only in recent times has attention been given to the care and preservation of the teeth. Now everybody has his favorite toothpaste and knows that he should visit the dentist at least twice a year. Much of this information comes through the advertising of worthless dentifrices and mouthwashes but it does impress upon people the importance of caring for the teeth.

In addition to the relationship of the teeth to the general health, there are other equally good reasons why the care of the mouth is important. Poor teeth and an unhygienic mouth constitute social and economic liabilities. They are unsightly and offensive. Furthermore, the cause of the well-known "halitosis" can frequently be found in decomposition of protein material in a cavity of a tooth or in accumulations of food between or around the teeth. To attempt to correct this by the use of mouthwashes is quite analogous to the use of powder and perfume instead of soap and water.

The Teeth of Primitive Man. Skulls of Eskimos buried for hundreds of years and excavated by Arctic explorers usually con-

[346]

tain complete sets of teeth with little or no evidence of dental decay. This has been true in general of the teeth of primitive people. On the other hand, skulls of Aztecs show abundant evidence of decay and root abscesses, as do skulls from the Nile Valley, where cereal grains constituted a major portion of the diet, and from the Hawaiian Islands, where the natives lived chiefly on poi, from taroroot, which consists largely of carbohydrates.

Dental Caries

Toothbrushes, dentifrices, and reparative dentistry belong to a modern era; so all primitive people were on equal footing in this regard. Their diets, however, were different, a fact which is frequently suggested as the probable cause for the differences in the condition of their teeth. Support for this view is found in the increase of dental decay among the Eskimos who live on American foods, and in the much greater prevalence of dental decay among American school children than among immigrant children from southern Europe. These immigrants, for the most part, are very poor and live on the simplest kind of food, yet they have almost perfect teeth. A generation in our "melting pot" and they are typical Americans, dental caries and all.

Early studies of the cause and prevention of dental caries suggested that there might be a single causative factor, but further results show that the problem is a complex one, with diet, heredity, internal secretions, mechanical factors, and oral hygiene of greatest importance.

Diet and Dental Caries. There is now general agreement that diet probably is the most important single factor in the maintenance of sound, healthy teeth and that an adequate diet is most essential during the period of most rapid growth. McCollum and Simmonds conclude from an experimental study that rats which are kept on a deficient diet during a part of the growing period have inferior teeth and early decay, even though an adequate diet is provided later. In the days before viosterol had been developed and before cod-liver oil was widely used, McCollum also reported that at the age of entering school 9 per cent of children who had been breast-fed for at least 6 months had dental caries,

22 per cent of children who were fed on cow's milk or on milk mixtures, and 27 per cent of those who were fed on oatmeal water and other prepared foods. This would indicate that the foundation of dental health is laid very early in life, but it appears that the prenatal period is also of great importance in this regard. Consequently emphasis is now being placed upon a proper diet during pregnancy. McCollum also states that a strictly carnivorous diet throughout life will prevent dental caries.

Important though diet admittedly is, there does not seem to be any single dietary factor which is responsible for dental caries. Calcium and phosphorus, the two minerals found in bones and teeth, and vitamin D, which regulates the utilization of these minerals by the body, are clearly essential. Of these, calcium and vitamin D were first thought to be of greatest importance, but the more recent work seems to indicate that phosphorus is of as great if not greater importance than calcium. Milk, certain vegetables, and fish foods are rich sources of both calcium and phosphorus. Vitamin D is very likely to be deficient in natural foods during the winter months but is easily administered in the form of cod-liver oil, vitamin D milk, or viosterol.

Children have long been denied candy because of the belief that sugar is related to dental decay, and certain studies carried out in institutions for orphans where the diet is strictly controlled suggest that the prevalence of dental caries is directly related to the amount of carbohydrate in the diet. Cereals from which the hull of the grain has been removed seem to have an unfavorable influence upon the development of the teeth, and several investigators believe that oatmeal contributes directly to the formation of caries. Carbohydrates and starches around and between the teeth form a favorable medium for the growth of acid-forming organisms.

On the other hand, it is reported that no caries were found in the teeth of 2,500 South African natives whose food consists largely of carbohydrates and who never clean their teeth. Osman[1] expresses the further opinion that the relationship of candy to

[1] Osman, A. A., "The Importance of Sugar in the Diet of the School Child," *Proceedings of the Royal Society of Medicine*, vol. 5, p. 1103, 1931.

[348]

dental decay may be due entirely to the fact that the excessive sweets dull the appetite for other necessary foods and that the harmful results of depriving children of this valuable source of energy may outweigh any possible harm that its inclusion in the diet might cause to the teeth.

Such divergent opinions concerning the relation of diet to dental health leave one rather confused. Apparently no one dietary factor is responsible for resistance to caries, but various elements are necessary for the proper development and continuing soundness of the teeth. For practical purposes a well-rounded diet, containing liberal amounts of milk, orange juice, fresh fruits, vegetables, and for children cod-liver oil or some other form of vitamin D, may be depended upon to supply the nutritional requirements of the teeth.

Some clarification of one aspect of this problem has been given by studies of the bacteria found in the mouth. If a particular germ called *Lactobacillus acidophilus* occurs in quantity, caries develop with great rapidity. This is because these bacteria act upon carbohydrates, particularly sugars, on and around the teeth to form acids which dissolve the enamel and the dentine. These studies have also shown that if persons have excessive numbers of lactobacilli in their mouths, the amount of caries can be reduced by the elimination of sugars and other easily fermentable carbohydrates from the diet.

Chewing gum is alternately praised and condemned by dentists. Best present opinion seems to be that any cleansing value that it may have is more than offset by the impetus to decay given by the sugar which it contains. Even worse are the hard candies which are held in the mouth while they dissolve.

Fluorides and Dental Caries. During the past several years investigations have taken another turn. It was determined that the only chemical difference between carious and noncarious teeth is that carious teeth contain less fluorine, a chemical element which is present in minute amounts in the bones and teeth. This was followed by an investigation by the U.S. Public Health Service of the fluoride content of the drinking water in areas in which dental caries are rare and areas in which they are prev-

[349]

alent. Here again a difference in fluoride content was found
(Table 25). From these studies it has been concluded that the

TABLE 25

FLUORIDES AND DENTAL CARIES

Frequence of dental caries in school children and natural fluoride content of drinking
water in 21 cities.

City and State	Number of Children Examined	Per Cent of Children Caries-free	Number DMF* per Child with Caries Experience	Fluoride, Parts per Million
Galesburg, Ill................	273	27.8	2.36	1.9
Colorado Springs, Colo......	404	28.5	2.46	2.6
Elmhurst, Ill................	170	25.3	2.52	1.8
Maywood, Ill................	171	29.8	2.58	1.2
Aurora, Ill..................	633	23.5	2.81	1.2
East Moline, Ill.............	152	20.4	3.03	1.2
Joliet, Ill...................	447	18.3	3.23	1.3
Kewanee, Ill................	123	17.9	3.43	0.9
Pueblo, Colo................	614	10.6	4.12	0.6
Elgin, Ill...................	403	11.4	4.44	0.5
Marion, Ohio................	263	5.7	5.56	0.4
Lima, Ohio..................	454	2.2	6.52	0.3
Evanston, Ill................	256	3.9	6.73	0.0
Middletown, Ohio............	370	1.9	7.03	0.2
Quincy, Ill..................	330	2.4	7.06	0.1
Oak Park, Ill................	329	4.3	7.22	0.0
Zanesville, Ohio.............	459	2.6	7.33	0.2
Portsmouth, Ohio............	469	1.3	7.72	0.1
Waukegan, Ill...............	423	3.1	8.10	0.0
Elkhart, Ind................	278	1.4	10.37	0.1
Michigan City, Ind..........	236	0.0	10.37	0.1

* Decayed, missing, or filled.

presence of approximately one part of fluorides per million parts
of drinking water results in a decreased prevalence of caries.

Proceeding on the basis of this information, several investigators have experimented with the application of fluorine to the
surface of the teeth of children. In this study Knutson and Arm-
strong reported that the application of 2 per cent sodium fluoride solution to the teeth resulted in 40 per cent less caries over
a period of a year in 289 children than developed in 326 untreated

controls. No healing effect was noted on teeth in which caries existed.

Of much greater potentiality for the prevention of caries than the application of a fluoride solution directly to the teeth is the addition of fluoride to the drinking water of municipalities whose water supply contains little or no fluorides. The initial experiment with this type of preventive measure was made by the U.S. Public Health Service in Grand Rapids, Michigan, in 1945. Sodium fluoride was added to the city's water to bring its content up to one part per million, the amount that occurs naturally in the water of Cincinnati and many other cities. At the end of 5 years the conclusion was that the development of caries in children six years of age who had been drinking fluoridated water since birth was reduced by 65 per cent. In older children the reduction was less but still substantial.

The technique of this study was to determine at the beginning and at the end of the experiment the amount of caries in school children of various ages in Grand Rapids, Michigan, Muskegon, Michigan, and in Aurora, Illinois. The city waters of Grand Rapids and Muskegon naturally contain no fluorides while the water of Aurora contains 1.2 parts per million. Sodium fluoride was then added to the water of Grand Rapids, but not of Muskegon. At the beginning of the study, the children of Grand Rapids and Muskegon had 65 per cent more caries than the children of Aurora. Five years later the caries rate in Muskegon and Aurora remained the same as before, but the rate in Grand Rapids dropped to essentially the same rate as in Aurora.

Subsequent studies in other cities have given similar results. In view of this one wonders why all municipalities with low fluoride content in their water do not adopt this measure for the reduction of dental caries. The reasons are many: some political, some financial, some inertia, and some because of organized opposition. The opponents of fluoridation point out that fluorides are used as poisons for rats and other rodents and question its safety. It is true that fluorides in sufficient quantity are poisonous, but so is chlorine which is regularly added to drinking water supplies to destroy disease-producing organisms, and so is

[351]

iodine which we add to table salt to prevent goiters. In some communities in which the natural content of fluorides in the water exceeds 2 parts per million a stained or flaked condition of the teeth, called mottled enamel or dental fluorosis, sometimes occurs. There is, however, no evidence or even suggestion that a fluoride content of drinking water of 1 part per million is in any way harmful or deleterious.

Opposition to new public health measures always occurs, but eventually the public insists upon having the protection which scientific progress makes available. A report as of November, 1952, shows that 479 communities with a total population of 9,972,000 were using water to which fluoride was added and that 353 other communities with a population of 17,280,000 had officially approved this action.

Cleanliness. It is frequently said that "a clean tooth never decays." Whether or not this is true depends upon the definition of cleanliness. If cleanliness implies freedom from bacteria, the statement probably is correct. But with bacteria constantly present in the mouth and in the food we eat, it is impossible to have the teeth bacteriologically clean.

The mechanism of decay is through the action of acids produced by bacterial decomposition of food, first upon the enamel and then upon the softer dentine of the tooth. The action of this acid upon the tooth structure may begin in any crevice, irregularity, or break in the enamel. The amount of decomposition and acid formation is greatest when there are gross accumulations of food substances. In fact, it is between the teeth, where it is difficult to prevent accumulations of food, that decay most frequently begins. Hence, although cleanliness of the teeth is not the only or even the most important factor in the prevention of dental decay, it is not without significance.

Other factors play a part in determining the health of teeth. That this is the case is evident from the fact that some persons remain immune from caries no matter how unbalanced the diet or how unclean the mouth, while others develop caries even though the diet, so far as we can tell, is entirely adequate and the care of the mouth perfect. One of these additional factors probably is heredity, and the functioning of the glands of internal secretion may be another.

In summary, a study of the occurrence and treatment of dental caries states:

Among the nation's school children, the caries attack rate, as shown by various studies, is between nine-twelfths and eleven-twelfths of a tooth per child per year. The only satisfactory method of combating the disease is to fill affected teeth during the early stages of decay. Unless this is done, the teeth attacked by caries will be lost in almost every instance. Thus, the logical present method of meeting the dental health need of school children is to fill all carious permanent teeth.[2]

To be most effective, routine dental care should begin at the age of two.

Apical Infections

The so-called "apical abscesses" which develop around the roots of teeth are the most dangerous type of mouth infection. Infective organisms usually reach these areas by traveling from deep cavities down the pulp of the tooth and along the root canal. On the other hand, abscesses occasionally occur around the roots of apparently healthy teeth.

An infection at the root of a tooth begins as a small inflammatory area in the bone in which the tooth is embedded. Unless an abscess forms and works its way to the surface, becoming a so-called "gum boil," these infections cannot drain. The result is that their toxic products and even the bacteria themselves may be absorbed into the blood and lymph stream to be circulated throughout the body. The toxic products cause fatigue, lassitude, and various aches and pains, while bacteria which are absorbed may set up infections in the joints, kidneys, or heart valves. Abscesses at the roots of certain teeth of the upper jaw may extend directly into the antrum, producing one of the most severe types of sinus infection. The development of these root abscesses is usually accompanied by pain, but they may develop,

[2] "A Study of the Occurrence and Treatment of Dental Caries Among School Children Aged 6–18 in the United States," *Journal of the American Dental Association*, vol. 31, March 1, 1944.

particularly at the roots of "dead" teeth, without any warning whatsoever. The only satisfactory treatment is free drainage obtained by the removal of the tooth.

Gingivitis and Pyorrhea

"Gingivitis" means an inflammatory condition of the gums, while "pyorrhea" implies that actual pus is present. The normal gums are pink or light red in color, thin and firm. If they become bright red or purplish, soft, swollen and spongy, or bleed easily, they should receive attention. The cause of an unhealthy condition of the gums may be faulty diet, mechanical irritation, or bacterial infection.

Vitamin C seems to be the dietary factor most directly related to the health of the gums. In scurvy, the disease due to vitamin C deficiency, a spongy, bleeding condition of the gums is a prominent symptom. Hanke reports that the addition of a pint of orange juice and the juice of one lemon to the daily diet leads to an almost complete disappearance of gingivitis.

Mechanical injury to the gums may result from the faulty use of the toothbrush or from the accumulation of tartar—limelike deposits—on the teeth at the gum margin. Such mechanical injury causes irritation and is frequently followed by secondary infection.

Exercise and massage of the gums by biting and chewing assist in the maintenance of an adequate circulation and a healthy condition. For this reason it is important that teeth be kept in proper repair so that they will be used regularly and uniformly. Missing teeth and poor fillings prevent the proper use of the teeth in chewing. Gentle massage of the gums with the fingers or the toothbrush, using a stroke *toward* the gum margin, is helpful in maintaining good circulation.

Pyorrhea is a more severe infection of the gums which demands expert treatment. There is no mouthwash, toothpaste, or powder that will cure it.

Trench Mouth. A severe form of gingivitis which received special study during the First World War has been called "trench mouth." This is caused by a specific germ and is easily communicated from one person to another, either directly or indirectly through drinking glasses or eating utensils. The treatment of trench mouth is a problem for a physician or a dentist.

Care of the Mouth and Teeth

Cleanliness of the mouth and teeth is important from an aesthetic as well as from a hygienic point of view. It is difficult to keep the mouth clean in view of the irregularities in the shape of the teeth and the crevices between them. Nevertheless, by the regular use of the toothbrush and dental floss the teeth may be kept relatively free from deposits of food and mucus. The mouth should be cleansed upon rising in the morning, after each meal, and before retiring.

The Toothbrush. A small or medium-sized brush with a straight or slightly convex brushing surface seems to give the best results. The bristles should be relatively short and stiff, with the tufts widely separated and containing bristles of different lengths. The expense of the brush is not necessarily a criterion of its value.

Cold water should be used in brushing the teeth, for hot water softens the bristles. After using a brush, it should be washed and hung up where it will become thoroughly dry before subsequent use. It is well to have several brushes which may be used alternately.

The teeth should be brushed on all surfaces which the brush can reach. Other surfaces should be cleaned with dental floss. A technique recommended for brushing the teeth is to place the brush against the teeth with the bristles slanting away from the gums. Then with a gentle, rotary motion work the bristles between as well as over the surface of the teeth. If there is a tendency for the gum margins to recede, the gums should be massaged with the brush when cleaning the teeth, using a gentle stroke toward the edge of the gum margin.

Toothpastes and Powders. The chief merit of dentifrices has been that they are pleasant to use and encourage regularity in the care of the teeth. They contribute but little to the cleansing and nothing to the preservation of the teeth. Nor do they prevent

[355]

pyorrhea and gingivitis. And the use of some dentifrices is actually worse than nothing at all, for they contain abrasive, gritty substances which wear down the enamel of the teeth.

Mouthwashes. The only merit which can be ascribed to mouthwashes is that they give a pleasing sensation of cleanliness. They have no antiseptic properties of any consequence. If the mouth is healthy, they are unnecessary; and if not, they are valueless.

There is some suggestion that the persistent use of some of the popular "antiseptic gargles" may be harmful. Whether or not this is correct, it is unintelligent for people to be cajoled into spending money for such preparations by the writers of advertising copy who know nothing about health and care less.

Halitosis. Disagreeable odor of the breath may come from decayed teeth, from collections of decomposing food between the teeth, from infections in the nose or sinuses, from plugs in the crypts of the tonsils, or from malodorous volatile substances eliminated from the blood stream through the lungs. The conditions affecting the teeth can be corrected by dentistry and dental hygiene; nose and throat infections by medical care; and the excretion of unpleasant odors from the lungs reduced if not eliminated by diets of low fat content. Mouthwashes may temporarily mask unpleasant odors but they never really eliminate the odor or remove its cause (see page 162).

Dental Care. The selection of a competent dentist is of first importance in the care of the teeth. Cheap, incompetent dentistry usually means one of several things: decay left under fillings to infect the pulp and give rise to apical abscesses, poorly prepared cavities from which fillings easily become loose, badly fitting fillings which permit of decay around their edges, difficult work neglected, and good teeth sacrificed to poor judgment. In dentistry as in other things one does not get something for nothing. The ultimate cost of poor dentistry is much greater than the cost of good work in the first place.

Teeth should be cleaned and examined at regular intervals of six or, better still, three months. The thorough cleaning aids in the prevention of decay and the examination discovers cavities when they are just beginning and as yet of minor importance. If cavities are properly filled when small, the progress of decay is arrested and the structure of the tooth saved. To postpone or neglect necessary dental work is no economy. Dentistry is expensive and even the most skillful reconstructive work is not nearly so satisfactory as sound, natural teeth.

DISCUSSION SUGGESTIONS

1. Discuss the possible reasons for the good condition of the teeth found in the skulls of certain primitive races.
2. Explain the mechanism of dental decay.
3. List the contributory causes of dental caries.
4. Discuss the relation of diet and cleanliness to dental caries.
5. What is meant by apical infections and what is their relation to health?
6. Discuss the cause and prevention of gingivitis.
7. What is meant by pyorrhea?
8. Outline the proper technique for brushing the teeth.
9. What is the value of dentifrices? What possible harm may result from the use of certain ones?
10. Explain why cheap dental work is poor economy.

REFERENCES AND READING SUGGESTIONS

1. Brekhus, Peter J.: "Your Teeth, Their Past, Present, and Probable Future," University of Minnesota Press, Minneapolis, 1941.
2. Hilleboe, Herman E., and David B. Ast: "Public Health Aspects of Water Fluoridation," *American Journal of Public Health*, vol. 41, p. 1370, November, 1951.
3. Yahraes, Herbert: "Your Teeth and How to Save Them," Public Affairs Pamphlets, New York, 1949.
4. "The Truth about Fluoridation," American Dental Association, Chicago, 1953.
5. Pamphlets on Dental Health, American Dental Association, Chicago.

Text-Films

The following McGraw-Hill Text-Film on Health Education is recommended for use with Chapter XVI of this text.

Body Care and Grooming (17 min sd MP). For description see page 373.

Chapter XVII

CARE OF THE SKIN AND HAIR

THE average person spends more time and money on the care of the skin, the hair, and the nails than on medical and health services. This is most illogical, for the appearance of the skin and hair is dependent more upon the general health of the body than upon the use of cosmetic preparations.

The appearance of the skin, hair, and nails is important. A careless unattractive appearance is a handicap in the business as well as in the social world. In addition, morale is improved and self-confidence bolstered by a good appearance.

The skin, of which the hair and nails are inert appendages, performs several important functions:

1. It protects underlying organs and tissues against injury. Very few germs can penetrate the unbroken skin. Blisters and calluses develop to protect underlying tissues from injury. Tanning keeps out the irritating rays of the sun.

2. It plays an important role in the regulation of body temperature. The various metabolic and vital processes of the body produce heat which must be eliminated. If this heat is accumulated in the body, heat stroke or heat exhaustion follow. Most of this heat is lost from the skin by radiation to the surrounding air or by the evaporation of perspiration.

Blood flow through the skin is important in controlling the rate of heat loss. When the body is hot and heat loss is essential, the blood vessels of the skin dilate, causing an increase in blood flow and a flushed or red appearance of the skin. The increased blood flow in turn causes an increase in radiation and a stimulation of perspiration. An individual who perspires easily is able to adjust to high temperatures better than the person who perspires with difficulty. Excessive heat loss or chilling causes constriction of the blood vessels, with blanching and discontinuance of perspiration.

3. It provides a sensory covering for the body. The nerve endings in the skin give rise to sensations of touch, pressure, pain, heat, and cold. As a result of these sensations, many bodily processes and actions are controlled.

4. It serves as an accessory excretory organ. Most metabolic waste products are picked up by the blood and eliminated through the kidneys. The skin, however, also contributes to this function. Under ordinary conditions and moderate activity two to three quarts of perspiration, containing salt and some urea and uric acid, are eliminated each twenty-four hours.

Care of the Skin

The most important factors in maintaining the health of the skin are those same factors important for maintaining the health of the rest of the body—adequate rest, exercise, proper diet, and cleanliness. Attention to these general rules of hygiene will do more to produce a clear, attractive skin than the application of the many different types of so-called "skin foods" advertised so freely. Of these hygienic practices, cleanliness is all-important in preserving a good complexion.

The face should be washed at least once daily with warm water and a mild soap. For those whose skin is unusually oily, a cleansing with soap twice a day may be necessary. The idea of cleaning the face with cold cream *only* is scientifically unsound. The skin of the face is constantly exposed to dirt which, with the fatty secretion from the oil glands in the skin, causes an accumulation of dirt and fat on the face. If oils and creams are used as a substitute for soap and water this accumulation of oily dirt on the face is never completely removed and may be a cause of skin disorders. For those whose skin is unusually dry, an application of cold cream at night after the face has been thoroughly cleansed with soap and water may be beneficial. It is not harmful even for the less dry skin but may be harmful for those who have a tendency to acne.

Chapping of the skin occurs most frequently in cold weather when the activity of the oil glands in the skin is reduced. Too frequent washing with strong soap removes oil from the skin and makes it more susceptible to chapping. Protection of the skin against wind and cold and the use of oil, cold cream, or glycerin reduce the likelihood of chapping.

Skin Disorders

Acne. Acne is one of the common skin disorders of young adults and may be a source of great discomfort and humiliation. Acne is an inflammation around the oil glands. During the adolescent and early adult life the oil glands and other glandular structures develop a new activity. A chief cause of acne is an excessive secretion of oil with the formation of blackheads. Only a few lesions may develop, or they may be numerous. They usually occur on the face, chest, and back. Because permanent scarring may develop in severe cases, it is wise for the person having acne to have treatment by an experienced physician. Thorough cleansing of the skin several times a day with soap and warm water is important. This should be followed by drying with a rough towel. Likewise the diet should avoid greasy foods, pastry, and large amounts of carbohydrates and chocolate. Some physicians think that the chocolate, rather than the sugar, in candy and ice cream is responsible for acne in susceptible persons. One can test for this by discontinuing all chocolate for a month to see if one's acne disappears. In other persons, certain drugs, such as iodine, may be responsible for acne. Improvement in such persons will result from the substitution of plain salt for iodized salt together with the avoidance of all sea foods.

The measures recommended for the prevention of acne are adequate sleep, a well-balanced diet, exercise and recreation, correction of constipation, cleanliness of the skin and scalp, avoid-

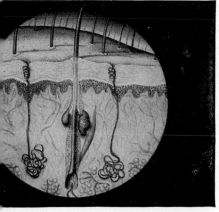

glands bring dirt to the surface of the skin.

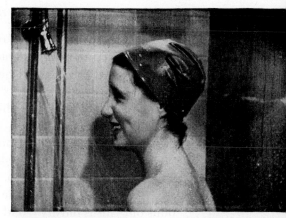

A daily shower is the first step in immaculate grooming.

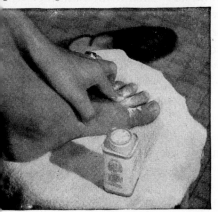

r rubbed between the toes when they are etely dry can help prevent athlete's foot.

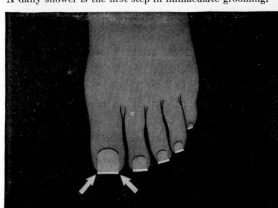

Toenails should be clipped straight across to avoid ingrown nails.

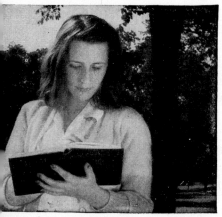

nattractive appearance is more often the of carelessness than any physical defect.

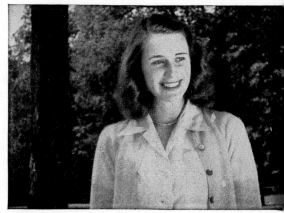

Shining hair, clean teeth, immaculate skin, and care and taste in dress add up to a charming appearance.

(From Body Care and Grooming, a McGraw-Hill Text-Film)

ance of creams and greases on the face, and the gentle removal of blackheads, using an "extractor" after soaking the face in warm, soapy water. Sunlight is beneficial to some people but bad for others. While acne may be very distressing during the early adult years, in most persons, the condition disappears in the early twenties.

Boils. Boils are infections that are usually caused by a staphylococcus that enters the skin along hair follicles. The common belief that boils are due to "bad blood" is erroneous. An excessive amount of sugar in the blood increases the susceptibility to boils but this is hardly "bad blood." Persons with boils should eat less sugar and starches and should have their urine examined by a physician. Occasionally this will lead to a diagnosis of diabetes.

Boils are infectious and may be spread from one part of the body to another or from person to person by contact, clothing, towels, etc. Boils should be covered and cared for by a physician.

Athlete's Foot and Ringworm. This widespread condition is caused by a fungus (mold) which penetrates the superficial layers of the skin. It occurs most frequently in the damp, warm skin between the toes. Early signs are areas of moist whitish skin between the toes and cracking of the skin. Unless secondarily infected, infections with this fungus are rarely incapacitating.

The fungus or mold which causes this disease is widespread. The infection is usually contracted from the floors of locker rooms, showers, bathrooms, and swimming pools, where people walk barefoot. Careful washing of the feet, including between the toes, with soap followed by thorough drying reduces the likelihood of infection. Individual towels, washcloths, and bath slippers should be used.

An analysis of forty-two advertised remedies for athlete's foot showed many of them to be exceedingly irritating and led to the conclusion that improper treatment causes more trouble than the disease itself. From such studies, as well as from widespread experience, only one conclusion is possible: that is, "do not treat your feet with home or patented remedies. They may only aggravate the condition or cause additional irritation. Consult your physician rather than your favorite advertisement."

Fig. 29

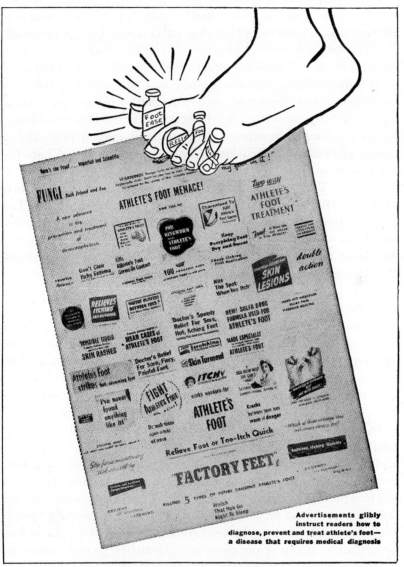

Advertisements glibly instruct readers how to diagnose, prevent and treat athlete's foot— a disease that requires medical diagnosis

(From Hygeia, November, 1946.)

A fungus known as "ringworm" may also become established on the skin or in the hair. On the skin it causes circular scaly patches which tend to heal in the center and extend peripherally. In the scalp the fungus may penetrate the shafts of the hairs, causing them to break off and to leave small, round bald areas, or it may produce only fine scaling in round areas of the scalp. Certain cases of ringworm are recognizable only under "Wood's light," a form of ultraviolet-light inspection. This condition is found commonly in school children. It is spread primarily by means of combs and brushes or by means of caps and hats that have been worn by infected persons.

Warts. Warts are caused by a specific virus which produces cauliflowerlike overgrowths of the horny layer of the skin. They may be spread from one part of the body to another by handling and from person to person by both direct and indirect contact. At times they appear and disappear without apparent cause. Warts may occur on the soles of the feet and may become so painful that removal is essential. The removal of a wart should be done by a physician.

Moles. Moles are an overgrowth of the deeper pigment layers of the skin. Most moles are harmless, but occasionally one develops into a malignant cancer. Chronic irritation from clothing, shaving, etc., may stimulate a mole to sudden growth activity. Most moles in a location where they are subject to irritation should be removed by a competent physician.

Birthmarks. A "birthmark" is a term applied to discoloration or pigmentation of the skin from an abnormal condition of surface blood vessels. The name merely indicates that these markings are usually present at or appear immediately after birth. The superstition that birthmarks are due to some prenatal influence or fright on the part of the mother is without foundation. Although birthmarks are rarely dangerous, they should not be irritated. Many of the so-called "strawberry type" disappear spontaneously; others persist throughout life.

Scabies (the Itch). Scabies, which used to be one of the most common of the skin diseases, is rarely seen today even in charity clinics and hospitals. It is caused by the itch mite, which burrows under the skin and lays its eggs. The mite is most frequently found between the fingers. Scabies is transmitted from one person to another by direct contact and indirectly by the use of bedding, gloves, or underclothing of an infected person. It is readily controlled by the exclusion from school and isolation of infected children and the disinfection of clothing and bedding. Certain drugs which destroy the itch mite can be applied to the infected person. Complete elimination of the mite usually requires several days of treatment.

Pediculosis. Pediculosis is an infestation with lice. There are three common types of louse which infest human beings: the head louse, the body louse, and the crab louse. The louse commonly is found in the hairy parts of an infected person. The presence of pediculosis is usually a result of uncleanliness. It is frequently said that it is no disgrace to get lice but it is to keep them. Pediculosis is transmitted by direct contact with someone infested or indirectly by contact with clothing or bedding of such a person. Pediculosis can be controlled by the recognition of the state of lousiness and proper measures to remove the lice and the nits (see typhus fever, Appendix D). Constant precautions are necessary to prevent the entry of lice into hospitals.

Impetigo Contagiosa. Impetigo is an infectious dermatitis which characteristically develops as small blisters, weeping sores, and crusts. It is most common on the face and hands. Impetigo is caused either by staphylococci or streptococci. It is transmitted from one person to another by direct or indirect contact. The person who has impetigo may spread the disease from one part of the body to another by scratching. While impetigo is more commonly found among children, especially in warm weather, it may also occur in adults. In the pediatric wards of hospitals great care must be taken to prevent the spread of impetigo, should a child be admitted with the infection. The treatment consists of local application of drugs. Ointments containing certain of the antibiotic drugs have been found to be very effective. The prevention and control of impetigo depend upon the recognition, isolation, and prompt treatment of infected individuals.

A somewhat similar infection with the staphylococcus or

streptococcus may occur on the face, where it is commonly known as "barber's itch." The transmission is by means of razors or towels.

Urticaria. Urticaria, commonly known as "hives," consists of small pink and whitish elevations of the skin which have the general appearance of insect bites. They are of various sizes, ranging from the size of the head of a large pin to a wheal of a half inch or more in diameter. They represent an allergic reaction to a substance, frequently penicillin or some other drug, that is either brought into direct contact with the skin or absorbed by the respiratory or intestinal tract and carried throughout the body in the blood stream. Itching is usually severe.

Localized urticaria may result from insect bites in case the subject is sensitive to the formic acid introduced by the bite of the insect. It may also be due to some substance such as wool, dyes, lacquers, etc., to which the individual is sensitive. Elimination of such substances from the environment is the most effective preventive measure. Emotional stress and disturbances are important factors in the development of urticaria in some people.

Poison Ivy. Several plants, such as poison ivy, poison oak, and poison sumac, give rise to inflammation of the skin (dermatitis) in susceptible persons. Individual susceptibility changes, so that a person who believes himself immune to ivy poisoning may later find that he is susceptible. The severity of the reaction varies from a few small red itchy spots to swelling and blister formation over large areas of the body.

The irritating substance from these plants is an oil or a resin. This may reach the skin by direct contact or through something which has touched the plant, such as clothing, shoes, tennis balls, garden tools, dogs, etc. The oil or resin may remain on such articles for long periods of time. Inflammation of the skin may appear in 6 to 12 hours or it may develop 4 to 10 days after exposure.

Very minute amounts of the oil are sufficient to cause severe reactions in sensitive persons. The spread from one part of the body to another occurs by means of hands, clothing, towels, etc., or by absorption and spread through the lymphatic system. Such spreading may occur before as well as after inflammation develops. The more frequently a person has been affected by poison ivy the earlier the symptoms appear.

The disease runs a course of one to several weeks, depending on its severity. Treatment, at least of severe cases, should be under the direction of a physician. If one has been in contact with these plants, washing the area immediately afterward with gasoline or alcohol and soap and water may remove the irritant oil and so prevent the development of the disease. Eating ivy leaves or drinking a "tea" made from them is sometimes suggested as a means of increasing one's resistance to ivy poisoning. Such procedures, however, are dangerous and should be avoided.

Cosmetics

A clear skin and attractive hair are assets to beauty and so desired by every woman, young or old. That the appearance of the skin and hair is related to the general health of the body is too frequently forgotten by many women. The advertising propaganda of the cosmetics industry has led many women to believe that the source of beauty is in a jar or bottle and that a good complexion can be acquired through the use of certain creams, powders, or rouge. The woman of today who refrains from using cosmetics is conspicuous. The intelligent woman must know, however, that cold cream or hair lotion cannot be a substitute for the attractiveness that good health gives to the skin and hair, and that they should be used only to complement the beauty with which Nature has endowed the healthy person. Marie Stopes has said, "You can take no credit for beauty at 16. But if you are beautiful at 60, it will be your own soul's doing."

Since training in the sciences has become so large a part of our educational system, it is amazing to find the widespread belief in the magic claims in advertisements made for products manufactured from quite ordinary ingredients. Just pick up the current issue of any of the so-called women's magazines and turn to almost any cosmetic ad. Whether it be rouge, lipstick, cold cream or turtle oil cream, you get the impression that all a woman has to do is invest in five or six essential cosmetics and she will in short order acquire the lure of an oriental houri plus the finish of a Hollywood actress. . . . These ex-

[367]

travagant claims, alas, have no basis in fact. The little brochures that read like the Arabian Night's entertainment and are illustrated with pictures of lovely women are the product of imagination, not science. There is no Santa Claus, no magic lamp or ring in real life that can grant one's fond desires in these matters. There are certain things that a few simple cosmetics will do.[1]

Cosmetics should be used to improve appearance. The commonly used types of cosmetics are face creams of various types, face powders, lipstick, and rouge. If these preparations are pure, they may be used without harm.

The function of a *face cream* is to lubricate the skin and to prevent roughness and chapping. Manufacturers of cosmetics advertise special creams that are so-called "tissue building" or "nourishing creams" or "skin foods," supposed to be of some particular value to the skin. The idea that one should use three or four different types of cream is merely a clever sales scheme. Ordinary plain cold cream is probably the safest and most satisfactory type to use. The cost of such a cold cream varies with the manufacturer. If the company has obtained the endorsement of well-known society women, the cost of such endorsement will be added to the cost of the cold cream. The formulas of the many special-purpose creams may be somewhat different from cold cream, but the physiological effect on the skin is only that of lubrication.

The type of cold cream called "vanishing cream" is actually a kind of soap. When such creams are rubbed into the face, it is merely the equivalent of leaving soap on the face after washing. Because of this, vanishing creams tend to dry the skin. For women who have an oily skin, usually no irritating effect from the vanishing cream will be noted, and the face powder will stay on for a longer period of time. For the dry skin, vanishing cream will increase the dryness and may cause actual scaling and roughness of the skin.

Face powders usually contain talcum, magnesium, French chalk, and starch or rice powder. A few years ago many face powders contained lead, mercury, or bismuth, all of which are definitely harmful. Face powders also have been made with orris

[1] Phillips, M. C., "Skin Deep," Vanguard Press, New York, 1934.

root, to which many individuals are allergic. At the present time few face powders made by reputable manufacturers contain any of these undesirable ingredients.

The sensible procedure to follow in selecting a face powder, provided you are not sensitive to rice or wheat, starch or orris root, is to buy the one whose color and perfume best suit you. There is no particular advantage in buying a high-priced powder unless you wish to pay an exorbitant price for a fancy container or a particularly appealing perfume. The less expensive varieties, such, for example, as the larger size boxes containing comparatively unknown and unadvertised brands found at the five-and-ten-cent stores, will serve equally well and will probably, with the exceptions already mentioned, be entirely safe to use. It is pathetic to watch girls employed at a very low salary skimp on their lunches or go hungry in order to buy an expensive, much advertised box of powder in the belief that they are purchasing something that will have a matchless or magical effect on their appearance. An adequate meal will have a far more beneficial effect on their general health, which is the most important factor in good looks.

One last word of caution—be sure your powder puff is clean, and never use another person's powder puff. Your neighbor's germs may be unfriendly to your complexion.[2]

Rouge and lipstick are also usually harmless cosmetics and if used skillfully may contribute much to one's attractiveness. The chief danger is in those which may contain certain anilin dyes to which some people may be allergic. Consumers' Research has had a number of popular brands of lipstick and rouge analyzed for dangerous ingredients, and several of the commonly advertised brands were found to be free from most undesirable substances. Even these, however, may not be safe for the occasional individual who may be sensitive to a certain perfume or dye which may be harmless for the majority of people.

Eyelash Dyes

The best way to be certain you avoid harmful dyes in eyelash preparations is to avoid preparations that are obviously dyes rather than the usual mascaras. Even if a product is not called a dye, you can identify it as such quite readily. The first indication will be in its advertising claims. It will be claimed to produce "permanent" color. This is a relative term meaning that the color will be unaffected by water, tears or abrasion for several months as compared with mascara, which must be reapplied at least daily. There are usually directions

[2] *Ibid.*

for application, and sometimes gadgets are included to protect the eyes during dyeing. Mascaras usually consist of a cake or cream accompanied by a brush for application; directions usually suggest a simple method of application. It is difficult to visualize how a chemical can be applied to the eyelashes without coming in contact with the eyes themselves, regardless of precautions.

One should assume nothing when such vital and irreplaceable structures as the eyes are involved. In any discussion of eye cosmetics, the safety of the eyes overshadows all other considerations. For this reason, the use of eyelash dyes is strongly discouraged.[3]

Depilatories. A depilatory is a substance that removes hair. For this purpose the common methods are shaving, scraping the skin with pumice stone or emery board, or the use of hair removers, of either the chemical or wax variety. None of the above methods removes the hair permanently, as they have no effect on the root of the hair, which is the source of growth. The only safe method of permanently removing hair is by electrolysis. In this method an electric needle is inserted into each individual hair follicle, thus destroying the hair root. Unless this is done by an expert, permanent removal of hair by electrolysis may cause scarring. Because each hair must be removed separately this is an expensive method of hair removal.

There is a common belief that shaving causes hair to grow out thicker and coarser than it was before. That this superstition has no foundation in fact was shown by a series of experiments conducted by Drs. C. H. Danforth and Mildred Trotter of Washington University School of Medicine. They had three girls shave the left leg from knee to ankle twice a week for eight months. After the hair had grown out again microscropic examination of the hairs of the left leg and the right leg which had not been shaved showed that there was no demonstrable difference between the hairs after shaving and the hairs on the leg which had not been shaved.

Chemical and wax hair removers are not entirely safe to use. In some individuals they cause irritation of the skin and may even cause a skin infection. Some of these preparations which are on the market claim to remove the hair permanently. Such claims are entirely false.

The only safe method which can be recommended for remov-

[3] Conley, Veronica, *Today's Health*, February, 1954.

ing hair is a razor. One can be sure that there is no danger of skin irritation or poisoning from any chemical and need have no fear that shaving will cause the hair to grow out coarser than it was before. Plucking the hair is also a safe method of removing hair but obviously is very time-consuming. Hair should never be plucked from a mole, as this may cause irritation of the mole.

Deodorants

Body odor is caused by fatty acids that are formed as a result of decomposition of sweat. For those individuals who perspire excessively the prevention of body odor may be an important consideration in personal hygiene. Since such body odor is caused by perspiration and the fatty acids formed from the sweat, the most important remedy in its prevention is frequent bathing, frequent changing of the clothes, and, in some instances, the use of a deodorant. There are two types of deodorant commonly advertised—those which deodorize the perspiration without restricting its flow, and those which both deodorize and stop the flow of perspiration. The first type depends for its action upon such ingredients as boric acid, benzoic acid, or zinc stearate, and may be obtained either in a dry or paste form. It is usually harmless to use. The second type, which also diminishes the flow of perspiration, depends for its value on aluminum chloride, tannic acid, or zinc sulphate. While many people may use this type of deodorant without harm, in some preparations the solution may be so strong that it will cause a skin rash or other discomfort in sensitive individuals. If this type of preparation is used, it should be used no oftener than is absolutely necessary.

The Hair

The same general principles of good hygiene which are used for the care of the skin also apply to keeping the hair healthy. The hair, as is true of all other structures of the body, gets its nourishment from the blood. If the general health is good, the hair and scalp will be healthy. Again, cleanliness is one of the most important aids in keeping the hair attractive. The hair, like the skin of the face and hands, is exposed to smoke and dirt. To keep the scalp and hair clean the hair should be washed at least once every two weeks with a pure, mild soap. For many people a shampoo each week or oftener is necessary. Daily brushing of the hair will aid greatly in preventing the accumulation of dirt and in keeping the hair attractive.

Excessive dryness, excessive oiliness, excessive dandruff or falling out of the hair are not normal and indicate that something is wrong. A physician should be consulted. Certain types of dandruff which cause a thick, oily scale to appear upon the scalp are due to a germ infection and should be treated as such by a physician. The more common type of dandruff, causing dry scales to appear upon the scalp, is usually a symptom of unhygienic habits of living such as lack of sleep or excessive nervous strain or sometimes of improper diet. Most of the so-called "dandruff cures" which are advertised are of no more value in curing dandruff than are soap and water, though they may improve the appearance temporarily. Hair oils may be used by those with dry hair and scalp if it is not due to disease. The oil need not be expensive. Mineral oil or olive oil, with perfume if desired, is satisfactory.

Bald and balding American men are spending millions of dollars for futile hair-saving and dandruff-curing treatments. Baldness in most persons is hereditary. In others the cause is unknown. Neither massage, "hair tonics," mechanical devices, ultraviolet light, hormones, vitamins, nor any other treatment will prevent baldness or cause hair to grow in bald spots.

Hair dyes of all types are to be avoided. While some of them may be used over a period of time with no apparent ill effects, others contain dangerous substances which may cause severe damage to the skin or eyes, and in some cases even may be absorbed and cause kidney damage. The bleaches that remove the color from the hair and enable a brunette to become a blonde at her pleasure are probably not harmful, although they may leave the hair dry and brittle.

The permanent wave is a method of curling naturally straight hair by the application of chemicals and heat. When carefully and skillfully done, the permanent wave probably has no harmful effect on the hair. The heat may make the hair dry, but this effect is usually not lasting. Specialists advise against using bleaches in any form previous to permanent waving and advise caution with waving hair that has been bleached by overexposure to sunlight.

DISCUSSION SUGGESTIONS

1. What are the important factors in maintaining a healthy skin?
2. Discuss the cause and control of impetigo, pediculosis, and scabies.
3. What is urticaria? How may it be prevented?
4. What are warts, moles, and birthmarks?
5. Of what value are face creams? When should they not be used?
6. What kinds of face powder may be harmful to some people?
7. Why are eyelash dyes dangerous?
8. Discuss the various types of depilatory.
9. Discuss the causes of body odor and its prevention.
10. Discuss the care of the hair.
11. What harmful effects on the hair may be caused by a permanent wave?

REFERENCES AND READING SUGGESTIONS

1. Behrman, H. T., and O. L. Levin: "Your Skin and Its Care," Emerson Books, Inc., New York, 1948.
2. Cole, Harold N.: "The Skin in Health and Disease" (special pamphlet), American Medical Association, Chicago, 1948.
3. Committee on Cosmetics: "Hair and Scalp Treatments," *Journal of the American Medical Association*, vol. 139, p, 840, March 26, 1949.
4. ————: "Hair-raising Business," *Reader's Digest*, July, 1949.
5. Greenbaum, S. S.: "The Facts on Sun Tan," *Hygeia*, vol. 27, p. 478, July, 1949.
6. Koven, A. L.: "Facts about Athlete's Foot," *Hygeia*, vol. 24, p. 828, November, 1946.
7. Phillips, M. C.: "Skin Deep," Vanguard Press, New York, 1934.
8. Smith, Austin: "Cosmetic Facts and Fancies," *Hygeia*, vol. 25, p. 856, November, 1947.

Text-Films

The following McGraw-Hill Text-Film on Health Education is recommended for use with this chapter and with Chapter XVI.

Body Care and Grooming (17 min sd MP). This film develops the theme that good grooming starts with daily personal care, and describes a routine of recommended health habits. Emphasis is laid on the desirability of good grooming as a basis for social acceptability among young people. Animated drawings explain basic health arguments for clean hair, nails, teeth, skin, etc.

Silent follow-up filmstrip based on material in the motion picture offers an opportunity for review, testing, and discussion.

Chapter XVIII

GLANDS OF INTERNAL
SECRETION[1]

FASCINATING research, momentous discovery, and fantastic speculation are among the terms which properly apply to recent work on the glands of internal secretion, the so-called "endocrine glands." On the one hand, some of the best of modern research has been done in this field, while, on the other, speculation runs rampant to suggest that these glands hold the secret of eternal youth and to describe Napoleon as a "pituitary type" and Charles Dickens as "the product of an exceptionally vigorous thyroid."

These mysterious structures exert an amazing influence upon the growth, development, and functioning of body and mind. They are called "glands" because they manufacture new substances called "hormones" out of materials which they take from the blood stream, and glands of "internal secretion" because the hormones which they manufacture are absorbed directly into the blood stream to be circulated throughout the body. In this regard they differ from ordinary glands, such as the salivary glands, the pancreas, and the liver, which have tubes or ducts to collect and to carry their secretions to the place of use.

---

[1] The paragraphs quoted in this chapter are from "The Physiological Roles and the Clinical Significance of the Endocrine Glands," University of Minnesota, Sigma Xi Lecture, by Dr. Irvine McQuarrie. (*Journal-Lancet*, vol. 56, pp. 254–270, May, 1936.)

The existence of these glands was known for centuries before their functions were understood. In fact, since they had no apparent secretions, one could not be sure that they were glands at all. Even yet our knowledge concerning their activities is far from complete, but great progress is being made. Modern chemical and research techniques are making it possible to obtain more and more of their secretions in pure form. Hence, they can be analyzed and their effects upon the body studied. It has even been possible after accurate determination of their chemical structure to manufacture some of these substances in the laboratory.

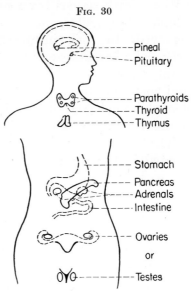

FIG. 30

The location of the endocrine glands. (*Northwestern National Life Insurance Company, Minneapolis.*)

The more important glands of internal secretion are the thyroid, parathyroid, pituitary, thymus, adrenals, the "islands of Langerhans" of the pancreas, the pineal gland, and the sex glands. These glands are located in different parts of the body but functionally are closely related. A deficiency of thyroid secretion retards growth through its effect upon the pituitary; pituitary secretions stimulate the development of the thyroid and of the sex glands; and adrenalin is antagonistic to insulin. There is evidence also that when the secretions of certain glands are deficient there is an effort on the part of complementary glands to compensate for this deficiency by increasing their secretions.

The Thyroid

We have more accurate knowledge concerning the thyroid than concerning any of the other glands of internal secretion. Thyroid enlargement, which is called a "goiter," has been recognized since remote antiquity, and almost a century ago the absence of the thyroid in cretins, the physiologically and mentally retarded dwarfs found in goiterous regions, was pointed out.[2] Then it was found that the feeding of thyroid glands of cattle or other animals to young cretins caused resumption of growth. Somewhat later surgeons began to operate upon the thyroids of patients with serious toxic goiters, such as hyperthyroidism or exophthalmic goiter, and occasionally too much of the gland was removed. In such instances, physical and mental changes occurred, characterized by diminished activity, gain in weight, scanty hair, thick, dry, scaly skin, coarse features, drowsiness, and mental retardation. This condition, now called "myxedema," is analogous to cretinism in children. Patients with it also improve when given thyroid by mouth.

The thyroid is a small gland weighing approximately an ounce located in the front of the neck just above the breast bone. Its secretion regulates the metabolism of the body, an excess causing a speeding up of the pulse, respiration, and other body functions and an increase in nervous irritability and activity. Carbohydrates, fats, and proteins are burned more rapidly; and glycogen which is stored in the liver is discharged into the blood stream. On the other hand, a deficiency of thyroid secretion results in a lowering of metabolism, a slowing of body processes, a lack of energy, and fatigue. In women absence of the menses and infertility are associated with moderate thyroid deficiency. Extreme deficiency gives rise to cretinism in children and myxedema in adults.

In spite of the great importance of the secretion of this gland upon health, the total amount of active thyroid secretion which is present in the body at one time amounts to only about 1/2,500 ounce. The active principle of this secretion is now prepared in pure crystalline form under the name "thyroxin," the administration of which is just as effective in increasing the rate of metabolism and in preventing cretinism and myxedema as is the whole gland.

[2] We now know that cretinism usually is due to a thyroid deficiency on the part of the mother and can be prevented by giving iodine during pregnancy.

Goiters. There have been times and places when goiters were considered marks of beauty, but we look upon them as abnormalities to be prevented.

Most goiters are simple enlargements of the thyroid gland, due to a deficiency of iodine in the food or drink and without effect upon health. Such goiters are not limited to man but occur also among domestic animals. In 1918 Marine found that 90 per cent of the dogs in Cleveland had goiters and Smith reports that in Montana a million pigs are lost annually on account of this condition. New-born pigs in goiter regions are stunted and hairless. Goiters are even found in fish in waters with an exceptionally low iodine content. Addition of iodine to the water is all that is necessary to prevent it.

Some difference of opinion exists among physicians as to whether iodine deficiency is the only factor in the development of goiter. Possibly it is not, because not everyone in goiterous areas develops goiters, while some goiters occur in regions where there is plenty of iodine in the soil and in the drinking water. It has been shown, however, that the administration of iodine is highly effective in preventing this type of goiter. Very little is needed and this may be supplied in any one of several ways. Practically, the use of an iodized table salt which bears the seal of acceptance of the Committee on Foods of the American Medical Association is a simple, convenient, and dependable method of supplying the iodine needs of the body.

The toxic, or so-called "exophthalmic," goiter is an entirely different condition. Its cause is not known, although there is some evidence that emotional shock may be a precipitating factor. In exophthalmic goiter the thyroid may or may not be enlarged, but the symptoms are typical of an excessive and abnormal thyroid secretion. The patient is nervous, hyperactive, even trembling; the eyes are staring and prominent; the pulse and respiration are rapid; and in severe cases there may be nausea and diarrhea. The metabolism is markedly increased and weight is lost.

Surgical removal of part of this hyperactive gland gives entirely satisfactory results in most cases. The administration of iodine will not prevent or cure this condition, but in sufficient dosage it does cause temporary improvement. In fact, iodine is frequently given to patients with hyperthyroidism to get them in better condition for operation.

Cretinism, or extreme childhood myxedema, is seen far more frequently in goiter regions than elsewhere but occurs sporadically in all parts of the world. The child born with an undeveloped or atrophied thyroid gland can be recognized at once because the signs of cretinism or infantile myxedema are unmistakable. The victim is a puffy and misshapen creature with a thick, protruding tongue, too large for his mouth. Because of this he is often unable to nurse and must be fed artificially. His cry has a coarse, brassy quality. If he lives but receives no specific treatment, his physical development is markedly retarded and the higher nervous system remains undeveloped functionally, so that his intelligence ranges between feeble-mindedness and complete idiocy. The face is wholly lacking in animation. The blunt nose becomes flat and somewhat saddle-shaped. The eyelids and lips thicken. The mouth gapes and drools saliva constantly. Deafness is not infrequently present. The skin becomes dry and thick with a dull, muddy tinge. The hands and feet are broad and clumsy. The abdomen protrudes. The breathing is slow but noisy. The pulse is slow. The body temperature is subnormal, because his metabolic fires burn low. X-ray examination of the bones shows their development to be extremely retarded. The teeth erupt late and are scraggly and of poor quality. Such is the picture of extreme thyroid deficiency in early childhood. When a similar misfortune comes to an adult who has previously been normal, retrogressive changes of both body and mind finally produce a similar clinical picture, already referred to as myxedema.

If the thyroid deficiency in such patients as these is made up by administration of thyroid extract or of pure thyroxin, the beneficial effects are usually phenomenal. The swollen tissues of the body give up their pathological stores of water and the cellular nutrition tends to return to normal, as shown by metabolism tests. Facial dullness is superseded by animation and the disposition improves immeasurably. Mental keenness returns and, in the case of a child, growth and development proceed very rapidly. The earlier treatment is begun in the case of childhood myxedema the greater are the chances for normal development. A condition of "masked hypothyroidism" or mild under function of the gland is far more common than these extreme cases. Thyroid treatment greatly benefits such persons.

The Parathyroid Glands

The parathyroids are tiny glands, usually four in number, attached to the undersurface of the thyroid, near what might be called its four corners. In the early days of thyroid surgery these were sometimes accidentally removed with the thyroid. When this occurred, symptoms which we now recognize as typical of parathyroid deficiency developed.

The chief function of the parathyroids seems to be to regulate the utilization of calcium by the body. In this respect their action is supplemented by vitamin D.

A deficiency of parathyroid secretion gives rise to a disease called "tetany." This condition is characterized by an abnormal excitability of the nervous system, which may cause spasms or cramps of the muscles. The spasms may be intermittent or constant and may affect only a few muscles or the entire body. A mild form of tetany which occurs in childhood is known as "spasmophilia."

An extract of the parathyroid glands, which was first prepared a few years ago, has made it possible to study their function more accurately and to treat patients in whom evidences of a deficiency of this internal secretion occur.

The Pituitary Gland

The pituitary gland is the most intriguing and probably the most important of all the glands of internal secretion. It is only about the size of a pea and is situated underneath the brain at the approximate mathematical center of the head. Anatomically this gland consists of three parts, the anterior, middle, and posterior lobes.

The *posterior lobe* . . . is known to produce two distinct hormones. . . . These have been isolated in sufficiently concentrated form to permit their use in medical practice. The chief physiological action of the first of these, *pitocin*, is apparently that of stimulating the uterus to contract during certain phases of its career, particularly during child birth. . . . Pitocin or pituitrin is employed by many obstetricians during the third stage of labor, if the uterus fails to contract normally.

. . . The second active principle, *pitressin*, is the more important of the two in that it evidently serves three different functions. It has a stimulating or toning effect on the involuntary muscle coats of the intestines and the blood vessels, causing these structures to contract when it is administered. This property makes it a valuable adjunct in the treatment of circulatory

[379]

collapse or shock and in gaseous distention of the intestines. When injected hypodermically, it causes a prompt rise in blood sugar. It thus serves as a potential antagonist to insulin. Finally, this hormone acts on the kidneys to inhibit excessive loss of water from the body.

Another effect of pitressin, as yet unexplained, is the remarkable relief which it gives to patients with diabetes insipidus. This rare disease, apparently hereditary, is characterized by enormous thirst, and the excretion of large quantities of very dilute but otherwise normal urine. Patients are reported to have drunk as much as 10 gallons of water in 24 hours and to have excreted a corresponding quantity of urine. Two to three gallons of urine per day are common in this disease. After injection of pitressin the thirst disappears and the quantity of urine becomes comparatively normal. This suggests that the disease is due to a deficiency of pitressin, but, queerly enough, complete removal of the pituitary does not produce it. To explain this paradox various theories have been advanced but the final solution remains for the future.

The *intermediate lobe* of the pituitary gland elaborates a separate hormone, *intermedin*, which causes expansion of certain pigment cells or chromatophore cells in frogs and other cold-blooded animals. When some of this hormone is injected into the lymph sac of a light-colored speckled frog, his melanophore or pigment cells expand until he is dark all over. While we do not know with certainty just what part this substance plays in human physiology, it has been suggested that it has to do with the function of pigment cells in the retina of the eye, aiding particularly in adjustments to darkness. This gland and the adrenal may play a special role in pigment changes in the skin but, so far, this relationship has not been determined.

The *anterior portion* of the pituitary produces several internal secretions and is even more mysterious and far-reaching in its effects upon the body than the middle and posterior portions. Its most marked effect is upon growth.

. . . Total removal or complete destruction of the gland in early life produces a state of infantilism or physical *dwarfism*. The midgets seen in circuses are usually of this type. Body growth is arrested. The thyroid glands, the adrenals, the gonads and other sex organs, the breasts and the parathyroids remain small and underactive. The victim ages prematurely. The body proportions are far more nearly normal than they are in cretinism, but the size of all struc-

[380]

tures is markedly reduced. Surprisingly, the mental development is often but little impaired. . . . Sufferers from this fortunately rare disorder show extreme wasting of the body, muscular weakness, loss of hair, loss of sex power and finally death, if treatment is not given. Administration of crude extracts of the whole anterior lobe is apparently capable of correcting these abnormalities to a large extent.

Overactivity of the anterior lobe causes the reverse picture, that is, overgrowth of the body, together with enlargement and increased activity of the adrenal cortex, the thyroid gland, the parathyroids and the sex glands. A form of mild diabetes mellitus is produced at the same time. Simple hyperplasia or tumor of the anterior lobe is now known to produce symmetrical *gigantism* in young individuals whose normal bone growth has not been completed. Such victims have been known to reach the height of nine feet.

This gigantism is due to an increase in the rate of growth and not to a prolongation of the growing period. Overactivity of the gland in adult life leads to bizarre enlargements of certain portions of the body—a condition known as "acromegaly." The bones of the face become prominent, the nose widens, the hands and feet enlarge, individual bones become thick with blunt, prominent ends. Muscular power and mental ability are usually undiminished.

Another abnormality of growth which has been attributed to a deficiency of anterior pituitary secretion is extreme adiposity. The fat boys and fat ladies of side shows belong in this group. Autopsies on such persons show degeneration of the pituitary gland, usually as a result of pressure from a tumor. Experimental work on animals, however, indicates that adiposity does not follow removal of the pituitary gland unless the brain tissue just above it is injured. Tumors in this region press on this brain tissue as well as on the pituitary gland. Another still more recent report indicates that there probably is a secretion of this anterior portion of the pituitary which directly affects the metabolism of carbohydrates and fats and may have some relationship to diabetes; all of which goes to show that investigation in this field is just beginning.

The anterior pituitary secretion also contains hormones which influence the activity of other glands of internal secretion. One of these regulates the activity of the thyroid. Others influence

[381]

sexual development, maturity, and function. The absence of this factor at the time of puberty results in sexual infantilism of the adult; and its disappearance, due to atrophy of the pituitary gland, after sexual maturity has been attained, in cessation of menstruation, impotence, and a regression of the typically male and female physical characteristics such as hair distribution, growth of beard, contour of the body, and development of the breasts.

It appears at the present time that the anterior lobe produces two gonadotropic hormones. One of these stimulates development of the Graafian follicle in the ovary and spermatogenesis in the testis, and the other stimulates the development of the corpus luteum of the ovary and probably stimulates the interstitial cells of the testis. In pregnancy, even as early as the first few weeks after conception, the blood and urine contain gonadotropic substances in such high concentration that their presence can be demonstrated in the urine. This fact is used to make a diagnosis of pregnancy before physical changes occur.

This test consists of injecting a small amount of urine into an immature female mouse or rabbit and observing its effect upon the ovaries. If these hormones are present, the ovaries show changes so characteristic that it is possible to make a diagnosis of pregnancy. An ingenious adaptation of this test is the use of Japanese fish, called "bitterlings." Apparently all that is necessary is to add a small amount of the urine to be tested to a bowl of water containing one of these female fish. If the hormones associated with pregnancy are present, the fish shows an enlargement of the tiny oviduct which protrudes from the undersurface of the body.

Another of these anterior pituitary hormones stimulates the activity of the mammary glands. And still another, called ACTH (adrenocorticotrophic hormone), is necessary for the normal functioning of the adrenal glands (see also page 389).

The Thymus and the Pineal Glands

The pineal gland is a small cone-shaped structure about a quarter of an inch in length located near the back of the brain;

the thymus is a rather flat, elongated, slightly irregular gland located in the lower portion of the neck and upper middle part of the chest. In calves and lambs the thymus is called the "sweetbread" or the "neck sweetbread." Both of these glands are present during childhood and disappear rapidly after puberty.

The chief function of the thymus has to do with body development and growth and the metabolism of lime salts. . . . When thymus substance is fed to young tadpoles they grow to unusually large size and their metamorphosis or change to the frog state is much delayed, whereas thyroid feeding has the opposite effects. That it is in some way connected with sex development in man is indicated by the fact that the secondary sex characters do not develop normally if the thymus does not undergo involution or shrinking at the usual time. The thymus does not atrophy or decrease in size at the age of puberty if the sex glands have failed to develop or have been removed previously. Destructive disease or extirpation of the adrenal gland causes an enlargement of the thymus. Overactivity of the thyroid has a similar effect.

As regards the influence of the thymus on calcium metabolism, the first convincing evidence was derived from studies on birds. It was early found that pullets, after having their thymus glands removed, laid eggs lacking in shells. Finding that certain pigeons without any such operation laid eggs devoid of shells, Riddle treated them with thymus extracts, with the result that normal eggs were produced.

Rowntree, Hanson and their co-workers have added a new and interesting chapter to our knowledge of this elusive gland. Following the daily injection of a relatively potent thymus extract into the peritoneal cavity of rats from the time of birth until they bore young, these workers observed the offspring to be unusually large and precocious in their development. This tendency in the offspring was markedly increased when the parent rats in succeeding generations continued to receive injections. In the later generations the offspring were as far advanced in size and development, both physically and in respect to behavior, at the age of three days as normal control rats are at the age of nearly three weeks. Whereas normal rats are born hairless, do not open their eyes until the fourteenth day and cannot be weaned before this time, the offspring of the fifth and sixth generations of thymus-treated rats were found to have heavy coats of fur, to open their eyes and to fend for themselves without nursing their mothers at the age of three or four days. The fertility of the rats was appreciably increased. The mortality rate of the offspring was greatly reduced and the onset of adolescence was hastened. The marked degree of speeding up of the latter process was illustrated by the performance of one mother rat which bred at the age of twenty-two days instead of the normal age of between seventy-two and ninety days and cast a litter of

[383]

precocious rats at the age of forty-three days. Four days before the birth of her offspring she weighed 102 grams. Her five baby rats together are said to have weighed 90 grams at birth! When instead of receiving injections of thymus extract, successive generations of parent rats had their thymus glands removed, it was found that their offspring, although born at the usual time, were much smaller than normal rats and were much slower in developing. . . .

It has been suggested that the normal function of the *pineal* is to prevent the too early development of the body and particularly of the sex organs. Hanson has recently obtained an extract from the pineal of animals which, when injected into parent rats in successive generations, apparently produced dwarfed offspring. In striking contrast to the effect of thymus extract under similar circumstances, this material results in an unmistakable delay in development. Much further experimental work will be required before we can tell what part this gland normally plays in animal economy.

The Pancreas

Less than thirty-five years ago, insulin was unknown. Today, it stands between life and death for hundreds of thousands of persons with diabetes the world over. The discovery and early preparation of insulin are a thrilling story of scientific investigation and discovery.

Insulin is the internal secretion of the pancreas, a wedge-shaped gland 3 or 4 inches long located just below and behind the stomach and called the "belly sweetbread" in the meat market. Its chief function is to secrete the pancreatic juice, which plays a major role in the digestion of proteins and fats. Scattered about throughout this glandular tissue which secretes digestive juice are small masses of cells, which are different in appearance and are unconnected with the typical pancreatic tissue. These were first described by Langerhans as "islands" of cells; hence, they came to be known as the "islands of Langerhans."

The disease, sugar diabetes, now known to be due to a deficiency in the internal secretion of the pancreas, was apparently known to the writer of the earliest medical document which we possess, the papyrus Ebers, dating from approximately 1500 B.C., *i.e.*, three centuries before the birth of Moses and a thousand years before Hippocrates, the father of medicine. Before the beginning of the Christian era Greek physicians had described some of the cardinal symptoms and signs of uncontrolled diabetes, *i.e.*, excessive thirst, drinking and passing of enormous amounts of water, marked loss of weight and feeling of weakness in spite of the inordinate consumption of

FIG. 31. THE HUMAN PANCREAS

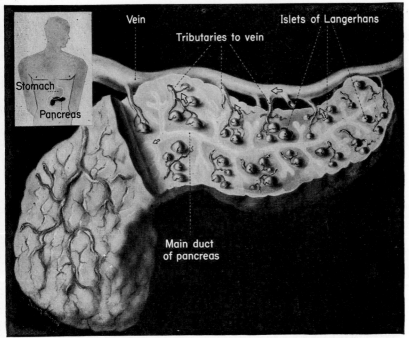

(*Northwestern National Life Insurance Company, Minneapolis.*)

food. Sweetness of diabetic urine was first mentioned in the sixth century
A.D. by a Hindu writer who called the disease Madhumcha, meaning "honey
urine."

In spite of many attempts to isolate the active antidiabetic principle
from the pancreas in sufficiently pure condition for treatment of patients,
no satisfactory method was devised until 1922. Banting and Best of Toronto
then took up the problem by making an extract of dog pancreas which had
previously been prepared by ligation of the ducts to destroy all but the islet
tissue. They succeeded in obtaining an extract which would reduce the
amount of sugar in the blood and urine of other dogs which had been made
diabetic by complete removal of the pancreas. With the aid of the biochemist,
Collip, they were soon able to prepare the hormone in a form which could
be injected under the skin of human diabetics. This final success was heralded
the world over and within a few years thousands of previously doomed sufferers
were daily employing this life-saving remedy which was given the name, insulin. Before the advent of this great boon, practically all children who developed
diabetes died within five or six years in spite of the most skillfully prepared
diets. Surgical operations on diabetic patients in the pre-insulin era were

[385]

attended with great danger. Today, however, neither of these special situations concerns the doctor seriously because he is enabled by the proper use of insulin to control the diabetic tendency. In the days before insulin was available, the majority of diabetic patients who died from the disease developed a severe form of acidosis due to accumulation in the body of acid products resulting from the incomplete or faulty burning of fats, which is a secondary manifestation of active diabetes. Even today this serious stage may be reached before the victim is aware that he has diabetes. The symptoms of this complication are deep, rapid breathing, excessive loss of body water and alkaline minerals and later uncontrollable drowsiness. Unconsciousness then supervenes and the patient ultimately dies in this comatose state, if insulin is not administered. One of the most dramatic and gratifying results that a practicing physician is privileged to experience is that of literally snatching such a patient from the brink of the grave by the proper use of insulin.

FIG. 32. INFLUENCE OF WEIGHT ON DIABETES MORTALITY

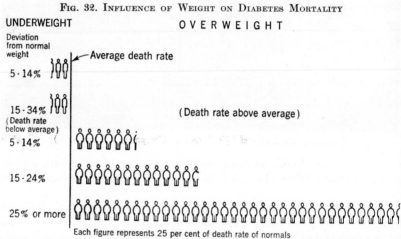

Each figure represents 25 per cent of death rate of normals

⟨Data from L. I. Dublin and A. J. Lotka, Twenty-five Years of Health Progress, Metropolitan Life Insurance Company, New York, 1937.⟩

The function of insulin is to control the metabolism, the burning, of carbohydrates. Just how this occurs is not known but, without insulin, carbohydrates are absolutely useless to the body. It seems almost as though insulin acts like a spark to set off their combustion.

In diabetes the production of insulin is reduced. The reason for this is a degeneration of the "island" cells, but the cause for the degeneration is still being sought. Heredity is a factor, and so is overweight, but other factors, possibly more important than

[386]

these, are as yet unknown. If the reduction of insulin is slight, modification of the diet is all that is necessary to control the disease; but if severe diabetes exists, life cannot continue without insulin injections. These injections do not cure the diabetes, but they make life possible for many who could not live long without it. In spite, however, of this dramatic effectiveness of insulin,

FIG. 33. DIABETES AND MODERN TREATMENT

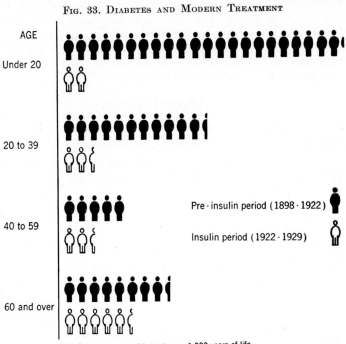

Each figure represents 20 deaths per 1,000 years of life

Decline in mortality of diabetes as the result of modern treatment. Death rates per 1,000 years of life, by age groups. Experience of Elliott P. Joslin, M.D., Boston. (*Data from L. I. Dublin and A. J. Lotka, Twenty-five Years of Health Progress, Metropolitan Life Insurance Company, New York, 1937.*)

diabetes remains an important cause of death, particularly in the United States, which has the highest death rate from diabetes of any country in the world (Tables 3 and 26).

Just as the thyroid is overactive in exophthalmic goiter, so the islands of Langerhans may show a hyperfunctional reaction to tumor or increased growth of its specialized cells. Under this condition, spoken of as hyperinsulinism, the amount of sugar in the circulating blood is decreased to such a low level only a few hours after a meal that the brain, muscles and other organs suffer from

[387]

a veritable fuel shortage. As a result, the victim develops a typical series of distressing symptoms, exactly like those produced by an overdose of insulin. These at first consist of a feeling of restlessness and weakness or "all goneness," which many people feel when excessively hungry. Later nervousness or irritability, trembling, cold perspiration and prostration follow. At this time such an individual may be irrational. If no treatment is given, epileptiform convulsions are likely to occur. Taking a lump of candy, a few ounces of orange juice or some other food containing sugar brings quick relief, if given when the first mild symptoms appear. The injection of adrenaline also gives prompt relief because, as pointed out before, this hormone from the adrenal gland increases the blood sugar. Permanent cure of this condition has been obtained in some instances by the surgical removal of a portion of the over-active gland tissue or a tumor, if such is found to be present.

The Adrenal Glands

The adrenals, or suprarenals, are small glands which fit like caps over the tops of the kidneys. Anatomically they are composed of two parts, the cortex, or outer part, and the medulla, or central part. The cells which compose these two portions of the gland and the functions which they perform are very different.

The adrenal cortex seems to have a close relationship to the reproductive system. In fact, in certain lower animals it functions as a sex gland. It enlarges during pregnancy and the nursing period. Feeding it to immature animals produces a marked stimulation in the growth of the reproductive glands; and precocious sexual development with accentuation of the physical characteristics of the male is frequently associated with tumor growths in this portion of the gland. Various instances have been reported in which young women have ceased menstruation and have developed hair over the face and body as a result of a tumor of the adrenal cortex. Removal of such tumors, when successful, has been followed by the disappearance of the hair and the reestablishment of menstruation. Full beards in girls of one, two, and three years of age have been caused by such tumors. This strongly suggests that the secretion of the adrenal cortex is stimulating to male and antagonistic to female sex characteristics. There is some suggestive evidence that the adrenal cortex may be related also to the destruction of the toxins of disease.

Atrophy of the adrenal cortex, occasionally produced by tuberculosis, results in an interesting though rare condition called "Addison's disease." Extreme weakness is the most prominent feature of this disease. The blood pressure becomes very low. Sexual power and desire are lost and in women menstruation ceases. Later the skin shows a marked yellowish pigmentation. In the past Addison's disease was considered a hopeless condition, but the recent isolation of a secretion, called "cortin," has already resulted in the restoration of health to patients who otherwise would have been doomed.

Recently over thirty different compounds have been isolated from the adrenal cortex. One of these, called cortisone, gives great, though temporary, relief to patients with certain types of chronic arthritis or rheumatism. Interestingly an anterior corticotrophic hormone of the pituitary gland, referred to as ACTH, gives similar benefit in chronic arthritis, in asthma, and in certain other conditions. This pituitary hormone apparently stimulates the adrenal cortex to produce cortisone.

The medulla of the adrenal gland secretes the well-known adrenaline, also called "epinephrine." This is released into the blood stream when there is stimulation of the sympathetic nervous system, its output being greatly increased by emotional states, such as fear, anger, excitement, and sexual stimulation. Its physiological effects are to increase the pulse rate, constrict the blood vessels, decrease the activity of the intestinal tract, and cause the liberation of sugar which has been stored in the liver. All of this is apparently a preparation of the body for intense struggle or effort; hence, the function of the adrenals has been interpreted to be one of self-preservation. As has been suggested, there seems to be some antagonism between adrenaline and insulin and a relationship between certain activities of the pituitary and the adrenal glands.

Adrenaline and its synthetic twin, ephedrine, which is now manufactured in the chemical laboratory, are both widely used in medical practice to stop bleeding from small blood vessels, particularly in nose and throat operations, to relieve asthma and other allergic conditions, temporarily to reduce nasal congestion, and occasionally to stimulate the heart and circulatory system.

[389]

The Sex Glands

According to the poet the beautiful emotion of love is centered in the heart, but the scientist prosaically ascribes it largely to the activities of the glands of internal secretion, and particularly to the reproductive glands. These glands, which are called the "gonads," comprise the testes of the male and the ovaries of the female. In structure and activity both of these are more complex than most glands of internal secretion because they produce not only reproductive cells, the sperm of the male and the ovum of the female, but also several internal secretions. In general the sex glands are concerned with the preservation of the race, the other glands of internal secretion with the preservation of the individual.

The internal secretions of these reproductive glands begin to function even before birth, stimulating differentiation of male and female sex organs. Then from birth to puberty they are relatively inactive, being held in check by the growth-stimulating hormone of the pituitary and by the secretion of the thymus.

During puberty the sex glands become active and the production of an internal secretion is revived. This secretion now seems to play a major part in the development of the physical, and probably the temperamental, characteristics of the mature man and woman. Among these are the development of the breasts and the onset of menses in the female, and the growth of a beard and the lowering of the pitch of the voice of the male. It is probable that the internal secretions of these glands are responsible also for the development of interest in the opposite sex and for sexual desire. Queerly, however, some of these so-called "secondary sex characteristics" have been observed in persons without testes or ovaries.

During pregnancy several of the hormones are increased and some additional ones, apparently produced in the reproductive organs, are found in the blood and urine.

In addition to producing the germ cells or ova by which the race is perpetuated, the female sex glands or ovaries produce two distinct regulatory hormones which prepare the female accessory sex organs for the successful carrying out of reproduction. Long before birth the ovaries contain numerous young or primordial egg cells, each surrounded by a layer of smaller less highly differentiated cells. . . . Even before birth some of these egg masses or Graafian follicles, as they are called, show signs of change. The smaller cells surrounding the ovum increase in number. Then, the follicular fluid which they secrete accumulates on one side of the follicle. . . . This fluid contains a hormone, *theelin*, which is gradually absorbed and distributed by the circulating blood to other parts of the body where it performs its specific functions. As the period of puberty is approached, this process of hormone production becomes more evident, that is, the young girl shows signs of development of her secondary sex characters.

One of the Graafian follicles, lying near the surface of the ovary, instead of regressing as all have done previously, becomes more distended than usual with the follicular fluid and ruptures outwardly. The contained ovum or egg together with the fluid is thus set free into the abdominal cavity, from which it makes its way into the uterus. A yellowish structure, known as the corpus luteum, develops from the inner layers of follicular cells. This produces a second ovarian hormone, *progestin* or *progesterone*. . . .

If the released ovum chances to meet and fuse with a male germ cell in passing to the uterus, the process of fertilization occurs and pregnancy follows. The follicular hormone contained in the fluid and the hormone produced subsequently by the corpus luteum successively stimulate the inner coat of the uterus or endometrium to develop in such a way as to provide an ideal nesting place for the future embryo. In the event that the ovum is not fertilized, all of the elaborate uterine preparation comes to naught and the thickened inner lining sloughs out. This constitutes menstruation. With the development of a new Graafian follicle under the influence of the pituitary gonadotropic hormone, the same process recurs at intervals of approximately four weeks up to the time of the menopause in late middle life, except when pregnancy intervenes. When pregnancy does not occur, the corpus luteum, whose hormone has been chiefly responsible for the changes in the uterine mucosa, begins to undergo absorption about two weeks from the time of ovulation or discharge of the egg from the follicle. It is at this time of withdrawal of the influence of the corpus luteum that menstruation occurs. In the event of pregnancy, however, the corpus luteum does not degenerate but enlarges and functions throughout pregnancy as an endocrine organ. Its hormone, progestin, has the effect of preserving the favorable physiological state of the placenta during pregnancy and prevents premature uterine contractions.

During pregnancy the estrogenic or follicular hormone, and probably the principle from the corpus luteum as well, exert a restraining influence on the secretion by the pituitary of the gonadotropic and the lactogenic hormones. At the same time they stimulate the growth and development of the secretory tissue of the mammary gland. With the termination of pregnancy and expulsion of all of the uterine contents, these sex hormones promptly decrease in

[391]

amount in the body, thus permitting increased secretion of the lactogenic hormone which alone can stimulate milk production. From this brief exposition, it is obvious that the harmonious functioning of these closely interrelated hormonal mechanisms is absolutely essential to reproduction. The successful preparation of the chemically related female sex hormones in essentially pure form . . . now offers many new lines of investigation. The significant discovery that the follicular hormone and its chemical allies derived from coal tar are capable of initiating the development of cancer, when applied to the ear of a mouse or rabbit, offers a new approach to the study of that dreaded disease. At the same time it warns against the haphazard clinical use of these new products.

In later life the activity of the sex glands declines. The ovaries ordinarily cease to function at forty to fifty years of age. After this an ovum is no longer discharged each month, the menses cease, the breasts shrink, body fat increases, and some growth of hair appears upon the face. Sexual desire may or may not be diminished. With this abrupt cessation of ovarian activity at the menopause, major readjustments in the activities of other glands of internal secretion and in certain body functions occur. These may be accompanied by disturbing physical sensations, nervous tensions, and emotional disturbances. Much of this unpleasantness, however, may be ameliorated by the administration of the ovarian hormone which nature has suddenly ceased to provide. The male experiences a gradual diminution in the activities of the sex glands rather than an abrupt cessation of the reproductive function. Associated with this, he too may have similar mental and nervous discomfort.

An interesting and important effect currently being studied of some of the internal secretions of the ovary and testis is the slowing and in some cases regression of certain cancerous growths. These preparations do not cure anyone with cancer, but in certain patients they relieve pain and prolong life.

Rejuvenation Operations

For more than a hundred years observations have been made of the effect of administering or implanting sex glands or injecting their extracts in castrated and normal animals of the same and of the opposite sex. In general the implantation of sex glands into castrated animals of the same sex has resulted in sexual development and temporary restoration of sexual activity. The effect upon animals of the opposite sex is less consistent: the implantation of ovaries into immature males gives rise to no feminine characteristics or behavior, while the implantation of testes into immature females is followed by the development of certain male characteristics.

Attempts to rejuvenate old men by implantation of the testes of young animals have resulted at best in only a temporary restoration of sexual power. There is no other evidence of rejuvenation or of improved body function. Many such operations have been performed, but most of them were unmitigated exploitation of silly old men trying to be "boys" again.

The Practical Aspect of Internal Secretions

This sketchy picture of the glands of internal secretion suggests the complexity of the problem and the difficulty of practical application even of established facts. Experimental work on animals with isolated hormones is difficult enough, but infinitely more complex is the problem in human beings with a whole series of interrelated glands, most of which produce multiple secretions that act both directly and through their effects upon other glands. In spite of these difficulties, however, great progress is being made in the diagnosis and treatment of glandular disturbances.

In some cases a portion of an overly active gland is removed by surgery. In others a deficiency in glandular secretion is made up by the administration of this gland or its extract. In others the removal of focal infection or the treatment of systemic disease improves the function of these glands. And in still others the supplying of substances which are deficient in the diet, such as iodine for the thyroid and calcium and vitamin D for the parathyroid, restores normal activity.

Beyond leading a reasonably normal life, there is little or nothing that one can do to keep these glands functioning properly. Of course, iodine is a preventive of simple goiter, and there is some evidence that intense emotional excitement may be a fac-

[393]

tor in the precipitation of toxic goiter. But of greatest importance is that one be endowed with a good set of these mysterious regulators of our lives and activities.

DISCUSSION SUGGESTIONS

1. Explain what is meant by endocrine glands; by hormones.
2. Define and explain the cause of cretinism and myxedema.
3. What is meant by simple or endemic goiter? What is the cause of it and how may it be prevented?
4. How does exophthalmic goiter differ from this?
5. Explain the cause of tetany; of spasmophilia.
6. Describe the location of the pituitary gland and its primary functions.
7. What is diabetes insipidus and how can it be treated?
8. Why is an extract of the pituitary gland injected in certain cases of childbirth?
9. Explain the cause of dwarfism; of gigantism; of acromegaly; of extreme adiposity.
10. Explain how it is possible to determine if pregnancy exists by testing the urine.
11. What is the thymus? Discuss its chief effects upon the body.
12. What are the symptoms of diabetes mellitus?
13. What is insulin and why is it useful in the treatment of diabetes? Is it a cure for diabetes? Explain.
14. What is meant by hyperinsulinism? How is it treated?
15. What are the adrenal glands? What are their primary functions?
16. What stimulates the physiological changes which occur at puberty? How is menstruation controlled?
17. Explain the reason for thinking that there may be a relationship between certain internal secretions and cancer.
18. Discuss the possibilities of rejuvenation by means of "gland operations."

REFERENCES AND READING SUGGESTIONS

1. Blakeslee, Alton L.: "Amazing Hormones," *Today's Health*, vol. 29, p. 19, June, 1951.
2. Braceland, F. J.: "Hormones and Their Influence on the Emotions," *Bulletin of the New York Academy of Medicine*, October, 1953.
3. Cannon, W. B.: "Bodily Changes in Pain, Hunger, Fear and Rage," Appleton-Century-Crofts, Inc., New York, 1929.
4. Collip, J. B.: "Hormones in Relation to Human Behavior," Harvard University Press, Cambridge, Mass., 1936.
5. Corner, George W.: "The Hormones in Human Reproduction," Princeton University Press, Princeton, N.J., 1942.

6. Dublin, L. I., and H. H. Marks: "Mortality from Diabetes throughout the World," American Diabetes Association, New York, 1952.
7. Hoskins, R. C.: "The Tides of Life, the Endocrine Glands in Bodily Adjustment," W. W. Norton & Company, Inc., New York, 1933.
8. Rubin, H. H.: "Your Life Is in Your Glands," Stratford House, New York, 1948.
9. Seale, Harris: "Banting's Miracle," J. B. Lippincott Company, Philadelphia, 1946.
10. Yahraes, Herbert: "Good News about Diabetes," Public Affairs Pamphlets, New York, 1948.

Text-Films

The following McGraw-Hill Text-Films on Health Education are recommended for use with this chapter of the text:

Hormones and the Endocrine Glands (about 15 min, available spring, 1955). In this film the structure and operation of the system of endocrine glands are shown, and the role of the hormones secreted by the endocrines in regulating our physical lives and influencing our behavior is demonstrated.

Human Reproduction (21 min sd MP). In this film models and animated drawings explain the reproductive systems of men and women and the process of normal birth. Emphasizes the importance of clear and objective understanding of these facts as the basis of successful marriage and parenthood.

Silent follow-up filmstrip based on the motion picture offers opportunity for review, testing, and further discussion.

I N SPITE of the widespread interest and instruction in sexual matters, psychiatrists, teachers, and physicians continue to encounter pathetic and tragic examples of ignorance and misinformation on this subject. It even seems that the educational procedures, the flood of "sex books" on the market, and our much-vaunted "free discussion" have hardly decreased the prevalence of erroneous and harmful information. On the contrary, they frequently serve to overemphasize what should be regarded as only one aspect of a normal life.

Investigation and study have thrown new light on this old subject. People have discarded traditional attitudes and ideas on sex and have embraced new ones. Modern youth is making dogma of sexual freedom, just as their Victorian parents made dogma of convention, secrecy, and restriction. But now the new ideas seem to be causing as many and as severe problems as the old. And there is evidence of a swing back toward more strict rules of conduct for both sexes. The reasons for this are obscure but probably are to be found in the psychological aspects of the sex instinct.

One has only to look at the sexual customs of primitive societies to realize that the sexual instinct may function successfully

[1] Prepared in collaboration with Dr. Ruth E. Boynton and Dr. E. M. deBerry of the Student's Health Service of the University of Minnesota.

and happily under a great variety of practices. It would seem that almost any pattern will do, provided it is accepted by the individual and by the group in which he lives. But in no society at any time do we find that man has regarded sex as a simple physiological necessity. He has always made it mean more to him than this. Modern teaching seems to run counter to this tendency, for we are told again and again that we should regard sex as a simple biological function, that we should strip it of all taboos, sentimentality, and mystery. But nobody has yet succeeded in doing this.

We have discovered a great many things about the mental side of sex, but as yet we have not been able to understand it completely. It is safe to say, however, that any system of behavior will be sounder and healthier if it is built upon an understanding of its physical aspects. In no other body function is information about physiology so important as it is in this field. Generally speaking, a person may be completely misinformed about the mechanism of the heartbeat, of respiration, or of digestion without in any way disturbing the functions involved. It is quite otherwise in sexual matters, in which erroneous ideas may cause as much difficulty as actual disease. For this reason menstruation, nocturnal emissions, masturbation, marital relations, and sex relations outside marriage will be discussed briefly in the following pages.

The Physiology of Sex

The sex organs of the male and female complement each other for the realization of nature's greatest purpose—the perpetuation of the species. In animals this is purely a physiological process, but civilized man encompasses his sex life with the tenderest of emotions and builds upon it love, home, family, and many other of the finest things in life.

The reproductive cells of the male, called "sperm," are produced in the testis, stored in the epididymis, and travel by way of the ductus deferens to the urethra through which they are discharged. The penis is the male sex organ which carries the urethra, a tube for the emptying of the urinary bladder and for the discharge of the fluid, called "semen," from the sex glands. The penis is composed largely of blood vessels which become engorged during sexual excitation, causing the penis to become firm and enlarged.

The reproductive cells of the female are produced in the ovaries and are called "ova." One ovum matures each month and as it attains full size bursts forth from the surface of the ovary.

FIG. 34

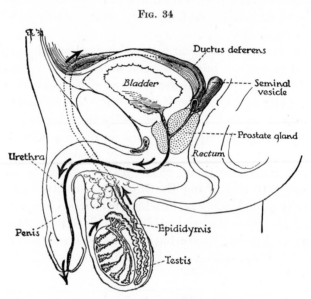

Male reproductive system. Arrows indicate route of spermatozoa.

This process is called "ovulation" and occurs approximately midway between menstrual periods. Upon leaving the ovary, one of which is located on each side of the pelvis, the ovum is free in the abdominal cavity. Very soon, however, it is drawn into the funnellike end of the oviduct (also called "fallopian tube" or "uterine tube"). It then passes downward into the cavity of the uterus, a muscular organ about the size and shape of a pear located in the center of the pelvis. In a day or two, if conception does not occur, the ovum loses its viability. The lower end of the cavity of the uterus, called the "cervix," protrudes into the upper end of a tubelike structure called the "vagina," which extends downward to the surface of the body.

During sexual intercourse the penis is inserted into the vagina and the semen discharged in the vicinity of the cervix. The sperm cells, which have the power of independent motion, then work their way up through the cervix and into the body of the uterus.

Fig. 35

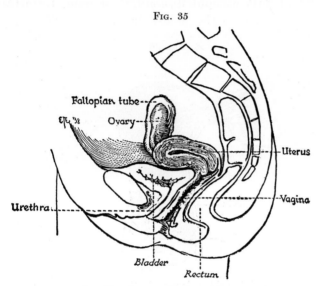

Female reproductive system.

If a sperm cell meets an ovum, fusion takes place and a new life is begun.

Menstruation

The onset of menstruation is a sign that a girl is sexually mature and that reproduction is possible. Once each month, the lining of the uterus, called the "endometrium," becomes thickened in preparation for the reception of a fertilized ovum. When fertilization does not take place, this thickened lining sloughs off and is discharged with some bleeding which we speak of as menstruation. This cycle is controlled by the internal secretions of several of the endocrine glands (see page 390).

The usual age of onset of the menstrual periods is between

twelve and fourteen years, although the periods may begin as early as ten years of age or as late as sixteen or eighteen. A girl should be told about menstruation so that the occurrence of the first period will not be unexpected and frightening.

Since menstruation is a normal process, one should expect but little inconvenience from it, and it actually does occur in about 85 per cent of girls without discomfort or pain. Unfortunately many mothers refer to the menstrual period as the "monthly

FIG. 36

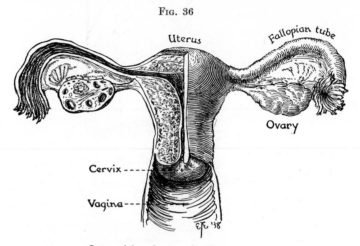

Internal female reproductive organs.

sickness." If girls are brought up with the idea that each menstrual period is a time when they should expect to feel ill, they are likely to become semi-invalids each month.

For the young woman who does have severe pain at each menstrual period, adequate medical advice should be sought. Usually by proper medical care it is possible to prevent this disability. The young woman whose general health and resistance are good is less apt to have painful periods than the girl who is greatly underweight or anemic. Likewise the young woman who gets plenty of exercise is less apt to have dysmenorrhea than the inactive girl.

The hygiene of menstruation should vary little, if at all, from one's usual routine. Except for strenuous exercise involving jumping, ordinary activity is beneficial at the menstrual period, for it increases circulation and prevents the congestion which is one of the causes of discomfort. For the normal healthy girl a mile walk on the first day of the period is of much more value than several hours in bed. Warm tub baths may be taken throughout the period as at any other time. Excessively hot or cold baths are not advised.

The aim of every mother should be to have her daughter intelligently informed about menstruation by the time she is eleven or twelve years old and through her own attitude toward this periodic natural process help the girl to live as normally as possible during these periods.

Nocturnal Emissions

Nocturnal emissions are an expression of development of the testicles and the accessory male organs of reproduction. Their occurrence is normal and should be regarded as such by both the boy and his parents. They may begin as early as the ninth or tenth year or as late as the sixteenth or seventeenth year. The age of onset appears to be without significance and to bear no relationship to the development of secondary sexual characteristics, such as growth of beard. In healthy boys their occurrence may be nightly for periods or not more frequently than once a month. Regularity or irregularity seems to have no significance, and no effort should be made to control it.

Much misconception exists about the meaning of nocturnal emissions. It is often stated or implied that they represent wasted energy and that their frequent occurrence results in loss of vigor. This is entirely erroneous, for the semen which is lost represents nothing which could be used by the body for other purposes. It is a secretion of several glands, which will be discharged in one way or another, regardless of the efforts of the individual to retain it. The supposed relation to general health probably is due to a confusion of this with the internal secretion of the testicles. The latter does affect growth and metabolism, but it comes from a different source and has nothing to do with the semen.

A boy should be prepared by his parents, or some other adult, for this occurrence by an explanation of its source, its nature, and its harmlessness. Unless interfered with by a severe emotional blocking, it will occur normally at more or less frequent intervals; but to regard it as dangerous may give rise to a sense of uneasiness and insecurity. Generally speaking, if the attitude of the parents is healthy, the child will ask questions about sexual matters, thereby presenting an opportunity to explain as much as seems necessary. It is unwise to make an occasion of this explanation or to force it on the child when he is indifferent.

If, as frequently happens, the pubescent boy fails to ask questions about nocturnal emissions or other sexual matters, it is generally wise to find out, by the simple method of asking him, how much he knows and what his ideas on the subject are. One may assume that his failure to ask indicates either that he is ashamed to do so or that he feels he has been sufficiently informed. In the first case it is necessary not only to give him the simple facts but to correct his emotional attitude. If he has been informed from other sources, such as the group of boys in the neighborhood, he will, in all likelihood, be misinformed. In either case the adult should make a convenient occasion for casual inquiry without embarrassment, and preferably when the question can be raised in relation to something else in the conversation. One may know that one has succeeded if the boy discusses the subject to the point of revealing his ideas. Directness, thoroughness, and frankness are more important than delicacy in such a discussion.

Masturbation

Masturbation[2] is said to be an almost universal practice among healthy boys and common among girls. It may begin at almost any age and has been reported in children under three. Frequently it is continued throughout adolescence, and occasionally into adult life, without any evidence of its being physically injurious. About 92 per cent of male college students admit masturbation, with the practice seemingly most common among healthy

[2] Self-stimulation of one's own sex organs, not "self-pollution," as given in some dictionaries.

and robust athletes. In more studious but physically less well developed types it may occur frequently or only at rare intervals.

Physically the habit as ordinarily practiced seems to be perfectly harmless and, unless it is regarded as dangerous by the individual, it gives no trouble. On the other hand, if a boy is taught or learns from reading out-of-date literature on the subject that masturbation causes a multitude of ills, that it undermines physical and mental powers, destroys the will, and weakens or destroys the sex powers, leads to insanity and other frightful consequences, he often develops a severe emotional conflict, which may make him asocial and self-conscious. The feeling of inadequacy which arises from this may affect injuriously his relations with other people and may decrease his efficiency in any work which he undertakes. It is important, therefore, that adolescent boys learn that masturbation is practically universal, and that, as far as we know, it is a harmless practice.

The boy who tries to inhibit this practice because he thinks it will do him harm fails in his good resolutions, whereas, if he knows that it is physically harmless, he usually masturbates infrequently and without emotional conflict, and begins normally to learn to gain positive satisfactions more acceptable to himself and society. It is always dangerous to warn boys against masturbation, even if the warning is a mild one, for they are apt to infer more than is said to them and to attribute to it all of their little failures and inadequacies until it becomes a really serious problem.

Among girls not only is this practice less frequent than among boys, but conflicts over it are less common and less likely to cause serious disturbances.

It is important to realize, however, that masturbation is not a desirable or adequate form of sex expression. In youth there is always a tendency to excess which may lead to the expenditure of energy on masturbation during the years that nature needs all her resources for building manhood and womanhood. Furthermore, in the presence of prevailing social and religious taboos the practice tends to psychic disturbances, conflicts, and the development of inferiority feelings which may have serious effects upon the growing personality.

Homosexuality

Another undesirable type of sexual expression is homosexuality; that is, sexual interest in persons of the same sex. Some interpret this as being an arrest and exaggeration of sexual development at an adolescent level when the gang spirit is strong among boys and "crushes" not uncommon among girls.

Early investigations either implied or stated explicitly that homosexuality was ingrained in the individual as a manifestation of structural peculiarity. Although this cannot be denied as a possibility, it can be shown that there is little evidence to support it. Structurally, anatomically, the homosexual does not differ from the heterosexual, and some homosexuals are cured of their homosexuality. Like other mental and emotional derangements it is probably a learned reaction and as such should be subject to reeducation. Whatever the deep sources of such behavior may be, the frequently expressed opinion that it is innate and unchangeable can do nothing but harm, since it closes the subject to further investigation and attempt at therapy.

It should be remembered that occasional homoerotic practices occur in the lives of most normal adolescents, probably as an expression of a stage in sexual development. Such passing episodes should not be occasion for alarm. The danger lies in their interpretation as expressions of deep pathology or innate peculiarity.

Sex Emotion

With the beginning of adolescence new and powerful forces enter to complicate the individual and social problems that grow out of sex. There comes a gradual awakening to sex consciousness—the awareness of sex. This awakening brings a psychic urge toward the opposite sex. This psychic urge is powerfully reinforced by a physiologic urge arising from the hormone activity of the sex glands. These inner factors of sex attraction together with the powerful and varied sex stimuli create for the adolescent youth a difficult problem of self-control. With the growth of the love-life in early adolescence there arises a new sex curiosity—curiosity about sex experience. This curiosity is natural and normal but obviously fraught with danger. . . . Adolescent curiosity calls for personal experience. It is largely this natural curiosity about sex experience that renders the lure of easily accessible prostitution in a community dangerous. A study of those who went in and out of a red-light district in a city a few years ago showed that a large proportion were boys of fourteen and fifteen years. Undoubtedly the lure of curiosity more than physiologic urge was the important factor.

Unstable and exaggerated emotions are characteristic of adolescent development. Swift changes from high elation to deep despair, are common. Usually this emotionalism centers largely in the now active mating instinct. The immaturity and instability of adolescent emotions mainly account for the numerous adolescent suicides, a large proportion of which occur for reasons that to an adult would seem trifling and silly. The most hopeful and potential characteristic in adolescent development is a strong undercurrent of idealism. . . .

The guidance of the new forces growing out of the mating instinct that manifest themselves progressively in the adolescent youth require *early* a philosophy of life in which the sex factor is soundly adjusted. As a basis for such a philosophy he needs a fuller understanding of the nature and significance of these forces and phenomena. For his peace of mind he needs to know that they are the normal manifestations of developing manhood or womanhood related to sex. The want of such understanding, and the appreciation which it brings, result in fears, worries and inner conflicts which are often seriously depressing and tend toward more or less permanent inferiority complexes. . . .

Modern knowledge of adolescent development indicates the importance of the youth's achieving emotional independence of his parents. The affectionate relationship between parents and child, especially between father and daughter and between mother and son, is essentially a sex relationship. Through overindulgence and misdirection this emotional relationship may, and often does, become so fixed so to hamper or make impossible the transfer of affection necessary for successful mating and married life. . . .

With the arrival of sexual maturity in puberty the individual experiences the urge to sex satisfaction. The normal satisfaction of that urge is attained in sex intercourse with a member of the other sex. In civilized society today this recurrent sex urge cannot be satisfied in sex relations with the opposite sex with social approval, for good and weighty reasons which have grown out of the accumulated experience of the human race. Early marriage is not usually feasible because of the years needed for schooling and preparing to bear the economic and social responsibilities of life. Even when physical and mental maturity is reached, in the early twenties, which would seem to be nature's indication that the individual is fitted for the responsibilities of mating and rearing a family, more years must be spent by many in further preparation for vocation and life, and marriage postponed. So, between sexual maturity and marriage in which the sex impulse may find normal satisfaction with social approval there is often a gap of eight to fifteen years. This situation creates sex problems of greater or lesser severity according to the individual and his training. This period is really one of biological abnormality. Whatever the answer may be, we must acknowledge the problem.

[**405**]

Insofar as this situation becomes a problem, every boy and girl and man and woman must face it, not to quarrel with it but to handle it intelligently and constructively. The essential question for each is, how shall I deal with the problem so as to keep it within bounds, so that my sex nature may contribute most to my ultimate happiness and welfare, and so that I may play fair with the society of which I am a part? No one need expect to escape all conflict and struggle in this sphere any more than in any other aspect of life, for conflict and the overcoming of resistance is in the essence of all life that is effective, and in this as in other areas one must not lose sight of the fact that it is not merely immediate but ultimate satisfactions that count.

At the outset youth needs to be aided to appreciate the fact that the years of deferred full sex satisfaction that civilized society imposes are by no means wholly a misfortune. They have brought tremendous compensations in that they have enabled us to reach a far higher type and level of love-life and sex-social relations than is possible on the primitive savage level. In savage life sex relations are mainly on the physical plane. They become the periodic gratification of a routine want like eating and drinking. The tender emotional component and the esthetic component of human sexuality which have so greatly enhanced, expanded and energized the love-life of human beings and largely woven the fabric of organized society are only rudimentary on the savage level.

In civilized life sex relations have risen to a vastly higher level. They have been given psychic and spiritual meaning and have been invested extensively with elements of beauty. Sex activity has taken on the service of love. It has become at its best the supreme love expression.

These psychic, esthetic and social qualities upon which enduringly happy marriage so largely depends do not come to us full-fledged in the early years of youth. They require time for growth and maturing. In the opportunity for their cultivation and the consequent enrichment of the love-life lies the compensation for such struggle as any deferring of physical sex relations during the years of youth may entail. In such cultivation lies the greatest assurance of achieving that kind and quality of married relationship to which we all aspire and as yet so few achieve. The refinements of civilization are bought at a price. In the sphere of sexual love at least the price is not too great to pay.

In relation to the sex ethics of youth it is important to bear in mind that the sex instinct is one of the most sensitive aspects of human personality and is extremely easily "conditioned" to certain lines of response. It becomes most easily bent to, and fixed in, a given line of reaction and behavior, and the attitudes and behavior patterns to which it becomes conditioned are tremendously significant in relation to marriage. An endless number of marriages become wrecked or move on low levels because adverse attitudes, ideals and habits acquired in youth have prevailed in marriage. This is one of the most frequent results from relations with prostitutes.

In a regimen for the wise handling of the sex problem the question as to the degree of physical intimacy a youth may wisely permit himself in his relations with the opposite sex arises. This raises the whole thorny question of petting. The impulse to indulge freely in physical intimacies is natural and it is strong in most of us. If the keen immediate pleasures which petting affords are to be limited or foregone, it must be for weighty reasons.

It may be readily admitted that a certain freedom in friendships and courtships is not only permissible but desirable, a freedom that is consistent with self-respect, with full respect for your partner and with the health and welfare of both parties concerned. We need, however, to face honestly certain facts which suggest limitations.

In the first place, the very nature of the sex impulse and the requirements of our social organization make rather definite limitations advisable. The sex impulse is a powerful and imperious force over which, beyond certain limits, we do not have full control. It easily becomes a tyrant. Give it an inch and it will take much more. Under the sway of these forces aroused in petting, especially of the heavier sort, judgment and control take wing and passion prevails. This is particularly true in men, in whom specific sex desire is naturally more easily and quickly aroused than in most women. For both young men and young women, however, indulgence in the more intimate forms of petting is for the most part playing with fire. However sincerely the petters may purpose to keep the indulgence within safe limits, nature has largely stacked the cards against them.

In the second place, petting is biologically and emotionally an abnormal experience. The intimacies of petting constitute the natural and proper approach to sex intercourse. . . . In petting the frequent arousal of the passions without their normal release tends to become physically and emotionally harmful. This is particularly true in women. The extent to which it may give rise to organic disease and functional disorders is becoming recognized and given attention by the medical profession.

In the third place, petting is frequently unfortunate in that it tends to exaggerate and overvalue the physical responses in relationships between the sexes. Enduringly happy marriage depends upon harmony between the whole of the two personalities—the physical, mental, emotional, temperamental, esthetic and social sides—and not upon passionate powers alone. Petting tends so to overemphasize and overvalue the physical side of the relationship as to warp the individual's judgment and experience and bring him to marriage ill-equipped to achieve the broader, richer basis of companionship which permanently happy marriage demands. The warped marriage ideal which he has acquired, the confusing of the limited, partial satisfactions of petting with the larger, richer satisfactions of the marriage relation at its best, often spell failure in marriage when it comes.[2a]

[2a] Quoted by permission from Exner, M. J., and W. F. Snow, "Sex Hygiene," The Practitioner's Library of Medicine and Surgery, vol. 12, "Hygiene and Preventive Medicine," pp. 149–155, Appleton-Century-Crofts, Inc., New York, 1937.

Sexual Promiscuity

Recent ideas about freedom in sexual matters have given rise to the belief in some places that sexual promiscuity is a harmless pleasure. The advocates of this new freedom generally hold that the sexual instinct is a natural force which should not be unnaturally dammed up by continence, and that inhibition may give rise to neurotic tendencies. This theory is not without basis, for undoubtedly certain neuroses and other personality maladjustments do result from the repression of sex. On the other hand, psychological repression and conscious control of one's actions are quite different.

Repression implies not only a refraining from sexual activity but also a refusal to recognize the existence of sexual desire, while conscious control admits the tendency but makes a conscious choice to refrain. In the case of repression the refusal to recognize the desire may lead to unhealthy emotional reactions. But promiscuous sexual intercourse is not a satisfactory solution even for inhibited people. On the contrary, it usually gives rise to a host of psychological difficulties, even in those who think that they are free from moral taboos and who have taken the necessary precautions against illegitimate pregnancies and venereal disease.

For this reason, we cannot justify current belief that promiscuity and free premarital relations are "healthy and natural." The emotional and psychic elements in sex are of far greater importance than its physical aspects; and as yet there is much that we do not know about these psychic results. So the wisest course for one to pursue is to avoid illicit sexual intercourse but at the same time to recognize the desire which one intends ultimately to satisfy. In this way one may avoid the danger incident to inhibition and repression, on the one hand, and the emotional conflicts which may arise from indulgence, on the other. The belief, occasionally found even among physicians, that continence is physically dangerous is unfounded.

The U.S. Children's Bureau reports that nearly 50 per cent of illegitimate births in this country are to girls between fifteen and nineteen years old. A

San Francisco clinic after studying 2,000 cases of promiscuity among girls concludes: "These girls don't enjoy sex. They are promiscuous because they are overwhelmed with problems." As a matter of fact, the girls who were most promiscuous reported that their experiences were definitely unpleasant. . . . Most promiscuity resulted not from "getting to know a boy too well" but from spur-of-the-moment acquaintances with strange boys that the girls rarely saw again. Love didn't enter into it. Most frequently the girl ended by hating the boy, blaming him and breaking up the relationship. . . . Promiscuity is related more to loneliness and friendlessness than to efforts to be popular. Most of these girls said that they had no friends at all. Contributing causes were frequently found in the family: lack of love, overstrictness, friction between the parents with divided loyalties on the part of the children. Treatment was based upon efforts to help the girl obtain an insight into her own personality; to gain some measure of self-respect; to understand that she can solve her own problems; and to get relief by "talking them out" with a skilled and understanding physician. The clinic's suggestions for prevention include constructive leadership in the home; the avoidance of both overstrictness and overlaxness; frankness in discussions of sex; efforts by parents to "put themselves in their daughter's place"; participation by children in the family life; and a strong association of sex with love and marriage.[3]

Two distinguished writers, one a woman and the other a man, have made such significant statements concerning chastity that we requested and were granted permission to reproduce excerpts from them here. The first is by Margaret Culkin Banning, who says:

If there is a case for chastity, it should be stated. Religion and obedience to moral codes still settle the question for many. But the increasing secularization of thought and the frequent denial that any moral issue is involved in sex conduct leaves uncounted thousands of young people today supposedly free to "make up their own minds," if such a phrase can be used concerning conduct which is nearly always the result of runaway emotion. . . .

We know that there are 50,000 unmarried mothers registered yearly in the United States; that through wealth and influence many unmarried mothers are not registered; that many couples marry after pregnancy is discovered; and that birth control and abortions prevent motherhood in most illicit affairs.

Nevertheless, we must remember that unchastity, common though it may be, is not the norm. That still is chastity. Society does not approve nor is it set up for the general practice of unchastity. Every adult must know, as I do, many young girls who are not troubled by this problem, and others whose

[3] Whitman, Howard: "What Makes Good Girls Bad," *This Week Magazine*, April 10, 1949.

[409]

lives offer no opportunity for it. They keep regular hours. They are pre-occupied with study, sports, domestic tasks and wholesome social activities. . . .

Dangers—disease, abortion, emotional disasters, and even death—surround every premarital relation. But many people run the risks and escape. If the girl does escape, is there still no case for chastity?

Each girl's chastity is the interweaving of her moral code, her nervous system, her physical being, and her mind. Does she realize how profoundly that interwoven fabric may be altered in a few yielding moments?

In the breaking down of chastity, her moral code is often violated. True, she may think she has none. Yet the great weight of tradition and poetry and romance is pressing on her, even if she is without a belief in orthodox religion. Hence many girls cannot but carry with them into early sexual experience a sense of sin which they never lose. This "guilt sense" is spoken of by almost all the doctors who have investigated such things. Even without a sense of actual sin against religion, the "guilt sense" persists in a large majority of cases. The girl who thus feels that she is doing wrong suffers shockingly. . . .

On the other hand, there are girls who have really cast off conventions—who feel no spiritual or moral connection with their sex conduct. How do they come out? Usually they are deserted. If a woman has this point of view, she almost always believes—and says so once too often—that she can look out for herself. In many cases that is what her lover ultimately allows her to do. And then she becomes an outlaw. Society provides no protection for her. She may have the bravado of the outlaw, but she also has his loneliness. . . .

Loudly as it may boast of its freedom, unchastity carries repression right along with it. There are places where it cannot go. The unchaste girl often lacks escort and open companionship. There are times when she may not speak to the one person she cares about. As long as passionate love or even excitement is growing and deeply shared, this may not matter. Secrecy is then a delicious privacy. But every recorded experience shows that such secrecy has the seeds of bitterness in it. The girl usually becomes resentful, hating to be hidden and unacknowledged, and yet more fearful of the discovery of her relation. If the adventure is, as it very well may be, casual in fact to the boy in the case, who passes on to other conquests, the consequences to the girl can only be torments of jealousy, frustration and despair.

Such breaks and the resultant sense of inferiority and pain often make a woman promiscuous. . . . The promiscuous woman is usually in doubt of her own attractiveness and is seeking reassurance by repeated and varied experience with men. The fact of inferiority is also true of promiscuous men, who in such ways prove a virility which they secretly doubt. It is bad for a man who ultimately wants a happy home relation because he soon becomes neither romantic nor patient enough to give his wife satisfaction. Also, the promiscuous man or woman finds adjustment to monogamy almost impossible.

An unchaste past is intrusive and a troublemaker. Sex loses charm, but the craving for satisfaction and the nervous search for it goes on. Promiscuity makes people lose the greatest experience in life—love. . . .

The thing to do is to help these young couples out, and, if their attraction is not casual, to encourage their marriage. As the authorities who were interviewed on this subject of chastity made their comments, the statement came again and again with repeated emphasis that the best solution was early marriage. This is not by any means synonymous with hasty marriage. But if a boy and a girl felt that they did not have to face an indefinite postponement of sex relations, their attitude would change. It is the hopelessness cast in their faces, the long gap between the awakening of their passions and its decently authorized expression which makes for rebellion against conventions and accepted rules. . . .

Finally, normal young men and women do not want unchastity. They are searching for an ethic to guide them. College investigations show that students believe in fidelity, want marriage. They want an emotional life with vitality in it, one that will wear. The case of chastity does not need much pleading before young people thus disposed. Given proper ideals, decent upbringing, half a chance, it is what girls and boys want.[4]

The second statement, which is supplementary to this, is by Donald Culross Peattie, who writes:

. . . Chastity *is* important, because it is right. And because it is beautiful, and something in which to take a pride such as nothing else can give you. . . .

How easy it is to lead youth to die for an ideal upon the advice of their elders, the cemeteries in France declare. It should not be more difficult to persuade a young man that chastity is an experience he owes himself, as well as owing some of its spiritual and bodily integrity to his bride and his babies. There are of course some boys, never trained to any sort of self-discipline, from whom it is already too late to expect any response to these ideas. And some girls also. . . . But are you going to hold up for the rest nothing in chastity to admire and desire? . . .

I have three sons. . . . My ideal is to make my sons good lovers, for love and chastity are facets of the same stone. . . . I want my sons to be good lovers, because the lover is, voluntarily and naturally, chaste. It is a corollary, of course, to this proposition, that I want my sons to be chaste because I want them to be good lovers. For I honestly believe that chastity on both sides before marriage is worth far more than any advantages possessed by the previously experienced lover.

When I say I want my sons to be good lovers I do not mean skillful seducers, or perennial ladies' men. By good lovers I mean good husbands. And

[4] Banning, Margaret Culkin, "The Case for Chastity," *The Reader's Digest*, vol. 31, p. 1, August, 1937.

[411]

something better than settled, faithful, and patient husbands. Someone, in short, who can make love well enough to get his wife to feeling like the Duchess of Windsor just when she knows she must be looking like the Witch of Endor. Somebody who slips a loving hand just under the weight of her heart, and so makes it perpetually feel a little lighter than it really is. . . .

I hope that my boys fall genuinely in love early, and stay in love—the best protection for their chastity. I shall not pretend that it is an easy thing to keep. Few of the best things in life are come by easily. Most take years of self-discipline and application. It is precisely the element of the difficult about chastity that puts the high value on it, and I am counting on my children's understanding this, because they are not moral softies who give up if a thing requires any exertion. . . .

The sex instinct propels us to seek a mate; mating is its only aim, and everything connected with sex has no other meaning. But man, I am going on to say to my sons, is not a thoughtless beast. Man stands up and directs his destiny. He cannot, in most cases, permanently deny the sexual instinct, nor should he, but he can pick his time and his partner. And if he cannot even perform so agreeable a task as this decently, he has every reason to be ashamed of himself. For life, I am going to repeat often to my sons, is holy ground, and we should all walk here with some reverence, grateful for the short time that we are allotted to till that ground and, mastering it, make it bear us fruit.

And that fruit is our children. So that it matters to a man not only out of whose womb they are going to be born, but also what sort of a father gives his blood to their blood. It is hardly reasonable of a man who "tore around" nightly for 10 or 15 years before he settled down to marriage with a decent girl, to be astounded if he should have a daughter with morals no better than his own. It need not surprise him, if he once succumbed to a wishy-washy girl and had to marry her, if she gives him wishy-washy sons. Such sons and daughters come by these qualities quite honestly, and their parents cannot reproach them.

I shall remind my sons that each one of them is the converging point of a vast number of hereditary lines. When they choose a girl they choose more than an armful of sweetness. They choose her family, living and all the way back.

And they are making this fateful choice, for all they know, when they are not proposing marriage at all but just trying a little experiment. Almost parenthetically, because I expect my children to be as sensible and decent as most young people, I shall remark that it is playing with fire to start intimacies; for after a certain point there is no turning back, and that point is reached far sooner than expected due to the fact that in sex pleasure-hunting one has always to go a little farther than the last time to revive the original thrill. I shall point out that the "easy girl" has lost the habit of faithfulness and never acquired the habits of wifely love. And the young man who doffs his chastity with a scornful laugh for it may not find that light and shining garment again.

I do not mean that one misstep must damn soul or body; I would certainly not want my boys to think that their parents would not forgive anything and try to understand. But missteps in love are steps going down, and everybody knows it in his heart. They lead down into bitter regrets that don't mend the situation, into shuddering revulsion that the chaste lover never has to know, into a hardening of the spiritual arteries, a relentless soul-coarsening. It is possible, for a very strong and determined spirit, to climb back up those steps again and scrape himself clean. But strong and determined souls are not, usually, the ones who can be persuaded to descend in the first place. They are the ones who have generally kept their chastity. And while it is kept, the rapture and the pride of sex remain enthroned.[5]

Marital Relations

Marriage and the family always have been and doubtless always will be the foundation of society among civilized people. Even Soviet Russia, which proposes to substitute the state for the family, still recognizes marriage.

The basic emotion which brings a man and woman together in marriage is sex; and compatibility in this regard is one of the requisites for a happy marriage. In fact, sexual satisfaction for both partners in marriage is almost essential for happy married life.

In spite of the importance of the sexual aspects of marriage, there is so much variation between individuals in the matter of psychosexual constitution that it is difficult to give general advice on the subject. When an individual has difficulty with sexual relations in marriage, it usually is due not to ignorance on the subject but to complicated emotional attitudes, the correction of which necessitates far more information than it would be possible to obtain from a general discussion of the subject. In individual cases of maladjustment, therefore, it is wiser to consult a psychiatrist than to seek aid from books that have been published on the subject.

From certain writings one gets the impression that sexual adjustment in marriage is exceedingly difficult, that it requires

[5] Peattie, Donald Culross, "A Way to Chastity," *The Reader's Digest,* vol. 31, p. 30, December, 1937.

a highly developed technique and constant care to prevent things from going wrong. This is an erroneous attitude, which may give rise to difficulties just as severe as those arising from ignorance.

There are certain things, however, about which a person should be informed. In the first place, general knowledge about the physiology underlying the sexual act is valuable, for it tends to allay fears which might arise from misconceptions. Then, too, there is the question as to frequency. Actually there is no established norm in this matter. But the probability is that unless one is motivated by some drive other than normal sexual desire, excesses will not occur. The best guide probably is inclination, controlled by consideration for the partner. There are great variations from individual to individual in habits of sexual expression, and even in the same individual over a period of time. For this reason it is unwise to lay down any rule governing the practice.

In very large measure the problems of sex adjustment which lead to maladjustment and failure arise out of the natural differences in the sexual constitutions of men and women. Even at best, when understood, these differences of themselves present more or less formidable adjustment problems. But with a sympathetic understanding of the natural sex differences there is large hope and prospect for making the adjustments successfully. It is the widely prevailing ignorance of, and misconception about, the differences in sexual make-up of men and women and, hence, the failure to take them into account that has caused such frightful mismanagement of sex relations and such widespread tragic consequences. . . .

Briefly stated, we may say that in men sex desire is fairly uniform, they do not vary as widely in regard to it as women do; in men sex desire lies close to the surface and is easily aroused and quickly satisfied, and man is always liable to sex desire in all its forms. In women sex desire varies much more widely, the extremes are farther apart; it lies deeper, and is more slowly aroused and more slowly satisfied; it is subject in most women to tidal rhythm related to ovulation and menstruation; and it is subject to development to full power gradually through experience.[6]

[6] Exner, M. J., and W. F. Snow, "Sex Hygiene," The Practitioner's Library of Medicine and Surgery, vol. 12, "Hygiene and Preventive Medicine," p. 157, Appleton-Century-Crofts, Inc., New York, 1937. See supplementary reading list (p. 420) for references to books and pamphlets which contain much excellent and sane information concerning sex relationships in marriage.

A sound understanding of contraception is part of the equipment for an intelligent approach to marriage. This is now widely recognized and such information is available to those who seek it. Birth control, if practiced, should be for the purpose of limiting the size and spacing of one's family in accord with the best interests of both children and parents. Religious groups which condemn artificial methods condone the limitation of pregnancy by attention to the so-called "safe period," when the likelihood of conception is minimized. The practice of contraception is physically harmless to the individual if proper contraceptive methods are used. On the other hand, practices which cause stimulation without complete satisfaction are to be condemned, as is contraception when used purely selfishly to gain gross satisfaction with no intent of fruition of function in family life and children. Such practices interfere with one of the normal and healthy forces of integration both for the individual and for society.

Venereal Diseases

The term "venereal," derived from Venus, the Roman goddess of love, is applied to those diseases which are contracted primarily through sexual relationship. Syphilis and gonorrhea are the two important diseases included under this term, although there are several others such as chancroid, lymphogranuloma inguinale, and venereal warts, which belong in the same general group. Both syphilis and gonorrhea have caused untold illnesses and deaths for hundreds of years; but only recently has it been possible to write about them in the public press, and even yet certain radio stations bar mention of them over the air.

*Syphilis,** sometimes called the "pox" or "lues," is caused by a living organism called the "treponema pallidum" or the "spirochete" of syphilis. Infection is usually acquired through sexual intercourse or congenitally from one's parents, although at certain stages it is transmissible through kissing or by contact with objects recently contaminated with discharges from an infected person. Common drinking cups and towels have been found to

*See also Appendix D.

[415]

transmit the infection, but fortunately the germ of syphilis is killed very quickly outside the body by drying, sunlight, or soap and water. Consequently, ordinary measures of sanitation and personal hygiene are adequate protection against the indirect transmission of syphilis.

Just how prevalent syphilis is, is not known. Routine blood tests for syphilis required in Selective Service examinations led to diagnosis of this disease in 3.4 per cent of over 3,000,000 white inductees; and 20.5 per cent of 800,000 Negro inductees. Among some groups the percentage is lower than this and among others, particularly those who might be considered on the fringe of society, such as criminals, prostitutes, and drifters, it is certainly much higher. In a series of 19,000 Wassermann tests performed as part of the routine physical examinations of University of Minnesota students, 39 cases of syphilis were found—one-fifth of 1 per cent. One might well ask whether the use of this test is justified when it leads to the discovery of so few cases. From a statistical point of view this might seem doubtful, but a consideration of the individuals involved can leave no doubt concerning its value. The infections of some of these students were acquired; others were congenital. None of the thirty-nine was under treatment, although in practically all cases the disease was still curable. Untreated, many of these young men and women would have had in store for them years of invalidism and early death. A report from the University of Wisconsin states that an article on syphilis in *Reader's Digest* brought 3,400 volunteers to the health service for Wassermann tests. When the student daily of the University of Kansas sent out 200 questionnaires to alphabetically selected students, 193 replied that they thought the Wassermann test should be a compulsory part of the physical examination. The director of the Health Service at the University of Iowa reports that routine Wassermann tests led to the diagnosis of congenital syphilis in one of their students and to the recognition of syphilis in both parents, a brother, and a sister.

A few years ago two physicians from Indianapolis reported that by the routine use of the Wassermann test they discovered

[416]

syphilis in between 2 and 3 per cent of presumably healthy men and women who came to them for physical examinations. These patients were about equally divided between those who would be called well-to-do and those in moderate circumstances. Such information leaves no doubt as to whether this test for syphilis ought to be included in every physical examination. Many states now have laws which require a blood test for syphilis of everyone who applies for a marriage certificate.

The U.S. Public Health Service estimates that approximately 3,000,000 people in the United States are infected with syphilis and that 150,000 additional persons acquire the infection each year. A large proportion of these persons are promiscuous in the sexual relationship and so spread the infection to numerous others. In 1952 some 6,000 persons died from syphilis and an equal number entered mental institutions because of this disease. Statistics also show that syphilis causes 10 per cent of all insanity cases, 12 per cent of "strokes," and 18 per cent of the diseases of the heart and blood vessels. Conservative estimates also state that at least 10,000 children each year are born with congenital syphilis. Congenital syphilis could be eradicated, or nearly so, by the adoption of two procedures: routine diagnostic blood tests for syphilis in all pregnant women, and adequate treatment of the syphilitic women during pregnancy. Syphilis is definitely on the decrease but is still far from eradicated in this country.

The first stage of syphilis, called a "chancre," is a local sore, relatively painless, at the point of infection. This usually appears from 12 to 40 days after exposure. It may be an ulcer of considerable size or merely a small blister or pimple or red spot which may be entirely unnoticed. This latter is particularly true in women. In a chancre the spirochete of syphilis can be detected by microscopic examination. At this stage the disease is highly communicable.

The Wassermann[1] test is a test of the blood to determine whether it contains antibodies against syphilis. Antibodies de-

[1] The Kahn, Kline, and Kolmer tests are simplified methods of performing this same type of blood examination.

[417]

velop only as a result of infection; so a positive test indicates, except for certain inaccuracies, existing syphilitic infection. Since it takes some time for antibodies to develop, this test usually does not become positive until about the third or fourth week after infection. It then tends to remain positive as long as infection exists except in some of the late degenerative stages of the disease. If treatment is started before the Wassermann test becomes positive, more than 90 per cent of those treated can be cured. After the blood test has become positive, the chance of cure is reduced. The disappearance of the chancre, which occurs in a short time with or without treatment, is frequently mistaken by the patient for the end of the disease.

Although syphilis is a continuously progressive disease, it frequently is spoken of as manifesting itself in three or four stages, the second of which is characterized by a skin eruption which may resemble measles or chickenpox and by sores in the mouth and throat. At this stage the patient may infect others through kissing. These secondary manifestations are often so mild and inconspicuous as to escape notice. Like the chancre, they too disappear after a time without treatment.

The late stages of syphilis, which follow in 2 to 20 or more years, are the degenerative effects of the disease upon the heart, blood vessels, brain, spinal cord, or other tissues or organs of the body. At this stage adequate treatment will still arrest the disease in approximately half of the patients, but the damage which has been done cannot be repaired.

Syphilis is one of the diseases over which we could have complete control. We know its cause and how it is transmitted. We have a simple test to aid in its diagnosis, and we have an effective cure. Scientifically, nothing more could be desired. Yet this disease will continue to be a major cause of illness and disability until the public and the medical profession make more intelligent application of the control measures which science has made available to us.

*Gonorrhea** is another venereal disease caused by a specific germ. It has no relationship to syphilis, although both are ac-

*See also Appendix D.

quired in the same way and may be contracted at the same time. Like syphilis, gonorrhea is usually contracted through sexual intercourse with a person who has the disease, although it may be transmitted by towels or toilet articles used by infected persons. If a mother has gonorrhea when her baby is born, its eyes frequently become infected and blindness may result unless proper preventive treatment is utilized. Female children are not infrequently victims of a gonorrheal infection as a result of coming in contact with the infective discharges of an infected parent or other person.

Gonorrhea is several times as prevalent as syphilis; in fact, it is estimated that there are more than a million new cases of gonorrhea in this country each year. Although gonorrhea is frequently considered as insignificant, in the aggregate it is responsible for an enormous amount of disability and invalidism.

The gonorrhea germ, called the "gonococcus," sets up a purulent infection of the mucous membranes of the genital tract. This causes a yellowish, purulent discharge from the genital organs. After several weeks this discharge stops, even without treatment, but the bacteria continue to live in the deeper parts of the reproductive tract. In the male an abscess may develop later in the prostate gland and the germs may be discharged during sexual intercourse, even though no symptoms have been present for some time. In the female the gonococci travel up the genital tract into the pelvis and frequently cause chronic and serious infections. In fact, gonorrhea is the most common cause of sterility and pelvic operations in women.

Gonorrhea responds well to treatment with sulfonamides and the antibiotics, but such treatment needs to be administered under competent medical supervision. Self-treatment or the ministrations of the quacks and fakers who promise quick and cheap cures merely lead to serious complications.

DISCUSSION SUGGESTIONS

1. Define testis, sperm, epididymis, vas deferens, urethra, ovary, uterus, fallopian tube, cervix.
2. What is meant by ovulation? Approximately when does it occur?
3. Trace the course of the ovum which does not become impregnated.

4. Explain the process of menstruation. What treatment is ordinarily required during the menstrual period?
5. What is meant by nocturnal emissions and what is their effect upon health?
6. Discuss the suggestion that masturbation leads to insanity.
7. Discuss the development of the sexual emotion and its influence upon behavior.
8. Discuss the arguments for and against sexual promiscuity.
9. What is meant by homosexuality? Is it, as generally supposed, a hopeless condition?
10. If you were about to be married, where would you turn for further information concerning marital relationships?
11. What is a Wassermann test? What does a positive test indicate?
12. What is the cause of syphilis and how may it be transmitted?
13. Discuss the prevalence of syphilis.
14. Outline a community program for the prevention of syphilis.
15. What is gonorrhea? How does it differ from syphilis?
16. What is the relation between gonorrhea and sterility?

REFERENCES AND READING SUGGESTIONS

1. Brown, Fred, and R. T. Kempton: "Sex Questions and Answers: A Guide to Happy Marriage," McGraw-Hill Book Company, New York, 1950.
2. Corner, George W.: "Attaining Manhood: A Doctor Talks to Boys about Sex," Harper & Brothers, New York, 1952.
3. Fishbein, Morris: "A Natural Method of Child Planning," *The Reader's Digest*, September, 1951.
4. Griffith, Edward F.: "A Sex Guide to Happy Marriage," Emerson Books, Inc., New York, 1952.
5. Marquardt, Martha: "Paul Ehrlich," Henry Schuman, Inc., Publishers, New York, 1951.
6. Richardson, F. N.: "For Girls Only: The Doctor Discusses the Mysteries of Womanhood," Tupper and Love, Inc., Atlanta, Georgia, 1953.
7. Sorokin, P. A.: "The Case against Sex Freedom," *This Week Magazine*, January 2, 1954.
8. Yahraes, Herbert: "Planning Your Family," Public Affairs Pamphlets, New York, 1948.
9. Pamphlets of American Social Hygiene Association, New York, and American Medical Association, Chicago.

Text-Film

Human Reproduction (motion picture 21 min). For description see page 395.

Chapter XX

MODERN PARENTHOOD[1]

IMPROVEMENT in obstetrical and infant care and the resultant decrease in the terrific death rates of mothers and infants are among the achievements to which modern civilization can point with greatest pride. The conditions which surround childbirth among most primitive people are almost unbelievable and are convincing evidence of backward civilizations. Often childbirth is considered not the glorious beginning of a new life but rather a repulsive animal function which the mother is supposed to perform under unspeakable conditions and without help or sympathy even from her husband or members of her family. The contrast between that and the modern birth of a baby in a hospital or properly prepared home is as great as the difference between night and day. Yet there are still far too many deaths—unnecessary deaths—among both mothers and infants occurring in our own country today.

The Course of Pregnancy

Conception takes place and pregnancy begins when the male reproductive cell, called the "sperm," finds and unites with the reproductive cell of the female, called the "ovum." This union normally occurs in one of the ducts or canals, called "fallopian

[1] Prepared in collaboration with Dr. Ruth E. Boynton, director of the Students' Health Service, University of Minnesota.

[421]

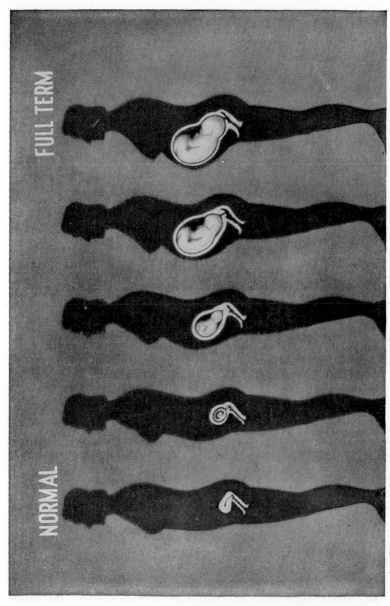

As the fetus develops from the first month to full term, the figure of the mother undergoes marked physical changes. (*From Human Reproduction, a McGraw-Hill Text-Film.*)

tubes," which conduct the ova from the ovaries to the uterus, or womb. First there is a single new cell, then as development begins, two, then four, then eight, and so on. Next cells differentiate into different tissues and organs with growth proceeding at an enormous rate. The relative rate of growth is never again so rapid as during these early months of beginning life, yet it is not

FIG. 37

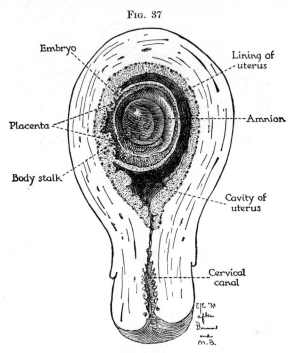

Uterus about one month pregnant.

until approximately four months after conception that it is possible to make a positive diagnosis of pregnancy by the ordinary examination. Two to three months earlier than this, however, an almost positive diagnosis of pregnancy can be made by means of the hormone test described in Chapter XVIII (page 382); and there are the well-known suggestive signs of pregnancy such as cessation of the menses, morning sickness, breast changes, and enlargement of the abdomen.

The average duration of pregnancy is 280 days—9 calendar

[423]

months or 10 lunar months—but there is no reliable means of estimating the exact date of the baby's arrival. The rule most commonly followed for estimating the probable date of birth is to add 7 days to the date of the first day of the last menstrual

Fig. 38

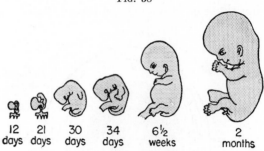

| 12 days | 21 days | 30 days | 34 days | 6½ weeks | 2 months |

Development of human embryo (actual size).

Fig. 39

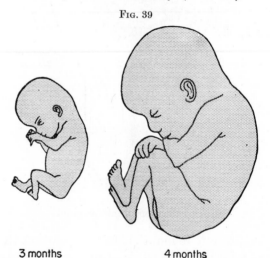

3 months   4 months

Development of human embryo into fetal stage (one-half actual size).

period and then to count back 3 months. The date thus arrived at will indicate within a few days the date in the future on which to expect the baby.

PRENATAL CARE

As soon as a woman suspects the possibility of pregnancy, she should consult her doctor, not only to be assured of her condition

[424]

but also to provide proper care for herself and for her developing child. It is true that childbearing is a natural process, but it is one which may very quickly become seriously abnormal. It is only by adequate medical care during pregnancy that the health of mother and child can be safeguarded. Every woman should

FIG. 40

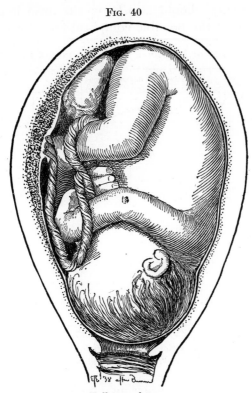

Full-term fetus.

have a complete and thorough examination at the beginning of pregnancy and a subsequent examination by her physician at least once a month during the first 6 months of pregnancy, and then every 2 weeks or oftener until delivery. Supervision of the pregnant woman, once she has placed herself under a physician's care, naturally is his responsibility, but it is up to her to put herself under his care at the beginning of pregnancy and to cooperate by following his advice and instructions thereafter.

[425]

Every pregnant woman and her husband should inform themselves concerning the physiologic changes which occur during pregnancy, labor, and the post-partum period. This information may be obtained from authoritative books on the subject, or from bulletins of the U.S. Children's Bureau or the state health department. They should also know the most important signs and symptoms of the possible complications of pregnancy, such

FIG. 41. TREND IN MATERNAL MORTALITY IN THE UNITED STATES

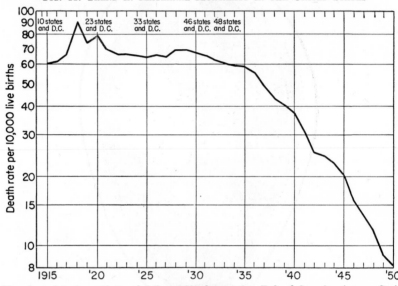

(*Based on data from National Office of Vital Statistics, Federal Security Agency, Social Security Agency, Social Security Administration, U.S. Children's Bureau.*)

as persistent headache, recurring vomiting, dizziness, disturbances of vision, swelling of the hands, face, or ankles, severe pain in the abdomen, vaginal bleeding, acute illnesses, obstinate constipation, and marked shortness of breath, and should report the appearance of any of these promptly to the physician.

THE HAZARDS OF PREGNANCY

During 1952 there were reported in the United States 2,530 deaths related to childbearing, one for every 1,500 live births. This is a decline of 83 per cent from the rate which existed in

1930, when 15,165 maternal deaths were reported. This is encouraging progress (Fig. 41), but we should do still better because most of these 2,500 deaths could have been prevented. In 1950 the maternal death rates by states varied from 2 per 10,000 live births in North Dakota to 24 per 10,000 live births in Mississippi (Fig. 42).

The causes of these deaths are shown in Fig. 43. An intensive 3-year study of the causes of maternal death in New York City

FIG. 42. MATERNAL MORTALITY BY STATES FOR 1950

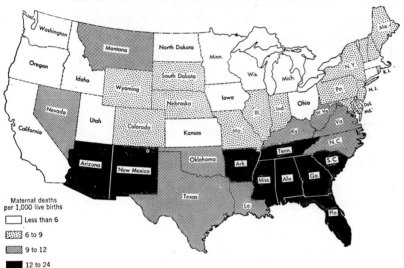

Maternal deaths
per 1,000 live births

▢ Less than 6

▨ 6 to 9

▧ 9 to 12

■ 12 to 24

(Based on data from National Office of Vital Statistics, U.S. Children's Bureau, Department of Health, Education and Welfare.)

concluded that 66 per cent of the women who died might have been saved if they had had proper treatment and care. The general causes for inadequate care may be grouped under three headings: poverty, ignorance, and inadequate or incompetent professional service during pregnancy and delivery.

Some of the accidents and serious hemorrhages of childbirth are unavoidable, but competent professional attention will prevent most of them. Infection in connection with childbirth, called "puerperal sepsis," is practically all preventable. In 1843 Oliver Wendell Holmes, physician and author, declared in a paper en-

[427]

titled "The Contagiousness of Puerperal Fever" that physicians, nurses, and midwives were responsible for most of the infections which occur during childbirth. That was before the days of Pasteur's discovery concerning the relationship of microorganisms to disease and prior to the introduction of asepsis and antisepsis by Lister. In those days infection and fever were the rule rather than the exception following childbirth, and most physicians believed that this so-called "childbed fever" was due to the will of God and not to the carelessness of man. (Abortions we

FIG. 43. CAUSES OF MATERNAL MORTALITY

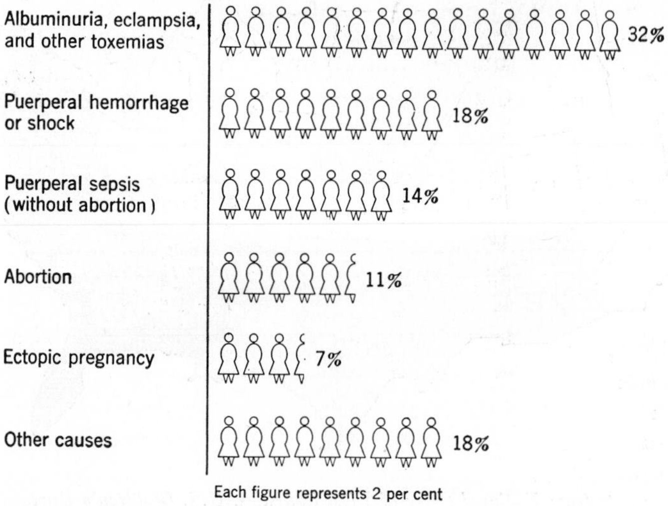

Albuminuria, eclampsia, and other toxemias	32%
Puerperal hemorrhage or shock	18%
Puerperal sepsis (without abortion)	14%
Abortion	11%
Ectopic pregnancy	7%
Other causes	18%

Each figure represents 2 per cent

shall speak of in a subsequent paragraph.) In addition to aseptic techniques for delivery, penicillin and the other antibiotic drugs are playing important roles in the reduction of deaths from puerperal infection.

The toxemias, or poisonings, of pregnancy, which cause damage to the liver and kidneys and may result in high blood pressure, vomiting, convulsions, and death, can be recognized in their incipiency and usually can be successfully combated by the program of prenatal care which has been outlined.

The Chicago Maternity Center reports a maternal mortality of less than one-fourth the rate for the country as a whole and its clients are among Chicago's poorest mothers. A few years ago, Cattaraugus County, New York, reported that mothers receiving prenatal care had a death rate less than one-fourth the rate for the nation as a whole.

PLACE OF DELIVERY

An increasing number of mothers are going to hospitals for delivery of their babies. Obviously there are definite advantages in the better facilities of the hospital delivery room, particularly if some unforeseen abnormalities or accidents should occur. On the other hand, hospital care increases the expense and unfortunately, in many hospitals, the danger of infection during delivery is greater than in the home. Instructions in regard to proper preparation for delivery in the home may be obtained from private physicians, public health nurses, or state and local health departments.

PROFESSIONAL CARE DURING DELIVERY

The U.S. Children's Bureau reports that in 1950, 88 per cent of births were attended by physicians in hospitals; 7 per cent by physicians in the home; 4.5 per cent by midwives; 0.5 per cent by other nonmedical attendants. Without question the most competent service at a delivery can be expected from a physician adequately trained and experienced in obstetrics. Physicians in general practice are trained to conduct normal and certain of the less seriously abnormal deliveries. Realizing their limitations to deal with some of the rarer and more serious complications, they are quick to call for whatever consultation is in the interest of the patient. Midwives in certain foreign countries are reasonably well trained to render obstetrical service in normal deliveries, but the vast majority of the midwives practicing in this country are old, careless, and dirty and have had little or no training. Exceptions to this are the trained nurse-wives who are rendering splendid service in the mountains of Kentucky and in certain other sparsely settled regions where medical service is not available.

NORMAL AND INSTRUMENTAL DELIVERY

The vast majority of deliveries will occur spontaneously and should be permitted to do so, because instrumental delivery increases the risk of infection, of hemorrhage, and of accidents to both mother and child. In probably not more than 5 per cent of deliveries is instrumental or operative interference really necessary. In the New York study the death rate from instrumental and operative deliveries was five times as high as that from spontaneous delivery. In this group of operative deliveries, of course, are included the seriously abnormal cases. On the other hand, this same study reports that 77 per cent of the deaths following operative delivery were judged avoidable, as compared to only 48 per cent of the deaths which followed spontaneous delivery.

Instrumental delivery is frequently a lifesaving procedure for mother or child, but it is uniformly agreed by the specialists in this field that instruments are used far too often. For this physicians are themselves in part to blame, but part of the responsibility must also be laid at the door of the patients who insist upon instrumentation to shorten labor.

Cesarean section is delivery of the child through an incision in the abdominal wall and in the uterus. There are many instances in which this operation has saved the lives of both mother and child, but, like instrumentation, it is an operation attended with greatly increased risk. Many of the Cesarean operations could be avoided by proper medical care during the prenatal period.

ANESTHESIA FOR LABOR

One of the greatest blessings that science has given to mankind is that of anesthesia. Dr. Crawford Long of Atlanta, Georgia, in 1844 was the first to use ether for anesthesia, but the real impetus for its use in surgery was given by Dr. W. G. T. Morton, who in 1846 demonstrated its effectiveness before a surgical clinic in the Massachusetts General Hospital. During the same year a Scottish physician, Dr. James Simpson, introduced anesthesia into the practice of obstetrics. For some time the relief of pain during childbirth was considered irreligious, but this opposition died down rapidly after Queen Victoria sanctioned its use on the occasion of the birth of Prince Leopold in 1853.

Today a woman has the right to expect some relief from the pain of childbirth, but no mother should demand relief at the risk of her own life or the life of the child. All substances which are used to produce anesthesia are toxic, and no single method or combination of methods is uniformly applicable. The time and degree of anesthesia must be determined by the physician and not decided on the basis of some magazine article on the subject.

In recent years many mothers have been giving birth to their babies with little or no great pain. The method is based upon studies which indicate that much of the pain of childbirth is due to fear, tension, and muscle spasm. Preparation for this type of delivery, which begins several months before the baby is due, consists of a thorough understanding of the birth process, exercises to strengthen the muscles which are needed for delivery, and practiced relaxation. To be successful teamwork is required on the part of the mother, the father, the physician, and the attending nurses. In some cases a bit of light anesthetic may be used, but the mother remains a conscious participant in this great miracle of the beginning of human life.

ABORTION

Abortion means the interruption of pregnancy before the child is sufficiently developed to be able to live outside the mother's body. Dr. Frederick J. Taussig, who has made a greater study of abortion than anyone else in this country, estimates that approximately 600,000 abortions occur yearly in the United States, and that thousands of women lose their lives from this cause every year. Many of these deaths are reported as due to other causes and so do not show in the mortality statistics. Two-thirds of these abortions he estimates are induced and one-third are spontaneous. The death rate following abortion is three times as high, and the invalid rate ten to fifteen times as high, as that following delivery of the child at term. The specific dangers of abortion are infection, subsequent sterility, and endocrine disturbances which may cause chronic invalidism.

[431]

Spontaneous abortion is a condition which needs careful medical study. Some cases are due to disease, such as syphilis, toxemia, and diabetes; some to deficiencies in the endocrine secretions related to pregnancy; some to deficiency of vitamin E; some to weakness inherent in the germ plasm of the sperm or ovum; and some to physical abnormalities of the pelvic organs. Obviously, most of these are preventable.

Induced abortion carries a terrific hazard to both life and health. Many abortions are self-induced by methods which would make anyone who understands physiology and asepsis shudder. Others are performed as illegal operations by "doctors." Some of these abortionists are unethical physicians; others belong to some of the cults; and still others are not licensed as any type of practitioner. The major reasons for abortions are poverty, large families—and, of course, poverty is a factor here—illegitimacy, marital difficulties, and selfishness. Very rarely the physician will need to perform an abortion to save the mother's life; and there are situations in which the limitation of offspring is advisable. The only safe way to accomplish this, however, is not by abortion but by the practice of contraception or by sterilization.

OBSTETRIC SUPERSTITIONS

There has long been a superstition that maternal impressions or emotional disturbances of the mother, such as anger, fright, grief, or horror, may cause her unborn child to be marked, injured, or deformed. Certain hereditary traits are transmissible from parents to offspring through the germ cells which unite to give rise to the new child; but after conception has once taken place, the mother's body merely provides warmth and nourishment for the baby until it has developed to a point that it is able to lead an independent existence. The only connection between the mother and the baby is through the umbilical cord. This cord carries arteries and veins but no nerves, and even the blood of the mother does not mix with the blood of the child, the exchange of nutrients and excretory products taking place through a membrane which separates the two circulatory systems.

[432]

Infant Care

Man achieves immortality largely through his children and his work. As soon as an infant has been born, its health and welfare become the first concern of both its father and its mother. This is one of the points of difference between man and most of the lower animals; and as culture and civilization advance, we

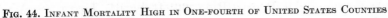

Fig. 44. Infant Mortality High in One-fourth of United States Counties

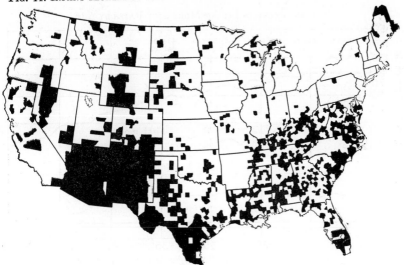

Counties in black have infant mortality rates between 38 and 120 per 1,000 live births. White areas cover other counties with rates ranging from 13 to 38 per 1,000. Ten thousand infants could be saved each year if the infant mortality were as low in the black-area counties as in counties with cities of 50,000 population or more. (*Children's Bureau, U.S. Department of Health, Education and Welfare, September, 1953.*)

find mankind attempting to provide better and better protection and educational and vocational opportunities for children. Sir Arthur Newsholme, leading English authority on public health, states: "Infant mortality is the most sensitive index of social welfare and of sanitary improvement which we possess. If babies were well-born and well cared for their mortality would be negligible." In some sections of the world the chances are not more than one in two that a newborn child will live to reach its first

[433]

birthday, and in some cities of our own country within the present century approximately one child out of three died during the first year of life. In the registration area of the United States 162 infants per 1,000 born alive died during the first year of life in 1900; by 1930 this number had been reduced to 64.6, and by 1952 to 29 (Fig. 45). In 1952 the corresponding rates for several other countries were as follows: Chile, 154; Indian, 127; Colombia, 111; Portugal, 94; Puerto Rico, 66; Italy, 64; Japan, 48; West

Fig. 45. Trend in Infant Mortality Rates by Age

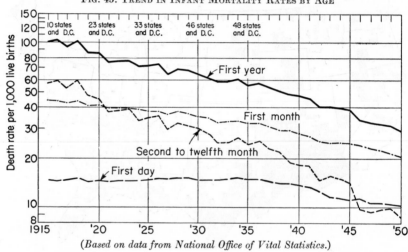

(*Based on data from National Office of Vital Statistics.*)

Germany, 48; France, 45; England, Scotland, and Wales, 29; Switzerland, 29; Norway, 27; New Zealand, 22; and Sweden, 20. In 1950 the infant mortality in the individual states ranged from 21.8 for Connecticut to 54.8 for New Mexico.

The direct causes of infant mortality among the white population of this country at the present time are presented in Fig. 46. The five leading causes are premature birth, congenital malformations, postnatal asphyxia and atelectasis, injury at birth, and pneumonia. Of premature births, the toxemias of pregnancy and syphilis are the primary causes. Adequate care during the prenatal period will prevent many toxemias of pregnancy. Congenital syphilis can be prevented by the examination of all mothers and treatment of those who are infected. Modern hospi-

[434]

tal facilities for the care of premature infants will reduce these deaths. The same may be said concerning some of the respiratory diseases. Bronchitis, pneumonia, and other respiratory infections are serious in infants because they have little resistance against them. Hence, all infants should be safeguarded in every possible way from exposure to children and adults who may transmit colds or other infections to them. Malnutrition and the deficiency diseases lower the infant's resistance and so contribute to the seriousness of these respiratory infections.

The diarrheal or intestinal diseases long occupied first place among the causes of infant mortality and still do so in certain

FIG. 46. CAUSES OF DEATHS OF INFANTS UNDER ONE YEAR OF AGE

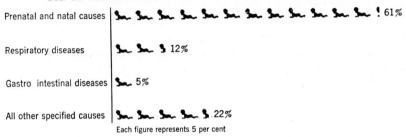

Prenatal and natal causes | ! 61%

Respiratory diseases | 12%

Gastro intestinal diseases | 5%

All other specified causes | .22%

Each figure represents 5 per cent

countries. The marked reduction in the deaths from these diseases which has taken place in this country has been due largely to sanitation and improved methods of infant feeding. Breast milk is the ideal food for a baby. Studies have shown that the death rate from intestinal diseases is three to ten times as high among artificially fed as among breast-fed children. The young women of today are physically superior to the women of previous generations and almost all of them are able to nurse their babies for at least the major part of the usual nursing period of 9 months. Breast milk is desirable not only because it is easily digested and is most nutritious for the child, but also because it offers protection against diarrheal and intestinal diseases and increases resistance against measles, scarlet fever, and other common infections of infancy.

Of the birth injuries some are unavoidable, but their number and seriousness can be materially reduced by proper prenatal

[435   ]

supervision, competent professional care during delivery, and fewer instrumental deliveries. Influenza, whooping cough, and accidents are all reducible, as we have seen in other chapters.

A few years ago a serious and frequently fatal blood disease of newborn infants was found to be caused by a certain incompatibility of the parents' blood. This is dependent upon what is known as the "Rh factor." Blood which contains this factor is called Rh-positive; blood without it is called Rh-negative. When the mother's blood is Rh-negative and the father's blood is Rh-positive, the blood of the mother sometimes destroys the red blood cells of the baby she is carrying. When this occurs, the baby may be born with hardly enough red blood cells to sustain life. In such cases, the only hope of saving the child is to drain the baby's blood from its body immediately after birth and replace it with healthy blood.

Tests can be made for the Rh factor in the father's and the mother's blood and also for the beginning of destruction of the baby's blood cells. If this occurs, the risk to the child can be greatly reduced by careful medical supervision and care during pregnancy.

The more important indirect causes of infant death are poverty and ignorance. Many studies have shown a direct correlation between low income of the wage earner and high infant mortality. One of these studies reports 168 infant deaths per 1,000 live births among families with an annual income of $500 or less as compared to a rate of 30 per 1,000 among families with incomes of $3,000 or more, and an increase of 20 per cent in the infant death rate in families of which the wage earner became unemployed during the depression years of 1929 to 1932.

The conditions of poverty are all adverse to the survival of the delicate life of the newborn infant. On the other hand, poverty, unemployment, and larger families than can possibly be supported are frequently the result of the same sort of ignorance and irresponsibility which contribute to a high infant death rate. It has also been shown that, by instruction of the mother concerning the proper care and feeding of infants, it is possible materially to improve nutritional status, even though the family's income be no more than relief allowance. The U.S. Children's Bureau in Washington and the state and local health departments make available bulletins of information, advice, and, if necessary, public health nursing service for maternal and infant care, so that there is no longer any justification for the ignorance and neglect which has been responsible for most of the deaths of mothers and infants in the past.

Heredity

Heredity is the major determining factor in the sum total of the qualities, characteristics, and traits which have been transmitted from generation to generation through the ages past and will continue to be transmitted to future generations still unborn. It is common knowledge that children frequently resemble their parents. This is evidence of the hereditary transmission of certain physical characteristics. Many other less evident but much more important traits are inherited, and these may come not only from one's parents but also from one or more of one's four grandparents or one's eight great-grandparents or sixteen great-great-grandparents, and so on for generations.

Some inherited traits do not appear in every generation even though they are transmitted through these generations to their children or their children's children. Furthermore, hereditary traits transmitted from one parent may be submerged or modified by the inheritance of opposite traits from the other parent.

Human heredity is a complicated mosaic, but science has begun to identify the elements in this picture and arrange the pieces so as to make for an increasing understanding of this all-important factor in our lives.

In sexual reproduction there is a union of the nucleus of the sperm with the nucleus of the ovum. In each of these nuclei are twenty-four minute structures known as "chromosomes." These chromosomes carry all the hereditary elements, called "genes," which are transmitted from parents to their children. The infinitesimal size of these genes can be appreciated from the fact that 10 million sperms may be contained in a single drop of seminal fluid. Upon the union of these reproductive cells the

[437]

chromosomes from the two parents unite in the nucleus of the cell which represents the beginning of a new life. This fertilized cell, its nucleus and its chromosomes, then divide and redivide innumerable times as the new child is developing. In time these cells become specialized to form the various tissues and organs of the body, including the ovaries and testes. In these are developed and stored the chromosomes, with their genes, to pass along the accumulated hereditary traits to future generations. Nothing that happens in the life of either men or women alters the genes which their children receive. And it seems to be merely a matter of chance as to what proportions and combinations of these all-important genes are contained in an individual ovum or sperm. For this reason children of the same parents do not necessarily show identical hereditary patterns.

Congenital Influences upon Health. Hereditary influences, as we have seen, are transmitted through the reproductive cells. In addition to this a newborn child may be influenced to a certain degree by the condition of the mother during the nine months that the child is developing in the uterus. The child's nervous system and circulatory system are entirely separate from those of the mother, but food and oxygen pass through the membranes which separate the blood of the child from that of the mother. In similar fashion certain poisons or infections may be transmitted from mother to child. Peculiarly, attacks of German measles (rubella) during the first four months of pregnancy seem to be related to an increase in congenital defects in the children. Influences of this sort exert their effect upon the child after its development has started and are called "congenital" in contrast to those hereditary influences which are inherent in the germ cells and transmitted from generation to generation.

The Mendelian Law. An Austrian monk, Gregor Mendel, was the first to demonstrate the specific operation of heredity. His experimental materials were two varieties of peas, one tall and one dwarf. He fertilized the blossoms of the tall variety with pollen from the dwarf variety. The seeds which developed from these cross-pollinated plants were then planted. All of the plants which grew from these seeds were of the tall variety. These plants

[438]

were then allowed to develop normally, fertilizing themselves, and the seeds they produced were planted. From these seeds there developed both tall and dwarf varieties, but there were three times as many of the tall as of the dwarf. When the self-pollinated seeds from this crop were planted only dwarf peas grew from the seeds which had come from dwarf plants, but the seeds from the tall variety again produced both tall and dwarf plants, with five times as many of the tall as of the dwarf variety. This proportion continued generation after generation. However, by selection Mendel was able to obtain from among the tall variety certain plants, the seeds of which would produce only tall peas.

From these observations it was obviously the rule that, whenever a pure strain, either tall or dwarf variety, was fertilized by pollen from the same variety, the seeds which developed produced only the corresponding variety; but that cross-fertilization between the tall and the dwarf varieties resulted in seeds which produced only the tall variety. From this it was concluded that, when hereditary elements which made for tallness or shortness were both present, the determinant for tallness always predominates.

This phenomenon, which has been found to obtain in a large number of hereditarily transmitted characteristics, gave rise to the designation of certain traits as "dominant" and others as "recessive." A simple example of this in humans is in the color of the eyes. It has been observed that brown eyes are dominant over blue. Consequently, if both parents have pure brown eyes all the children's eyes will be brown, or if both parents have pure blue eyes all the children's eyes will be blue. However, if one parent has pure brown eyes and the other pure blue eyes, the children will have brown eyes or a mixture of brown with blue with the brown predominating. On the other hand if the parent has these "mixed"—hybrid—brown eyes the children may have either brown eyes or blue eyes.

Experimentally one can demonstrate the operation of this so-called "Mendelian law" by breeding black rats with white rats. In this case black is dominant over white, with the result

[439]

that the first generation of hybrid rats will all be black but they will be hybrid black, that is, carrying the genes which make both for black and for white fur. If rats of this first generation of hybrid blacks are bred together the next generation will be one-fourth pure black, one-fourth pure white, and one-half hybrid black or mixed. Among small numbers of offspring these proportions may not hold but in large numbers these ratios will invariably hold true.

Among the more important human traits and conditions influenced or determined by heredity are the following:

1. Conditions the inheritance of which seems to follow the Mendelian pattern with the trait dominant in character: diabetes insipidus; telangiectasis (purple areas in the skin, frequently accompanied by serious nosebleeds); hypospadias (abnormal opening in male ureter); allergies; migraine headache; Huntington's chorea (progressive mental deterioration beginning about middle age); mirror reading, cataract in young persons, glaucoma, optic-nerve atrophy, hereditary night blindness, drooping eyelids, opaque ring over iris, absence of iris; progressive inner-ear deafness, word deafness, absence of ear; defective enamel of teeth; stub fingers, extra fingers and toes, stiff joints, webbed fingers or toes; brittle bones; deformed spine; dwarfism; progressive muscular atrophy, muscle stiffness; Friedreich's ataxia; pigment spots on skin, lack of pigmentation in skin and hair, fatty growths in skin (frequently on eyelids); horny skin, cysts on scalp, baldness (men only); defective hair (beaded, infantile, excessively long, woolly, prematurely gray); defective nails.

2. Conditions which are hereditary according to the Mendelian pattern but recessive in character—that is, they develop only if inherited from both parents: diabetes mellitus;[2] jaundice of the newborn; certain types of feeble-mindedness; nearsightedness and extreme farsightedness, complete color blindness, blurred vision in strong light; albinism, skin and hair dead white with pink eyes; small fatty growths on face and scalp; skin sensitivity to light; absent nails.

[2] A diabetic can now be told that the chance that each one of his offspring will become diabetic is between 10 and 15 per cent.

3. Conditions which are transmitted according to the Mendelian patterns but are sex-linked—that is, they act as dominant traits in males and as recessive in females, appearing in males if inherited from either parent but in females only if inherited from both parents: hemophilia (defective blood clotting, "bleeders"); red-green color blindness; pink eyes without other albino effects.

4. Conditions the inheritance of which is probably Mendelian in character but whose dominance is uncertain or imperfect: cleft palate, harelip; otosclerosis; double row of eyelashes; astigmatism; missing teeth, extra teeth; thick nails; imperfectly developed male sex organs; tendency to produce twins; left-handedness.

5. Conditions which are hereditary but seem to follow a pattern of blending of dominant and recessive characteristics: general body size; stature; weight; skin color; hair form; shape of head and facial proportions.

6. Conditions which apparently are subject to heredity but it is uncertain to what extent they are hereditary and how they are inherited: general mental ability, memory, temperament, musical ability, literary ability, artistic ability, mathematical ability, mechanical ability, longevity; liability to hernia; some types of epilepsy and insanity; high blood pressure; cancer; psoriasis; thick or shedding skin; deaf-mutism; gout; certain defects of the glands of internal secretion; pernicious anemia; paralysis agitans; birthmarks; resistance to disease.

EUGENICS

The practical application of the established principles of heredity to the improvement of the human race is called "eugenics." In animals scientific knowledge in this field has been extensively utilized for the improvement of the stock. In humans similar application is infinitely more difficult. Our inheritance is so complicated and human life and liberty of action are so highly valued that it is difficult to formulate scientifically sound programs of action and still more difficult to enforce restrictive measures even upon the subnormal and delinquent portion of the population. In some states sterilization of individuals with certain hereditary defects, such as familial feeble-mindedness, has been legalized in the hope of reducing the number of children who are likely to become public charges in institutions for the feeble-minded, jails, or reform schools. More hopeful is the increasing public interest and information on this subject. Young people are coming to realize "that each one of them is a converging point of a vast number of hereditary lines" and that when they choose a life partner they are choosing more than an attractive young man or charming girl. They are choosing also his or her "family, living and all the way back."[3]

DISCUSSION SUGGESTIONS

1. What is meant by conception? Where does it take place?
2. Discuss the reasons for having examinations during pregnancy.
3. How frequently should such examinations be conducted?
4. What are the major causes of maternal deaths?
5. What evidence is there that these can be reduced?
6. What are the suggestive symptoms of beginning complications of pregnancy?
7. Discuss the values and the hazards of instrumental deliveries.
8. What is puerperal fever? How may it be prevented?
9. Explain what is meant by "Cesarean section."
10. What are some of the causes of spontaneous abortions?
11. Discuss the dangers of induced abortions.
12. Discuss the influence of maternal impressions upon the unborn child.
13. Define the term "infant mortality."
14. Discuss the differences in the infant mortality rates of the various countries of the world.
15. What are the major causes of infant mortality in the United States?
16. How can each be prevented or reduced?
17. Discuss the relation between social and economic conditions and infant mortality.
18. Discuss the Mendelian law.
19. What are sex-linked characters?
20. Discuss human eugenics.

REFERENCES AND READING SUGGESTIONS

1. Baumgartner, Leona: "Nation-wide Plan for Reduction of Premature Mortality," *Journal of the American Medical Association*, vol. 146, p. 893, July 7, 1951.

[3] Peattie, Donald Culross, "A Way to Chastity," *The Reader's Digest*, vol. 31, p. 30, December, 1937.

2. Breckinridge, Mary: "Wide Neighborhoods," Harper & Brothers, New York, 1952.
3. Duvall, Evelyn: "Building Your Marriage," Public Affairs Pamphlets, New York.
4. Gruenberg, S. H.: "The Wonderful Story of How You Were Born," Hanover House, Garden City, New York, 1952.
5. Guttmacker, A. F.: "Having a Baby," The New American Library of World Literature, New York, 1950.
6. Kenyon, Josephine H., and Ruth Russell, "Healthy Babies: A Complete Handbook for Modern Mothers," Atlantic Monthly Press, Little, Brown & Company, Boston, 1951.
7. Landis, Paul H., and Helen Bond: "Your Marriage and Family Living," McGraw-Hill Book Company, Inc., New York, 1946.
8. Metropolitan Life Insurance Company: "Information for Expectant Mothers," New York.
9. Potter, Edith: "Fundamentals of Human Reproduction," McGraw-Hill Book Company, Inc., New York, 1948.
10. Potter, Edith L.: "Saving Premature Babies," *Today's Health*, vol. 30, p. 38, December, 1952.
11. Read, G. D.: "Childbirth without Fear: The Principles and Practice of Natural Childbirth," Harper & Brothers, New York, 1953.
12. Spock, Benjamin: "The Pocket Book of Baby and Child Care," Pocket Books, Inc., New York, 1946.
13. Thompson, Morton: "The Cry and the Covenant," Doubleday & Company, Inc., New York, 1949.
14. Thomas, Herbert: "Training for Childbirth," McGraw-Hill Book Company, Inc., New York, 1950.
15. U. S. Children's Bureau: "Prenatal Care" and "Infant Care," Pamphlets, U.S. Department of Health, Education and Welfare, Washington, D.C.
16. Pulford, G. S.: "The Rh Factor," American Medical Association, Chicago.

HEREDITY AND HEALTH

1. Cook, Robert, and Barbara Furks: "How Heredity Builds Our Lives," American Genetic Association, Washington, D.C., 1946.
2. Osborn, Frederick: "Preface to Eugenics," Revised, Harper & Brothers, New York, 1952.
3. Pfeiffer, John: "Genetics: The Science of Heredity," Public Affairs Pamphlet, New York.
4. Scheinfeld, A.: "You and the New Heredity," J. B. Lippincott Company, Philadelphia, 1950.
5. Snyder, L. H.: "The Principles of Heredity," D. C. Heath and Company, Boston, 1951.

Text-Films

The following McGraw-Hill Text-Film on Health Education is recommended for use with this chapter of the text:

Human Reproduction (21 min sd MP). In this film models and animated drawings explain the reproductive systems of men and women, and the process of normal birth. Film emphasizes the importance of clear and objective understanding of these facts as the basis of successful marriage and parenthood.

Silent follow-up filmstrip based on the motion picture offers opportunity for review, testing, and further discussion.

Chapter XXI

HEALTH PROBLEMS OF
ADVANCING YEARS

THERE comes a time in life when it is good to sit by the fire and contemplate the future. Youth, with its successes and its failures, its joys and its heartaches, has been a thrilling, glorious adventure. But those stores of exuberant energy, of hope and enthusiasm, are fast diminishing. The first half is over; what of the future? Should one press on for prestige, power, success; or will peace of mind and the cultivation of intellectual, artistic, and human interests give more satisfaction in the years to come?

Life after forty may be spent in a futile effort to perpetuate youth or it may contain the richest, fullest, most interesting years of all. Up to this time one has been occupied with growing up, obtaining an education, establishing a home, raising a family, acquiring a position in the world. These earlier years have been filled with strong emotions, impetuous action, and intense struggle. To carry on the same type of life in the future puts an enormous strain upon a waning vitality. Long before our high-pressure modern era Seneca wrote: "Man does not die; he kills himself," And Moscowitz, discussing the increasingly important problem of high blood pressure, speaks of the "tragedy of the successful man." In contrast to this, a few years ago every member of the United States Supreme Court was over sixty years of age and five of the nine members were over seventy years. In 1932 one of its most distinguished members of all time, Justice

Holmes, retired at the age of ninety in physical health and mental vigor. These men and others like them have so modified their lives that while they conserve their physical and nervous energy they grow in wisdom, intellectual interests, and breadth of vision. A readjustment of objectives, of point of view, is essential to an appreciation of maturity.

Fig. 47. Sickness Increases with Age

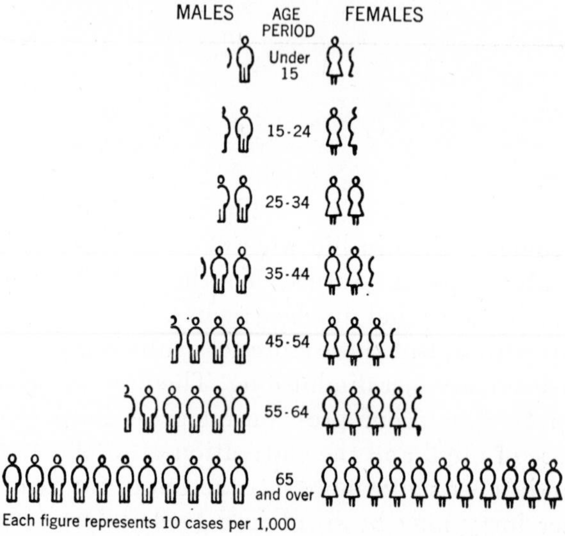

Each figure represents 10 cases per 1,000

Sickness on day of survey among 1,000 white persons. Metropolitan Life Insurance Company. (*Data from Dublin and Lotka, " The Money Value of a Man," The Ronald Press Company, New York, 1930.*)

As the diseases and conditions which destroy life prematurely are brought under control, an increasing number of persons reach advanced years. In 1900 there were approximately 3,000,000 people in the United States over sixty-five years of age. By 1940 this number had increased to 9,000,000, and it is estimated that by 1960 this number will be 14,000,000, and that by the year 2000 it will be 21,500,000

This increase in the proportion of older persons means an increase in the importance of the health problems of advancing years. Medical terminology calls this "geriatrics." Literally, this means the medical care of aging persons; more poetically, it has

[446]

TABLE 26

LEADING CAUSES OF DEATH BY AGE GROUPS

Cause of Death	Deaths	Death Rate*
45–54 years:		
Heart disease	52,610	293
Cancer	30,940	172
Apoplexy	12,740	71
Accidents	10,190	57
Tuberculosis	4,940	28
Cirrhosis of liver	4,200	23
Pneumonia	3,440	19
Suicide	3,340	18
Diseases of circulatory system (except heart)	2,730	16
Nephritis	2,680	15
55–64 years:		
Heart disease	108,110	783
Cancer	56,310	408
Apoplexy	26,470	191
Accidents	10,010	73
Diabetes	6,050	44
Diseases of circulatory system (except heart)	5,330	39
Pneumonia	5,210	37
Tuberculosis	4,730	34
Nephritis	4,400	32
Cirrhosis of liver	4,400	32
65–74 years:		
Heart disease	157,290	1,763
Cancer	62,740	703
Apoplexy	48,880	548
Diseases of circulatory system (except heart)	11,400	128
Accidents	10,140	114
Diabetes	8,490	95
Pneumonia	7,630	75
Nephritis	5,080	57
Cirrhosis of liver	5,020	33
Tuberculosis	4,510	51
75 and over:		
Heart disease	202,890	5,200
Apoplexy	75,650	1,755
Cancer	50,470	1,295
Diseases of circulatory system (except heart)	30,230	776
Accidents	16,560	437
Pneumonia	14,580	387
Nephritis	7,180	217
Senility	6,790	205
Diabetes	6,770	204
Diseases of prostate	2,600	70

* Rates per 100,000 white population in each age group for the United States in 1952.

[447]

been defined as the science of helping older people enjoy life longer.

Each decade after forty carries increasing hazards to health and life. The best insurance that one can have against these, according to Dr. Raymond Pearl, is to have long-lived ancestors. Next in importance comes temperament; the calm, contented type live longer than those who are nervous, irritable, and inclined to worry. Strenuous exercise and heavy muscular work after forty are liabilities to long life. Even robust health is not so important as one would suppose, for a considerable number of individuals in Pearl's series who lived to a ripe old age reported that they had been sickly or frail throughout a part of their lives.

Degenerative Diseases of the Heart and Blood Vessels

Of particular importance after forty are the degenerative diseases of the arteries, as they ramify in all parts of the body. Their inner walls break down and in them a fatty material is deposited, and this in time further breaks down and is replaced by deposits of a bony substance, called "calcium." The result is the condition known as "arteriosclerosis." In places where arteries run close to the surface, as in the wrist and over the temples, these hardened slatelike vessels may be felt. Such arteries will not permit the usual amount of blood to pass through them; hence, whatever organ or group of cells was supplied by such weakened arteries must then suffer from a diminished supply of blood. When these changes take place in the pancreas, we have the diabetes of middle-aged people; when the brain suffers by such derangements in its blood supply, we get the dementias and personality disorders of old age. And when the vessels of the kidney become sclerotic, we have a type of the well-known chronic Bright's disease.

Interference with the flow of blood also occurs when there is constriction of the small arteries due to spasm. This spasm is the result of an overactive nervous system. If life is to continue, an adequate flow of blood must be maintained. When the size of the opening through which the blood must pass is reduced, the flow can be kept up only by having the blood come up to the obstruction under greater pressure from behind. A greater "head" is needed. Nature provides for this by increasing the blood pressure. This means, however, more work for the heart. To meet this increased demand the heart enlarges and thereby

FIG. 48. DEATHS FROM HEART DISEASE BY COLOR, SEX, AND AGE

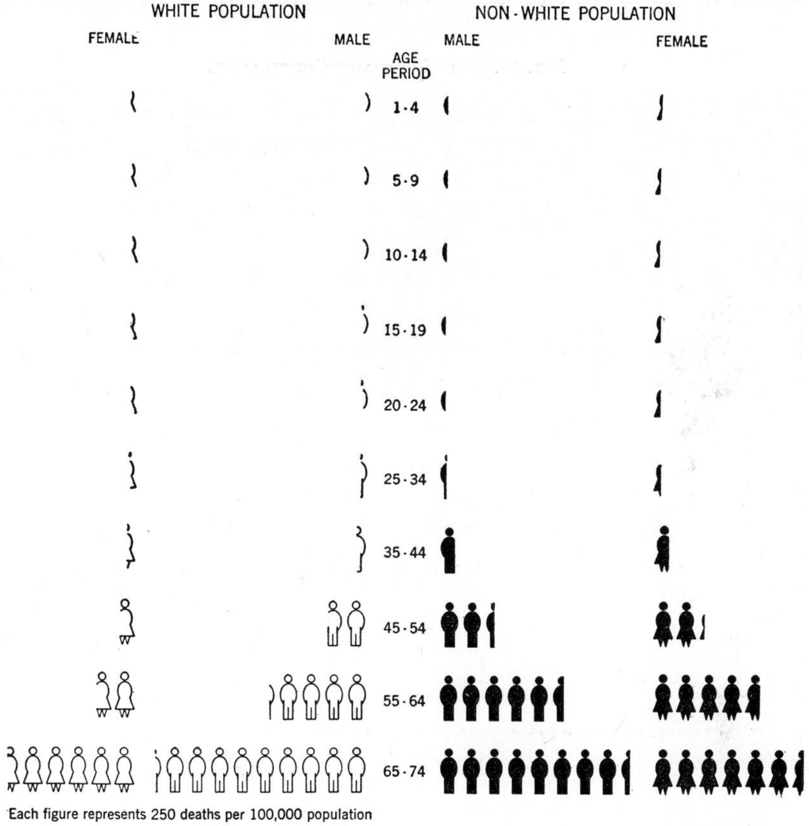

Each figure represents 250 deaths per 100,000 population

Averages of annual death rates for organic diseases of the heart per 100,000 persons by color, sex, and age. Ages 1 to 74 years. (*Data from National Office of Vital Statistics.*)

has its reserve diminished. For a time this is not serious but eventually the reserve becomes so greatly reduced that a sudden strain may cause the heart to fail.[1]

Still another cause for the final destruction of the individual

[1] Note records of your blood pressure during your college years, Appendix C.

[449]

may arise on the basis of these narrowed and obstructed vessels. Blood can no longer course through them readily and rapidly; it slows down. There is then a tendency for clots to form inside of the vessels. These clots are called "thrombi." When thrombi occur in the blood vessels which supply the heart muscle, we speak of the condition as "coronary thrombosis." The obstruc-

Fig. 49. The Coronary Circulation

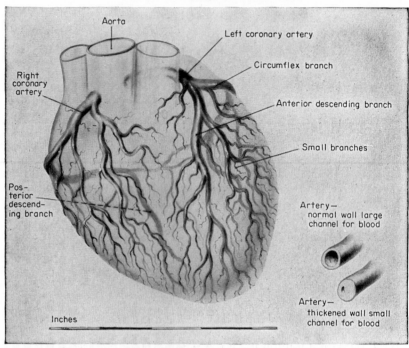

(*Northwestern National Life Insurance Company, Minneapolis.*)

tion, partial or complete, of these blood vessels is frequently accompanied by severe attacks of pain, called "angina pectoris." This pain usually originates in the region of the heart and radiates to the left shoulder and down the left arm. Coronary thrombosis is the most common cause of death from heart disease and seems to be considerably more frequent among individuals in occupations involving primarily mental work than among man-

[450]

ual workers and more frequent among physicians than among any other occupational group.

Sometimes clots float about in the blood stream. They are then called "emboli." Floating along, one may reach a vessel too small for it to pass through and it stops. Whatever tissue may lie beyond it awaiting a blood supply will thereafter be cut off and the tissue of which it is composed will die. Emboli thus may destroy large areas of tissue in kidney, spleen, lungs, liver, and brain.

Sometimes the small, weakened, brittle arteries of the brain break and hemorrhage occurs into the surrounding tissue. This is called "apoplexy." The paralysis which usually follows a stroke of apoplexy is due to the pressure of the hemorrhage upon the brain cells. If the hemorrhage is large and not promptly absorbed, disintegration of these brain cells with permanent paralysis may follow.

These degenerative diseases of the circulatory system represent the end results of accumulated injury from excesses or inadequacies of diet, physical and nervous strain, or infections and poisons in constitutionally susceptible individuals.

No single factor has been identified to which we can point as the cause either of arteriosclerosis or of high blood pressure. Some investigators believe that diets with a high content of fat are related to arteriosclerosis, and it seems that heredity, overweight, and nervous and emotional strain are related to high blood pressure. There are, however, no specific diets or other measures that can be recommended for the prevention or cure of either of these diseases. Drugs are helpful in certain persons; surgery in others. More important for most people, however, is the reduction of weight and a modification of the habits of life so that the strain upon the circulatory system is reduced to a minimum. By these measures a long and useful life is usually made possible.

Cancer

The fear of cancer is prominent in the minds of most persons past middle life and well it may be, for one woman out of every eight and one man out of every fourteen over forty years of age will die of cancer. Cancer is not a germ disease but a condition in which the cells in certain tissues of the body begin to reproduce wildly and without limit. For example, cells in the breast, in the stomach, in the skin, or in some other tissue grow beyond their natural limits and invade other tissues and organs. Cancer is not, as many believe, an ulcerating process, although, because

Fig. 50. Skin Cancer

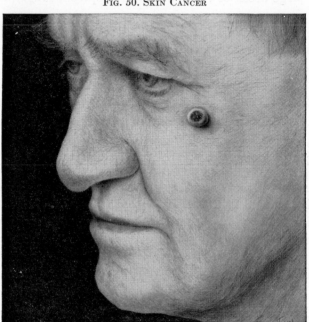

(*Northwestern National Life Insurance Company, Minneapolis.*)

of its low vitality, cancer tissue easily becomes infected if exposed to injury.

Cancer has been likened to a vicious, fast-spreading weed that invades a healthy lawn. The first tiny shoot is so similar to grass that it may escape detection. As it grows and spreads, it devours the nourishment of the soil and chokes the roots of the grass. When they first start to grow such weeds are easily destroyed, but as they spread they erode and kill everything around them. The same is true of cancer.

[452]

FIG. 51. CANCER DEATHS BY COLOR, SEX, AND AGE

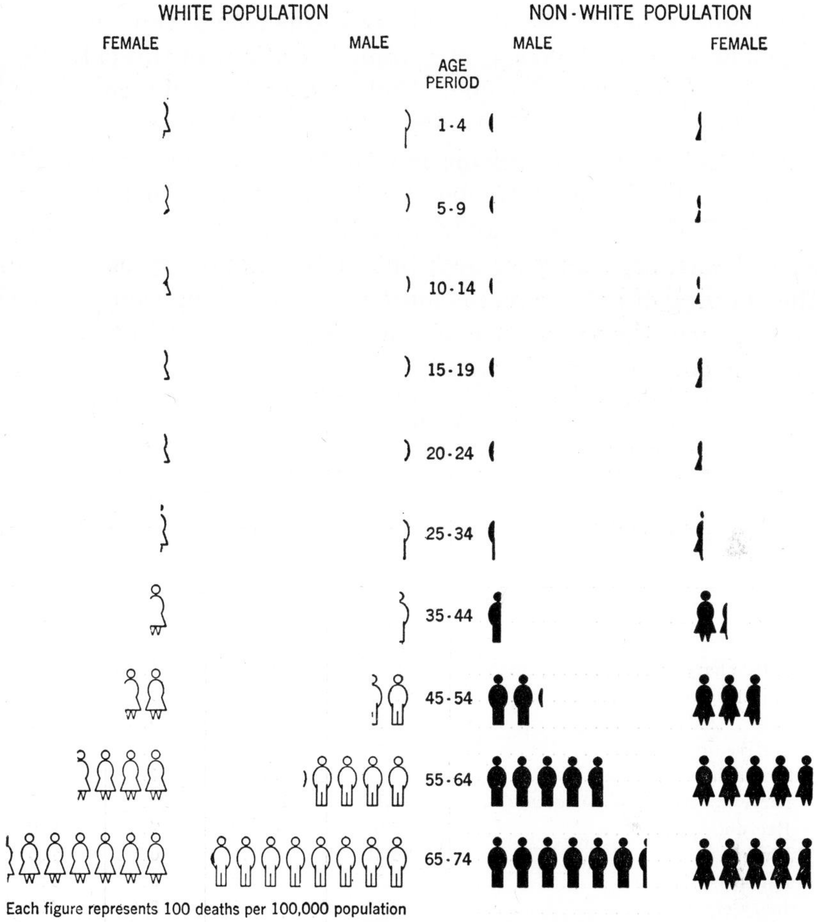
WHITE POPULATION
NON-WHITE POPULATION
FEMALE
MALE
MALE
FEMALE
AGE PERIOD
1-4
5-9
10-14
15-19
20-24
25-34
35-44
45-54
55-64
65-74
Each figure represents 100 deaths per 100,000 population

Averages of annual deaths from all forms of cancer per 100,000 persons by color, sex, and age. Ages 1 to 74 years. (*Data from National Office of Vital Statistics.*)

There is no occasion for worry because a parent or a grandparent has developed cancer. The unusual prevalence found in certain families suggests a familial susceptibility but is not conclusive evidence that the disease is hereditary. Members of such families are naturally concerned about cancer and should inform themselves about the disease, its diagnosis, treatment, and prevention.

The prevention of certain types of cancer is distinctly within the realm of possibility. Particularly is this true of those cancers which develop as the result of chronic irritation. In this category belong cancers of the tongue, cheek, lip, and certain cancers of the skin and female genital organs. Tobacco chewing and smoking, jagged teeth, unhygienic mouths, alcohol, and syphilis all favor the development of cancer of the tongue. In this country, cancer of the tongue is approximately ten times as prevalent among men as among women; but in India and Ceylon, where the chewing of betel leaves is more common among women than among men, the prevalence of cancer of the tongue in the sexes is reversed.

TABLE 27

CANCER DEATHS BY ORIGIN AND SEX, UNITED STATES, 1952

Place of Origin	Deaths		Rate per 100,000	
	Male	Female	Male	Female
Total................................	114,000	110,130	148.3	139.6
Mouth, pharynx....................	3,750	1,100	4.9	1.4
Respiratory organs.................	20,152	4,100	26.2	5.2
Breast............................	170	20,200	0.2	25.6
Digestive organs...................	45,510	37,840	59.2	48.0
Stomach......................	15,700	9,200	21.5	12.2
Large intestine (except rectum).....	10,100	12,200	13.5	16.1
Rectum.......................	5,900	4,550	7.8	6.0
Liver.........................	4,500	5,600	6.0	7.5
Pancreas......................	5,100	3,700	6.8	4.8
Urinary organs....................	6,760	3,820	8.8	4.8
Genital organs....................	13,350	22,330	17.4	28.3
Blood and lymphatic systems.........	11,280	7,750	14.6	9.8
Nervous system...................	2,450	1,600	3.2	2.1
Skin.............................	2,050	1,500	2.7	1.9

Cancer of the lip is many times as frequent among men as among women and particularly common among smokers. On the other hand, nonsmokers may develop it and many who have smoked for years never do. It usually appears on the lower lip at a point which is subjected to continual irritation as from a broken or decayed tooth, a rough, hot pipe stem, a hot cigar, or cigarette smoke. No one should neglect persistent sores or unusual spots, crusts, or growths on the tongue, lips, or cheek.

Cancer of the skin may develop as a result of irritation by burns, infections, soot, coal tar, petroleum, and aniline dyes. Any sore that does not heal within a month should be investigated for the possibility of cancer. Moles or pigmented warts which are located where they may be irritated by clothing, shoes, or shaving should be removed, for they may begin to grow and, when they do, they become among the most malignant of cancers.

Cancer of the lung, which is rapidly increasing in frequency, with 6,732 deaths in 1938 and 16,450 deaths in 1948, is believed by many investigators to be related to cigarette smoking. Unfortunately this disease causes few symptoms in its early stages, and these are usually masked by a "chronic cigarette cough." An x-ray examination of the chest every 6 to 12 months of all persons, particularly men past forty who have smoked heavily, is recommended for the early diagnosis of this serious disease. Early symptoms are chronic cough, wheezing, voice change, or chest discomfort.

Cancers of the stomach and upper portions of the intestinal tract also are difficult to diagnose early (page 150), but cancers of the lower bowel frequently cause bleeding and cancers of the rectum can usually be discovered by a rectal examination. Such examinations therefore should be included in physical examinations of persons past middle age.

Cancer of the breast can be discovered early if looked for regularly and carefully. Examination by a physician is necessary for diagnosis, but self-examination techniques as developed by the American Cancer Society can be exceedingly helpful in the early discovery of lumps which should be investigated.

Cancer of the female genital tract usually gives early symptoms of bleeding or discharge. In the male genital tract the most common early symptoms are enlargement of the testicle or urinary obstruction.

Cancer of the female genital tract frequently develops from chronic irritation produced by an injury which occurred during childbirth. Hence, repair of such injuries is a preventive measure against cancer.

The successful treatment of cancer depends upon its complete removal by surgery or destruction by x-ray, radium, or cautery. In its early stages cancer is a local collection of cells and is easily removed. Later, when the cancer cells have invaded surrounding tissue or have spread through the blood or lymph vessels to other parts of the body, complete removal becomes impossible. Hence, cancer can be treated successfully only when it is diagnosed early.

Reports on follow-up studies of cancer patients lead to the conclusion that at least 75 per cent of breast cancers and up to 95 per cent of other "external" or "accessible" cancers can be cured if diagnosed and properly treated early. In internal or "inaccessible" cancer the possible cure rates are much lower, probably 25 to 50 per cent, because symptoms frequently are not present or at least not recognized early; diagnosis is more difficult and treatment less effective. Certain hormones are useful in retarding the growth of some types of cancer (page 392) but they never cure the disease.

Early diagnosis would be facilitated if everyone in the cancer age would have a thorough physical examination once a year or, better still, once in six months. Such examinations would discover some early and unsuspected cancers and lead to the correction of other conditions which physicians recognize as precancerous. Furthermore, many deaths from cancer will be prevented if the public ever learns that chronic indigestion or abnormal bleeding from the bowel or genital tract should be investigated; that every woman who notices a lump in the breast should consult a physician—usually these lumps are unimportant but in case of doubt they should be removed and examined microscopically; and that a sore of the skin, lip, cheek, or tongue which persists for more than a month or six weeks may be cancer.

There is no medicine, diet, or serum that will cure cancer. Ointments and plasters are worthless and massage and manipulation tend to disseminate cancer cells throughout the body. The cancer quack is the most despicable of all the vultures who prey upon human misery. He alleges to cure cancer without surgery, to take it out by the "roots," using electrical treatments, salves, light, diet, etc. His treatment is worthless, but worse still, while the patient relies on his treatment, the cancer progresses until even the best of medical care is unavailing.

Rheumatism

Rheumatism causes more illness and disability than any other chronic disease. In fact, at least one in every twenty Americans— more than 7,000,000 in all—suffers from some form of rheumatic disease. Rheumatism does not kill, but it disables most of its victims for long periods of time. Compared with an average of 18 work days lost for each accident, rheumatic patients lose an average of 80 days out of each year.

The term "rheumatism" covers a host of aches and pains which, although rarely fatal, cause an enormous amount of discomfort and disability. If joints are involved, the more specific term "arthritis" is used. In childhood and early adult life an acute type of rheumatism (page 48) with involvement of the heart is the rule, but in later life the chronic type predominates. This may be merely annoying, partially handicapping, or completely incapacitating over a few months or many years. Devastating, demoralizing pain and greater or lesser deformity are its outstanding features.

The cause of chronic arthritis may be an infection at the root of a tooth, in a sinus, tonsil, or some more remote portion of the body. Metabolic disturbances are responsible in certain cases, as also are severe physical or emotional shock, fatigue, injury, exposure, abnormal weight, inadequate diet, and constitutional or hereditary predisposition.

Treatment of arthritis should be based upon a determination of its type and a thorough search for its cause. The removal of foci of infection, vaccines, dietary measures, etc., are of benefit in selected cases. Drugs, such as sodium salicylate and aspirin, reduce the pain and sometimes seem to be beneficial. Heat, whether applied by baking, hot applications, electricity (diathermy), or various types of baths, relieves pain and in some cases produces lasting improvement.

Researches by Drs. Hench and Kendall of the Mayo Clinic indicate that the injection of Cortisone, a substance from the cortex of the adrenal gland, gives dramatic relief to many persons long crippled by rheumatism. Similar results are obtained with ACTH (see page 389). These preparations do not cure rheumatism, but they give relief so long as patients continue to receive them. This suggests that, as with insulin in diabetes, the substance given is replacing a similar substance which the body needs but which is either absent entirely or present in insufficient amounts.

Rheumatism is one of the most lucrative fields for all sorts of irregular medical practitioners. The methods which they employ are legion, including various kinds of baths, manipulations, electrical treatments, diets, foot twisting, and mental healing. Yet each one has its cures and some of them number their adherents by the thousands. This is largely because there is a big nervous element in arthritis, the pain causing nervous irritation, and the nervous irritation aggravating the pain. Then, too, arthritis normally goes through cycles of improvement and relapse. Consequently, any treatment in which the patient has confidence is likely to be of some benefit; and if this happens to be applied at a time when improvement is about to occur anyway, "miraculous results" are obtained. There is no panacea for arthritis, but intelligent, individualized, and patient treatment will give considerable relief in most cases and lead to permanent improvement in some.

Respiratory Illnesses

Respiratory illnesses occupy a position of major importance among the causes of illness and death in every age group but become increasingly important in the upper decades of life. With advancing years common colds become less frequent, but chronic bronchitis, asthma, and pneumonia are more common and more serious. All too often these are accepted as an inevitable accompaniment of age and the possibilities of obtaining relief are neglected. The cause of asthma frequently can be determined and eliminated. Bronchitis may be secondary to sinus infection, to excessive smoking, or to some other remediable general condition. Or what is thought to be chronic bronchitis may be a low-grade chronic tuberculosis. Many an elderly person with tuberculosis is in reasonably good health himself and yet is a danger to others. No aged person with "chronic bronchitis" should be permitted in a home with young children unless it has been demonstrated that this chronic bronchitis is not tuberculous.

Digestive Disturbances

Many digestive disturbances make their appearance or assume major importance in adult life. The effects of dietary indiscretions, nervous tension, indigestion, and ill-advised efforts to correct constipation accumulate over the years to produce distress and disability.

Weight

Excessive weight is disadvantageous to health and longevity throughout adult life, but its hazard becomes greater with increasing age. According to life insurance computations the lowest death rate among persons over forty-five to fifty years of age occurs in those who are 10 to 20 pounds *under average weight.* This does not mean that weight loss is necessary but merely that the weight which is desirable at the age of thirty should be maintained.

Diabetes

Diabetes has already been considered (page 384) but it becomes of such greatly increased importance with advancing years that it should be mentioned again in this chapter. It is estimated that there are a million unknown diabetics in the nation. Most of these are overweight and are the relatives of diabetic persons. If this disease is discovered early, as it can be by urine examinations, its progress can be controlled and life prolonged by restriction of fats and carbohydrates in the diet and by the injection of insulin prepared from some other animal.

Sexual Adjustment

Most of the reproduction of the race takes place during the first twenty or thirty years of adult life. During this period the sex glands are active and the sex emotion prominent. Then between forty and fifty there is a cessation of reproduction by women and a diminution of sexual activity on the part of men.

This change, the so-called "menopause," is anticipated with dread by most women. It is said to involve unpleasant physical and mental changes; and it pronounces with finality that youth is passed. Physiologically what occurs is that the ovaries cease to discharge an ovum once each month. This makes unnecessary the continuance of menstruation, which is the preparation of the uterus to receive this ovum. Simultaneously, the internal secretions which are related to sexual activity and reproduction are diminished.

During the period in which readjustments of glandular activities are taking place there may be physical and emotional disturbances. Irritability, jealousy, despondency, and self-pity may make life almost intolerable. During this stage, temporary though it is, sympathy and understanding by those who are near and dear are essential to happiness and peace of mind. Ordinarily no medical treatment is necessary but the counsel of the family physician is helpful. Anxiety and unnecessary worry may thus be obviated, and occasionally special treatment with the glandular secretion which is diminishing too rapidly may be indicated.

The passage of this period is followed by a stability and poise never before attained. The impetuous years of life are over but the future holds broader interests, greater sympathy, and maturity of understanding. And sex life is not necessarily ended, for with the burden of childbearing and the hazard of pregnancy removed, some women, according to an eminent gynecologist, experience a more satisfactory sex life after fifty years of age than before.

The reproductive life of men does not cease so abruptly as does that of women. There is instead a gradual diminution of sexual urge and activity. Failure to recognize and adjust to this may give rise to serious emotional conflicts and psychological situations.

Periodic Health Examinations

The money value of the average male of forty, according to computations of Dublin, is $25,794 if he is in a $2,500 maximum income class, and $45,500 if he is in a $5,000 maximum earning class. Anyone with an automobile or a piece of machinery worth $25,000 or $45,000 would give it the best of treatment and care, particularly if he knew that he could never have another one. The suggestion that one should have a periodic health examination is merely saying that one should bestow upon the only body that one will ever have as much care and intelligence as one would give to a piece of fine machinery.

Many defects and diseases do not produce recognizable symptoms until they become advanced, but thorough, careful physical examinations performed periodically will discover many of these conditions at a time when their progress can be arrested. Life insurance companies have found that such examinations pay big dividends in the prolongation of the lives of their policyholders and so provide such examinations free of charge. For children periodic examinations are recommended semiannually, and for young adults annually or biannually. But with advancing age examinations should be more frequent, for this is the period in which degenerative processes make their appearance and become rapidly progressive (see Appendix C).

When Does Old Age Begin?

This important question was well answered some years ago by an anonymous writer who said:

Youth is not so much a time of life as it is a state of mind. It is not a matter of ripe cheeks, red lips and supple knees; it is a temper of the will, a quality of the imagination, a vigor of the emotions; it is a freshness of the deep spring of life.

Youth means a temperamental predominance of courage over timidity, of the appetite of adventure over the love of ease. This often exists more in a man of fifty than in a boy of twenty.

Nobody grows old merely by living a number of years; people grow old only by deserting their ideals. Years wrinkle the skin, but to give up enthusiasm wrinkles the soul. Worry, doubt, self-distrust, fear and despair—

[461]

these are the long, long years that bow the head and turn the growing spirit back to the dust.

Whether seventy or sixteen, there is in every being's heart the love of wonder, the sweet amazement at the stars and the starlike things and thoughts, the undaunted challenge of events, the unfailing child-like appetite for what next, and the joy and the game of life.

You are as young as your faith, as old as your doubt; as young as your self-confidence, as old as your fear; as young as your hope, as old as your despair.

In the central palace of your heart there is a wireless station; so long as it receives messages of beauty, hope, cheer, courage, grandeur and power from the earth, from men and from the infinite, so long are you young.

When the wires are all down and the central palace of your heart is covered with the snows of pessimism and the ice of cynicism, then you are grown old indeed and may God have mercy upon your soul.

How to Live after Forty

Health after forty is determined largely by heredity and by what has transpired in the years before forty. Inherent traits cannot be modified nor can damage already done be repaired.

> The Moving Finger writes; and having writ
> Moves on: nor all your Piety nor Wit
> Shall lure it back to cancel half a Line
> Nor all your Tears wash out a Word of it.

The foundation has been laid and the structure built, but much can be done to keep it in repair and to prevent unnecessary strain and wear and tear upon it. Periodic health examinations provide information concerning the state of health and make possible minor adjustments and the successful treatment of many major diseases before they become serious. Reduction of strenuous physical activity and emotional tension reduces the strain upon the circulatory system and lessens the danger of both functional and organic disorders. The limitation of the diet to the needs of the body removes the hazard of obesity. It is possible also that liberal amounts of the so-called "protective" foods—milk, eggs, fresh fruits, and vegetables—will result in improvement in some of the degenerative diseases.

This is the time of life for intellectual interests, friendships, travel, recreation. Maturity and experience open new vistas of interests and pleasures which become richer as the years go by. An active physical and mental life may be continued, but now as never before it is essential to live intelligently.

The late Dr. C. Eugene Riggs in his seventy-third year presented in the following paragraphs[2] his conception of the changes and adjustments which occur with advancing age:

The middle years bring their definite and distinctive stress. The life impulse gradually wanes and the forces of disintegration begin their predetermined task. Hereditary tendencies, ofttimes quiescent in the developmental period, now awaken into activity. Involution is a normal physiological process—it is the reaction of personality to definite biological and environmental conditions that constitute the period of the middle years; it is Nature's readjustment period of the organism. Changes in the ductless glands tend to nervous instability; overeating and lack of exercise open Pandora's box and the degenerative diseases which cause an alarming mortality spring forth.

The middle years are also a testing time of personality. The restraints of the childhood home, the influence of parents long since dead, brothers and sisters scattered, constitute a waning force. Not only may physical efficiency be impaired but in addition to this organic stress there is great perturbation in the psychic sphere due to unhappy marriages, disappointment in children, the loss of the ideals and aspirations of the early years and embitterment because actual accomplishments have fallen so far below hopes and ambitions. The outstanding dynamic at this time is the home, children and friends—a sustaining and stabilizing power. The delinquencies of the riotous forties arise not from caprice or lawless impulse, but are due to the harboring of the antisocial thought in the subconscious whose activities determine the issues of life—a glorious consummation or an ignoble defeat.

Old age is the final epoch in the life cycle. It is inevitable; one can honor and dignify it, but cannot escape it. Many are born old; some old are young; one has said, "At forty, old age is in its infancy; the fifties are its boyhood and girlhood; the sixties its youth; and at seventy it attains its majority." The Greek language possesses great flexibility of expression. "Bios" means both life and death—a subtle suggestion that we achieve life through death. When one reaches the sixtieth year, he can be called old; the senium has been reached. Even in the normal senium, where degenerative change has not become pathologic, to be swept aside willy nilly causes a tinge of bitterness—a feeling of injustice that strength and virility should so lack in appreciation and graciousness.

"It is only those rarely serene souls," says Myerson, "who reach an elevated resignation." The rarely serene souls, I believe to be the rule rather than the

[2] Riggs, C. Eugene, "The Dynamics of Personality," *Minnesota Medicine*, vol. 9, p. 291, June, 1926.

exception. To youth, age is afar off; the joy of life enthralls. Ofttimes it is critical, even harsh—age has had its day; as for death it is an event too remote to interest. Age realizes the inevitable; it revels in the glories that are past; like Alan Seeger, it keeps its rendezvous with death undismayed. Age is life's crown of glory; the past has made possible this culmination of nature's foreordained purpose. It is man's last opportunity—so have the great souls regarded it. Said Clara Barton to a gathering of friends in her ninetieth year, "My working hours are fourteen out of twenty-four. It is my duty to work for the good of my kind; while the strength is given me I have no right to lay it down." Conrad wrote his first novel when he was fifty years of age. Gladstone took up Greek in his sixtieth year and was made Premier of England in his eighty-third year. Charles the Fifth summoned Titian to Augsburg to court to paint portraits when he was seventy years old and he was still painting them when over ninety, dying in his ninety-ninth year. Michelangelo was made architect of St. Peter's in his seventy-second year; he then planned the great dome immortalizing himself and his art. Marion Harland at eighty-eight broke her wrist; unable afterwards to use her pen, she learned typewriting; later, becoming blind, she dictated her articles. She died in her ninety-third year. Of her it is said, "The ardor for study and expression never burned low in her heart." James Bryce made his masterly address at the Williamstown Conference in his eighty-fourth year. William de Morgan was sixty-five years of age when he wrote his first novel. It is said the girls who typed the manuscript were moved to tears and laughter as they did their mechanical work. He died at eighty-seven while working on one of his most interesting stories. Julia Ward Howe, endeared to the American people because of her beautiful poem, The Battle Hymn of the Republic, wrote the reminiscences of her life when eighty years of age. The founder of the Red Cross, Clara Barton, gave an address in her eighty-ninth year, before six hundred people, standing during its delivery, and after its close greeted graciously her audience. She died in her ninety-first year, mentality unimpaired. Joshua, the ancient hero, was already old and stricken in years when he received his Lord's message, "There remaineth yet very much land to be possessed." With splendid courage and efficiency he completed the divine commission. The master of modern medicine, Sir William Osler, contracted in October, 1919, a cold, which gave him, as he described it, "a bad knockout." In one of his last letters he wrote, "The confounded thing drags on in an unpleasant way and in one's seventy-first year the harbour is not far off—and such a happy voyage and such dear companions all the way!— and the future does not worry."

Age has its desires, its aims, its ambitions; it is selfless, sagacious, disillusioned. With magnificent courage, it says with Browning:

> "Grow old along with me!
> The best is yet to be,
> The last of life, for which the first was made."

DISCUSSION SUGGESTIONS

1. What are the major factors which determine longevity?
2. What are the major causes of death after fifty years of age?
3. Explain what is meant by "arteriosclerosis" and what its effects are.
4. Explain the mechanism of the development of high blood pressure.
5. What is coronary thrombosis?
6. What is meant by "emboli" and what is their effect?
7. Explain the mechanism of apoplexy.
8. Just what is a cancer? A tumor? Are all tumors cancers? All cancers tumors?
9. Discuss what is known concerning the cause of cancer.
10. Outline a program for reduction of deaths from cancer.
11. Discuss the importance, the cause, and the treatment of rheumatism.
12. Discuss the importance of respiratory diseases in old age.
13. Explain the relation of obesity to length of life after fifty.
14. Discuss the physiological and emotional changes and adjustments which occur at the menopause.
15. Discuss the value of periodic health examinations.
16. Check ages of your ancestors and review findings on your own health examinations, Appendix C.

REFERENCES AND READING SUGGESTIONS[3]

1. Alvarez, Walter C.: "How to Live with Your Blood Pressure," Wilcox & Follett Company, Chicago, 1951.
2. ———: "How to Live with Your Heart Condition," Wilcox & Follett Company, Chicago, 1951.
3. Blakeslee, Alton L.: "Arthritis and the Miracle Drugs," Public Affairs Pamphlets, New York.
4. ———: "Know Your Heart," Public Affairs Pamphlets, New York.
5. Crosby, Alexander: "Your Blood Pressure and Your Arteries," Public Affairs Pamphlets, New York.
6. Giles, R.: "Begin Now—Enjoy Tomorrow," Mutual Benefit Life Insurance Company, Newark, N.J., 1951.
7. Grant, Lester, "The Challenge of Cancer," U.S. Government Printing Office, Washington, 1950.
8. Johnson, Dallas: "Facing the Facts about Cancer," Public Affairs Pamphlets, New York.
9. Keys, Ancel: "Prediction and Possible Prevention of Coronary Disease," *American Journal of Public Health*, November, 1953.
10. Lawton, George, and Maxwell Stewart: "When You Grow Older," Public Affairs Pamphlets, New York.

[3] See also Major Health Problems, Chap. II.

11. Lerrigo, Charles H.: "The Better Half of Your Life," John Day Company, New York, 1951.
12. Perrott, G. St. J., *et al.:* "Illness and Health Services in an Aging Population," Public Health Service Publication No. 170, Washington, 1952.
13. Potter, Robert D.: "Arthritis: What You Can Do about It," Dodd, Mead and Company, New York, 1951.
14. "Looking Forward to the Later Years," U.S. Public Health Service, Washington, 1953.
15. Stieglitz, E. J.: "The Second Forty Years," J. B. Lippincott Company, Philadelphia, 1946.
16. Bulletins of the American Cancer Society, the National Tuberculosis Association, the Arthritis and Rheumatism Foundation, the American Heart Association, the National Health Council, and the United States Public Health Service. For addresses see p. 590.

Text-Films

The following McGraw-Hill Text-Film on Health Education is recommended for use with this chapter of the text:

Diseases of the Heart and Circulatory System (about 15 min, available spring, 1955). This film explains the various kinds of damage to the heart and circulatory system, commonly grouped together under the general term "heart disease." Emphasis is placed on the high degree of normal activity available to persons having heart ailments, provided that good habits of healthful living are followed.

Chapter XXII

CHOOSING A HEALTH ADVISER

Nowadays there's little meaning
For a person to be gleaning
    When a man attaches "doctor" to his name.
He may be a chiropractor
Or a painless tooth extractor,
    He's entitled to the title just the same.

Or perhaps he is a preacher
Or a lecturer or teacher
    Or an expert who cures chickens of the pip.
He may keep a home for rummies
Or massage fat people's tummies
    Or specialize in ailments of the hip.

Everybody is a "doctor"
From the backwoods herb concocter
    To the man who takes the bunions from your toes.
From the frowning dietitian
To the snappy electrician
    Who shocks you loose from all the body's woes.

So there's very little meaning
For a sufferer to be gleaning
    When a man attaches "doctor" to his name.
He may pound you, he may starve you,
He may cut your hair or carve you,
    You have got to call him "doctor" all the same.[1]

[1] "Tonics and Sedatives," *Journal of the American Medical Association.*

THERE are times when everyone needs a doctor. One may postpone calling him as long as possible but sooner or later his services become indispensable.

For minor or imaginary illnesses any sort of medical service may seem satisfactory, but when major illnesses occur everybody wants the best. This is as it should be, but it is frequently more important to have expert service for minor conditions and for periodic health examinations. The diagnosis of tuberculosis, cancer, and other diseases is easy after they become advanced but by that time even the best of care is usually unavailing. Of far greater value is the recognition of these conditions when they are just beginning. At this stage diagnosis is difficult, but it is the time when most can be done for the patient.

Scientific Medicine

Scientific medicine is built not upon unproved theory or untenable hypothesis but upon careful observation and research. The admonition of the ancient Greek physician Hippocrates to his pupils "to observe and record for mankind" has been followed through the ages. From time to time theories have been propounded to explain observed phenomena, but each one has been thoroughly tested and tried, and any found wanting has been discarded.

Concerning the development of medicine Oliver Wendell Holmes wrote that "medicine learned from a monk how to use antimony, from a Jesuit how to cure ague, from a friar how to cut for stone, from a soldier how to treat gout, from a sailor how to keep off scurvy, from a postmaster how to sound the Eustachian tube, from a dairy maid how to prevent smallpox, and from an old market woman how to catch the itch-insect. It borrowed acupuncture and the moxa from the Japanese heathen, and was taught the use of lobelia by the American savage."[2]

The progress made in scientific medicine during the past century has exceeded that of all earlier time. Patient research and brilliant observation have unraveled the mysteries of one disease

[2] Fishbein, Morris, *Proceedings of the Staff Meeting of the Mayo Clinic*, October 14, 1936.

after another and have pointed the way to their prevention and cure. Much that seemed impossible has been achieved. But the end is not yet, for research and investigation are being carried forward as never before. New discoveries, observations, conclusions, and techniques are constantly being presented to physicians in order that they may deal more effectively with the health problems of mankind.

Charlatans and quacks maintain that the medical profession is unsympathetic to new ideas, new forms of treatment, and new discoveries. Nothing could be farther from the truth, as is evidenced by the ready acceptance of insulin for diabetes, liver therapy for pernicious anemia, Cortisone and ACTH for rheumatism, and the antibiotics for various infections. On the other hand, the public would be in a sorry plight if physicians adopted every proposal which is made in the name of health. Medical science has never been static. Physicians are more than willing to use any form of treatment that will benefit their patients. All that they ask is reasonable evidence that the treatment is safe and has real merit.

The training of physicians is carried on primarily in the great universities of the country, some of which are privately endowed, others state supported. This is particularly notable in view of the fact that all the schools for the training of the practitioners of the healing cults are without university affiliation.

Approximately forty years ago there were 162 medical schools and 5,750 medical graduates annually in this country. Most of these schools were privately owned proprietary institutions with no support other than the fees paid by students. A few were good, some indifferent, and many poor. Realizing that inferior medical schools and inadequately trained physicians are a hazard to the public health, the Council on Medical Education of the American Medical Association requested the Carnegie Foundation to make a survey of medical education. On the basis of this survey standards of an acceptable medical school were formulated and individual schools rated. Soon after this, individual states began to require that to be eligible for licensure to practice medicine physicians had to be graduates of "approved" medical schools.

The result was closure of practically all the inferior schools—until now there are in this country only approved medical schools, 78 complete schools and 7 schools of the basic medical sciences (these schools offer the first two years of the medical course, the students transferring to other schools for their last two or "clinical" years).

Although there are only half as many medical schools in this country today as there were forty years ago, the annual number of medical graduates, after dropping to approximately 2,500 in 1922, gradually increased to 6,400 in 1953. This is almost 50 per cent more than the number of physicians who die each year and represents an annual net increase of 2,000 physicians for the country as a whole.

Practically all medical schools require three or four years of premedical college training as a prerequisite for admission, and 98 per cent of the students admitted to medical schools in 1953 had completed three or more years of college work. The purpose of premedical requirements is to provide medical students with a sound foundation in the sciences on which medicine is based, a familiarity with the social sciences concerned with human relationships, and an acquaintance with other fields of knowledge which contribute to a liberal education. In recent years the number of applicants for admission to medical schools has been several times the number of students accepted. The result has been that only students with superior qualifications have been admitted to accredited medical schools. This in turn means better physicians for the country.

It is not enough, however, for a physician to have a good medical education and hospital training before starting practice. In these days of rapid advances in medical knowledge, he will be hopelessly behind the times in a few years unless he is able to keep abreast of progress. A physician does this in various ways. He reads medical books and journals. He attends medical meetings and postgraduate courses. In addition, an alert physician learns from every patient. To him each one is a problem for special study and research, and he soon learns that no two are exactly alike. He learns also by consultations with other physicians, by observing operations upon his patients, and by post-mortem examinations of those who die.

Some persons are reluctant to request or even to permit post-mortem medical examinations[3] on their relatives. This shows a lack of understanding of the purpose and value of medical examinations. Physicians are able to practice better medicine because of what they learn from post-mortem examinations. Occasionally, a medical discovery, such as insulin, of value to millions of persons, grows out of observations made in connection with such examinations. Abraham Lincoln in his Gettysburg address expressed the hope that "these dead shall not have died in vain." This same statement could well be applied to post-mortem examinations; one's death is not in vain if it contributes to the life and health of others.

Choosing a Physician

The casual way in which most people go about the selection of a physician to act as personal or family health adviser suggests that they little appreciate the importance of this choice.

The standards of training for physicians and the ideals of service set up by the medical profession are of the very highest, but, after all, physicians are only human and so practice their profession with various attitudes and various degrees of proficiency. Against incompetent and dishonest physicians, medical licensing boards of the various states are providing the public with considerable protection. Before one is licensed to practice medicine one must present evidence of graduation from an approved medical school, of good moral character, and, in most states, of hospital experience. Then one must pass examinations in the various branches of fundamental science and medical practice. Another safeguard is set up by the county medical society, which has its own qualifications for admission and occasionally refuses membership to a physician, even though he be licensed to practice in the state.

In small communities, where everybody knows everybody else, the choosing of a physician is rarely difficult. But in larger cities

[3] Also called "autopsies."

[471]

there are many general practitioners and specialists about whom one knows little or nothing. It then becomes a problem to know how a wise choice may be made.

Several years ago a letter was sent to the deans of the leading medical schools of this country asking them how they would advise a person who was new in a community to select a competent physician. Some of the deans replied that there is no way in which this can be done, but others made interesting suggestions. Among these was that one should ask the superintendent of a leading hospital for recommendations. This is sound advice, for the better hospitals choose carefully the physicians on their staffs; hence, one would be quite certain to get a competent physician if one made a selection from this group. Another suggestion was that one get a list of physicians from the secretary of the county medical society, with the school from which each graduated, his hospital experience, postgraduate training, and length of time in practice. Another suggested that one ask one's friends what physician they would call if their own doctors were not available. Such recommendation would be free from the element of personal friendship which so frequently exists between patient and physician. Still another suggested that one inquire as to who takes care of certain doctors' families when they are ill. Physicians rarely care for members of their own families for fear that personal concern and anxiety may interfere with sound medical judgment. That same anxiety, however, leads to the careful selection of another physician to assume this responsibility.

If there is a medical school in the community or even in the state, an inquiry addressed to the dean should result in helpful suggestions. Or if one who already has a trustworthy physician is moving to a new community, he can ask his physician to make inquiries as to whom he should select in the place to which he is moving.

The size of a physician's practice is not always a dependable criterion of his medical ability; for personality, self-confidence, salesmanship, and similar qualities may enable a mediocre physician to build up a big practice. In general, however, ability is rewarded in the practice of medicine just as in other fields of human endeavor. One possible objection to the selection of a physician with a large practice is that he may be too busy to give adequate time to the minor illnesses and health problems of those who are in reasonably good health. Neither is the doctor who "puts on the best show" or makes the most positive diagnoses always the safest physician. The charlatan specializes in impressing his patients with ceremony, x-rays, and other scientific-looking equipment and is never in doubt about a diagnosis.

Additional informal standards by which the physician can be judged include lack of advertising on the part of the physician of his name, specialty, methods, cures, or low fees in any commercial way; the dignity, sobriety, and modesty with which he conducts himself before his patients; the neatness and cleanliness of his office and of his person; the efficiency with which he keeps his case records, and the amount of respect he receives from other doctors.

A good doctor will not charge you too much. . . . Always ask the doctor his fees for any medical care he proposes to give you and always tell him your financial status. Doctor's fees are more or less standardized according to the patient's income, and the best is not likely to charge you more than the worst for a given treatment or operation. . . .[4]

The General Practitioner. The good old general practitioner, who diagnosed all of the family ills, brought the children into the world, pulled grandfather and the babies through pneumonia and father through typhoid fever, removed tonsils and appendixes, and served as veterinarian, priest, and mailman, belongs to a past generation. Medical science has advanced too rapidly and too far for one man to be proficient in all fields. This has led inevitably to specialization in medical practice.

This does not mean that the family physician is an institution of the past. On the contrary, in this age of specialization the need for a family health adviser is greater than ever before. This modern family physician, however, no longer attempts to do everything himself. He knows his patients, provides most of the medical care they need, and advises the services of specialists when necessary. Such is the family physician of today and tomorrow.

Specialists. Specialization in the practice of medicine has been developed to such a degree that it is becoming confusing to

[4] Williams, Greer, "How One Should Select a Physician," *Hygeia*, June, 1942.

physicians as well as to laymen. A few years ago we had the surgeon and the internist. Then the obstetrician, the pediatrician, the orthopedist, the dermatologist, the neurologist, the gynecologist, the urologist, the oculist, the rhinologist, the otologist, the laryngologist, and the psychiatrist made their appearance. But even this was not the end, for we have in addition the roentgenologist, the gastroenterologist, the proctologist, the bronchoscopist, and specialists in tuberculosis, diabetes, blood diseases, metabolic diseases, and the diseases of internal secretion; and surgeons who specialize upon the brain, the chest, the bones, and upon children.

Such an array of queer names seems bizarre, but for each of these specialists there is adequate justification. The more a physician concentrates his attention upon one particular system of the body or upon one diagnostic or therapeutic procedure, the more proficient he will become in that field. For the broad specialties of internal medicine, surgery, obstetrics and gynecology, pediatrics, and diseases of the eye, ear, nose, and throat there is frequent need. The services of the others are less frequently necessary, but the skill of the highly specialized bronchoscopist or brain surgeon occasionally means the difference between life and death.

But when should one go to a specialist and how is one to know which specialist can best render the service needed? On these points the family physician can give valuable advice. Many conditions for which patients go directly to specialists could be treated just as satisfactorily and in some cases more satisfactorily by the family physician. The specialist makes an invaluable contribution to the health of the community, but one needs advice as to when and how best to utilize his expert service.

The services which specialists are called upon to render make it obvious that special training and experience are necessary, and it is important for the patient that the specialist whom he selects be thoroughly competent in his special field. State licensing boards do not set up specific requirements for practice of the specialties of medicine, but physicians in the various specialties are doing so themselves. In general three to five years of special graduate study and actual experience in an approved institution are required in order to qualify for the rigorous examinations by the specialty boards. The physician who meets all of the requirements is granted a certificate by the board before which he has qualified, such as the American Board of Ophthalmology, of Surgery, of Obstetrics and Gynecology, of Internal Medicine, of Urology, and of Roentgenology. One can be certain that a physician who possesses a certificate of one of these boards is thoroughly qualified for the practice of that particular specialty.

Clinics. Physicians in various parts of the country are grouping themselves together into clinics in order to practice medicine on a cooperative basis. These clinics usually contain physicians in general medicine as well as surgeons, pediatricians, obstetricians, nose and throat specialists, etc. By frequent consultations and the pooling of laboratory and x-ray facilities the group hopes to provide better service than the patient would ordinarily receive if these same physicians were practicing independently.

There are clinics to which I would be perfectly willing to send members of my family for medical care, even if I were not acquainted with any of the physicians in them. This is because I know that the quality of service which they render is of the best and that no physician would be on the staff if he were not thoroughly competent. On the other hand, clinics are no better than the physicians of which they are composed, and there is a possibility that in the clinic type of organization personal interest in the patient may be submerged to efficiency in the functioning of the organization as a whole.

What to Expect from a Physician

Having selected a physician, what should one expect from him? In the first place, he should render careful, conscientious, interested service during illness, utilizing such facilities and obtaining such consultations as are necessary to arrive at a diagnosis and provide adequate treatment. In some diseases it is possible to make an accurate diagnosis upon first examination, but others require careful study and observation before the nature of the illness can be determined. In addition, he should

[475]

give advice on minor problems of health and illness. He should advise and administer vaccinations and immunizations of established value; and he should perform periodic examinations of each member of the family.

A noted specialist told me that he demands three things from his fellow physicians and surgeons in this order:

1. Honesty. Faith in one's doctor is often more important to recovery than the treatment he prescribes, but it is false security if the physician is dishonest in his claims, intent, diagnosis, treatment, or fees. . . .

2. Service. Careful examinations take time. You want a doctor who will give you enough attention to leave the smallest possible likelihood that he has missed some significant sign or symptom, as well as to relieve your psychologic anxieties.

3. Knowledge. When you see a physician, you want everything that is known in medical science about the detection, prevention, and cure of your ailment to be brought to bear on your case. Some might place knowledge first, but the specialist put it third because you cannot get the benefit of existing knowledge unless the physician is honest (keeps within the limits of scientific knowledge) and gives you service (allows himself to apply his knowledge). . . .[5]

With confidence in the physician of one's choice, the wisest procedure is to follow his advice concerning diagnostic and treatment measures. He will not perform miracles but will steer one on the best known course back to health. If one is not completely satisfied, a consultation may be requested; or if confidence is completely lacking, a change of physicians may be made.

All too frequently people take pride in boasting that they have not consulted a physician for 10 or for 20 years. The following letter, which appeared in "B. L. T.'s" column, is an illustration of this attitude:

Dear Alf:

Your letter came. Glad you bought a team of horses. Hilda is sick. She has diphtheria and she will die I think. Clara died this eve. She had it too. We are quarantined. 5 of Fishers family have got it. My wife is sick. She hasn't got it yet. If this thing gets worse we may have to get a doctor. Them trees are budding good. Everything is O.K.

                                                                              Dan.

As a result of procrastination, physicians are called upon chiefly to repair damage which has already been done. This is

[5] Williams, *loc. cit.*

unfortunate, for the most valuable service that physicians can render lies in the field of prevention. The physician of today has infinitely more to offer as a health adviser than did the traditional family doctor of the past. Given an opportunity in this capacity he will render the most distinguished service of all.

One hears complaints from time to time about difficulties in obtaining the services of a physician, particularly to make house calls and at night. Most of this could be avoided if people would select the physician of their choice and get acquainted with him before illness strikes. The physician would then know the patient and his family and would feel a special responsibility for their welfare. The response to a night call from a regular patient is quite different from that to a call from a total stranger.

Healing Cults

Irregular systems of medical practice exist in every land, but in no enlightened country do they find such ready acceptance as in the United States. Possibly this is because we have been following unbeaten paths to find material wealth in unexpected places and so are hopeful that we may discover the secret to health in a similar manner. Possibly it is because we like to gamble and dislike to face reality, or possibly it is because we believe in giving everybody a chance. At any rate we are the most credulous people in the world on medical matters.

The criterion of the healing cult is that it propounds a single theory as the explanation of disease and offers a single form of treatment for its cure. The ideas upon which cults are based are not developed by careful study or investigation but usually come as a vision to one with little or no training in biological science. Such phantasies occur to many people, but only occasionally are they put into practice by one who has the personality and good fortune to obtain a following.

Why Cults Flourish

Healing cults flourish when a considerable portion of the population lacks an understanding of the fundamental principles of health and disease. This does not necessarily imply an ignorant population, for many people who are intelligent and well informed on other subjects regard health as they regard life hereafter, a matter for conviction and belief rather than for study and investigation.

The reasons why the cults are able to hold patients and build reputations are several. One is that they promise a cure if the patient takes an adequate number of treatments. The number considered adequate is variable, but the duration is always sufficiently prolonged to give plenty of time for recovery. Most of man's illnesses are acute and self-limited, with recovery occurring in the natural course of events. For such recoveries during the course of treatments the cults take full credit.

Another reason for their success is that many persons who go from one doctor to another have nothing organically wrong. Their complaints may be very real but they are occasioned by emotional disturbances and made worse by the concentration upon them. Improvement in such cases frequently follows elaborate, mystical, and suggestive treatments which take the patient's mind off himself and his troubles. But this is only temporary and then the pathetic victim drifts on, groping blindly for some other miraculous cure.

During the Second World War, as in every war, many soldiers became partially paralyzed, unable to speak, to sleep, and occasionally even to hear and to see. Many such cases developed under terrific bombardment; hence, the condition was called "shell shock." Yet the same condition is sometimes found among recruits who have never heard a gun go off. Physical examinations reveal no organic disease, so it is frequently said that these individuals have nothing wrong with them, that they are merely malingering. This is far from the truth. The pain, the suffering, the paralysis are just as real as though they had been caused by shrapnel wounds. Fear, nature's instrument for protecting the individual from danger and destruction, can be just as overpowering as physical illness.

Under the conditions of private life the same mechanism operates to provide an escape from unpleasant situations or unwelcome responsibilities or to compensate for personal shortcomings and inferiorities. The neglected child is given attention and has its way when it is sick; the ineffectual parent dominates the family by illness. Indigestion or headache is produced by trying situations. If such reactions to emotional situations become habitual, real illnesses may develop on a purely functional basis. Such patients frequently are improved temporarily by any form of treatment which takes their minds off themselves and in which they have sufficient faith. In fact, it is with such cases that charlatans, by promising cures, obtain their most miraculous results. The psychiatrist, on the other hand, attempts to obtain more permanent improvement by recognizing the emotional problems involved and seeking to determine and remove their basic cause.

Other patients who, for a time, sing the praises of the cults are those with chronic illnesses which go through alternating periods of improvement and relapse. The physician, understanding the condition, may advise the patient that there is nothing that can be done for him. But the "cultist" in his ignorance is optimistic and when improvement occurs both he and the patient are jubilant. Relapse comes in due time; but this may occur after treatments have been discontinued, in which case arrangements for another series are hopefully made.

Still other cures obtained by irregular methods of treatment are cures of diseases which never existed. It is easy to cure a "pneumonia" which is nothing more than the grippe, or an "appendicitis" which is only indigestion. Most such incorrect diagnoses are made by cultists themselves who examine the patient, possibly even with the x-ray, and then announce that some serious condition exists. In so doing the cultist may be entirely sincere. He was told certain things during his training and, having no scientific or educational background for critical thinking or sound judgment, he accepts them unquestioningly and in all sincerity applies them in his practice.

Medical Quacks

The medical quack may be a physician, a practitioner of one of the cults, or may lay no claim to any sort of medical education whatsoever. His only purpose is to exploit human misery for personal gain. His technique may be to promote a dietary fad, sell reducing salts, give electrical treatments, or twist feet; or he may proclaim himself a "specialist" in cancer, in "diseases of men," or some other condition.

The quack usually claims to employ a secret form of treatment with which he obtains miraculous cures. This in itself should be a warning that his motive is selfish personal profit. Otherwise he would not keep his treatment secret but would publish his discovery, as is the custom of physicians and scientists, so that it might be utilized to relieve the suffering of mankind everywhere. But this he dare not do, for he knows that his methods will not stand the light of day, and that they are of value only to him and then only so long as they are kept secret.

A few years ago an extensive piece of quackery was perpetrated on the American public with the aid of a machine which was said to adjust radioactive waves of the body which were out of harmony, thereby giving rise to disease. Diagnosis and treatment consisted merely of turning some dials. These machines, which were supposed to cure everything, were sold or leased only on condition that they would not be opened. A few physicians fell for this racket, but its mysteriousness appealed particularly to the cults, by whom it was widely used and still is used to some extent.

An investigation of the machine by one of Mr. Ford's electrical engineers revealed only a storage battery, a few simple coils, a buzzer, and a meaningless jumble of wires. This "marvelous invention" was developed by a physician in California, who must have chuckled at the gullibility of human nature as a fortune came pouring in.

Self-medication

People have always had a blind faith in medicines, and until recently the more complicated and bad-tasting a medicine was, the better it was supposed to be. A home-doctor book of about a century and a half ago prescribed for vomiting a powder consisting of "crab's eyes, red coral, ivory, burnt hartshorn, cinnamon, and red saunders." To stop nosebleed it recommended, "take a dried toad, sew it up in a silk bag, and have it at the pit of the stomach a considerable time. This hath performed the cure when other medicines have failed."

Today we no longer use crab's eyes and dried toads but we waste millions of dollars on medicines and "health products" that are just as worthless as these primitive cure-alls. Actually, the amount of money spent in this country for self-medication is several times as much as that which is spent for drugs prescribed by physicians. The magazine called *Drug Topics* reports that the sale of "home medicaments" in 1947 amounted to $547,597,000. Nobody knows exactly what all this money is spent for, but probably the big advertisers get most of it. It is certain that the public gets little value from it.

The preparations used for self-medication vary enormously in content, purpose, and importance. Some are standard drugs of known composition, such as aspirin, soda, and Epsom salts, the use of which in general is safe and in some cases unobjectionable. Claims that aspirin will prevent or cure colds are unfounded, but it relieves pain and headache, lowers fever, and is somewhat sedative. On the other hand, even aspirin causes severe allergic reactions, such as asthma, rhinitis, and urticaria, in some people. Epsom salts is a good cathartic but should not be used regularly.

Antiseptics, such as tincture of iodine or merthiolate, for use on cuts and abrasions, have a proper place in the home medicine cabinet. So also has aspirin for headaches and a mild cathartic; but these and others which might be added should be selected and used according to the advice of one's physician.

Preparations of unknown composition with copyrighted names belong to a different category. Some are harmless but entirely worthless—just plain fakes. Others consist of standard drugs packaged to sell at fancy prices. Still others contain drugs that are actually dangerous, such as pyramidon (page 238) and the potentially toxic and habit-forming acetanilid found in certain headache and cold remedies.

Furthermore, it is important to realize that—except for the sulfonamides and the antibiotics in certain bacterial infections; chloroquine, primaquine, and quinine in malaria; emetine and arsenic in amebic dysentery; penicillin, bismuth, mercury, and arsenic in syphilis; chaulmoogra oil in leprosy; and antimony in certain tropical diseases—the drugs we use are not specific cures for disease but are of value because they control undesirable reactions, support some body function, or alleviate suffering. The physician who prescribes them does so for specific reasons in an individual case. One patient with abdominal cramps may be relieved by a cathartic, while another may suffer a ruptured appendix from the same treatment.

The following comments on the business side of the treatment of colds are indicative of the type of advice one may expect from the prescribing druggist when one turns to him with one's medical problems:

The best pharmacists do not prescribe for their patients. Physicians have maintained that the best interests of the patient demand that prescribing be done by medically trained persons only; the ethical pharmacist should limit himself to compounding and purveying. If anyone believes seriously that counter prescribing is not a standard trade practice in drug stores, attention should be called to an article in the November 1937 issue of the *American Druggist* under the title "A Billion Dollar Sneeze." This article presents many correct, pertinent and useful facts about colds, their infectiousness, the relation of metabolism and exposure to their occurrence, their cost, and what science knows about their prevention. Then tucked away at the end, next to advertisements of Adex Tablets and Smith Brothers' Cough Drops, are five steps to cold prevention by means of which the druggist is assured "your preventive products sales will increase." The first step is vitamins. "Science," it seems has proved "that the vitamin A and D content of these (fish liver) oils helps in the treatment of colds, the laity terminology being that they help build up the resistance." The Council on Pharmacy and Chemistry (of the American Medical Association) does not allow such claims, but the council is not a sales organization. The second step is a laxative! "The laxative treatment you recommend can be a 10 cent item or a $1.25 sale. . . ." The third step has to do with sales possibilities in nose drops, jellies, sprays and inhalants, and the fourth step cashes in on "any one of a number of mouth washes and gargles." In the fifth step the customer gets over on the alkaline side with milk of magnesia, antacid powders and tablets. And the climax:

"Clerks should be taught the practical advantage of solicitous inquiries about the customer's symptoms. Muscular pains, sore throat, headache, clogged nasal passages, chills, chest pains, and coughs each may be the basis

for the sale of a product over and above what the customer came in to buy
. . . get your share of this billion dollar business. . . . and you will make
money out of sneezes and sniffles in 1937–38 . . . Ah-choo."

So pharmacy à la the *American Druggist* is a science and a profession. The
science is salesmanship—but the profession is the practice of medicine. And for
practicing medicine the druggist needs a license in medicine.[6]

At least five patent medicine concerns have each paid more than a million
dollars a year for newspaper advertising. The radio has brought an entirely
new problem. The broadcasts reach an enormous audience. In 1935, the drug
manufacturers spent $15,986,507 on radio advertisements. That they can
afford to spend such vast sums shows the profits derived from the business.

We may be perfectly certain, as these lines are being read, that groups of
shrewd men, here and there around our fair land, are busy sharpening their
wits to try to find loopholes in the new Food, Drug, and Cosmetic Act that
will let them continue to thimblerig, bamboozle, dupe, dope, and poison innocent sufferers, and make millions out of it.[7]

The principle of self-medication is unscientific and unsound,
as is well expressed by the maxim "He who hath himself for a
doctor, hath a fool for a patient."

DISCUSSION SUGGESTIONS

1. What is meant by modern scientific medicine?
2. Discuss the advantages and disadvantages of medical practice on a
   private-patient basis.
3. Discuss the advantages and disadvantages of the systems of socialized
   medical practice in operation in certain European countries.
4. What factors should be taken into consideration in choosing a physician?
5. If you were moving to a new community, how would you select a competent physician?
6. Discuss the function of the general practitioner and of the specialist.
7. What are the advantages and disadvantages of medical clinics?
8. What is reasonable and what unreasonable to expect of a physician?
9. What is meant by "healing cults"?
10. Discuss the basic theories of the major cults in this country.
11. Explain why cults flourish.
12. Discuss the hazards of self-medication and of the widespread advertising
    by "patent medicine" companies.

[6] "Current Comment: Why Druggists Prescribe," *Journal of the American Medical
Association*, vol. 110, p. 290, January 22, 1938.

[7] Editorial, "Patent Medicines and Advertisers," *American Journal of Public Health*,
vol. 28, pp. 1332–1333, November, 1928.

13. What medicines would you select for inclusion in your family medicine cabinet? Why?

REFERENCES AND READING SUGGESTIONS

1. De Kruif, Paul: "Introducing the Personal Physician," *Today's Health*, March, 1953.
2. Dorin, D. M.: "Patient Doing Fine: Know Your Doctor and Your Hospital," Vantage Press, Inc., New York, 1951.
3. Fabricant, N. D.: "Why We Became Doctors," Grune & Stratton, Inc., New York, 1954.
4. Haggard, H. W.: "Devils, Drugs and Doctors," Harper & Brothers, New York, 1929.
5. Health and Welfare Division: "12 American Health Heroes," Metropolitan Life Insurance Company, New York.
6. Janet, Pierre: "Psychological Healing, A Historical and Clinical Study," The Macmillan Company, New York, 1925.
7. Miller, Benjamin F.: "You and Your Doctor," McGraw-Hill Book Company, Inc., New York, 1948.
8. Moon, G. R.: "How to Become a Doctor: A Complete Guide to the Study of Medicine, Dentistry, Pharmacy, Veterinary Medicine, Occupational Therapy, Chiropody and Foot Surgery, Optometry, Hospital Administration, Medical Illustration and Other Services," 2d ed., The Blakiston Company, New York, 1950.
9. Smith, Austin: "The Drugs You Use," Revere Publishing Company, New York, 1948.
10. Solomon, Charles: "The Traffic in Health," Navarre Publishing Company, New York, 1937.
11. Spencer, Steven M.: "Wonders of Modern Medicine," McGraw-Hill Book Company, New York, 1953.
12. Thomson, Morton: "Not as a Stranger," Charles Scribner's Sons, New York, 1954.
13. Williams, Harley: "The Healing Touch," Charles C Thomas, Springfield, Ill., 1951.
14. "A Doctor for You," American Medical Association, Chicago, 1953.
15. "Is There a Future Doctor in Your House," *Today's Health*, September, 1953.
16. Woglom, William H.: "Discoverers for Medicine," Yale University Press, New Haven, Conn., 1949.

Chapter XXIII

COMMUNITY HEALTH

THE conditions of modern life make it impossible for the individual acting alone to provide for himself and his family either adequate protection against disease or the advantages of modern medical care.

The Eskimos, the early American Indians, the natives of Tibet, and people in other remote sections of the world were isolated for generations, but today few sections of the globe which are habitable to man are without some contact with the outside world. Such contact inevitably brings exposure to the communicable diseases of the rest of the world. Because of this the American Indians were decimated by the smallpox and tuberculosis of the white man; and whenever trading ships put Eskimo villages in contact with civilization epidemics of respiratory infections are likely to follow. In 1875 a sailing vessel brought measles to the Fiji Islands and in 4 months 40,000 of the 150,000 population died.

Life in urban communities and modern methods of transportation contribute enormously to the comforts and advantages of life, but they also bring with them health hazards which can be minimized only by group action. For this reason a discussion of healthful living would be incomplete without some consideration of community health problems and practices.

[485]

Looking Backward

The progress which civilization has made from primitive tribal life to the modern society of our Western world has been dependent in large measure upon man's ability to prevent and control the diseases which always before had taken a terrific toll of life and lowered the vitality of those who remained.

It is almost impossible today to believe that for many centuries man existed under conditions in which it was accepted that more than half of the children born would die in infancy; that fever (infection) after childbirth was considered normal; that diseases such as smallpox, typhoid fever, tuberculosis, venereal diseases, and even leprosy were present in every community and in almost every household; that body discharges and other wastes were scattered broadcast; and that periodically major epidemic diseases, such as plague, cholera, and yellow fever, would wipe out a large percentage of the population.

Progress in the control of these diseases was slow until about a hundred years ago. Only after the cause and the method of spread of a disease is determined can specific measures for its prevention be developed. The discovery by Louis Pasteur about seventy-five years ago that microscopic forms of life called microorganisms or "germs" cause disease was the first solid foundation upon which scientific control measures could be based.

Many centuries before this, occasional keen observers had noticed the apparent relationship of diseases to certain practices and situations. They noted that people who associated with persons ill of certain diseases frequently contracted these diseases; also that certain diseases seemed to be related to food or to drinking water. These observations led to the formulation of certain health rules or codes, such as one finds in the early Mosaic law; to the emphasis of the Greeks upon cleanliness and clean living; and to the efforts of certain cities to provide pure mountain water for their people.

Also before the work of Pasteur, which represents the beginning of the era of scientific disease control, Dr. Edward Jenner, by careful observation and thoughtful experiment, developed

[486]

vaccination against smallpox and proved its value for the prevention of this dread disease (page 265).

With the development of effective methods for disease control, intelligent and responsible citizens began to ask how the public could benefit by these discoveries. Some things the individual could do for himself; others required group action.

Group Action for Health

Among the more important health services which can be provided only by group action are the control of communicable diseases, the provision of adequate and safe water supplies, the sanitary supervision of milk and other foods, waste disposal, school health services, industrial hygiene, hospitalization, and medical, dental, and nursing education. Most of these subjects have already been discussed from the viewpoint of the individual. The remaining chapters of this book will consider them from the point of view of the community.

In addition to the specific health services listed above, experience has demonstrated that group action can be helpful in other ways. Among these are the conduct of health education and the dissemination of health information; the provision of clinic services for prospective mothers and for infants; the development of rehabilitation services for the physically handicapped; and the organization of special programs to combat major health problems such as accidents, mental illnesses, cancer, and heart disease.

Health Education

Scientific medical progress contributes little or nothing to better health until it is utilized for the benefit of the individual. Unfortunately, as Dr. William H. Welch has said, the application of scientific discoveries is discouragingly slow:

When a Koch discovers the tubercle bacillus, a Banting discovers insulin for the relief of diabetes, or a Von Behring an antitoxin for the cure of diphtheria, or a Park demonstrates the value of the toxin-antitoxin for the prevention of diphtheria, the world draws a long breath as if saying to itself, "Now we are rid of that terror which has haunted the human race for centuries." It then straightway forgets and goes on its way comfortably assuming that of course the great discovery, or invention, is being carried into effect.

The actual facts are quite different. A few people, those of unusual initiative, or ample means, or who happen to be under the care of exceptionally alert physicians, or within the jurisdiction of exceptionally competent health officers, receive the benefits of the new discoveries; but the great mass of the human race goes on as before, and the death rate from these diseases is reduced slowly and over long periods of time.

In fact, the health field has a woefully ineffective distribution service, as compared with the laboratories of the world. We know how to do a lot of things which we do not do, or do on a wretchedly small scale. Few of the great discoveries of preventive medicine, except the prevention of yellow fever are anywhere nearly fully applied.

Medical schools, medical societies, and medical journals keep physicians abreast of medical progress but only as the individual citizen becomes intelligently interested in and accurately informed about health matters, and then does something about them, will real progress be made.

It makes no difference how good a vaccine we have against smallpox or diphtheria, if parents do not have it given to their children. It makes little difference how skillful a surgeon is, if the patient does not come to him until after an appendix has ruptured or a cancer has spread to other parts of the body. It makes no difference how effectively pasteurization destroys the disease-producing organisms in milk, if people persist in using raw milk. It makes no difference how safe sanitary engineers can make water supplies, if we do not insist that our governing bodies pass the legislation and make the appropriations necessary to apply these engineering developments to the water supplies of our individual communities.

Health information is something people always get. Unfortunately, much of what they get "just ain't so." Such misinformation may come from well-meaning friends or neighbors or from advertisers or promoters with something to sell. To counteract this and to provide the public with sound information on health matters, health agencies and organizations are devoting an increasing amount of time and effort to health education. This reaches the public through magazine and newspaper articles; through special magazines, such as *Today's Health*[1] and *The Child;*[2] through motion pictures and radio; and through special pamphlets and bulletins published and distributed, mostly free of charge, by state and city health departments, by the U.S. Public Health Service, the U.S. Children's Bureau, the American Medical Association, life insurance companies, and such national organizations as the American Cancer Society, the National Tuberculosis Association, the American Heart Association, the National Foundation for Infantile Paralysis, the American Red Cross, the National Committee for Mental Hygiene, etc.[3]

Maternal and Infant Health

The health of mothers and infants is of such great importance that both the Federal Government and the individual states have special bureaus or departments devoted to the health problems of these two groups. In Chapter XX we have analyzed these problems in considerable detail.

Few medical conditions are so surrounded with ignorance and superstition as childbirth. In fact, ignorance is responsible for a large proportion of both maternal and infant deaths. Group action in the interest of maternal health therefore is largely educational.

Instruction as to how to improve the health of mother and child and how to minimize the potential dangers of childbirth and infancy is offered by health departments, by the U.S. Children's Bureau, and by other health agencies in the form of special pamphlets, bulletins, and monthly letters. To be most effective these materials should be supplemented by personal instruction and medical supervision. This is usually and preferably given by one's private physician; but public health nurses, special classes, and community clinics for mothers and children render invaluable service to those unable to afford private physicians. Infant welfare clinics frequently offer not only instruction

[1] Published by the American Medical Association, Chicago, Ill.

[2] Published by the U.S. Children's Bureau, Department of Health, Education and Welfare, Washington, D.C.

[3] The addresses of these organizations as well as the names and addresses of others which publish various types of health pamphlets can be obtained from the National Health Council, 1790 Broadway, New York 19, N.Y.

on child care and nutrition but also physical examinations and immunizations.

Another important service rendered by health departments is the collection and analysis of data concerning births and deaths. These data show whether the maternal mortality rate and the infant death rate are increasing or decreasing, how these rates compare with those of other communities, and what the specific causes of the deaths are. Certain health departments make a special investigation as to the cause of every maternal death and try to decide whether it might have been prevented and, if so, how. They then use this information as the basis of a program for the improvement of maternal health in the community.

In 1930 there were in the country about 70 maternal deaths for every 10,000 live births. By 1952 this rate was reduced to 6.6 per 10,000 live births. This meant at least 23,000 fewer deaths of women from causes associated with childbearing in the United States than would have occurred if the rate of 1930 had continued to the present time. Stated another way, the dangers of death from these causes are today only about one-tenth as high as they were two decades ago. This is splendid improvement, but the fact that 15 states had rates of less than 6 and at least one state had a rate of 2.4 per 10,000 live births is evidence that still more lives can be saved by individual and group effort.

Infant death rates also have been reduced from approximately 100 per 1,000 live births in 1915 to 29 per 1,000 live births in 1952. The factors responsible for this have been better medical service, improved sanitation, particularly of milk and other infant foods; the control of communicable diseases, and the instruction of mothers in the better care of children. Group action has provided education, well-baby clinics, improved sanitation, and the control of communicable diseases. Further improvement will depend upon the expansion of these public health services, particularly into rural areas.

Mental Health Programs

After years or even centuries of neglect, the colossal problem of mental illness is finally beginning to receive the attention that

[490   ]

it must have if society is to avoid being continuously and increasingly burdened by it. In 1952 there were in this country more than 800,000 hospitalized victims of mental disease, and the estimated cost of mental illness in this one year alone, exclusive of the loss in wages and productivity, approached $1,000,000,000. Even so, there are probably ten times as many persons in need of treatment for mental illnesses outside of hospitals as there are in them. And expenditures for care of patients in most mental hospitals are so pitifully inadequate that many patients stay on and on who with proper treatment might be returned to their homes to lead useful lives in the community.

In the past mental illness has been considered such a private and personal problem that all the public attempted to do about it was to provide hospitalization for those who could not be cared for in any other way. However, the mushrooming demand for hospitalization for the mentally ill is finally causing responsible citizens to ask whether there is not something that society can do to prevent or to cure it.

The answer is definitely in the affirmative. By group action we can accomplish four things:

1. We can bring about the cure or improvement of a much larger proportion of the patients with mental illnesses. This will mean shorter hospitalization, less need for hospital beds, and the return of large numbers of people from a parasitic existence to productive life. To accomplish this we need more psychiatrists and more and better-trained auxiliary personnel for the treatment of mental patients, more attractive employment opportunities for the personnel, and better hospital and outpatient-clinic facilities for the treatment of persons with mental illnesses.

2. We can reduce the number of persons who need to be hospitalized for mental ailments. Many persons who by their associates are considered normal suffer emotional instabilities and sensitivities that interfere with their work and their happiness. Such persons seldom need hospitalization but they do need psychiatric treatment. Yet little is being done for them. This is unfortunate because, if mild cases are neglected, they tend to become worse. Furthermore, unhealthy emotional and behavior

[491]

patterns frequently become the basis for mental illnesses in later life. So, to keep more people out of mental hospitals, we need treatment facilities for persons with mild mental illnesses; we need more education for parenthood, more teachers, school counselors, and probation officers trained to recognize mental disturbances; we need special facilities for retarded children in public schools; more psychiatric services to assist juvenile courts in dealing with offenders, more clinics for the psychiatric care and treatment of serious behavior-problem children, and separate mental hospitals for children requiring hospital treatment.

3. We can push forward the search into the causes, effects, prevention, and treatment of mental illnesses. This will require increased appropriations by governmental bodies for the support of research. Any contribution to our knowledge about mental illnesses is worth many millions of dollars; yet appropriations for the study of these illnesses have been distressingly hard to obtain and woefully inadequate.

4. We can inform the people generally, and particularly parents, about the basic principles of mental health and the prevention of mental illnesses. Many of the unhealthy emotional habits of children could be prevented by understanding on the part of parents.

Nutrition

America has long been considered such a land of plenty that only in recent years has nutrition been a matter for public concern. In fact it is shocking to read the conclusions of a recent nutritional survey by the U.S. Public Health Service which states that the diets of 20 per cent of American families cannot be rated as better than poor by accepted nutritional standards.

During the Second World War foods were scarce and the vitality of the nation became of paramount importance, and a federal commission, the Food and Nutrition Board, was established. This board recommended the enrichment of flour to improve nutrition and the establishment of food-rationing policies to provide a reasonably adequate and balanced diet for everyone. The result was a general improvement in nutrition.

Group action for better nutrition can be effective in several ways. It can provide warm, nutritious school lunches. For some children this is the best meal of the day; for practically all, it is far better than the lunches they carry with them. Group action can be effective also in securing legislation that is in the interest of better food and nutrition. And, most important of all, group action can provide the information which every mother needs concerning the nutritional requirements of her family and how to meet them. Bulletins and pamphlets prepared by the Bureau of Human Nutrition and Home Economics of the U.S. Department of Agriculture provide valuable and practical information as to how one can plan nutritionally adequate meals on various income budgets.

Accidents

The great importance of accidents as a public health problem was presented in a new way recently by an analysis of the number of working years lost by death from the leading causes of death. This analysis is based on the assumption that the working years for the average person are from the age of 20 to the age of 65. The results (Table 28) show that accidents take a greater toll of working years than any other cause of death except heart disease.

Group action for the reduction of accidents includes the passage and enforcement of laws that are in the interest of safety; the provision of conditions on the highway and in industry that will reduce accident hazards, and the education of children and adults alike in safe habits and practices. Schools can contribute to safety education by providing instruction in driving for teenage boys and girls and by directing safety surveys of the school buildings of the community and particularly of the homes in which the children live. Industry has a great responsibility to provide instruction for employees in safety practices. Health departments and other community agencies could profitably take a much more active part than they have in the past in reducing the tragic and increasing toll of life and of health which accidents are taking in this country.

[493]

TABLE 28

TOTAL WORKING YEARS LOST BY WHITE MALES AND WHITE FEMALES AS RESULT
OF PREMATURE DEATHS FROM CERTAIN CAUSES, 1952

Disease	Deaths	Average Working Years Lost per Death	Total Working Years Lost
Male:			
Heart disease........	498,000	4.1	2,041,800
Cancer.............	105,130	4.8	504,624
Apoplexy...........	72,820	2.8	203,896
Accidents..........	58,970	19.9	1,173,503
Nephritis...........	8,880	4.3	43,516
	1,240		
Pneumonia..........	19,280	14.7	283,416
Tuberculosis........	12,740	14.7	187,278
Female:			
Heart disease........	296,890	3.0	896,670
Cancer.............	100,410	6.5	652,665
Apoplexy...........	76,350	2.7	206,145
Accidents..........	25,950	13.5	350,325
Nephritis...........	7,560	4.3	36,163
	950		
Pneumonia..........	13,980	15.6	218,088
Tuberculosis........	5,430	21.8	118,374

Rehabilitation of the Physically Handicapped

Estimates of the number of people in the United States with handicapping conditions of varying types and degrees of severity have ranged as high as 23 million. Some 8 million of these, who are so seriously disabled they cannot work or are employed on a part-time basis, are males of working age. Some have been blind, deaf, dumb, paralyzed, deformed, or otherwise crippled from birth. Others have handicaps resulting from accidents or war injuries. Still others—and by far the largest group—have disabling conditions arising out of disease.

During the Second World War, there were 17,000 amputations among members of the Armed Forces. During the same period of time, there were 120,000 major amputations among our civilian population.

Although many of these disabled people cannot be restored

through rehabilitation, the best available estimates indicate that about 2 million could be rehabilitated and returned to work. Probably an additional two to three times that number could be restored to the point where they would be able to move about and care for their personal needs, even though they could not enter employment. For the latter, being able to feed and wash themselves, use the bathroom, and get into and out of bed and chairs by themselves greatly lightens the family's burdens; it reduces the cost of nursing and attendant care; and gives to the individual hope, happiness, and self-respect where only gloom and despair existed.

The economic loss to society which these handicapped persons represent, as well as the financial burden of their care, is staggering. It is clearly not only a humanitarian service to provide rehabilitation, but also, for the community, it is a financial investment which yields enormous returns in increased production, reduced expenditures (public and private) for care, and an increase in federal, state, and municipal taxes paid.

The U.S. Office of Vocational Rehabilitation has demonstrated how rehabilitation pays off economically. Of the 61,308 persons rehabilitated during the fiscal year 1953, about three-fourths were unemployed at the time they were accepted for rehabilitation. Nearly 1 out of 5 (11,355) was receiving public assistance at the time services began or at some time during the course of rehabilitation. To maintain these disabled recipients of public assistance on relief for just one year would cost an estimated 8 million dollars. But the cost of their rehabilitation was only about 6.4 million dollars, or about four-fifths of what it would cost to maintain them at public expense for only one year.

It is estimated that the 61,308 persons rehabilitated during 1953 earned at an annual rate of 16 million dollars before rehabilitation compared with 112 million dollars after rehabilitation. The federal income tax payments which they will make are estimated at 10 million dollars a year. Thus the 30 million dollars in federal income taxes that they are expected to pay in the next three years exceeds the entire 1953 federal investment in the rehabilitation program by more than 30 per cent. Furthermore,

[495]

it has been estimated that over his work life a rehabilitated person will return $10 in federal income taxes for every $1 of federal funds invested in his rehabilitation.

This state-federal program of vocational rehabilitation is financed by both federal and state funds. It provides vocational counseling, medical services, job training, and placement as well as other services, depending on the disabled individual's requirements. While the Federal Government shares in financing the program, it is carried out by state agencies.

In addition, many nongovernmental organizations are helping with this work. The National Foundation for Infantile Paralysis has had a profound influence on the care of poliomyelitis victims in this country. The foundation has financed extensive medical care and rehabilitation services, has provided funds for a large-scale program of specialized training for physicians, therapists, medical social workers, and others, and has launched a program of financial support for schools and individuals in both undergraduate and graduate training. The National Society for Crippled Children and Adults, and its state and local affiliates, conduct a nationwide program providing various services for the physically handicapped. The Shrine builds and operates hospitals throughout the nation for the care of crippled children. In addition, local charitable organizations in many communities operate clinics for the physically handicapped and help them find suitable employment.

This is excellent as far as it goes, but unfortunately all these agencies together reach only a small proportion of the disabled persons who could be benefited by rehabilitation. The Office of Vocational Rehabilitation and the Bureau of the Census have developed estimates indicating that, in addition to the 2 million people who could be rehabilitated but are not being reached, some 250,000 become disabled each year and in need of rehabilitation services.

Clearly, therefore, rehabilitation programs need much greater support from both governmental and nongovernmental sources. Vigorous group action is needed to obtain this support and to see to it that rehabilitation centers are developed wherever they are needed.

Chronic Diseases

Heart disease, cancer, and other chronic diseases have long been recognized as leading causes of death and disability, but only recently have health departments attempted to do anything about them except to collect statistics concerning their frequency as causes of death. This was not due to any lack of interest in these diseases. Their importance was appreciated, but they were considered as personal health problems rather than as community responsibilities.

Fortunately, some physicians and laymen felt differently about it. They believed that certain things could be done about these diseases. Their interest and initiative led to the formation of the American Society for the Control of Cancer in 1913 and the American Heart Association in 1922.[4] Both these organizations now conduct nationwide campaigns for funds which they use for research and for educational work in the control of cancer and heart disease.

The Federal Government took its first official action concerning these diseases in 1937 when Congress created the National Cancer Institute as an integral part of the U.S. Public Health Service. By similar action Congress subsequently created the National Heart Institute, the National Institute for Neurological Diseases and Blindness, and the National Institute for Arthritis and Metabolic Diseases. These institutes now receive appropriations for the support of research and for the control of these diseases. Some of the funds appropriated are expended for work conducted directly by these institutes, but most of them are distributed to the individual states for the conduct of control programs and to medical schools and research institutes for research and teaching.

[4] The name of the American Society for the Control of Cancer was later changed to the American Cancer Society and the names of state organizations to State Division of the American Cancer Society.

Control programs are largely educational and are directed toward getting people to understand the nature of these diseases and the importance of securing proper medical care during their early stages when the chances of cure are greatest. Periodic medical examinations are urged as aids to early diagnosis.

Group action can be helpful in reducing these diseases by supporting voluntary campaigns for funds and by urging governmental appropriations for researches concerning their nature, prevention, and treatment. Sustained educational effort through group action will be helpful in reducing the disability and the lives lost unnecessarily from these diseases through ignorance or procrastination.

For patients with these chronic diseases who need institutional care adequate medical and nursing services can be provided through specialized hospital facilities and programs in a more satisfactory manner and at lower cost than is possible in general hospital wards or rooms. Most of these patients are not acutely ill and are therefore able to provide for themselves some self-care. This improves patient morale and reduces the nursing and auxiliary services required. In these days of high costs and shortages of hospital personnel this is exceedingly valuable, but important also is the happier situation for these patients who in cooperation with others in similar circumstances are doing something for themselves and for their associates. Community interest and planning can provide specialized institutions or, better still, special wards or wings of general hospitals for this type of service.

DISCUSSION SUGGESTIONS

1. How have changes in modes of life influenced health problems and made community action for health protection necessary?
2. Why is the work of Pasteur considered as the beginning of a new era in medicine and health?
3. What are the more important health services that can be provided only by means of group action?
4. Discuss the increasing importance of health education in future health programs.
5. How can the community reduce maternal and infant deaths?
6. What can be accomplished by group action in the field of mental health?

[498]

7. Discuss nutrition as a community health problem.
8. Outline a community program for accident prevention.
9. Why is rehabilitation of the physically handicapped considered of importance to the community?
10. Discuss cancer and heart disease as community health problems.

REFERENCES AND READING SUGGESTIONS

1. "All Their Powers," Health Information Foundation, New York, 1951.
2. Buell, Bradley, and Associates: "Community Planning for Human Services," Columbia University Press, New York, 1952.
3. Burney, L. E.: "Community Organization—an Effective Tool," and K. I. E. Macleod: "Working with Your Community," *American Journal of Public Health*, January, 1954.
4. Maisel, A. I.: "Your Neighbor's Health Is Your Business," Public Affairs Pamphlets, New York, 1953.
5. Norwood, W. D., P. H. Fugea, and R. R. Sacks: "Community Health Planning: Study of Atomic City (Richland, Wash.)," *Journal of the American Medical Association*, vol. 154, p. 44, January 2, 1954.
6. Patterson, Robert G.: "Foundations of Community Health," McGraw-Hill Book Company, New York, 1950.
7. Shepard, W. P., C. E. Smith, R. R. Beard, and L. B. Reynolds: "Essentials of Public Health," 2d ed., J. B. Lippincott Company, Philadelphia, 1952.
8. Smiley, D. F., and H. G. Gould: "Your Community's Health," The Macmillan Company, New York, 1952.
9. Yahraes, Herbert: "Something Can Be Done about Chronic Illness," Public Affairs Pamphlets, New York, 1952.
10. "A Doctor for Your Community," American Medical Association, Chicago, 1953.
11. Pamphlets and bulletins of the National Committee for Mental Hygiene, the American Cancer Society, the National Foundation for Infantile Paralysis, the American Heart Association, the U.S. Public Health Service, the Health Information Foundation, the National Tuberculosis Association, the National Health Council, etc. For addresses see page 590.
12. Health Resources Advisory Committee: "The Disabled Can Work," Office of Defense Mobilization, Washington.

Chapter XXIV

CONTROLLING
COMMUNICABLE DISEASES

MODERN science can point to no more brilliant achievement than its conquest of communicable diseases during the past half century. Had the death rates of 1900 prevailed in 1950, there would have been in the United States in that one year not 96 but 47,168 deaths from typhoid fever; not 8,352 but 210,825 deaths from enteritis and diarrheal diseases, mostly of children; not 410 but 60,731 deaths from diphtheria; not 35 but 14,467 deaths from scarlet fever; not 1,118 but 18,385 deaths from whooping cough; not 468 but 20,043 deaths from measles; and not 33,959 but 292,956 deaths from tuberculosis. This makes the astounding total of more than 600,000 lives saved in one year as a result of the reduction which has occurred since the beginning of the century in the death rates of these seven communicable diseases. And this saving of lives has been chiefly in the younger age groups which mean most to national strength and vitality.

Many diseases, which a generation ago struck fear into the hearts of parents in every community are little more than names to the youth of today. This represents almost unbelievable progress toward the goal of preventive medicine and public health. Yet in spite of it all, there is a distinct hazard in the current widespread feeling of security and lack of concern about these epidemic diseases. Sources of infection of these diseases are still present throughout the country, and, like a fire, they will spread

[500]

into a major conflagration if inflammable material exists and control measures are relaxed.

A communicable disease[1] is one which may be transmitted from one person or animal to another in any manner whatsoever. When such diseases occur singly they are said to be *sporadic;* when a communicable disease is present more or less continuously in a community or region it is said to be *endemic.* If it attacks large numbers of people in a community or region it is said to be *epidemic.* And, if it spreads over a large region or over the world, it is called *pandemic.*

Causes of Communicable Diseases. The communicable diseases are all caused by living microorganisms, commonly spoken of as "germs." Some of these microorganisms are bacteria, some viruses, some animal parasites, and some other types of living organisms. Most of the microorganisms which cause diseases of man have become adapted to living under the conditions that exist in the bodies of humans or of animals. Consequently, they are able to survive only a relatively short time outside the body, except when cultivated in the laboratory under conditions which approximate the conditions of the body.

Sources of Infection. Practically all communicable diseases, therefore, are contracted from human or animal sources. In fact, the greatest source of infection of man is some other person. This person may be one who is actually sick with the disease; or one who, although infected with the disease, has such a mild attack that it is not diagnosed, in which case he usually continues about his duties exposing others; or the source of infection may be one who has recently convalesced from the disease; or one who, although well, harbors the germs of disease in his body and scatters them about to infect others. This last type of individual is commonly called a "carrier."

For thousands of years, long before microorganisms were known to exist, there was some realization that persons who were in contact with patients ill with certain diseases were themselves likely to develop these diseases. Lepers have long been considered

[1] For outline of communicable disease control measures recommended by the American Public Health Association see Appendix D.

as outcasts. The book of Leviticus in the Old Testament outlines definite rituals for the purifying of the body after certain illnesses. In the Middle Ages the Venetians, observing that epidemics, particularly of bubonic plague, followed the arrival of ships from certain foreign ports, passed a law requiring that ships with cases of pestilence aboard be held in the harbor 40 (*quaranta*) days. From this we get the modern word "quarantine."

Routes of Dissemination. Infective germs are obviously of no danger to anyone else so long as they are retained within the body of the person who is a patient or carrier. It is the germs which get out of the body that cause the infection of others. The routes by which these germs escape from the body depend upon the portions of the body infected. Most common of all routes are the nose and mouth, the discharges from which are responsible for a large number of diseases and are most difficult to control. Among the more important of the diseases spread through the discharges of the nose and mouth are colds, influenza, pneumonia, tonsillitis, scarlet fever, diphtheria, measles, whooping cough, mumps, meningitis, tuberculosis, and leprosy.

Diseases disseminated through discharges of the intestinal tract are for the most part those which enter the body with the food and drink and localize primarily in the intestinal tract. Most important among these are typhoid fever, paratyphoid fever, dysentery (amebic and bacillary), cholera, hookworm, and other intestinal parasites.

Among the intestinal parasites hookworm differs from the others in that its usual portal of entry is through the pores of the skin between the toes. In this manner hookworm larvae get into the blood stream. By the blood they are carried to the lungs, but, being too large to pass through the tiny capillaries, they burrow through the thin membranes into the alveolar sacs; thence, they pass up through the bronchial tubes and trachea to the mouth to be carried with the saliva to the stomach and to the small intestine, where they set up the infection which is characteristic of the disease.

The venereal diseases are most commonly disseminated by discharges from the genital tract. Streptococci infections, in-

cluding scarlet fever, may be disseminated by the pus from infections which discharge to the surface of the skin or mucous membrane or from infected middle ears or sinuses. Trachoma and the
various types of conjunctivitis are disseminated by the infected
discharges from the eye. From infected areas of the skin itself
numerous diseases are contracted; most common among these
are boils, impetigo, pediculosis, scabies, and ringworm, one type
of which is called "athlete's foot."

Bloodsucking insects are responsible for the transmission of a
large group of diseases through the unbroken skin. These include
malaria, yellow fever, tularemia, and bubonic plague.

Principles of Prevention

The prevention of communicable diseases in general depends
upon three types of measures:

1. The prevention of the dissemination of infected material
from the person who is the source of infection. This involves
isolation, quarantine, and disinfection of bodily discharges and
objects which may have been contaminated.

2. The blocking of the usual routes of transmission of infected
material. This is the purpose of most of the measures of modern
sanitation, such as water purification, sewage disposal, pasteurization and sanitary handling of milk, use of individual drinking
cups, sterilization of dishes, glassware, and other eating utensils,
and washing of hands.

3. Immunization of the susceptible individuals. Artificial
immunization constitutes an important preventive measure
against certain diseases (Chapter XII).

Quarantine and Isolation

By definition of the American Public Health Association,
quarantine means "the limitation of freedom of movement of
persons or animals who have been exposed to communicable diseases for a period of time equal to the longest usual incubation
period of the disease to which they have been exposed." A similar
public health measure called "isolation" provides for "separating
of persons suffering from a communicable disease, or carriers of

[503]

the infective organism, from other persons in such places and under such conditions as will prevent the direct or indirect conveyance of the infectious agents to susceptible persons."

In practice both isolation and quarantine are frequently modified by the specific application of scientific knowledge concerning the diseases in question. For example, malaria and yellow fever are controlled by preventing people from being bitten by infected mosquitoes; a case of smallpox is of little or no danger in a thoroughly vaccinated community; bubonic plague is spread by fleas from infected rats; typhus fever by body lice or by rat fleas; Rocky Mountain spotted fever by wood ticks; etc. Intelligent isolation of patients with these diseases must take such basic facts into consideration.

Disinfection

Disinfection, strictly defined, is the destruction of all organisms and their products which are capable of producing disease, while *sterilization* is the destruction of all microorganisms, saprophytic as well as disease-producing. *Antiseptics* prevent the multiplication of microorganisms but do not destroy them. *Deodorants* destroy and neutralize unpleasant odors but many of these have no disinfecting powers. *Fumigation* is the use of fumes or gases to destroy microorganisms, vermin, or insects.

Disinfection may be accomplished by physical or chemical means. Physical methods of disinfection are chiefly dry heat, steam, boiling, drying, ultraviolet light, etc. Chemical disinfectants for the most part are applied in liquid form but may be gaseous.

The manner in which disinfectants destroy bacteria is through physical or chemical changes of the cell substance of the organisms; consequently *time* and temperature are important in all disinfection. Usually the stronger the solution the more quickly the disinfectant will act, but *none acts instantly*. The presence of organic and albuminous matter interferes seriously with the action of practically all disinfectants except chlorinated lime and potassium permanganate.

The relative efficiencies of the many disinfectant solutions on the market are usually expressed in terms of "phenol coefficients," which means their ability to destroy bacterial life in comparison to a 5 per cent solution of phenol. In general, disinfectants with phenol coefficients of less than 1 have relatively little value.

In connection with the care of patients with communicable diseases we speak of concurrent disinfection and terminal disinfection—*concurrent disinfection* pertaining to the disinfection of hands, clothing, linen, body discharges, food, drink, etc., during the period that the patient is in isolation, and *terminal disinfection* being that which is carried out upon completion of the case, either by recovery or by death. Of these two, concurrent disinfection is by far the more important, and upon its being carried out *to the minutest detail* will depend the effectiveness of isolation.

TECHNIQUE OF DISINFECTION

Although a wide variety of disinfectants may be satisfactory, the following are the most frequently used for the purposes specified:

For the hands and body, a 5 per cent solution of carbolic acid diluted with an equal amount of water or a 1 to 1,000 solution of bichloride of mercury. The hands or soiled portions of the body should be washed in one of these solutions, then washed with soap and water, and then immersed again in the solution.

Soiled linen, for example, towels, bedding, clothing, should be immersed immediately in 2½ per cent solution of carbolic acid in the sickroom and allowed to soak one or more hours.

Food from the sickroom should be burned. Liquids should be treated in the same manner as bodily discharges.

All *discharges* from nose, mouth, bowels, and bladder should be received into vessels containing a solution of carbolic acid (5 per cent) or milk of lime (1 quart of dry, freshly slacked lime to 4 or 5 quarts of water) of at least twice the volume of the discharge, or the discharges should be collected on pieces of cloth which are immediately burned or immersed in one of these solutions. After standing for an hour these discharges except feces may be thrown into the toilet. Feces are difficult to disinfect and must be allowed to stand in the above-mentioned solutions for 12 hours or thoroughly stirred in the solutions and allowed to stand for at least 1 hour. These special precautions for feces are necessary only in cases of typhoid fever, cholera, dysentery, and hookworm.

Sputum from consumptives is the source of infection the importance of which cannot be overestimated. It should be received into covered cups containing the carbolic acid or lime solution. Handkerchiefs soiled by sputum should be soaked in carbolic acid and then boiled.

Closets, sinks, etc. Discharges should not be emptied into closets until they have been thoroughly disinfected. A quart of carbolic solution should be allowed to remain in the pan. Sinks and closets should be flushed with disinfecting solution at least once daily.

Dishes, knives, forks, etc., used by the patient should be kept exclusively for him and not removed from the room. Before being taken from the room they should be washed first in the carbolic acid solution, then in boiling hot soapsuds, and finally rinsed in hot water.

The body, in case of death, should be completely wrapped in several thicknesses of cloth wrung out in the carbolic or bichloride solution. The body should be prepared for burial by a licensed embalmer only.

Terminal disinfection procedures in cases of communicable disease are:

1. Everything which is in the sickroom or has come in contact with the patient and is of no particular value (newspapers, magazines, paper, wooden or cloth toys, etc.) should be burned.

2. Before removal from patient's room washable clothing, sheets, etc., must be immersed in 5 per cent carbolic acid solution or be wrapped in a sheet or other suitable cover which is saturated with a 5 per cent carbolic acid solution. To complete the disinfection such clothing must remain in a 5 per cent carbolic acid solution for at least ½ hour or be boiled for ½ hour.

3. Certain not-too-thick articles presenting free surfaces, such as blankets, can be made safe by exposure in the open air to direct bright sunlight for a period of 4 or 5 days so that the actual exposure to the sun's rays shall be not less than 24 hours. Such articles as carpets and rugs treated in the same way should in addition be sponged and brushed with a 5 per cent solution of carbolic acid or a 1 to 1,000 solution of corrosive sublimate (bichloride of mercury).

Recent experiments show that sunlight and skylight will kill bacteria in 2 hours in the middle of the day. Even if windows are closed, bacteria will be destroyed if sunlight and skylight are allowed to enter. In order to give a sufficient margin of safety 4 or 5 days of sunlight and airing are usually recommended.

4. Thorough scrubbing of woodwork and wood and metal furnishings, etc., combined with disinfection through the use of 1 to 1,000 solution of corrosive sublimate, or a 5 per cent solution of carbolic acid, of doorknobs, open cracks and crevices, and such room furnishings as may come in direct contact with the patient, patient's discharges, or hands of patient's attendants may be relied upon to protect against reinfection from the room. At the discretion of the health officer, re-papering, painting, calcimining, etc., may be necessary.

Fumigation, although valuable in the destruction of vermin and insects, and in preventing the spread of insect-borne diseases, is unnecessary after the usual communicable diseases, provided that disinfection has been properly carried out.

Community Action

The control of communicable diseases is truly a teamwork job. Scientists make their contribution by searching for additional information that will be helpful in prevention or cure. Physicians, nurses, public health engineers, and other health workers apply this information to the practical problems of disease control. Individual citizens must provide the necessary cooperation and support for these efforts.

In the interest of effective teamwork, our Federal, state, and local governments have established health departments with responsibilities for communicable disease control. These departments receive reports from physicians concerning the communicable diseases occurring in the area and investigate those which seem to be of importance. For example, a report of a case of typhoid fever is immediately investigated to determine, if possible, where the patient got the infection, to appraise the possibility of others getting the infection either from the patient or from the same source from which he got it, and to outline a plan of control measures. This type of specialized service is called epidemiology.

As further aid in communicable disease control, most health departments provide bacteriological laboratory services to assist physicians in the diagnosis of communicable diseases. Many also provide vaccines for prevention and antitoxins or other serums for treatment. Health department physicians sometimes administer these vaccines, particularly for those unable to afford the services of private physicians. Health departments also inform the people about the prevalence and the seriousness of communicable diseases and about preventive measures that can be taken to avoid them. It is depressing to see the list of deaths, particularly of children, that would not have occurred if their parents had utilized the preventive measures that are available to all.

In other sections of this book (Chapters II, VII, XII, XIII, XXV, XXVI, XXVII, Appendix D) we have considered or will consider the more important of the communicable diseases. Two of these, however, seem to merit special mention at this point both because of their widespread importance and because a major national health organization is devoted to the control of each of them. These diseases are tuberculosis and the venereal diseases.

TUBERCULOSIS CONTROL

In 1900 tuberculosis caused over 200 deaths for every 100,000 of the population. In 1920 the rate was still over 100. Today it is about 16. This is such a splendid achievement that we are apt to forget that there are still about 500,000 active cases of tuberculosis in the United States; and that every day of the year more than 200 new cases are diagnosed and 70 persons die from tuberculosis in this land of ours. These deaths are said to be unnecessary because authorities believe that it is possible to virtually eliminate tuberculosis as a cause of death in our country within a generation. To accomplish this, well-coordinated and vigorous action both by individuals and by the community is necessary.

We have already considered the prevention of tuberculosis from the standpoint of the individual (pages 34 to 42). To be completely effective this program must be supplemented by community action along the following lines:

1. Diagnostic facilities and services must be provided so that the disease may be recognized early when the possibilities of cure are brightest and the danger of spreading the disease to others least. During the Second World War every individual who joined the armed forces had an x-ray examination of the chest before induction. This was the greatest case-finding program ever undertaken. The record of 1.2 hospital admissions for tuberculosis per 1,000 men in the Second World War as compared to 9.4 in the First World War could leave no doubt as to its value. Since the war, similar programs for the x-ray examination of whole communities—even up to half a million population, as in Minneapolis, Minnesota—have been shown to be practical. These programs have been organized and supported jointly by health departments and by local tuberculosis associations. Other diagnostic services are offered by school health services (page 546),

[508]

by community clinics, by private physicians, and by health department laboratories. Everyone who has been found by a tuberculin (Mantoux) test, by x-ray, or by other examination to have had a tuberculosis infection should have a chest x-ray and a physical examination at least twice a year. All persons over fifteen years of age should have a physical examination, including a chest x-ray or tuberculin test, once each year. A person who has special exposure to tuberculosis should be examined more frequently as his physician advises.

2. Whenever persons are discovered to have tuberculosis, epidemiologists should search for others whom they may have infected and for the source from which they contracted the disease. The name "family disease" is sometimes given to tuberculosis because it is spread mostly by close contact. This contact is frequently in the home, but it may be at school, in the factory, or in the office. For the protection of others, persons who are potential sources of infection must be discovered and isolated. To accomplish this, adequate local health departments are essential.

3. In some areas additional hospitals need to be provided for the care of patients with tuberculosis. Early hospitalization saves lives, shortens the period of disability, and prevents the infection of others. Hospitals should have adequate staffs and facilities. Patients should have access to hospital care reasonably near home. Rehabilitation services need to be provided in most institutions. Home-care programs must be under proper medical and nursing supervision.

4. Instruction concerning the cause, methods of spread, symptoms, early diagnosis, treatment, and prevention of tuberculosis must be carried even more effectively to all groups of the population. High infection rates are associated with ignorance and poverty. The National Tuberculosis Association and its 3,000 affiliates throughout the nation, supported by Christmas seal sales, are doing a magnificent job of informing people about tuberculosis, but there are still millions of people in this country who ignore symptoms and refuse treatment, thereby infecting others and reducing their own chances for recovery.

[509]

5. Research needs to be continued and expanded. We know a great deal concerning tuberculosis but we still do not have a satisfactory preventive or treatment. BCG vaccine for prevention and certain drugs for treatment (page 40) are helpful in certain situations, but neither is completely satisfactory. It is most important, therefore, that funds be provided for increased research for a uniformly effective vaccine and treatment for tuberculosis.

6. Improvement in standards of living means a reduction in tuberculosis. Poor housing, overcrowding, inadequate nutrition, all favor the spread of tuberculosis. Therefore, any campaign for the reduction of tuberculosis must be an integral part not only of a general community health program but also of a program to improve the social, economic, and educational levels of the population.

VENEREAL DISEASES

From the point of view of the scientist it should be possible to completely eradicate the venereal diseases. All of them—syphilis, gonorrhea, and chancroid (page 415)—are contracted, almost without exception, from intimate personal contact with an infected person. Such contacts can be avoided if one has the intelligence and the will to do so. In addition to knowledge as to how to prevent venereal disease, we now have available methods of treatment which, if properly utilized, will cure almost all of them. With such effective control measures available, it is a serious reflection upon our society that these diseases remain an important cause of death and disability in this country.

Control measures, well known to health officials, are handicapped by the strong biologic urge which often leads to exposure, by the complicated moral and social problems involved, and by the ignorance, misinformation, and "hush" attitude of a large part of the public about them. Prostitution, which is still tolerated in all too many communities, increases opportunities for infection of men, who in turn infect other women.

Group action for the control of the venereal diseases includes the following measures:

[510]

1. *Education.* Ignorance is an important factor in the spread of the venereal diseases, yet only a few years ago one was not permitted even to mention them over the radio or in "respectable" magazines. That situation has changed materially, but even yet health courses in the secondary schools rarely consider them, and a large proportion of adults have very fuzzy ideas about them. Effective programs for eradication of these diseases require widespread understanding of their importance and of the control measures applicable against them.

2. *Case finding.* Routine blood tests for syphilis were performed on all the men examined for the armed forces in the Second World War. These led to the discovery and treatment of more than 200,000 cases of syphilis. Similar routine blood testing is performed in many college physical examinations, in most prenatal examinations of pregnant women, and in many hospitals, clinics, and physicians' offices. Most patients with gonorrhea and chancroid and many with syphilis are first discovered when they go to see a physician because of symptoms.

3. *Contact finding.* Physicians who diagnose a venereal disease are required to make a report to the health department. It then becomes a problem in epidemiology to find the source from which the patient became infected and to search for others who may have been infected by him or by the source from which he got the infection. Such investigations frequently uncover a veritable chain of infections.

4. *Isolation of infective persons.* This is difficult but, if the spread of the infection is to be controlled, persons who are sources of infection must be isolated, either voluntarily or involuntarily, until they are no longer infectious.

5. *Treatment facilities.* Since effective methods of treatment are available, it is essential that persons with these diseases receive proper medical care and receive it early. Such treatment can be obtained from private physicians or reputable clinics. Since venereal.diseases are most prevalent among the lower social and economic groups, the maintenance of public clinics for treatment is essential. Otherwise these patients patronize advertising quacks or attempt to treat themselves with patent medicines.

[511]

6. *Reducing exposures.* Religious training, moral standards, self-respect, and respect for one's future life partner deter many young men and young women from exposing themselves to venereal infection. This can be further aided by group action for the elimination of prostitution and by the provision of desirable social and recreational facilities for young people. Complete eradication of the venereal diseases is not too high a goal for community action.

DISCUSSION SUGGESTIONS

1. Discuss the progress that has been made in the control of communicable diseases.
2. What individuals may disseminate to others the germs of communicable diseases?
3. Define quarantine; isolation.
4. List the major routes by which disease-producing germs leave the body and the more important diseases disseminated through each route.
5. Explain the manner in which the hookworm usually reaches the intestinal tract.
6. What are the general measures upon which the prevention of communicable diseases depends?
7. Define disinfection; concurrent disinfection; terminal disinfection; sterilization; antisepsis; fumigation.
8. What are the major methods of disinfection? What particular precautions must be observed in carrying out disinfection?
9. What are some dependable and inexpensive chemical disinfectants?
10. Of what practical value is fumigation?
11. Explain why community action for protection against communicable diseases is necessary.
12. Outline a community program for the prevention and control of tuberculosis.
13. Of what elements should a program for the control of the venereal diseases consist?

REFERENCES AND READING SUGGESTIONS

1. Anderson, Gaylord W., and Margaret G. Arnstein: "Communicable Disease Control," 3d ed., The Macmillan Company, New York, 1953.
2. Burnet, Macfarlane: "Natural History of Infectious Diseases," 2d ed., Cambridge University Press, New York, 1953.
3. Chadwick, Henry D., and Alton S. Pope: "Modern Attack on Tuberculosis," Commonwealth Fund, Division of Publication, New York, 1946.
4. Collins, S. D., and Josephine Lehmann: "Trends and Epidemics of

Influenza and Pneumonia, 1918–51," *Public Health Reports*, vol. 16, p. 1487, November 16, 1951.

5. Eberson, Frederick: "Microbes Militant; A Challenge to Man; The Story of Modern Preventive Medicine and Control of Communicable Diseases," The Ronald Press Company, New York, 1948.

6. Myers, J. A.: "Tuberculosis among Children and Adults," 3d ed., Charles C Thomas, Springfield, Ill., 1951.

7. Parran, Thomas: "Shadow on the Land," Reynal & Hitchcock, Inc., New York, 1937.

8. Smith, Geddes: "Plague on Us," Commonwealth Fund, Division of Publication, New York, 1941.

9. U.S. Public Health Service: "VD Fact Sheet," U.S. Department of Health, Education and Welfare, Washington, D.C., 1951.

10. Vonderlehr, R. A., and J. R. Heller: "The Control of Venereal Diseases," Reynal & Hitchcock, Inc., New York, 1946.

11. Winslow, C.-E. A.: "The Conquest of Epidemic Disease," Princeton University Press, Princeton, N.J., 1944.

12. Winslow, C.-E. A.: "Man and Epidemics," Princeton University Press, Princeton, N. J., 1952.

Chapter XXV

ANIMALS, INSECTS, AND DISEASE

WHEN we speak of animals, we usually think of those animals which range in size from mice to elephants. By definition, however, animals include all living things endowed with sensation and independent motion. The animals related to diseases of man are not only the larger animals, such as rats, rabbits, swine, cattle, goats, horses, etc., but also an extensive group of tiny animals known as arthropods. The arthropods include all small animals with articulated body and limbs, such as insects, spiders, ticks, mites, etc.

Larger animals are associated with disease of man primarily because man is susceptible to certain communicable diseases of these animals. The arthropods are important primarily because they serve as a means of transmission of disease-producing germs from man to man or from animal to man.

Animal Diseases Transmissible to Man

The more important of the animal diseases transmissible to man are brucellosis, bovine tuberculosis, trichinosis, rabies, tapeworm, plague, tularemia, anthrax, psittacosis, and equine encephalitis.

Brucellosis. Much the greatest menace among the animal-borne diseases in this country today is brucellosis—also known as undulant fever, Malta fever, Bang's disease, and contagious

[514]

abortion of cattle. In humans brucellosis is a prolonged debilitating disease with recurrent periods of fever.

Man becomes infected from cattle, swine, or goats; rarely, if ever, from humans. It is estimated that 5 per cent of the cattle of breeding age in this country have Bang's disease. Infection occurs from the use of raw (unpasteurized) milk or milk products or from contact with infected animal tissues or their secretions during butchering, working with infected animals, or handling infected meat.

Treatment of brucellosis has until recently been completely ineffective. Fortunately, however, some of the newer antibiotic drugs, notably aureomycin, are curing a large proportion of the patients with this disease.

Prevention depends upon the eradication of the infection among domestic animals (vaccination is helpful in accomplishing this); upon the pasteurization of all milk before drinking or before processing into milk products; and upon the use of rubber gloves and antiseptic measures in handling diseased or potentially diseased animals or their products. By observing these simple precautions some thirty or forty thousand people each year can avoid this infection which saps the vitality and produces prolonged invalidism and disability.

Bovine Tuberculosis. A generation ago children crippled from tuberculosis of the bones and carrying scars from tuberculosis of the lymph nodes were common sights. Today in this country both conditions are exceedingly rare. This is because these infections were produced by tuberculosis germs that cause the disease in cattle. Children contracted it by drinking raw milk from infected cattle.

The attack on bovine tuberculosis began about fifty years ago, when 10 to 50 per cent of the cattle in many sections of the country were infected. The incentive to eradicate tuberculosis was primarily an economic one. Cattle were tuberculin-tested and those found to be infected were killed. Some state legislatures even provided money to reimburse the owners of destroyed tuberculous cattle. In 1924 only very few counties in the United States could be certified by the U.S. Department of

Agriculture as having less than 0.5 per cent of their cattle infected. Today every county has been thus certified and in very few of them are there any infected animals at all. This remarkable achievement demonstrates what can be done by an all-out scientific attack upon a disease.

The eradication of tuberculosis among the dairy herds was the chief reason for the disappearance of this infection in children. Another public health measure, however, which contributed to this is the pasteurization of milk. Pasteurization kills tubercle bacilli, so that one can use pasteurized milk with safety, even though there is no assurance that the milk comes from dairy herds that are free from tuberculosis. In most foreign countries tuberculosis still exists among the cattle. Therefore, when traveling abroad one should be careful to use only milk which has been pasteurized.

Trichinosis is a disease primarily of swine and of rats. Man gets it by eating inadequately cooked pork or pork products from infected hogs. Refrigeration for three weeks at 5 degrees Fahrenheit or lower kills the trichinae but the only reliable precaution is not to eat pork or pork products unless they have been thoroughly cooked. It is not practical to examine meat for trichinae; therefore, the use of government-inspected meat is no protection against trichinosis. (See also page 755.)

As a nationwide program for the control and ultimate eradication of trichinosis in man and animals the National Conference on Trichinosis makes the following recommendations: (1) the passage of state laws requiring that all garbage and offal fed to hogs be cooked at licensed cooking establishments where adequate recording controls are maintained; (2) enforcement by the U.S. Public Health Service of the section of the Interstate Quarantine Regulations that prohibit the shipping of uncooked garbage across state lines for the purpose of feeding swine; (3) the prohibition by federal law of the moving of live hogs or raw pork out of any state that does not have and enforce garbage-cooking regulations; (4) the education of the farmer to remove all raw pork scraps and offal from his own household garbage to be fed to swine for his own use; (5) the dissemination of information on incineration and alternative methods for garbage disposal; (6) the prohibition by state law of the sale of garbage-fed hogs for slaughter at plants not having federal inspection or its equivalent; (7) continuation of the program of informing housewives and other food handlers of the necessity for cooking all pork and pork products thoroughly; (8) promotion of further research on the use of ionizing radiation and quick freezing methods for the destruction of Trichinella in pork; (9) improvement of diagnostic procedures to reveal the number of infections in man and hogs.[1]

Rabies or hydrophobia is a uniformly fatal disease, primarily of dogs, and to a less degree of cats, wolves, foxes, and other animals. Its cause is a virus which sets up an infection of the brain. This is accompanied first by excitement, then by paralysis and death. The virus is present in the saliva of infected animals and is transmitted primarily by the bites of these animals. In a few cases infection has been reported to have occurred from the saliva of an infected dog or cat getting into a scratch or tiny break of the skin.

Dogs with rabies are commonly called "mad dogs." In the stage of excitement they may run great distances and snap at everything they meet. In the stage of paralysis, which may occur without the period of excitement, the animals drool and appear "drunk." The name "hydrophobia," meaning "fear of water," is given to this disease because when paralysis of the muscles of swallowing occurs, the animals cannot drink and therefore avoid water.

After the rabies virus gets into the body, it travels along the nerves to the brain. For this reason the length of the incubation period depends upon the location of the bite, bites on the face having a much shorter incubation period than bites on the hands or the legs. In general, rabies has a long incubation period, varying from 2 or 3 weeks up to 6 or 10 weeks or occasionally even longer.

This long incubation period makes it possible to treat persons with a vaccine even after they have been bitten by rabid dogs and in many instances to build up a good resistance or immunity

[1] *Journal of the American Medical Association,* vol. 152, p. 241, May 16, 1953.

before the disease develops. The vaccine, which consists of killed virus, is given hypodermically in a series of injections. It is essential that these injections begin at the earliest possible moment because once rabies develops in man nothing can be done to prevent a fatal outcome.

Eradication of this disease depends upon the elimination of stray dogs and upon the restraint, muzzling, and immunization of all dogs whenever rabies is present in the area. The vaccination of dogs gives neither complete nor lasting immunity, but it is a valuable procedure when used in connection with other control measures.

Every person who is bitten by a dog known to be rabid or suspected of being rabid should receive preventive treatment without delay. In case of doubt as to whether a dog is rabid, it should be kept under careful observation. If it has rabies it will show symptoms and probably will die within 2 weeks.

Tapeworm infestations are contracted by eating inadequately cooked beef, pork, or fish containing the larvae of these parasites. Prevention is accomplished by thorough cooking. (See also page 175.)

Plague is a disease which swept Europe in epidemic waves over a period of more than a thousand years. The most serious of these epidemics, called the "Black Death," occurred in the fourteenth century, with a death toll estimated to have been in excess of 25,000,000 people, one-fourth of the total population. The last great European epidemic of plague occurred in London in 1664–1665, when approximately one-third of the population of that city died in a period of a few months.

After this epidemic, plague rapidly decreased until it seemed to have almost disappeared. However, it reappeared in Hong Kong in 1894 and was rapidly carried by rats on trading ships to all corners of the globe. Today this disease persists primarily in India, where more than 10,000,000 deaths were reported between 1898 and 1923. In this country plague has become entrenched among the ground squirrels of the west coast and is gradually spreading eastward, infected animals having been found recently in Montana and Utah.

Plague is caused by a germ called the *Bacillus pestis* and is a disease primarily of rats and other rodents and only secondarily of man. The infection is spread from rat to rat and from rat to man by the bite of the rat flea.

In man the disease may take one of two forms, the bubonic or the pneumonic. In the bubonic form the lymph nodes, usually in the groin, which drain the area of the flea bite become swollen and filled with pus. Such nodes are known as "buboes," from which the disease derives its name. When the plague germs are carried to the lungs and cause a pneumonia, the condition is called pneumonic plague. Bubonic plague has a fatality rate of about 75 per cent, and the pneumonic form, of nearly 100 per cent.

Bubonic plague is transmitted only by the bite of a flea which has fed on an infected rodent or human. In the pneumonic form of the disease, the germs are present in the sputum. This form is communicable directly from person to person, in the same way as pneumonia, influenza, and other respiratory infections.

A vaccine of value has been developed against plague, but the control of the disease depends primarily upon the control of rats. Ships which come from plague-infested ports are routinely fumigated to destroy all rats and rat fleas. In areas where plague occurs, special attention should be given to the construction of ratproof buildings and to the destruction of all rodents. In countries where, because of poverty, rat control is impossible, plague will doubtless continue to spread. In the United States, in spite of the reservoir of infection among the wild rodents, it is improbable that plague will ever reach epidemic proportions.

Tularemia is a highly fatal, infectious disease of wild rabbits and to a less extent of certain other wild animals such as field mice, squirrels, opossums, skunks, and coyotes, with occasional accidental transmission to man. Occasionally tularemia becomes so widespread as almost to wipe out the rabbit population. Bloodsucking insects, such as wood ticks and deer flies, transmit the infection from animal to animal in nature. Infection of man may occur from the bite of infected ticks or biting flies, but it usually results from handling infected rabbits.

Reports of this disease are increasing in various parts of the country, although it can easily be prevented. Since 90 per cent of human tularemia infections come from rabbits, hunters should not bring home or even pick up rabbits which appear weak, sick, or sluggish or which have been found dead. Rubber gloves should be worn by everyone who handles, skins, or dresses rabbits. Wild game should be cooked until no "red juice" remains around the bones. These are simple but effective precautions against a serious disease.

Anthrax is a serious disease primarily of cattle, horses, and sheep and secondarily of man. The germ of anthrax, which is a large bacillus, was the first disease-producing germ ever seen under a microscope. Anthrax was also the first disease against which animals were successfully vaccinated. This vaccination was accomplished by Pasteur in 1881, when this disease threatened to wipe out the sheep and cattle in France.

Today anthrax is rare in this country, although it still occurs in certain countries of the world. Infection of man occurs from contact with diseased animals or with their hides or wool. In some places anthrax is known as "wool sorters' disease." Occasionally infections have been traced to shaving brushes made of horsehair.

Psittacosis or parrot fever is a disease of birds which may be transmitted directly to man. Its cause is a virus which in man produces an infection that resembles severe influenza, frequently with complicating pneumonia.

People contract this disease by inhalation of the virus from infected birds or their cages. Parrots, parakeets, and lovebirds are the most common sources of infection, although canaries and pigeons are occasionally infected.

Prevention depends upon recognition of the danger of making pets of birds of the parrot family, particularly when the birds have been recently imported or may have had recent contact with other birds, especially sick birds. Several outbreaks in this country have been caused by lovebirds purchased at county fairs.

Equine encephalitis is a virus disease which produces an inflammation of the brain in horses, pigeons, pheasants, prairie chickens, domestic fowl, and probably other species of animal and bird life. It is occasionally transmitted to man by any one of several varieties of mosquitoes and possibly in other ways. The name "equine encephalitis" was applied to it in 1937 when over 70,000 horses in the United States, most of which died, were diagnosed as having this disease. More recent researches suggest that birds may be the principal reservoir of infection and that the disease may be only secondarily transmitted to horses, as to man, by mosquitoes. No control measures are known to be effective against this disease.

Insects and Disease

A considerable number of diseases of man and the lower animals are transmitted by insects, some mechanically, others biologically.

"Mechanical transmission" implies that the insect carries the infective microorganisms from one place to another but is not an essential link in the transmission of infection. Infective material may be carried on the body of the insect or on its proboscis, or it may be taken into the insect's intestinal tract and regurgitated or discharged with the excreta. The common examples of the mechanical transmission of disease by insects are typhoid fever, bubonic plague, and tularemia.

Typhoid fever is transmitted by the housefly. The habits of flies are such that they are very likely to carry infective material from excreta to foods if they have access to them.

Bubonic plague is transmitted by the fleas of rats or other rodents. The fleas take the *Bacillus pestis* into their stomachs with the blood of infected animals, then regurgitate the organisms into wounds caused by biting other animals or human beings.

Tularemia is transmitted by the rabbit tick, wood tick, horsefly, deer fly, etc. These insects pick up the *Bacterium tularense* with the blood of infected animals and inoculate other animals or human beings in much the same manner that the *Bacillus pestis* is transmitted by fleas.

"Biological transmission" means that the microorganism undergoes some stage of its development within the body of the insect; that is, the disease is not transmitted naturally from one person or one animal to another except by passage through the insect, which acts as its intermediate host. The more important among the diseases transmitted biologically by insects are malaria, yellow fever, typhus fever, and Rocky Mountain spotted fever.

Malaria is the most widespread tropical disease in the world. In the United States only 7,203 cases were reported in 1952 as compared to 62,763 cases in 1945. Once contracted, the disease frequently becomes chronic. It is reported that during the Civil War more than 1,000,000 cases of malaria occurred among the Northern armies.

In the Second World War, during the battle for Sicily, more American and British soldiers were put out of action by malaria than by weapons of the enemy. In the battle areas of the South Pacific the malaria rate was terrific, reaching during the early years of the war 750 cases per 1,000 men per year.

Malaria is caused by a tiny parasite which lives inside the red blood cells and is transmitted by the Anopheles mosquito. The name "malaria," which means "bad air," was given to this disease centuries ago by the Romans, who noticed that the disease was prevalent in the swamps and lowlands and rare in the mountains. The typical symptoms of malaria are a severe chill followed by a high fever which lasts for several hours; hence the name "chills and fever" or "ague." These attacks occur with great regularity at intervals usually of 24 to 48 hours. Although few attacks of malaria result fatally, a person with malaria is half-sick all the time.

The malarial parasite is transmitted only by the female mosquito, which breeds chiefly in natural collections of water, such as swamps, streams, lakes, open pools, and puddles. The Anopheles is a large brown mosquito which is nocturnal in its habits, biting but rarely in the bright part of the day. It takes approximately 12 days from the time that the Anopheles mosquito has its meal of blood containing malarial parasites for the development of the parasite in the body of the mosquito to be completed and the mosquito to become infective.

[522]

One of the great triumphs of modern medicine and sanitation was the control of malaria among the armed forces of our country during the Second World War. Hundreds of thousands of our men lived and fought in areas of the world so badly infested with malaria that never before had white men been able to survive in them. The enemy made a serious miscalculation in believing that this could not be done. A similar determined attack upon malaria in this country is assuring vastly better health to millions of people of our Southern States.

Prevention depends upon (1) elimination of the breeding places of mosquitoes by the drainage of swamps; (2) destruction of mosquito larvae with oil, insecticides, or fish; (3) safeguarding of patients from mosquitoes until their blood is free from parasites; (4) blood examinations of persons living in malarial districts to determine which ones are infected so that they may be treated and cease to be reservoirs of infection; (5) screening of porches and houses and taking particular caution against being bitten by mosquitoes at night; (6) the use of insecticides (such as DDT) to destroy mosquitoes in or around human habitations; and (7) administration of small doses of quinine, Atebrine, or better still, the new drug chloroquine during periods of probable exposure.

After the Japanese captured the quinine-producing areas of the South Pacific, malaria prevention was possible only because the chemists were able to manufacture Atabrine with speed and efficiency. At first the value of Atabrine was in doubt, but large-scale use proved it to be just as effective as quinine. We now have in chloroquine a more effective drug for the prevention and in primaquine a more effective drug for the treatment of malaria.

Yellow fever is a serious disease caused by a virus and transmitted by the Aëdes mosquito. In 1793 yellow fever caused panic among the citizens of Philadelphia, taking a death toll of one-tenth of the population of that city in the space of a few months. Periodically thereafter it made sections of the Gulf coast almost uninhabitable. It drove the white man out of the Canal Zone. Then its spread by the Aëdes mosquito was proved by the United States Army Yellow Fever Commission, headed by Dr. Walter

Reed. Acting on this information, General Gorgas conquered it in the Canal Zone and construction proceeded. Thereafter, one by one, its strongholds were attacked, until today yellow fever has been eradicated from the face of the earth except for a few isolated regions in South America and Africa.

The virus of yellow fever is present in the patient's circulating blood only during the first 3 or 4 days of the disease, and it takes 12 to 14 days after ingestion of the virus by the mosquito before the insect becomes infective. Yellow fever is highly fatal, but those who recover have a high-grade immunity. An effective vaccination has been developed against this disease. Prevention of yellow fever, at least in civilized communities, depends primarily upon the extermination of the Aëdes mosquito, by which it is transmitted. This task, compared to the extermination of the Anopheles mosquito, is relatively simple because the Aëdes mosquito breeds almost exclusively in artificial containers of water located in the vicinity of human habitations. A second effective preventive measure is careful screening of the patient from mosquitoes, particularly during the first week of the disease.

Typhus fever, otherwise known as "camp fever," "jail fever," "ship fever," etc., is an acute infection, accompanied by high fever and a rash. This is a disease that has prevailed for centuries under conditions of poverty, overcrowding, and personal uncleanliness. It has been well said that "the history of typhus is the history of human wretchedness." There are at least three forms of this disease: louse-borne or epidemic typhus; flea-borne or endemic typhus; and mite-borne or scrub typhus.

Louse-borne typhus has always accompanied wars, causing an enormous amount of illness and death among both the military and the civilian populations. It was an important contributory factor to Napoleon's defeat in his attempted Russian campaign of 1812–1813. During the First World War it killed hundreds of thousands of people on the eastern front. By the time of the Second World War much had been learned about typhus, but even so it occurred in epidemic proportions among refugee groups and in many camps for war prisoners and displaced persons.

After the louse has had a meal of blood on a person with typhus fever, a developmental period of 4 or 5 days is necessary before the louse becomes infective. From then on until its death it will infect any susceptible person it bites.

Typhus fever disappears spontaneously with the observance of personal cleanliness. Specifically its prevention depends primarily upon the avoidance of lice. To aid in this some extraordinarily effective insect repellants and insecticides, most notably DDT, were developed and utilized in the Second World War.

The effectiveness of DDT in controlling typhus was demonstrated most dramatically during an outbreak among the civilian population of Naples in 1943–1944. Dusting the civilian population with DDT powder completely and promptly stopped what started out to be a serious epidemic. Never before under similar conditions had an epidemic of typhus fever been brought under control.

In addition, between the First and Second World Wars, a vaccine against typhus was perfected in this country and was given to all American military personnel sent into typhus areas. The result of these measures was that practically no typhus occurred among American troops, even though it was present in the civilian populations and among the unvaccinated troops of other armies in the same areas.

Flea-borne typhus, which has been reported in several states along the Gulf of Mexico and along the South Atlantic coast, is much milder than epidemic typhus. Its reservoir is primarily the domestic rat, from which it is occasionally transmitted to man by the rat flea. Control measures are directed principally to the destruction of rats or at least to keeping them out of human habitations. Typhus vaccine is effective also against this form of the disease.

Mite-borne or scrub typhus was a serious problem among our troops in certain areas of southeastern Asia during the Second World War. The mites get onto people from jungle grass or underbrush. Vaccines are of no value. If at all possible one should avoid areas in which the disease occurs. If this cannot be done, the danger of infection can be reduced by wearing clothing treated to be mite-repellant.

Rocky Mountain spotted fever is an infectious disease very similar to typhus fever. It occurs in various parts of the country but is of particular importance in Montana, Idaho, Wyoming, Colorado, Utah, Nevada, Oregon, Washington, California, South Dakota, and British Columbia. In Utah the disease has been mild and in Montana virulent, having a fatality as high as 90 per cent. This disease has been especially studied in the Bitter Root Valley of Montana, where the occurrence of the malignant form is limited to the western slope of the valley. During the past few years, a so-called "Eastern" type of Rocky Mountain spotted fever has been described. Both types are transmitted by ticks: the Western type by the wood tick, the Eastern type by the dog tick. In fact this seems to be a disease of ticks that is transmitted occasionally and accidentally to man. The prevention is directed entirely to the destruction of ticks and the careful removal of ticks without crushing. Bites of ticks in infected regions should be immediately cauterized with strong carbolic acid. An effective vaccine has recently been developed against this disease.

Other biologically transmitted insect-borne diseases, which are less common or less serious in this country, are dengue (breakbone) fever, transmitted by various Aëdes mosquitoes; trypanosomiasis (African sleeping sickness), transmitted by the tsetse fly; trench fever, transmitted by the body louse; and relapsing fever, transmitted by lice and by ticks. (See Appendix D.)

Most of the insect-borne and animal-borne diseases constitute definite community health problems, and their eradication depends upon community action. Yellow fever, plague, bovine tuberculosis, and rabies are examples of what can be accomplished. Others can be just as effectively controlled if we will apply the preventive measures which science has made available to us.

DISCUSSION SUGGESTIONS

1. List the diseases of animals which are transmissible to man, indicating the animal or animals involved and the mode of transmission.
2. Discuss the importance and the prevention of brucellosis.

3. How has bovine tuberculosis been eradicated and what effect has this had on the disease in humans?
4. Discuss the control of rabies.
5. Consider the possibilities of an epidemic of plague in this country.
6. Discuss the distribution and prevention of tularemia.
7. Why is anthrax called "wool sorters' disease"?
8. What is the importance of psittacosis and how can it be prevented?
9. Discuss equine encephalitis.
10. Define mechanical and biological transmission of disease by insects.
11. List the diseases transmitted by insects, indicating the insect or insects involved and the mode of transmission.
12. Discuss the importance and the prevention of malaria.
13. Discuss the distribution and the prevention of yellow fever.
14. Discuss the distribution and the prevention of typhus fever.
15. Discuss the distribution and the prevention of Rocky Mountain spotted fever.

REFERENCES AND READING SUGGESTIONS

1. Camus, Albert: "The Plague," translated from the French by Stuart Gilbert, Alfred A. Knopf, Inc., New York, 1948.
2. DeKruif, Paul: "Undulant Fever," *The Reader's Digest*, January, 1949.
3. Duran-Reynals, M. L.: "The Fever Bark Tree," Doubleday & Company, Inc., New York, 1946.
4. Faust, E. C.: "The History of Malaria in the United States," *American Scientist*, vol. 39, p. 121, January, 1951.
5. Francis, Edward: "Sources of Infection and Seasonal Incidence of Tularemia in Man," *Public Health Reports*, vol. 52, p. 103, January 22, 1937.
6. Gibson, John M.: "Physician to the World: The Life of General William C. Gorgas," Duke University Press, Durham, N.C., 1950.
7. Hampton, B. C.: "Plague Infection in the United States Reported during 1944 and a Summary of Human Cases, 1900–1944," *Public Health Reports*, vol. 60, p. 1361, November 16, 1945.
8. ——— and H. G. Eubank: "Rocky Mountain Spotted Fever; Geographical and Seasonal Prevalence, Case Fatality, and Preventive Measures," *Public Health Reports*, vol. 53, p. 984, June 17, 1938.
9. Muller, Edwin: "The Black Death," *The Reader's Digest*, January, 1949.
10. Myers, J. A.: "Man's Greatest Victory over Tuberculosis," Charles C Thomas, Springfield, Ill., 1940.
11. Soper, Fred L.: "The Newer Epidemiology of Yellow Fever," *American Journal of Public Health*, vol. 27, p. 1, January, 1937.
12. Spink, Wesley W.: "Today's Knowledge of Undulant Fever," *Hygeia*, vol. 27, p. 474, July, 1949.

[527]

13. Stage, H. H.: "Saboteur Mosquitoes," *National Geographic Magazine,* vol. 85, p. 163, February, 1944.
14. Stone, W. S.: "The Role of DDT in Controlling Insect-borne Diseases of Man," *Journal of the American Medical Association,* vol. 132, p. 507, November 2, 1946.
15. Wheeler, C. M.: "The Control of Typhus in Italy 1943–44 by Use of DDT," *American Journal of Public Health,* vol. 36, p. 119, February, 1946.
16. Zinsser, Hans: "Rats, Lice, and History," Little, Brown & Company, Boston, 1935.

THE splendid achievement which has been made in the control of certain of the communicable diseases has been possible not only because of scientific progress in the biological sciences but also because of the advances which engineering has made in the application of this knowledge to the prevention of disease. In general, the diseases against which engineering methods have been most effective are those that are transmitted by drinking water, notably typhoid fever, cholera, and the dysenteries. However, engineering techniques are becoming increasingly important in other fields of environmental sanitation, including industrial health, food supplies, and insect and rodent control.

Environmental sanitation is defined by the World Health Organization as the control of all those factors in man's environment which exercise or may exercise a deleterious effect on his physical development, health, and survival. It is the application of environmental sanitation to the control of diseases such as malaria, yellow fever, cholera, typhoid fever, the dysenteries, and intestinal parasitism that gives dramatic results in the many areas of the world in which these diseases are prevalent. Public health engineers are the specialists who are trained to apply modern engineering methods to the improvement of health.

Among the diseases which have been virtually eradicated in

[529]

this country by sanitation, but which still constitute important health problems in many countries of the world, are typhoid fever, cholera, and the dysenteries.

Typhoid fever is caused by a bacillus which sets up an infection in the intestinal tract and then enters the blood to be carried to all parts of the body. During the course of this disease, ulcers of the intestine develop which may lead to severe bleeding or to perforation of the wall of the intestine, permitting the intestinal contents to get into the abdominal cavity, with resulting peritonitis. Unless treated with antibiotics 10 per cent of typhoid fever patients die.

In the past typhoid fever was an exceedingly prevalent disease in this country, but improved sanitation has almost completely eradicated it. The danger of typhoid fever, however, will remain for many years and outbreaks can be expected whenever sanitary precautions are relaxed.

Most outbreaks of typhoid fever are caused by typhoid carriers. These are individuals who, although apparently perfectly well, harbor the germs in their bodies and discharge them with their excreta. One or two per cent of persons who recover from typhoid fever become carriers of typhoid bacilli for years or for life. Some of these contaminate water or milk supplies. Others engage in food handling and through soiled hands contaminate food which may serve as a source of infection for others. Some carriers have been responsible for repeated outbreaks and many deaths.

The control of typhoid fever has been one of the great achievements of public health, but nowhere has the effectiveness of control measures properly applied been so well demonstrated as in the army. During the Spanish-American War, out of every 100,000 men taken into the army, 19,265 got typhoid fever and 1,463 died. During the four years of the Second World War only 3 men per 100,000 got typhoid fever, and only 29 deaths occurred among almost 10,000,000 men.

In 1950 in the United States there were about 2,500 cases and 96 deaths from typhoid fever. Therefore, we must assume that sources of infection still exist, and take precautions accordingly.

All sewage must be considered infectious and all rivers which pass through urban communities must be considered contaminated. Under conditions such as exist in the armed forces or when traveling in foreign countries, individual resistance to typhoid should be increased by the use of typhoid vaccine (page 273). In addition, we should use only milk or milk products which have been pasteurized or boiled. Water not known to be safe, such as one encounters when touring or camping, should be boiled or otherwise disinfected (page 536).

Paratyphoid fever is similar to but milder than typhoid. It is transmitted and controlled in exactly the same way.

Dysentery. Dysentery is an inflammatory disease of the intestines, usually accompanied by severe diarrhea and blood in the stools. There are two major types of dysentery: amebic and bacillary. Amebic dysentery is caused by a single-cell organism called *Amoeba histolytica*. It is contracted from food or drink that has been contaminated with intestinal discharges containing the infective organism. The distribution of amebic dysentery is probably worldwide, but it is much more common in the tropics and subtropics than in temperate regions. Where sanitary conditions are poor the occurrence of the disease may be high. At the time of the World's Fair in Chicago in 1933, the water supplies of two large hotels became contaminated with *Amoeba histolytica*. The result was 185 cases and 19 deaths from amebic dysentery in Chicago and an additional 800 cases infected in Chicago but diagnosed later in other parts of the country.

Prevention depends upon providing safe drinking water and avoiding raw fruits and vegetables which may have been contaminated with the organism. Many of the army and navy personnel who served in tropical and subtropical regions during the Second World War contracted this disease.

Bacillary dysentery is caused by a microorganism, the dysentery bacillus. Like amebic dysentery it occurs most frequently in tropical and subtropical regions and is transmitted by food and drink which have been contaminated by the intestinal discharges of patients or carriers. Prevention depends upon the same general sanitary measures as are employed for the prevention of amebic dysentery. There is no vaccine that is effective for the prevention of dysentery.

Cholera is a severe and highly fatal disease of the intestinal tract, with such violent diarrhea and vomiting that the body literally shrinks from the loss of water. The cholera germ is spread almost entirely through drinking water and its spread is effectively controlled by adequate purification and sanitation of water supplies.

Over the years cholera has counted its victims by the millions as it swept around the world on several occasions. In this country it stalked the camps of the prospectors in California in the fifties, became established among the Indians and gave rise to tribal movements and wars, kept reappearing in the United States until the seventies, and in 1921 took half a million lives in India. Today cholera persists only in India, China, and other countries which do not have the benefits of modern sanitation.

Travelers to countries where cholera exists can by means of vaccination obtain considerable protection against this very serious disease.

Safe Drinking Water

Over the years, drinking water has been the most serious source of epidemic disease in urban communities, particularly transmitting typhoid fever, paratyphoid fever, dysentery, and cholera. In 1900 there were only about 3,200 municipal water-supply systems in the United States and most of these were of doubtful sanitary protection. In that year 23,000 persons died of typhoid fever, much of which was water-borne. Today there are about 16,000 public water supplies, and water-borne typhoid is extremely rare. This is splendid progress, but there is a danger that communities may feel so secure in this regard that they become lax about maintaining adequate safeguards against infection. Several fairly recent epidemics are convincing evidence that we dare not become careless. In the first 4 months of 1924, Santa Ana, California, a city of 30,000 population, had 620 cases of typhoid fever, 222 of which were due to pollution of the water supply on December 27, 1923, and 143 to a second pollution on

February 7; 200 cases were due to contaminated milk and 51 to personal contact. In 1929 the city of Olean, New York, population 22,000, had 230 cases of typhoid fever traceable to the city water supply. The city accepted full responsibility for the epidemic and appropriated over $350,000 to pay damages and other costs growing out of the epidemic. In December, 1932, and January, 1933, 282 cases and 29 deaths from typhoid fever occurred in Chamberlain, South Dakota, a city of 1,500 population. This terrific epidemic, with an infection rate of approximately 20 per cent of the population, was due to improper operation of the water works, which permitted inadequately treated Missouri River water to get into the city's water system.

In 1944 in Newton, Kansas, some 3,000 cases of bacillary dysentery occurred as a result of sewage entering the citywater system through frostproof hydrants and water-closet valves. This and the amebic dysentery epidemic which occurred during the World's Fair in Chicago (see page 531) are illustrations as to the hazard of inadequate, antiquated plumbing installations.

Economic considerations have usually been the determining factor in the establishment of the water supply systems of the larger communities. Without a public water supply our present-day urban civilization would be impossible. Industries have depended upon adequate water for their operation. Industrial demands frequently led to the establishment of public water supplies. It is not surprising, therefore, that in many of the public systems water was originally obtained from grossly polluted sources and was unsafe for human use. To the extent that they made water of known pollution readily available to the public these early systems, up to a certain point, may have been even a detriment to the public health.

Although the actual conduct of water supply systems has usually rested with a special board or with a privately owned company, the power to regulate the sanitation of these systems has been placed upon state or local health departments and in some cases upon public utility boards. Whatever body may have carried out this supervision the effect was the same, *viz.*, protection of the supplies so that the water furnished was safe for human use. As a result there has been quite uniform reliance upon public water supplies for domestic use.

The effect of education and regulation in this field has been a striking decline in typhoid fever that has paralleled the improvements in the water supplies. Although other factors such as sanitation of milk and shell fish and regulation of typhoid carriers have played important roles in this decline, the principal factor has been the improvement of the sanitary quality of the public water supplies. Without this improvement other influences would probably have been powerless to make substantial or lasting reductions in the incidence of typhoid fever.[1]

For public health purposes water supplies may be divided into two general groups: surface and underground. Surface water supplies are those obtained from lakes and streams and are not considered safe for drinking purposes unless purified. Underground water supplies are those from wells and springs. Such supplies are practically always safe, provided they are properly located, properly constructed, and properly operated.

The water supplies of large communities are usually obtained from lakes and streams and unless too grossly polluted may be rendered safe for drinking purposes by adequate treatment. The usual method of water purification is as follows:

Water is taken from the source of supply and a small amount of alum solution added. This, when thoroughly mixed with the water, reacts with some of its chemical constituents, producing a slightly gelatinous precipitate. This precipitate envelops the suspended material and carries it to the bottom of the coagulation basin. From this basin the water passes on to the filters. These usually consist of approximately 3 feet of sand, gravel, and crushed rock, with the fine sand on the surface and the gravel and crushed rock at the bottom. The treatment up to this point removes the suspended material and a large part of the color from the water and materially reduces its bacterial content. As the water leaves the filter, chlorine, usually in the form of gas, is added to the water to destroy any bacteria that may have passed through the filter. If the source of the water supply is badly contaminated, chlorine is added before as well as after filtration.

Underground water supplies are those obtained from dug, bored, driven, or drilled wells and from springs. If wells are located in limestone subsoil, they may be polluted by seepage from cesspools or privies located even at a considerable distance. With other types of subsoil, if a well or spring is so located that it is

[1] Anderson, Gaylord, "Regulation in Public Health, Regulatory Administration," John Wiley & Sons, Inc., New York, 1939.

not subject to flooding with surface water, so constructed at the surface that there is no opening through which surface water from the immediate surroundings of the well or waste water from the pump may get into the well, and if it is located at a distance of at least 50 feet from any source of contamination such as a privy vault or cesspool, the possibility of its becoming polluted is very remote.

When an individual is contemplating construction of a home on a lot where he must both derive his own water supply and develop his own sewage-disposal system, it is essential that he consider not only the location of his own sewage-disposal system but also the location of the sewage-disposal systems of his neighbors. Under this condition in order to provide satisfactory separation between his water supply and the sewage-disposal systems of his neighbors as well as his own, he should plan on a minimum lot area of approximately half an acre. Advice should be secured from local health authorities prior to planning a home which utilizes a private water supply and a private sewage-disposal system.

The most common defects of underground water supplies are (1) a location where it is subject to flooding with surface water during high-water periods; (2) the improper construction of well casings and covers and lack of adequate provision for drainage away from the well at the surface; (3) construction of well pits around the source of supply in which all or part of the pumping equipment is located—it is difficult to prevent surface and waste water from collecting in such pits and from gaining access to the well through leaks which may occur in the casings and pumping equipment; (4) connection of well pits with sewer or drainage system—such connections make it possible for polluted water and sewage to back up into the pit and thus pollute the water in the well.

Sanitary supervision of water supplies is necessary in order to ensure their safety for drinking purposes. Investigation of small individual sources of supply is a simple procedure and their safety can usually be determined by careful observation without examination of the water. Local officials or the owner, with the

[535]

aid of the information which is furnished in health department bulletins on the location, construction, and operation of private supplies, can usually pass upon the safety of small private wells, springs, etc. The more complicated water supplies should be investigated by a public health engineer who is competent to make correct field observations and interpret results.

Water from unknown or questionable sources, such as the camper or traveler must use, can be rendered safe for drinking purposes by boiling for a few minutes or by treatment with chlorine or iodine. Boiling drives off the dissolved air and gases, with the result that the water has a flat taste. Shaking the water in a bottle, stirring it with an egg beater, or exposing it to the air overnight will correct this. Boiled water should be kept in covered pails or well-stoppered bottles. If one wishes to use ice to cool the water, this should be placed around the container, not in it.

For chlorine disinfection of clear water one can use either chloramine water-disinfecting tablets, which are available at many drugstores, or 10 to 15 drops of common bleaching solutions, such as Clorox or Hi-lex, to a quart of water.

For the purification of small quantities of drinking water the Army is now using iodine tablets, each of which gives 8 parts per million of iodine when added to a canteen containing approximately a quart of water.

Travelers to tropical countries should not depend upon chlorine for the disinfection of drinking water since small amounts of chlorine will not destroy the cysts of amebic dysentery. They should either boil their drinking water or treat it with iodine in the dosages used by the Army.

Milk Supplies

Milk and milk products are commodities which are so susceptible to contamination and adulteration that the only way of obtaining protection against fraud and against the diseases which may be transmitted through milk is by community action.[2] The first step in the accomplishment of this is education, followed by

[2] For a consideration of the principles and problems of milk sanitation, see p. 175.

the passage of a satisfactory milk ordinance. It would seem that there should be no difficulty in passing such an ordinance, but entrenched interests in the marketing of milk, particularly the small milk dealers who wish to continue peddling raw milk because the volumes of their businesses do not justify installation of pasteurization plants, have been able to block the passage of satisfactory milk ordinances in some large and many small cities and towns.

After passage of an adequate milk ordinance the next step is to make sure that this ordinance is enforced. Most milk dealers are honest, but there are some who will take short cuts in the pasteurization process to save money if no one checks up on them. A catastrophic epidemic of typhoid fever occurred in Montreal in 1927, with 5,042 cases and 488 deaths as a result of milk that was labeled pasteurized but either was passed through and distributed from the plant without being subjected to pasteurization treatment,[3] or was contaminated from insanitary handling after pasteurization.[4]

In 1935 an even larger epidemic occurred in Rome, Italy, when about 6,000 cases of typhoid fever resulted from "pasteurized milk." Contamination of milk was caused by the infiltration of sewage from a leaking sewer pipe into a water cistern from which the washing water for utensils, bottles, etc., was drawn.

Milk inspection begins with the cow, prescribing definite conditions as to health and care. The government regulates the manner in which the milk is handled from the minute it leaves the cow until it is delivered to the ultimate consumer. These regulations relate to cleanliness of utensils, temperatures at which the milk shall be stored, health of the milk handlers and cleanliness of all milk plants. Further regulations establish miminum chemical standards as to fat and mineral content, and maximum bacterial content. All of these regulations are designed to protect the product against accidental contamination with disease-producing germs and to safeguard the consumer against adulteration through "watering" or "skimming."

The advent of pasteurization made available a powerful weapon for further protection of the milk supply, through destruction of those harmful germs

[3] "Report of the U.S. Public Health Service on the Montreal Typhoid Fever Situation," *Public Health Reports*, vol. 42, July 22, 1927.

[4] Pease, H. D., "An Investigation of Epidemic Typhoid Fever in Montreal in 1927," The Provincial Bureau of Health, Quebec, Canada, 1931.

that might have found their way into milk in spite of the precautions required by the sanitary regulations. It is true that economic considerations such as the delay in souring were the most potent factors in the adoption of pasteurization by many of the larger milk companies. This economic end might have been served, however, by a simpler process than pasteurization. When it became apparent to health departments that this process, if properly performed, could be a powerful protection to the sanitary quality of the milk, the police power of the state was quickly exercised so to regulate the process as to promote the public health. This has meant elaborate regulation as to temperature and time of heating, construction of machinery, and cleansing of equipment. Almost without exception these regulations have been upheld by the courts as proper exercise of the authority of public health agencies.[5]

Food Sanitation

The foods, other than milk, which constitute the chief potential hazards to health and the infections and food poisonings which may result from them have been considered in Chapter VIII. Against most of these hazards the individual must provide his own protection rather than rely upon society to do so. There is, of course, federal inspection of meats sold in interstate commerce. This provides considerable assurance that the animal is free from anthrax, actinomycosis, and gross evidences of tuberculosis and other infections. This inspection, however, applies only to meat which is butchered and sold by companies that do an interstate business. Some states and a few cities have their own meat inspection laws; but these are not general, nor usually considered very effective.

The licensing of restaurants and hotels by state or local departments of health gives considerable health protection to the public if adequate standards of sanitation are required and efficient inspection and law enforcement are provided. The same holds true for manufacturing plants and stores, wholesale and retail, which process or sell foods.

Waste Disposal

An important duty of every community is the satisfactory removal and disposal of waste matter. Improper disposal of domestic sewage and industrial waste not only endangers the public health, but it may destroy fish and other aquatic life and become such a public nuisance as to result in

[5] Anderson, *loc. cit.*

[538]

depreciation of property values. Pollution of lakes and streams may render them unfit for recreational purposes and for domestic and industrial uses.

The use of streams for the disposal of sewage and industrial wastes introduces problems which are essentially of intercommunity concern. Usually the pollution occurs down stream from the municipality whence the wastes are derived. Hence the nuisance so created is of no concern to the community responsible for the nuisance but may be of vital concern to the communities down stream. Frequently these rivers pass into another state so that stream pollution acquires an interstate aspect. It is obvious, therefore, that a satisfactory solution to the problem of stream pollution requires exercise of the regulating authority by a larger unit of government than the local municipality. Many state health departments are invested with varying degrees of authority over this aspect of sanitation. Important and desirable as this may be, it does not attack the difficult interstate problems. The solution of the latter requires either interstate compacts or the investment of a federal agency, preferably the Public Health Service, with authority to regulate the pollution of interstate waters.[6]

The basis for this has been laid in recent national water pollution legislation.

Sewerage systems collect domestic and industrial wastes and carry them to a sewage-treatment plant or directly to a point of discharge. Usually the discharge is into a river or large lake, but rarely is there sufficient dilution to permit this without serious objection. This means that in most situations sewage treatment is necessary. Such treatment may be no more than a settling process which removes the solids from the sewage and permits the liquid part to drain off into a lake or river. On the other hand, the sewage treatment may be so complete that the end product is neither objectionable nor dangerous to health. Complete sewage treatment involves first a settling process, then oxidation, filtration, and finally chlorination of the liquid effluent.

In the absence of sewerage systems, cesspools, chemical toilets, or privies may be utilized.

Cesspools. A common type of cesspool is built somewhat like a large well with the sides made of bricks or stones but laid so that the water may pass between them into the surrounding soil. Solids which accumulate at the bottom are greatly reduced in volume by the action of bacteria. If cesspools of this type are

[6] Anderson, *loc. cit.*

[539]

properly constructed in porous soil and located so as to avoid any possibility of contamination of drinking water, they will serve as a satisfactory method of sewage disposal for a long period of time.

Chemical closets may be used inside the house in the absence of running water. They consist of a jar or an iron tank. The excreta are received into a strong solution of caustic soda which liquefies and disinfects the material. Tanks which permit several months' storage are emptied by drainage into a cesspool or into a scavenger wagon. These closets, which are nearly free from odor, are sold by many manufacturers and can be used as a temporary expedient until a water-carriage system can be installed.

Privies. A sanitary privy requires a pit of proper depth and capacity, a tight building so constructed as to protect the excreta from flies, chickens, domestic animals, rats, etc., a floor above the ground level, a tight door that closes automatically, seat covers that close when not in use, and durable screens over all openings for ventilation. The provision of such elementary conditions of sanitation and decency would seem simple enough, but the primitive, insanitary conditions of waste disposal which still exist throughout this country are almost unbelievable.

Garbage Disposal

The disposal of animal and vegetable wastes, commonly called garbage, is accepted as one of the responsibilities of the community. This is usually accomplished either by collection of the garbage and disposal by incineration or by hog feeding, or by the disposal by individual citizens through the use of a garbage grinder which discharges into the sewer.

Garbage grinding in individual homes is entirely practical. However, communities must anticipate increasing the size of their sewage-treatment plants if garbage grinding becomes widespread.

Recent outbreaks of a serious disease of hogs, called vesicular exanthema, have focused attention on the dangers of feeding uncooked garbage to hogs. It is hoped that a result of this will be the elimination of the danger of human trichinosis from pork which has been infested by the feeding of uncooked garbage to hogs (page 755).

Failure to provide adequately for the proper disposal of garbage and other wastes gives rise to conditions which are conducive to the multiplication of rats, mice, and other animal and insect pests. Bubonic plague and endemic typhus fever can be transmitted by rats. Important also is the terrific amount of damage which they do to food supplies, a loss estimated to be hundreds of millions of dollars per year.

Soil and Disease

Soil may be related to health because of the absence of some essential food element, such as iodine, or because it contains disease-producing bacteria or parasites. Decomposition of animal and vegetable matter in fertile soil is the result of bacterial action, but the organisms are harmless to man. The ones which produce disease reach the soil with the intestinal discharges of man or animals.

Most of these organisms produce bacterial diseases of the intestinal tract, such as typhoid fever or dysentery, or intestinal parasitic infections. Except for hookworm, the larvae of which most commonly enter the body through the skin, man can become infected from the soil with these diseases only through contamination of his food or drink. If human excreta are used for fertilizer, as is the custom in the Orient and certain sections of the tropics, contamination of vegetables is likely. Otherwise, the danger of contracting disease from the soil is slight.

The germs of tetanus and gas gangrene are found in soil which contains animal excreta. They produce disease only when they gain access to wounds of the body (page 750).

Air Sanitation

Scientists are working to devise practical methods to reduce air-borne infections. In the interest of health the air we breathe should be free of harmful germs, dusts, smoke, gases, pollens, and other substances which cause illness. Much can be accomplished in this regard if as community groups we have sufficient interest to apply the measures that are available to us. (See also Chapter XI.)

Problems Remaining

In spite of all that has been accomplished in providing our people with the benefits of modern sanitation, there are many localities where much remains to be done. A nationwide inventory of sanitation needs made by the U.S. Public Health Service reveals the following serious deficiencies:

Over 2,000,000 persons live in 5,700 communities of over 200 population with no public water supply system, and 79,000,000 persons live in 15,000 towns and cities that have systems needing extensions or improvements. In rural areas 27,000,000 persons need new or improved water supplies.

Nine thousand towns and cities, with a total of 6,000,000 population, need complete sewerage systems; and nearly 10,000 cities and towns with 80,000,000 persons need improved systems. In rural areas the homes of 33,000,000 persons need new or improved sewerage systems.

Twenty per cent of the fluid milk sold in this country is still not pasteurized. And the eradication of insect-borne diseases still lags in spite of the new and tremendously effective insecticides.

As to the future, the U.S. Public Health Service points out that

. . . technological advances which have helped to conquer most infections also have created other problems. These relate to occupational and household hazards; international rather than local control of infection; ionizing radiations; the stresses and strains of noise, speed, light, congestion, and associated stimuli in the modern environment; chemical contamination; food processing; environmental influences which affect an aging population particularly; protection for travelers; application of sanitary measures in areas suffering disaster; air pollution; recreational improvements; water uses; popular education in modern health techniques; air conditioning; substandard housing; and the volume and healthfulness of the water supply. On the whole, modern problems are less bound up with preventing sickness than with promoting health.[7]

The responsibility for providing the sanitation facilities needed to protect the health of the people rests almost exclusively on local communities and states. In rural areas the responsibility for adequate sanitation rests largely upon individual home owners.

To extend the benefits of modern sanitation to all the people will require education as to why improvements are desirable and

[7] "Environment and Health," U.S. Public Health Service, Washington, D.C., 1952.

how they can be obtained. Out of this should develop group demands (1) for the enactment of state laws and local ordinances which set high standards for water, milk, and food supplies, for sanitation of public places, and for the elimination of disease-bearing animals and insects; (2) for well-trained state and local staffs of public health engineers and sanitarians to maintain standards, instruct responsible persons, and inspect establishments; and (3) for the enforcement of laws and ordinances promptly, fully, and without favor.

DISCUSSION SUGGESTIONS

1. What evidence is there that the danger of water-borne epidemics still exists?
2. What body should have the power to regulate the sanitation of water supplies?
3. Outline the methods of rendering surface water supplies safe for human consumption.
4. Enumerate the most common defects of underground water supplies and the precautions which should be taken to render them safe for drinking purposes.
5. How may the camper or traveler be certain that his drinking water is safe?
6. What are the diseases most commonly spread by milk?
7. Explain the approved method of milk sanitation.
8. What has been the chief value and what are some of the shortcomings of the Federal Pure Food and Drug law?
9. Discuss the methods which may be employed for the sanitary disposal of sewage under various conditions.
10. What precautions should be observed in the construction of cesspools; of privies?
11. Discuss the possible relation of soil to disease.

REFERENCES AND READING SUGGESTIONS

1. Adams, H. S.: "Milk and Food Sanitation Practice," Commonwealth Fund, Division of Publication, New York, 1947.
2. Ewing, Oscar R.: "The Nation's Health—A Report to the President," Federal Security Agency, Washington, D.C., September, 1948.
3. Staff Article: "Cholera in New York State, 1832," *The New Yorker,* October 18, 1947, p. 82.
4. "Nation-wide Survey of Sanitation Needs," Supplement 204, *Public Health Reports,* Washington, D.C., April, 1948.
5. "Environment and Health," U.S. Public Health Service, 1951.
6. "Clean Water Is Everybody's Business," Government Printing Office, Washington, D.C., 1950.

[543]

Chapter XXVII

HEALTH IN SCHOOL AND
ON THE JOB

PRACTICALLY every boy and girl in this country spends 8 to 12 years, and those that go on to college and professional schools 4 to 8 additional years, in school. These years are of vital importance, not only for education and learning, but also for health. It is during these years that some of the most serious of the communicable diseases, such as tuberculosis and rheumatic fever, are frequently contracted. Furthermore, the health intelligence, health attitudes, and health practices developed during this period are important factors in determining future health not only for oneself but also for one's family.

School Health Programs

For many years the National Education Association together with other educational groups has proclaimed that health is the first objective of education. This is splendid, but as yet few of the children of this country have the benefit of anything approaching a complete school health program.

Society requires that children attend school, crowded together in large numbers for hours at a time, under conditions quite unnatural for the growing boy and girl. All of this increases enormously their liability to fatigue and their exposure to communicable diseases. In so doing society assumes a heavy responsibility, but it is also provided with a unique opportunity. The responsibility is to make conditions in the schools as healthful as possible; the opportunity is to do something constructive for the health of the many children who could not be reached except through the schools.

The activities included in a school health program may be summarized somewhat as follows:

1. Health protection
   a. Sanitation of the school plant
   b. Health examinations—physical and psychological
   c. Communicable disease control—particularly, tuberculosis control
2. Correction of defects
   a. Follow-up work by the school nurse who visits the home to see that steps are taken for the correction of defects
   b. Special classes (for children with heart disease, cerebral palsy, poliomyelitis, defective hearing, defective vision, etc.)
   c. Clinics for correction of physical defects of children whose parents cannot meet the expense
3. Health promotion
   a. Hygienic arrangement of the daily study program
   b. Physical activities (physical-training program)
   c. School lunches
   d. Health education and motivation (including training in health habits)

The sanitation of the school plant begins with the selection of a site and the construction of the building and includes the provision of proper lighting, ventilation, seating, fire protection, safety devices, hand-washing facilities, safe drinking water made available in a sanitary type of drinking fountain, an adequate number of sanitary toilets, and sanitary supervision of food served in the school cafeteria.

Health Examinations. Physical examinations serve a number of purposes. They call attention to conditions such as defective vision or hearing, which may be handicaps in school work. They discover physical inadequacies or defects, such as malnutrition,

[545]

poor posture, flat feet, etc., which may be corrected. They discover more serious defects, such as rheumatic heart disease, which need attention. They appraise the status of immunity against those diseases for which effective vaccinations are available. And they serve as an effective instrument of health education. From an interest in one's own health it is easy to proceed to an interest in healthful living in general. Also the experience of having health examinations in school should lay the basis for the continuation of this practice into later life.

Health examinations, to be of value, must be carefully done by competent physicians and dentists with the assistance of nurses and teachers. One or both parents should be present, if possible. Physical handicaps which are discovered should be discussed with the parents and, if necessary, adjustments made in the child's program of school work. Physical inspections, and in some cases physical examinations, should be made of children who are returning to school after illness and those who appear to the teacher to be below par. Special periodic examinations should be given to those who wish to participate in strenuous athletics.

Psychological examinations aid in the proper placement of children in the educational situation and so help to prevent the emotional maladjustments which result from children getting into classes for which they are intellectually unfitted.

Communicable-disease control depends upon the immunization of children against those diseases for which practical immunizing methods have been developed; the exclusion from school of children who are sick or have a communicable condition such as ringworm, impetigo, or pediculosis, and of those who have been exposed to communicable diseases; the daily inspection of children by teachers and when necessary by nurses; the examination by physicians of children who are ill or are returning to school after having been ill; and the investigation by the school nurse of children who are absent on account of illness.

When a communicable disease is diagnosed in a school child, not only must that child be immediately excluded from school but the school nurse and the teacher must be observant for symptoms of the same illness among other children, particularly among those who have been exposed to the known case. It used to be common practice to close the schools when outbreaks of communicable diseases occurred. That obviously put an end to the epidemic in the school; no school, no epidemic in the school. The result, however, was that the epidemic continued in the community through uncontrolled exposures and contacts which the children had in their homes and the homes of their friends, as well as on the streets, playgrounds, and other places of amusement. It is now generally conceded that outbreaks of communicable diseases can be dealt with more effectively if the children continue in school where they can be kept under careful observation.

Tuberculosis control can be carried on with particular effectiveness through the agency of the schools. In fact programs are being formulated for certifying schools with reference to tuberculosis-control activities. In the state of Minnesota the qualifications for certification are as follows:

CLASS "A" CERTIFICATE

1. 95–100 per cent of the children have been tested every other year with tuberculin of adequate dosage with the following subsequent procedures:

   a. Children of grade school age who react to tuberculin need no other phase of the examination unless symptoms or signs are present. However, their family physicians and the local health department should be notified in order that the source of their infection may be sought among their adult associates.

   b. All tuberculin reactors shall have X-ray inspection of the chest during the freshman and senior years of high school, and whenever a shadow is found, complete examination shall be made to determine the etiology of the lesion causing the shadow.

   c. All nonreactors to tuberculin from kindergarten through high school shall be retested at least every two years, and preferably every year. Those who become reactors since the last testing shall be dealt with in the same manner as those who reacted to the first test.

2. All members of personnel of a school or system to be certified shall have the tuberculin test administered with the same dosage as for children. This includes teachers, engineers, cooks, bus drivers, and all others employed by the schools.

   a. All nonreactors shall be retested every two years.

   b. All reactors on first or subsequent testing shall have X-ray film inspection of the chest. Whenever a shadow is found, the examination shall be completed to determine whether the lesion casting the shadow is tuberculous and, if so, whether it is of present clinical significance.

c. All reactors, regardless of X-ray findings in the chest, shall be examined with reference to tuberculous lesions in other parts of the body which might be discharging tubercle bacilli.

Fig. 52

TUBERCULOSIS CONTROL AWARD

AMERICAN SCHOOL HEALTH ASSOCIATION

This is to certify that

Northfield Public Schools

have fulfilled the minimum requirements of the
American School Health Association
for the control of tuberculosis, in consideration
for which a Class "A" Certificate is granted

E. A. Meyerding, M.D.   S. B. M. Rueters, M.D.
TUBERCULOSIS CHAIRMAN   PRESIDENT
FOR MINNESOTA

                                         A. O. DeWeese, M.D.
October 15, 1945   SECRETARY

CLASS "A" CERTIFICATE

---

3. All students and members of personnel who are found to have progressive tuberculosis in any part of the body, that is, in the contagious stage or threatening to become so in the near future, shall be removed from school until adequate treatment has been administered and the danger of contagion is remote.

4. An educational program shall be required to make sure that the teaching staff understands thoroughly the underlying principles of tuberculosis control. This can be accomplished by devoting one period of the weekly staff meeting each semester to this subject. A short questionnaire to determine whether or not correct impressions are received to follow the lecture. The questionnaire

to be discussed openly so that the teachers can carry the information concerning tuberculosis to their students.

CLASS "B" CERTIFICATE

The same as for Class "A" but when only 80–95 per cent of the children from kindergarten through high school are tested with tuberculin.

CLASS "C" CERTIFICATE

In schools where the tuberculin test is not administered for such reasons as a high percentage of infected individuals, at least 95 per cent of the high school students and members of personnel shall have X-ray film inspection of the chest. Those whose films present shadows shall be completely examined to determine the etiology of the disease.

A complete physical examination, in addition to the X-ray inspection of the chest, shall be done to detect those who may have sinuses, etc., discharging tubercle bacilli.

CLASS "D" CERTIFICATE

Schools which have a regular program for tuberculin testing and X-raying of specified grades and school personnel, but do not comply with the requirements for Class "A," "B" or "C," may be awarded a Class "D" recognition certificate.

In four counties in Minnesota containing 277 schools a tuberculosis-control program along the lines outlined above was started in 1930. At that time 14 per cent of the children in these schools reacted to tuberculin. In 1947 only 2.7 per cent of the children in the same schools reacted. And in 219 of the 277 schools, not a single child reacted to tuberculin, indicating that tuberculosis had been completely eradicated in those communities.

Correction of Defects and Follow-up by Nurse. School health examinations, if well done, discover many physical defects which constitute potential handicaps. Experience has shown, however, that a very small proportion of these defects are corrected unless effective follow-up is done by the school nurse. In case the parents cannot afford the necessary medical or dental care, the school nurse frequently arranges for this through the appropriate local agencies.

Special classes for children with defective vision, defective hearing, and various physical handicaps are an important part of the school health program in the larger communities.

Clinics. Clinics for the correction of the physical defects of children whose parents cannot meet the expense occasionally are provided by the school health service, but more commonly provision is made to secure these services through established clinics or hospitals in the community.

The hygienic arrangement of the study program so as to avoid fatigue is important but all too frequently neglected.

Physical Activities. The provision of play facilities and the inclusion of physical and recreational activities in the school program have been making rapid progress in recent years, but in most schools these facilities are still inadequate and the program planning even worse.

School lunches are being provided with increasing frequency as part of the school health program. Well-planned, nutritious, warm lunches not only increase the efficiency and well-being of children in school but also, for many, make an important contribution to general health and growth. In addition, the best way to teach children to eat adequate and well-balanced meals is to provide such meals for them.

Health education and motivation are two of the greatest but most neglected opportunities which schools have to make a lasting contribution to the health of the children and the community. In the lower grades desirable health habits should be developed by example, practice, inspection, and special procedures. In the upper grades systematic health instruction should be planned to provide an understanding of the essentials of healthful living and community hygiene. Subjects such as accident prevention, home nursing, and mothercraft should be included at appropriate places in the curriculum.

Health service and health education in the schools have been splendidly developed in a few communities, but in general school health work has been sadly neglected. This must be changed if we wish our children to have the benefits of health service and health information which modern science should make available to them.

Health on the Job

A leading industrialist recently said that "during the past 10 or 15 years especially the industrial manager has been reminding himself that the most important element in any enterprise is people, and that the most amazing instrument yet devised is man himself."

The conditions under which our millions of employed men and women work are of major importance not only to health but also to productivity. Yet

. . . for years after the development of the modern industrial system, little attention was given to the potential health hazards of such work. All thought was directed toward production. Labor disputes hinged around wages and hours of labor with rarely any mention made of hazards of employment. It was not until the development of systems of industrial compensation and of insurance for illness or accidents that serious attention was directed to these hazards. This early attention was devoted to prevention of accidents, largely through guards about certain forms of machinery. More recently with the rapidly expanding use of chemical processes, industry and labor have become increasingly conscious of the existence of industrial diseases due to exposure to or contact with dangerous chemicals, usually in the form of fumes or dusts that are inhaled. This field of public health has thus expanded from one of mere accident prevention to an increasingly important program of occupational hygiene, or the prevention of occupational diseases.

Both of these fields of industrial safety are based in large part on regulations, imposed in part by the government as an exercise of the police power and by the insurance companies as a condition to low rates for coverage. The latter, while a potent force in the prevention of accidents or disease, are not true expressions of regulating power as they are a part of the insurance contract. It would be grossly unfair, however, to underestimate the force that they have exerted in this field.

The need for industrial insurance has arisen from the enactment of workmen's compensation acts. These have provided for payment to the worker for loss of time due to illness or accident incurred in the course of his employment. Death benefits have also been provided for the dependent. Although the compensation laws vary widely from state to state, the fundamental principle of reimbursement from the employer to the worker is common to all. The employer therefore seeks protection by some form of insurance. The risk to the insuring company quite obviously depends on the nature of the work and the precautions observed by the employer to reduce the hazards attendant upon the industry. A potent force which operates to reduce risks is thus introduced by a law which in its original intent was one of mere compensation for damages.[1]

Absenteeism of industrial workers due to sickness causes the loss of 400 to 500 million man-workdays per year. A rough esti-

[1] Anderson, Gaylord, "Regulation in Public Health, Regulatory Administration," John Wiley & Sons, Inc., New York, 1939.

mate is that this means a loss of at least 4 billion dollars in wages and probably a greater loss to industry in reduced production. Industrial accidents resulted in the loss of another 250 million man-workdays and an estimated 2.9 billion dollars in 1952.

The chief objective of occupational hygiene is to protect the health of the worker, whether in mines, factories, shops, stores, construction, transportation, farming, lumbering, or domestic work. Rarely is the individual employee, acting alone, able to change the conditions under which he is required to work. This requires group action, with employers, employees, and society working together.

The conditions in industry which most frequently affect health are dusts, fumes, temperature, humidity, light, sanitation, fatigue, hours of labor, medical service, physical examinations, industrial poisons, and accident hazards. From this list it is obvious that industrial hygiene becomes the application of general principles of hygiene to conditions in industry.

In addition to general hygienic considerations such as fatigue (page 232), medical care (page 467), and sanitation (page 529), which are applicable to every industry, there are certain special health hazards which occur in selected industries. Among these are extremes of temperatures and air pressure, which have been discussed (page 251), and a few others which merit special mention even in a brief consideration of the subject.

Dusts. Most dusts are not harmful because of the body's natural mechanisms of protection. A few dusts, however, are dangerous because they are irritating and carry disease-producing bacteria. Others, particularly those containing silica and to some degree asbestos, are responsible for serious lung diseases.

A disease commonly known as "silicosis" and frequently mistaken for tuberculosis occurs among workmen in any occupation in which the inhalation of high concentrations of finely divided silica dust is continued over a long period of time. This is most frequent among granite workers, sandblasters, and miners of any type of ore that happens to be mixed with sandstone or granite. Silica does not produce symptoms for years, but the disease once established is usually progressive and frequently associated with tuberculosis. Prevention depends upon the use of adequate exhaust systems to remove the dust, appropriate masks, or water sprays or other means of preventing dust accumulation.

Lead poisoning is one of the best known and most widespread of all the occupational diseases. It is due to the absorption of small quantities of lead or lead compounds which are stored in the body over long periods of time. Painters, pottery workers, printers, workers in storage-battery factories, and those in numerous other occupations may come in contact with sufficient lead or its fumes or dust particles to produce serious poisoning.

The chief symptoms of lead poisoning are loss of appetite, loss of weight, constipation, colic, weakness, and paralysis. Young people are more susceptible to lead poisoning than older persons, and women more susceptible than men. In a reported series of 212 pregnancies among women lead workers, only 61 living children resulted.

In nearly all the industries using lead it is possible to prevent lead poisoning, but the cooperation of both employer and employee is necessary. Lead usually reaches the worker in the form of dust and fumes or is carried directly to the mouth by the hands. Hence, the prevention of inhalation of dust and fumes laden with lead by means of adequate ventilation, respirators, or masks will do much to protect the worker. In addition the workers must be instructed to wash their hands frequently and always before eating, to take many baths, and to change clothing as soon as they have finished work.

Shoe-dye Poisoning. Nitrobenzene, which is often found in shoe dye, is capable of causing serious illness. It may be absorbed through the skin or its fumes may be inhaled. It produces marked cyanosis, which appears suddenly, often within a few hours from time of exposure. The symptoms are shortness of breath, weakness, dizziness, occasionally nausea and vomiting. These are caused by the reduced oxygen-carrying power of the blood, so that in fatal cases death really occurs from suffocation. Usually if the cause is detected and the recently dyed shoes, as well as the stockings, are removed at once, the symptoms disappear within 24 hours.

Prevention consists in using shoe dye that is free from poisonous chemicals, or in allowing all shoes which have been dyed to dry in the sun and wind for at least 3 days before they are worn. After this the feet should be kept dry—even dampness from sweat should be avoided—and stockings should be changed daily until there is no longer danger of absorption.

Other chemical poisons occur in certain industries, such as arsenic in the smelting of certain ores and in the curing of furs, hides, skins, and feathers; and mercury by spilling in the laboratory and in the manufacture of thermometers, barometers, incandescent lamps, felt hats, etc. Poisoning from these chemicals is relatively infrequent and the danger is constantly being reduced.

Carbon Monoxide Poisoning. Carbon monoxide is formed by the combustion of carbon compounds in an inadequate supply of oxygen. It is found in highest concentration in the burning of gasoline, coal, illuminating gas, coke, etc. This deadly gas can be neither seen nor smelled.

The poisonous effect of carbon monoxide is due to the fact that it forms a compound with hemoglobin which is from 100 to 200 times as stable as oxyhemoglobin. Therefore when carbon monoxide hemoglobin is present, it reduces the oxygen-carrying capacity of the blood, and if present in sufficient quantity, will prevent oxygen from reaching the tissues. The chief sources of carbon monoxide poisoning are coal fires, leaky gas fixtures, and automobile exhausts. A running motor in a small closed garage will produce a sufficient concentration of carbon monoxide to cause death in a few minutes.

Most industries now provide protection of their workers against carbon monoxide poisoning. This is done primarily by adequate ventilation. In domestic life the hazards have not been correspondingly reduced. Improperly adjusted gas burners, leaky gas pipes, rubber hose connections, room or water heaters without proper exhaust outlets, inadequate drafts in coal stoves and furnaces, and automobiles running in closed garages are the chief sources of poisoning.

Industrial accidents, briefly discussed on page 29, have been greatly reduced in recent years but are still responsible each year for approximately 15,000 fatal and 2,000,000 nonfatal accidents, almost 100,000 of which result in permanent disability. The National Safety Council reports that the highest accident rates occur in the following industries: lumbering, mining, marine transportation, quarries, construction, wood products, air transport, meat packing, foundries, clay products, transit, paper and pulp industries, food, petroleum, metal products, sheet metal, and public utilities.

In Korea from June, 1950, to June, 1953, the daily average battle casualties of killed and wounded was 114. During the same period the daily average of killed and injured in United States coal mines was 178.

A study of fatal accidents in Pittsburgh several years ago showed that, when it was possible to place responsibility, the victim or a fellow workman and the employer were responsible with about equal frequency. Employees contribute to accidents because of emotional upsets, improper clothing or protective devices, carelessness, ignorance, physical handicaps such as poor vision and defective hearing, intemperance, fatigue, certain illnesses such as epilepsy, and general unfitness for the job. The more important contributory factors to industrial accidents for which the employer is responsible are inadequate illumination, the lack of safeguards for machinery, working conditions which result in excessive fatigue, poor housekeeping in the plant, improper upkeep of the building, neglect of safety education of the employees, poor morale, and uninterested and inadequate supervision. Employee and employer working together can do much more to reduce the unnecessary toll which industrial accidents are still taking.

According to the National Safety Council small industries, usually without good safety and medical departments, have accident rates 50 per cent higher than large industries with good

[555]

safety programs and medical departments. These are the industries upon which the greatest efforts for improvement need to be centered not only because they have the highest accident and illness rates but also because 70 to 75 per cent of the nation's workers are employed in small plants with less than 500 employees.

Farm Accidents. An occupation which in recent years has become increasingly hazardous is farming. In fact, because of the large number of farmers in comparison with other industrial groups, the number of workers in agriculture killed is greater than in any other occupation. The farmer and members of his family operate powerful and complicated machinery without special training and with little or no supervision. They forget that a tractor is top-heavy; that loose clothing or gloves can pull them into gears, corn pickers, corn shredders, or buzz saws in a fraction of a second; that kerosene and gasoline sometimes explode in stoves with fatal results; and that horses, hogs, and bulls must always be handled with care. Since machines have become necessary to many farm operations, training in their safe operation offers the best means of reducing the toll of farm accidents.

MEDICAL SERVICE IN INDUSTRY

It has long been considered good business practice to provide for the maintenance, repair, and depreciation of industrial plants and machines. But only recently have any real efforts been made to keep the workers in good physical condition, or to make any provisions for their disability and retirement. In part through the interest of farseeing, responsible employers, in part through the efforts of labor unions, and in part through the passage of federal and state laws, not only do most employees now receive disability and retirement benefits, but in addition most of the larger industries and some smaller ones now provide a certain amount of health service.

Medical service in most industries began with the provision of emergency care for accidents. Today in some industries it is still no more than that. In others, complete medical and hospital care

are provided for the worker and the members of his family. In most industries the medical service is somewhere between these two extremes.

That good health services in industry pay dividends both to the employee and to the employer is clear from the report that during the Second World War sickness absenteeism in industrial plants with poor medical services varied from 4 to 6 per cent daily, as compared to 2 to 3 per cent in plants with good medical services.

The objectives of industrial medical service have been well summarized[2] as follows: (1) the care or supervision of those diseases or conditions—such as silicosis, lead poisoning, accidents, etc.—for which the employer is largely responsible; (2) the physical examination of applicants for work and, at intervals, of those already at work; (3) the maintenance of satisfactory sanitary and hygienic working conditions; (4) cooperation with the safety department in the prevention of accidents; (5) the protection of workers against the spread of communicable diseases in the plant; (6) the care and supervision of minor abnormal physical conditions, even though the cause is unrelated to employment, to the end that the affected worker may be kept at his duties; (7) cooperation in the placement of workers at the tasks for which they are physically and mentally suited; (8) the education of the work force in matters of health, sanitation, hygiene, and the like; (9) the giving of advice to workers regarding health matters unrelated to work, the treatment for which is properly within the domain of the family physician or the specialist, and the establishment of relations with the family physician for the purpose of handling these private matters to the best interest of all concerned.

In general the illnesses and accidents of industrial workers are the same as those of other groups. Employment, however, provides unusual opportunities both for the reduction of these illnesses and for the improvement of health. The diseases and accidents directly due to the conditions of employment constitute

[2] McCord, C. P., "The Economics of Industrial Medicine," *Journal of the American Medical Association*, vol. 98, p. 1237, 1932.

only a small fraction of the total illnesses of industrial workers. These conditions, however, are practically all preventable as well as compensable by law.

The president of a large manufacturing company recently said that the industrial nurse is the best contact the company has with the man and the man's family. Her interest in the problems of the family will open the door of friendship which makes possible a contribution to the lives of many families.

Among the more general areas in which industrial medical service is able to make particularly valuable contributions are:

1. Preemployment examinations to ensure proper job placement.

2. Periodic examinations of all employees to guard against wear and tear of the job.

3. Periodic inspection of the plant to discover and eliminate unsafe practices and uses of hazardous materials.

4. Tuberculosis control, utilizing x-ray examinations of the chest, the exclusion from employment of persons with a communicable form of the disease, and epidemiological follow-up of contacts and of sources of infection.

5. Reduction of fatigue, employing methods to improve morale and provide incentive, rest periods, an optimum work week, the reduction of unnecessary strain and repetitious movements, etc.

6. Improved nutrition, utilizing the services of a nutritionist to supervise the cafeteria, restaurant, and other eating facilities.

7. Employment of the physically handicapped, utilizing medical examinations and ability tests to determine physical and mental capacities and special skills, and then giving workers special training and work assignments in accord with their capacities. In this way not only will employment be provided for a large number of handicapped persons who would otherwise be dependent and public charges but also, as experience has shown, industry can obtain many unusually competent and conscientious employees.

8. Psychiatry, utilizing modern testing techniques and psychiatric counseling services to aid workers to adjust to their jobs

[558]

and to advise management in making promotions, particularly to supervisory positions. Also much unrest and dissatisfaction among employees, both as individuals and as a group, could be prevented by cognizance and treatment of personality peculiarities or emotional states.

9. Health education, utilizing talks, conferences, posters, pamphlets, and movies. Industry has a unique opportunity to reduce accidents and improve the health not only of employees but also through them of their families and the community.

Financing Industrial Health Service. The costs of health service in industry are sometimes borne completely by the employer, sometimes jointly by the employer and the employees, sometimes by voluntary or compulsory insurance plans, sometimes by insurance or other plans controlled by unions, and sometimes by adding the cost directly to the price of the product, as in the case of the addition of a fixed amount to the price of each ton of coal to support the United Mine Workers Health and Welfare Fund.

However industrial medical service is financed, there is general agreement that it pays big dividends to all concerned. In fact, a survey of results by some 1,600 industries, which have been providing health and medical services for their employees and improving the conditions under which they work, concludes that a reduction of 63 per cent has occurred in occupational diseases and a 30 per cent reduction in absenteeism due to sickness.

DISCUSSION SUGGESTIONS

1. What are the objectives of a school health program?
2. What activities are ordinarily included in school health programs?
3. Discuss the value of school health examinations.
4. What role should schools play in the prevention and control of communicable diseases?
5. Discuss the requirements and values of the Tuberculosis Control Award of the American School Health Association.
6. What positive health values can come out of a good school health program?
7. Discuss the necessity for industrial hygiene.
8. Enumerate and discuss the conditions in industry which most frequently affect health.
9. Define silicosis. How may it be prevented?
10. What are the chief symptoms of lead poisoning? How may it be prevented?

11. Why does carbon monoxide act as a poison? What are the major hazards of carbon monoxide poisoning?
12. What are the objectives of industrial hygiene?
13. Discuss the areas in which industrial medical services can make their greatest contributions.

REFERENCES AND READING SUGGESTIONS

SCHOOL HEALTH

1. Chenoweth, L. B., and T. K. Selkirk: "School Health Problems," 3d ed., Appleton-Century-Crofts, Inc., New York, 1947.
2. Grout, Ruth E.: "Health Teaching in Schools," 2d ed., W. B. Saunders Company, Philadelphia, 1953.
3. Nyswander, Dorothy B.: "Solving School Health Problems," Commonwealth Fund, Division of Publication, New York, 1942.
4. Turner, C. E.: "School Health and Health Education," The C. V. Mosby Company, St. Louis, 1947.
5. Wilson, C. C., ed.: "School Health Services: Report of Joint Committee on Health Problems in Education of the National Education Association and the American Medical Association," 4th ed., National Education Association, Washington, D.C., 1953.
6. Wheatley, George, and Grace T. Hallock: "Health Observation of School Children," McGraw-Hill Book Company, New York, 1951.

HEALTH ON THE JOB

1. Baetjer, Anna M.: "Women in Industry," W. B. Saunders Company, Philadelphia, 1946.
2. Bloomfield, J., and J. M. Dallavalle: "The Determination and Control of Industrial Dusts," *Public Health Bulletin* 217, U.S. Public Health Service, Washington, D.C., 1935.
3. Brody, M.: "The Dynamics of Mental Hygiene in Industry," *Industrial Medicine*, vol. 14, p. 760, 1945.
4. Doppler, W. S.: "Tuberculosis, Labor and Management: A Guide to Industrial Relations for Public Health Workers," National Tuberculosis Association, New York, 1943.
5. Gafafer, W. M., *et al.:* "Manual of Industrial Hygiene," W. B. Saunders Company, Philadelphia, 1943.
6. Hamilton, Alice: "Exploring the Dangerous Trades," Little, Brown & Company, Boston, 1943.
7. Harvey, V. K., and E. P. Luongo: "Physical Capacity for Work," *Occupational Medicine*, vol. 1, p. 1, 1946.
8. Health Resources Advisory Committee: "The Worker and His Health," Office of Defense Mobilization, Washington, D.C., 1953.

9. McGrath, B. J.: "Nursing in Commerce and Industry," Commonwealth Fund, Division of Publication, New York, 1946.
10. Vonachen, H. A., *et al.:* "A Comprehensive Mental Hygiene Program at Caterpillar Tractor Company," *Industrial Medicine*, vol. 15, p. 179, 1946.
11. "Physical Examinations in Industry," *Industrial Health Series* No. 2, Metropolitan Life Insurance Company, New York.
12. Roueché, Berton: "Eleven Blue Men and Other Narratives of Medical Detection," Little, Brown & Company, Boston, 1953.
13. Williams, Huntington, *et al.:* "Lead Poisoning in Young Children," *Public Health Reports*, vol. 67, p. 230, March, 1952.

Chapter XXVIII

GOVERNMENT AND HEALTH

CONCERTED group action for any purpose can be attained only through some type of organization. Governmental bodies, local, state, and national, have been formed for this purpose and in the field of public health their accomplishments have been magnificent. Unbelievable gains have been made in the control of disease and the prolongation of human life, but in spite of this there are still in the United States annually more than 100,000 deaths from communicable diseases, 2,500 deaths due to childbirth, 80,000 deaths in early infancy. All these are concerns of the health department and many of them may be prevented through prompt and adequate service. In addition, the amount of illness caused by the communicable diseases is enormous. Four of these, which we know how to control, produce approximately 265,000 new cases annually: typhoid fever, 2,500 cases; diphtheria, 5,800; tuberculosis, 120,000; and syphilis, 135,000. The cost of the care of these illnesses, conservatively estimated, amounts to over $100,000,000 annually.

More than this, public health authorities estimate the annual economic loss in wage-earning and preventable sickness directly attributable to lack of reasonably efficient rural health service is over one billion dollars. On the other hand, where a reasonably effective health program has been developed, it has been demonstrated that the expenditures for carefully planned health programs, executed by trained workers, yield large dividends.[1]

[1] Hiscock, Ira V., and F. W. Walker, "Public Health Organization and Budget,"

Official Health Activities

The average citizen expects the government to provide certain services which directly concern his welfare, such as protection of the country from invasion, police protection, fire protection, public education, mail service, and certain health services. That distinguished statesmen of the world have recognized the responsibility of the government for the health of the people is evident from quotations such as the following:

Theodore Roosevelt: "Our national health is physically our greatest asset. To prevent any possible deterioration of the American stock should be a national ambition."

Lloyd George: "I solemnly warn my fellow countrymen that you cannot maintain an A-1 empire with a C-3 population. You cannot bring up healthy people in unhealthy homes."

If a government is to function efficiently in the interests of public health, the following basic principles must always obtain: (1) Services rendered must be based upon need and upon the ability of the people to support them. Theoretically, it would be desirable to prevent every single case of typhoid fever, but to do so would be exceedingly expensive. In fact, the amount of money required to prevent the few scattered cases of typhoid fever which at present occur in most states could be used to much better advantage for other health services. (2) Public health work must be in the hands of trained, competent personnel who have chosen and prepared themselves for careers in this field. (3) Political consideration must not be permitted to enter into appointments of public health personnel or into the determination of public health policies. (4) The public should be informed as to what they have a right to expect in the way of public health service. (5) Public health programs should be planned so as to get the greatest possible returns for the money expended. (6) Public health services must be adequately supported. In spite of the fact that public health has long been recognized as one of the primary functions of government, it

The Practitioner's Library of Medicine and Surgery, vol. 12, chap. 28, Appleton-Century-Crofts, Inc., New York, 1937. (Quoted with permission of authors and publisher.)

receives a relatively small share of local, state, and national appropriations, frequently only a few cents out of the tax dollar— much less than is spent for roads, for military preparedness, for relief, for the custodial care of defective individuals, etc.

THE NATURE OF THE PUBLIC HEALTH AUTHORITY

The power of the state in matters of public health is an exercise of the fundamental police power. Society says to its members that they may not commit acts which will result in detriment to the health of the entire group or any individual member of the group. The people through their legislatures enact certain rules of conduct which are designed to eliminate or restrain conditions which may promote ill health; and health departments are created to enforce these laws. These departments in turn may be vested with power to adopt and enforce certain rules and regulations which have the force of law. Usually these rules are of a technical nature, too detailed and in need of too great flexibility, to be enacted as statutes.

The public health law governing any community is thus composed of those statutes which have been enacted by the legislative assembly, supplemented by regulations promulgated by the legally appointed executive body. How much of this legal control is of local origin and how much is imposed on the community by a more powerful central agency varies with different states. Both state and local assemblies (legislatures, county courts, municipal councils, boards of aldermen, town meetings, or other deliberative bodies according to the local form of government) may enact health laws or ordinances, and these in turn may be supplemented by rules of state or local health departments. In some states the major portion of the public health authority rests with the state government. Such a plan carried to its logical conclusion would envision the local boards as little more than agencies to enforce a state law, at least so far as their regulating activities are concerned. The opposite plan delegates the greatest possible authority to the local governmental unit. Between these two extremes can be found all degrees of division of authority between state and local units.

Each of these plans has its advantages and disadvantages. The older system of local authority, best seen in New England, is a natural outgrowth of the colonial era. It was ideally suited to meet the needs of the times for which it was devised. This was a period of relative isolation of communities, so that most public health problems were of purely local concern. Each community was self-contained to a degree that a person of the present day can hardly appreciate or understand. Public health theory placed chief reliance on community sanitation which was at that time essentially a local problem. Traveling from one town to another was at a minimum. There were comparatively few public health problems of an intercommunity nature. It was, therefore, logical to empower each community with a high degree of autonomy.

Changes in the social structure and new ideas of medicine and public health have introduced new problems and transformed old ones from local into intercommunity affairs. The distribution of water, food or milk in a single town involves problems that may affect several other communities and even other states. The river used as a source of water supply for one city may receive the sewage of many other cities further upstream. The milk sold in a large municipality may come from farms scattered in hundreds of communities in several states, whereas the food supply is derived from every state in the union and many foreign countries. Methods of rapid transportation have resulted in widespread travel with resultant possibility of spread of communicable diseases. Even the personal health problems have acquired their intercommunity aspect, as a school child neglected in one locality may in a few years be a problem to a distant municipality to which the family may have moved. Because of these considerations many of the regulating powers that were formerly local have been transferred to a larger governmental unit, *viz.*, the State.

The problem of the proper or desirable division of public health authority between federal, state and local agencies is one that cannot be solved to the satisfaction of all interested, and depends in large part upon controlling political thought. By federal constitution the state is the ultimate repository of power. America's political thought, therefore, holds that each state should have the highest possible degree of autonomy in matters pertaining to public health. Thus it need occasion no surprise that the federal government has the least power of the official agencies in the field of public health.

General usage commonly assigns regulatory powers as follows to federal, state and local health agencies.

A. Federal
    (1) Maritime and international quarantine
    (2) Supervision of health of immigrants
    (3) Regulation of interstate problems
B. State
    (1) Establishment of minimum standards for the state
    (2) Supervision of local health administration
    (3) Enforcement of state laws
    (4) Regulation of intercommunity problems
C. Local
    (1) Establishment of local ordinances
    (2) Local enforcement of state and local ordinances

Although these headings are broad and general ones, they indicate the difference in the scope of the federal, state, and local regulating power as commonly applied to public health.[2]

[2] Anderson, Gaylord, "Regulation in Public Health, Regulatory Administration," John Wiley & Sons, Inc., New York, 1939.

[565]

Health Activities of the Federal Government

The national government has only certain limited powers granted to it by the Constitution. The following are the more important of these related to public health: (1) Regulation of foreign and interstate commerce. Under this authority the Federal Government acts to prevent the introduction of communicable diseases from foreign countries and the spread of diseases between the states; it supervises the preparation of vaccines, serums, and certain medicinal products sold in interstate commerce, the working conditions in factories which manufacture materials sold in interstate commerce, and the sanitation of drinking water on interstate carriers. (2) Taxation. By levying special taxes the Federal Government can control the sale of such products as narcotics; it can also distribute funds raised by taxation to the states for public health work or other purposes on condition that the individual states meet the terms or requirements specified by the Federal Government. This is the method used for the development of health work throughout the states with the aid of complete or partial federal subsidies. (3) Education and research. Activities in these fields are based upon the power of the government to "provide for the common defense and general welfare of the United States." Public health work, health education, and scientific research are supported under this function of the government.

The recognized, and to a degree already provided, responsibilities of the Federal Government affecting health are:[3]

1. The study of international health conditions and the protection of the country from international hazards,

2. The study of internal health conditions and control of interstate transmission of disease by regulation of the movement of persons and goods,

3. The promotion by all educational means of public interest in disease prevention and control, safeguarding the lives and health of mothers and children, and the attainment of more complete physical and mental health,

4. The promotion of the study of health as a recognized part of education,

5. The stimulation of state and local governments to organize health work to insure more effective service to all people,

[3] Quotations concerning health activities of federal, state, and local governments are from Hiscock and Walker, *loc. cit.*

[566]

6. The providing of personnel to state and local health departments for consultation, educational and demonstration services; the training of workers for all aspects of public health service is necessarily a part of this responsibility,

7. The development and promotion of standards of performance of technical services in the several fields, including general administration,

8. The conduct and support by grants of research in any or all aspects of public health, particularly those problems beyond the capacity of local and state organizations relating to disease prevention, control of the incidence of morbidity and mortality at all ages, the influences—physical, social, economic and mental—affecting or contributing to a more healthy people,

9. The provision of direct grants in aid to states: to encourage the organization of state and local health services for all people in accordance with current knowledge; to equalize the tax burden of the public health program to the ability of the state to support it.

These responsibilities are now met through the services of a number of different bureaus in several governmental departments. The services which have to do, for the most part, with the problems and administration of state and local health work are:

The Public Health Service in the Department of Health, Education and Welfare

The Children's Bureau in the Department of Health, Education and Welfare

The Bureau of the Census in the Department of Commerce

The Bureau of Vital Statistics in the Department of Health, Education and Welfare

The Office of Education in the Department of Health, Education and Welfare

The Food and Drug Administration in the Department of Health, Education and Welfare

The Office of Vocational Rehabilitation in the Department of Health, Education and Welfare

The Bureau of Animal Industry in the Department of Agriculture

The Federal Trade Commission

Other divisions having certain public health aspects and responsibilities, yet not directly nor uniformly concerned with the promotion and administration of local health work are: Bureau of Labor Statistics, Women's Bureau, Employees' Compensation Service, Consular Service, Office of Indian Affairs, National Park Service, Bureau of Mines, Veterans Administration, Bureau of Dairying, and Bureau of Home Economics, in addition to the health services of the United States Army, United States Navy, and the United States Air Force. These federal services have grown up in response to the recognized public need and each, within its field, contributes markedly to public understanding and appreciation of health and to the improvement of the national health status.

[567]

The major operating health agency of the Federal Government is the U.S. Public Health Service. This agency was established in 1789 as the Marine Hospital Service to provide medical and hospital care for American seamen. Today one of its divisions still operates a series of hospitals for this same purpose. However, the organization and the other functions of this service have developed and expanded so greatly that today the U.S. Public Health Service is one of the most important and efficient public health agencies in the world. The organization of the Public Health Service is semimilitary in character, under the direction of the Surgeon General.

In 1953 the Congress created the Department of Health, Education and Welfare with Cabinet status. The U.S. Public Health Service, the Children's Bureau, the Food and Drug Administration, and the Office of Rehabilitation constitute the major health agencies of this department.

Pure Food and Drug Law

The first Federal Pure Food and Drug Act was enacted in the year 1906. In 1912 it was amended to forbid false and fraudulent therapeutic claims on labels of patent-medicine containers, and in 1938 to include cosmetics and contrivances for diagnosis or treatment. Anderson says:[4]

While this law has been a powerful weapon used in certain situations and held as a potential threat, its actual use has been but one of the forces leading to a vastly improved food supply. Probably the most potent force has been the work of the federal food and drug administration in cooperation with the food manufacturers and processors. The technical experts of the government have aided the industries in the studies of those factors which lead to deterioration of the product. Thus with the elimination of these factors much of the incentive to adulteration has been removed and at the same time the industry has gained an increased public confidence. There has thus developed a system of voluntary policing of these industries by the manufacturers themselves in cooperation with the federal authorities. From the standpoint of public health this can be considered as the ideal form of exercise of the regulatory power as it rests upon public understanding of the economic and social values of those procedures which best serve the public end.

[4] Anderson, *loc. cit.*

In spite of the good that it has accomplished, the average citizen assumes that he is receiving more protection under this law than it actually provides. The 1912 law was worded so as to require the government to prove claims fraudulent before any action could be taken against the producer. He could not be convicted under this law unless it could be proved that he actually knew that the claims were false. If he could convince the jury that he himself believed in the value of his products, he would be acquitted. The new law does not make it necessary to prove fraud. If the court decides that a product is falsely labeled or adulterated, the manufacturer can be fined. The Wheeler-Lee Amendment to this law makes false and misleading advertising illegal. The Federal Trade Commission, which is responsible for enforcement, can issue a "cease and desist order." If this is violated, the Department of Justice brings the manufacturer to trial. For first offenses, fines up to $5,000 may be imposed. If dangerous drugs or fraud are involved, the offense is criminal and six months in jail is added to the fine. For second offenses, penalties are doubled.

The present act provides no protection, except labeling, against many potentially dangerous drugs which are contained in certain "patent medicines." Serious toxic results and several deaths have been reported from the use, according to directions, of various nationally advertised and widely sold medicinal and cosmetic preparations. It is illuminating to see detailed reports of the constituents, the claims, ownership, and promotion methods of many of America's most famous remedies, such as Crazy Crystals, Cascarets, Jad Salts, Tanlac, Marmola, Fleischmann's Yeast, Cherry Pectoral, Vick's Vaporub, and Lydia Pinkham's Vegetable Compound. The advertising and sale of vitamins are the newest and among the most profitable lines ever entered by the patent-medicine trade. Studies of the subject present startling disclosures concerning the adulteration, mislabeling, and false claims made for many foods which effective and persistent advertising has led the American public to accept as standards of excellence. Clearly the consumer needs to take more interest in sound food, drug, and cosmetic legislation and education.

State Health Work

In many states

. . . the function of the state department has become that of stimulating local areas to recognize their health problems and of organizing the necessary facilities to handle them adequately. The state assists in providing those

FIG. 53. ORGANIZATION CHART OF TYPICAL STATE HEALTH DEPARTMENT

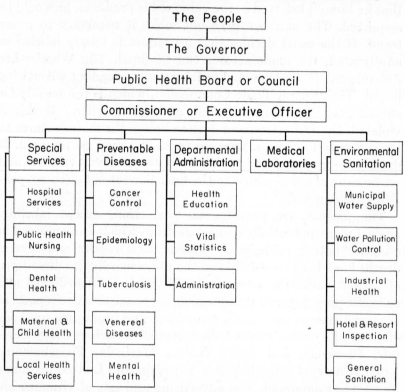

services which it is uneconomical for the local community to provide for the sole use of a small population unit. This may include laboratory facilities, special technical services in the handling of problems of sanitation, water supply and sewage disposal, of occupational diseases, facilities for the institutional care of tuberculosis, *et cetera*. Many states also wisely provide advisory and supervisory service to the local administrators and through standards of performance of professional service assist the local health officers in keeping local work at an effective level. The training of public health personnel for work in the local area should be as much a state responsibility as is the training of teachers in education. Only in limited fields and under unusual circumstances should the state department become an agency functioning directly in the local community dealing personally with the public.

Every state health department should be directed by a well trained and especially qualified commissioner or state health officer supported by a board of health or advisory council, appointed without political regard and solely for the knowledge and contribution which the members can bring to bear upon the health problems of the state. Such a body should assist the state health administrator in policy forming and in the preparation of the sanitary code. The bureaus of the state health department should be headed by especially trained and qualified individuals devoting full time to the service. A plan of organization which has been found effective in practice, and which conforms to the plan of local organization, would provide for a commissioner of health with supporting advisory body appointed by the governor and a department comprising a major division of central administration having to do with the stimulation, guidance and supervision of county and other local health work. Auxiliary divisions would provide services for the control of preventable diseases including epidemiology, maternal and child health, laboratory service, and sanitary engineering. A division concerned with the collection, tabulation, and analysis of vital statistics completes the organization of the department. As the function of the department is largely advisory and supervisory, the number of subordinate personnel is relatively small.

Since at the present time less than one-quarter of the counties of the country have organized full-time health departments and nearly 50 per cent of the population are without full-time health supervision, state departments have a major responsibility in acquainting local governmental officials and the public at large with the importance and advantages of effective local health service. It is conservatively estimated that not more than 25 per cent of the counties have organized full-time health departments and not more than 50 per cent of the cities have as yet developed their departments to include efficient service in the mimimum essentials of health protection and promotion here set up. The state's responsibility for effective health service extends to such areas as well as to the at present unorganized territory. In fact, it must assume a continuing responsibility for the stimulation of the local departments to avail themselves of newer knowledge of public health protection.

An equally important function of the state department is that of aiding poorer counties and local areas through direct subsidy to obtain a satisfactory health program. Not all counties within the state will be in position to raise the necessary funds for a satisfactory program from local taxes. It frequently happens that the magnitude of local health problems is overwhelming and the responsibility for the solution of these problems does not rest entirely upon the local community. The state then, through its general taxing power, must act as an equalizer and through services rendered or direct monetary

[571]

contributions to such areas or both, insure the conduct of a satisfactory program and the protection of the citizenry as a whole.

The guiding and supervisory functions which have already been discussed as responsibilities of the state are much easier and more effectively administered if the state assists the local area financially in carrying its health service. However, not all states are able, within their local resources, to meet the demand of health work and there is a national problem of adjustment which must be met through Federal aid to states in the organization of state administrative services and assisting the states to carry the burden of the poorer counties.

The duties and responsibilities of state health departments are established by laws enacted by their respective state legislatures. Many states have sound basic health legislation and make such changes from time to time as are necessary to enable their health departments to carry on efficient and progressive health programs in the interest of all the people. Other states, unfortunately, due to lack of good leadership or to a political spoils system, still are way behind in the effectiveness of their state health departments.

Local Health Organization

The basis of a satisfactory health service in a community is a well organized health department, adequately financed, with trained personnel, supported by suitable laws and ordinances, by favorable public opinion, and by all professional groups. Recognition of the need of a suitable population and the importance of a full-time trained administrative head led away from the establishment of services on the town or village basis to the county or district (city or groups of cities, part of county, or combination of counties) of 50,000 population or more, in a reasonable compass, as the unit of organization.

The basic principles of organization of such service in a community are: that the health administrative agency be a recognized part of the government of the area and be correlated with the government of the state; that, in view of the responsibilities which must be placed upon the health officer or administrative head of such services, a board of health or advisory council is an essential factor in the administrative plan to advise the health officer regarding policies and otherwise bring a broader community viewpoint to the administration of the service; that such a body include physicians, members of other public health professions, and representatives of the general public; that the health officer be appointed on professional qualifications and secured against political interference; that he be adequately compensated, commensurate with the public responsibilities placed upon him and devote his full time to the duties of his office; that his responsibility be either directly to the board which may have the appointing power or to the chief governmental executive of the area; that the major divisions of the department likewise be directed by full-time trained persons responsible to the health officer.

[572]

The physicians in a community, whether in private offices, clinics, hospitals or homes, perform a service in the treatment of disease whether as individuals or in organized groups which is the usual form of medical care in this country for those able to pay for such services. Because of their training, numbers and relationships to their clientele, physicians in private practice constitute the group which is potentially most capable of applying the lessons of preventive medicine to the habits and circumstances of the individual. The public generally, however, is not yet accustomed to demand or privately pay for such guidance in the application of preventive medicine to their own or their community's health problems. The program of local health work must therefore, provide for activities which will (*a*) carry out the legal responsibilities in disease control imposed by law; (*b*) provide those facilities for

Fig. 54. Organization Chart of typical County or District Health Department

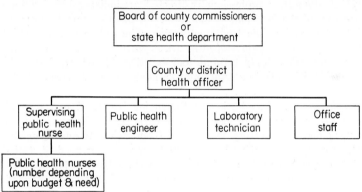

institutional care (communicable disease and tuberculosis), laboratory service, and diagnostic aid, which the individual patient cannot provide for himself alone; (*c*) stimulate a public demand for preventive health services, (*d*) supplement the services of the private physician in the community; and (*e*) aid in developing the interest and ability of physicians to render preventive health services.

A comprehensive local health program will include: services aimed at the control of preventable diseases (the acute communicable diseases, syphilis and gonorrhea, tuberculosis, heart disease, cancer, industrial disease, and mental diseases), care of crippled children, the improvement of nutrition, the promotion of maternity, infant and other child health services, the supervision of general sanitary conditions of the community, services for diagnostic aid (laboratory services and expert consultants), and service for the collection, tabulation and analysis of vital statistics. . . .

While in certain situations particular items of service listed above will not be necessary, it is the responsibility of the health department to study the community health problems in the several fields and provide the necessary facilities wherever the need exists, either through the local department, by use of state or voluntary aid, or by a combination of resources. . .

In the conduct of the local health program the health officer should be assisted by the following personnel:

Physicians and Dentists. The medical and dental aspects of the program should in every instance be under the direction, preferably full-time, of a competent person with special training or aptitude for the work in which he is engaged. In certain departments, medical and dental assistance will be needed in many of the fields beyond the capacity of one full-time worker. It is believed to be desirable in such circumstances to draw the best qualified local physicians and dentists interested in this field for service on a part-time basis.

Public health nurses, professionally directed, are indispensable for the proper performance of the functions of communicable disease control, maternity and child hygiene and public health education. The public health nurse is the backbone of every well-developed health department whether state or local, but the nurse whose only training and experience has been that of bedside care will find difficulty in attempting to render service in terms of the individual plus the community. . . .

Other Personnel. In addition to the major groups of personnel already listed, all departments will have need in carrying on the service, for public health engineers, laboratory technicians (bacteriologists and chemists), and clerks. Departments serving large populations will have need of statisticians and persons experienced in social service work. All personnel in these categories, it is believed, should be full-time and be especially trained or experienced in the work of their particular field.

Vital Statistics. The registration of births, marriages, and deaths should be localized in the health department since the sound conduct of health work is governed by information obtained from the careful analysis of material from these sources. Through intimate contact with these vital data, the health administrator is enabled to visualize his problem more accurately and to chart his course of procedure more intelligently than might otherwise be possible. The value of this work will be greatly increased when the reporting of illness from important causes becomes a routine practice with sufficient thoroughness to permit the health administrator to know more accurately the real state of sickness and health of his community. . . .

Local health services, both in urban and rural communities, indicate that the minimum essentials of service, as outlined here, will require at least $1.50 per capita, that a comprehensive program will require in addition facilities for the hospitalization of certain acute and chronic diseases discussed elsewhere. Unusually acute health problems of great community interest and demands for service may require additional services not provided in this program and budget. Some cities and rural areas have demonstrated that as much as $2.50 per capita can be wisely and profitably expended.[5]

A great need for the further improvement of the public health is for more adequate local, and particularly rural, health units. The Department of Health, Education and Welfare reports that 40,000,000 people live in some 1,200 counties without a public health department, or with inefficient departments that have only a part-time health officer; that 96,000,000 people in the rest of the country are served by inadequately staffed public health departments; and that only 7,000,000 people in the entire country are served by public health staffs that fully meet the minimum standards laid down by experts in this field.

A good community health program can be had for approximately $9 per family per year. The average American family spends 30 cents a day for tobacco and 60 cents a day for alcoholic beverages. Is it too much to ask that we spend 3 cents a day per family for a reasonably adequate public health service?

To improve the present situation more trained personnel and more adequate health department budgets are essential. And these two requisites can be provided only by community interest and support under the leadership of informed and public-spirited citizens. This part of the job can be done only by the people themselves in their own homes and in their own communities.

The World Health Organization

The World Health Organization was established following the Second World War to promote better health on a worldwide scale. It functions as a specialized agency of the United Nations. Its assembly consists of representatives of all the leading nations of the world. Russia, which was a charter member, has not participated in the past few years.

The logic behind the establishment of the World Health Organization and the reason for its support by the member nations is that today bad health conditions in one part of the world are almost certain to have an impact on the health of other areas. This may occur directly, or indirectly through the contri-

[5] Hiscock and Walker, *loc. cit.*

bution of ill health to poverty and to the social and economic conditions that breed unrest, revolt, and communism.

Without health man cannot produce according to his need. He cannot improve his standard of living. He is condemned forever to be the slave of his environment.

Given health, his labour can reap the fine reward which it merits. He can grow more, make more, sell more and eat better. He can achieve and maintain a state of complete wellbeing.

The records of man's fight against preventable sickness drive home these facts with compelling force. They show, for example, how in one region of South Africa the control of malaria increased the amount of land under agricultural production from 700 acres to 12,000 acres within ten years, while in another area the crops increased fourfold. The list of such successes grows year by year.

The lesson is simple and clear: if sickness and poverty go hand in hand, so also do health and prosperity. The way to world health and prosperity is through international action, for the evil we fight is the enemy of us all—and in this battle there can be no neutrals.[6]

The support of the World Health Organization by the member nations is by assessments based upon the population of the member country, the national income of the member country, and the amount of damage done to the country as a result of the Second World War. Six member nations, Australia, Canada, New Zealand, Sweden, the United Kingdom, and the United States, all pay approximately 2 cents per person per year toward the support of the World Health Organization.

The activities of the World Health Organization fall into three general groups:

1. Advisory services to governments with special emphasis on control and eradication of communicable diseases, public health services, and training of public health workers for national public health service. By the end of 1952, 2,680 fellowships had been awarded for such training.

2. Central technical services in such fields as epidemiology, health statistics, standardization of therapeutic substances, and health research.

[6] Chisholm, Brock, Director General of the World Health Organization, "Health Is Wealth," Pamphlet of the World Health Organization, 1953.

3. Emergency aid to governments (*a*) in dealing with epidemics, such as typhus fever (Afghanistan), meningitis (the Sudan), malaria (India, Pakistan, Thailand, Afghanistan, Cambodia, the Philippines, Iran, and Central America), tuberculosis (Afghanistan, Burma, Ecuador, Egypt, India, Indonesia, Iran, Iraq, Pakistan, El Salvador, Syria, and Thailand; (*b*) in meeting special health problems, such as the reconstruction of South Korea and the care of more than 850,000 refugees in the Palestine area.

Today along the whole long line of the world health front, international teamwork for higher levels of health and well-being for all people is being effected and constantly improved through the World Health Organization.

DISCUSSION SUGGESTIONS

1. What evidence is there that further progress is possible in the reduction of illness and death in this country?
2. What are the basic principles upon which governmental health activities should be based?
3. Discuss the nature of public health authority.
4. In general, what powers in the field of public health are assigned to the Federal Government? To the state government? To the local government?
5. Discuss the major health activities of the Federal Government.
6. What functions should a state health department be expected to perform?
7. Outline the organization and the activities of your own state health department.
8. What functions should a local health department be expected to perform?
9. Outline the organization and the activities of your own local health department.
10. Analyze the total budget and the average per capita expenditure of your local health department.
11. What is meant by vital statistics? What are their chief values?

REFERENCES AND READING SUGGESTIONS

1. Baumgartner, Leona: "Now They Live," New York City Health Department, 1953.
2. Hiscock, Ira V.: "Community Health Organization," 3d ed., Commonwealth Fund, Division of Publication, New York, 1939.
3. Milbank Memorial Fund: "The Next Steps in Public Health," Milbank Memorial Fund Publications, New York, 1936.

4. Mustard, Harry: "Rural Health Practice," Commonwealth Fund, Division of Publication, New York, 1937.

5. ————: "Government in Public Health," Commonwealth Fund, Division of Publication, New York, 1945.

6. ————: "An Introduction to Public Health," The Macmillan Company, New York, 1953.

7. National Health Assembly: "America's Health: A Report to the Nation," Harper & Brothers, New York, 1949.

8. Shyrock, R. H.: "The Origin and Significance of the Public Health Movement in the United States," *Annals of Medical History*, vol. 1, p. 645, 1929.

9. Smillie, W. G.: "Public Health Administration in the United States," The Macmillan Company, New York, 1947.

10. U.S. Public Health Service: *Annual Reports*, Washington, D.C.

11. U.S. Children's Bureau: *Annual Reports*, Washington, D.C.

12. "The State Health Department Services and Responsibilities," an official statement of the American Public Health Association, *American Journal of Public Health*, vol. 44, p. 235, February, 1954.

13. "World Health Organization: What It Is; What It Does; How It Works," Regional Office of World Health Organization, Washington, D.C.

Chapter XXIX

VOLUNTARY HEALTH SERVICES

I N TOTALITARIAN countries the government assumes complete responsibility for all health and welfare services. In democracies, on the other hand, it is traditional—and, many people feel, essential to the democratic way of life—that some of these services be conducted and supported by citizens on a voluntary basis.

In this country a vast amount of excellent public health work is being done by agencies with no governmental connections. Some of these are endowed philanthropic foundations; others are voluntary health organizations supported by contributions or membership dues; others are professional organizations; others are large business enterprises, such as insurance companies and the great corporations; and still others are local organizations of various types and purposes, such as hospitals, educational institutions, community chests, etc.

Philanthropic Foundations

Most of the philanthropic foundations have been established and endowed by individuals of great wealth. Some operate in local areas or in special fields; some are national or even international in scope. The larger ones have millions of dollars annually to spend or distribute. These foundations make large contributions each year for medical research, medical education, the training of public health personnel, the evaluation of public

[579]

health measures, experimentation with new public health procedures, health education of the public, the support of actual public health services in special situations, etc. The following are examples of the better-known foundations operating in the health field:

1. The Rockefeller Foundation, which supports medical and public health education, research, and service all over the world. This foundation has pioneered in the establishment of schools of public health both in this country and abroad and has aided in the improvement of medical education and given support to medical research in all parts of the world. The International Health Division of this foundation has played an important role in the control of yellow fever, malaria, and other epidemic diseases on a worldwide basis.

2. The Commonwealth Fund, which for years has been supporting medical research and the improvement of medical education, particularly in special fields such as psychiatry and child guidance. This foundation gave impetus to the improvement of health services by demonstrating in various parts of the country what an adequately supported and efficiently administered local health department, or child guidance clinic, or rural hospital, could accomplish. The Commonwealth Fund has also conducted a fellowship program to permit medical scientists of this country to study abroad and to bring health workers of other countries to America.

3. The Kellogg Foundation, of Battle Creek, Michigan, which has as its primary interest the improvement of medical service in rural areas. Its funds have been used to improve local health departments, to construct and support hospitals, to provide special diagnostic services, such as x-ray departments and laboratories; and to make available to physicians, dentists, and nurses continuation study courses on the newer developments in medicine. This foundation for a number of years functioned exclusively in the state of Michigan but is now providing support for programs of this type in other states and even in some of the Latin American countries.

Other major foundations which devote their funds primarily

to various aspects of medical and health work, include the Markle Foundation, the Milbank Memorial Fund, the Kress Foundation, etc.

Voluntary Health Organizations

It is characteristic of a democracy that people in natural groups will band together for the purpose of aiding the unfortunate. This cannot and should not be discouraged. Such groups have supreme advantages in our political structure. They are without ulterior motives. They transcend political lines and partisan politics. They are frequently made up of highly respected community leaders whose support is attractive to politicians. When banded together for health purposes, these leaders can rally the support of practically all factions in the community since no one objects to reasonable efforts to improve community health.

The voluntary organizations of all kinds in this country are distinctive American institutions, and the health agencies are no exception. The health agencies arise especially from the urge to do something to help the unfortunate. A few leaders with a vision of what can be done in a given direction gather some friends about them, discuss and define the problem, pass the hat to raise a little money, and a new local voluntary health agency is born. If their efforts are successful, the news spreads and other communities form similar organizations. This paves the way for a state or national organization with constitution, by-laws, budgets, regulations, directors, officers, conventions and head tables. Nevertheless, much of the nation's health progress is attributable to these voluntary health agencies. When official health departments are weak, they are bolstered, stimulated and supported by the voluntary agencies. When serious community and national health problems occur, it is often the voluntary agencies who first see and commence to remedy the situation.[1]

Outstanding among the health organizations supported by voluntary contributions or membership dues are the following, most of them national organizations with state and local branches or chapters:

1. The American Red Cross. This organization provides an invaluable supplement to the medical services of the armed forces in wartime. In peacetime it is the agency best equipped and always called upon for disaster relief. During the Second

[1] Shepard, W. P., C. E. Smith, R. R. Beard, and L. B. Reynolds, "Essentials of Public Health," J. B. Lippincott Company, Philadelphia, 1948.

World War and the war in Korea the American Red Cross collected and processed whole blood and blood plasma which saved the lives of thousands of American boys in field hospitals, in dressing stations, and on the fields of battle in all parts of the world. Since the end of the Second World War the Red Cross has been developing its "blood program" on a peacetime basis in order to make blood and blood products available for use when needed in civilian hospitals. The Red Cross is the leader also in teaching first aid and is active in improving nursing services and nutrition and health education of the public.

2. The National Tuberculosis Association. This association, which is supported by the Christmas seal sale, has played an important role in the reduction of tuberculosis from first place to ninth place as a cause of death in this country. It conducts a continuing campaign to educate people about tuberculosis; it supports research on all aspects of the disease; and through its local associations it promotes early diagnosis, and the best of treatment, and rehabilitation services for those who contract tuberculosis.

3. The National Foundation for Infantile Paralysis. This foundation, which was started by the late President Roosevelt and is financed by the March of Dimes, liberally supports all aspects of research and service concerned with poliomyelitis. In fact, the local chapters of this foundation pay the hospital and medical bills in whole or in part for most of the victims of this disease.

4. The American Cancer Society. This society collects funds by means of a well-organized nationwide campaign and disburses these funds primarily for cancer research and cancer education.

5. The American Heart Association. This association is developing a program of fund raising and of service similar to that of the American Cancer Society.

Prominent among the many other voluntary health organizations which operate in this country are the National Committee for Mental Hygiene, the American Social Hygiene Association, the National Society for the Prevention of Blindness, and the Society for Crippled Children and Adults, with its Easter seal sale. Such voluntary health organizations provide service, demonstrations, and experimentation, and stimulate interest in and support for specialized programs. They are more free to try new procedures and to concentrate on special health problems than are governmental agencies. Almost without exception these agencies serve a valuable purpose in our over-all health program and merit public support. However, if they are to function efficiently and make the best possible use of the money which is entrusted to them, public-spirited citizens must not only give them support but also participate in their activities and administration.

Professional Health Organizations

Various groups of professional workers in this country have formed organizations to promote their professional interests. Among the organizations of this type in the health field are the American Public Health Association and the American Medical Association.

1. The American Public Health Association includes in its membership the various professional workers in the field of public health; that is, health officers, epidemiologists, public health engineers, sanitarians, public health nurses, health educators, public health laboratory workers, etc. The purpose of this association is to improve public health practice by the establishment of standards, by the support of research and experimentation, and by keeping their members informed through meetings and publications of new knowledge in their fields. Closely related organizations with similar purposes are the National Organization for Public Health Nursing; the American Epidemiological Society; the American College Health Association; the American Association for Health, Physical Education and Recreation; the American School Health Association, etc.

2. The American Medical Association is an organization of reputable licensed physicians. This association, like many other similar professional organizations, is based upon local county units called county medical societies. The elected representatives of these county societies make up legislative bodies of state

[583]

societies; and representatives from the state medical societies constitute the legislative body of the American Medical Association. The purpose of this association is to improve the quality of medical service to the American people. This is accomplished by insisting upon high standards in medical education; by aiding physicians to keep abreast of advances in medical knowledge and practice; by the support of research; by publishing the results of the investigations of medicines, foods, and appliances advertised and promoted for sale on the basis of alleged medical or health values; by education of the public on health matters and by promoting special areas of health service, such as industrial hygiene, nutrition, emergency medical service, hospitals, and rural health. The American Medical Association is concerned not only with the cure of disease but even more with its prevention. It is for this reason that medicine has been said to be a profession that labors to destroy the need for its own existence. During the past few years the American Medical Association has been subject to criticism from certain quarters because of its opposition to proposals for a federal system of compulsory sickness insurance. It is claimed that this opposition is based on selfish interests on the part of physicians. There may well be some truth to this, but the overwhelming majority of physicians are interested above everything else in the welfare of their patients. Their stand on this issue, as on others, is based primarily on this consideration.

Other professional associations with similar purpose and types of organization are the American Dental Association; the American Nurses' Association; the American Society of Medical Technologists; the American Physical Therapy Association; the American Occupational Therapy Association, etc.

Hospitals

As medical science has progressed, the provision of medical care has become increasingly complex and involved. A generation ago most patients were cared for in their own homes. The family physician called to make the diagnosis and to supervise treatment. The instruments and most of the drugs which he used were carried in his "little black bag." Members of the family or neighbors provided nursing care.

Today the situation is vastly different. Although many patients with minor illnesses are still cared for, and properly so, at home, the utilization of modern scientific procedures for diagnosis and for treatment requires facilities that are available only in doctors' offices or hospitals.

For example, a generation ago when most patients with pneumonia were cared for at home, the physician based his diagnosis upon symptoms and upon his findings on examination of the patient. Treatment consisted of fresh air, good nursing care, and various drugs to relieve specific symptoms or to support the patient's general condition. Today in making his diagnosis the physician still considers symptoms and physical findings, but in addition he asks for an x-ray examination to determine the exact location and the extent of the pneumonia and to observe from time to time its extension or recession. And he calls upon the laboratory to find out what kind of germ is causing the pneumonia and to learn how the patient is reacting to the infection, as indicated by an increase or decrease in white blood cells. This information is important in deciding upon treatment; some kinds of pneumonia are benefited by penicillin and the sulfonamides, while others are not. In prescribing treatment the physician relies on the laboratory also to help him decide how much penicillin or how much of a sulfonamide drug should be given and whether or not the patient is in need of oxygen. To carry out these modern diagnostic and treatment procedures requires not only special facilities but also various types of specially trained personnel— radiologists, nurses, bacteriologists, medical technicians, x-ray technicians, pharmacists, dieticians, etc.—that are available only in hospitals.

Hospitals have existed since ancient times, but until recent years they were looked upon as places to be avoided. They were "pest houses," insane asylums, and places where people went to die. Today the situation is completely changed. In 1951 more than 18,000,000 persons, 12 per cent of the total population, were admitted as patients to the hospitals of this country. These

[585]

patients were cared for in 6,637 registered hospitals with a capacity of 1,529,988 beds. The average daily occupancy of these hospitals was 1,293,653 patients, or 44 per cent of the people estimated sick for any one day of the year. Almost 3 million births occur annually in these hospitals.

In some areas, available hospitals are adequate to meet the needs; in others, additional hospitals should be built. Competent hospital authorities recommend that on a state-wide basis there should be 4.5 beds in general hospitals per 1,000 population; 5 beds in nervous and mental hospitals per 1,000 population; and 2.5 beds in tuberculosis hospitals per average annual deaths from tuberculosis. These figures are useful in estimating needs for hospitals over large areas but they are not applicable to every community. In many situations better medical care will be provided by driving to a hospital 25 or even 50 miles away than by attempting to build a small hospital in every community. For the best medical service a hospital must be large enough to provide all the necessary facilities and equipment and in addition to have on its staff physicians, nurses, laboratory and x-ray technicians, and the other specially qualified personnel needed to properly utilize these facilities.

Hospitals are community assets and community responsibilities. Some are supported out of public (tax) funds; others by churches, fraternal organizations, or other groups. Good citizens should be interested in the support and the management of their community hospitals.

Pharmacies and Pharmacists

The manufacture and distribution of drugs is a big and exceedingly important business and public service. The discovery of insulin and penicillin would have been of no benefit to those who needed them if large and responsible drug manufacturers had not developed methods for their production in such quantities and of such quality that physicians everywhere could obtain them and use them with complete confidence in their purity and strength. The same is true concerning vaccines, serums, drugs, and all other types of pharmaceutical products.

For the protection of the public, drugs can be sold only by

licensed pharmacists. Pharmacy, from a Greek word meaning "the use of medicine," is the science and art of preparing drugs and medicines. Pharmacists are educated in schools of pharmacy conducted by many of the leading universities of the country. The modern trend of the so-called "drugstore" to offer for sale a varied line of merchandise, often specializing in soft drinks and light lunches, is a long way removed from the true meaning of the term "drugstore" and the original purpose of a pharmacy.

Teaching and Research Institutions

Education for the health-service professions, such as medicine, dentistry, nursing, public health, etc., as well as research in the health fields, was inaugurated in this country by privately endowed and supported universities and research institutes. In recent years tax funds have come to play an increasingly important role in the support of medical research and in education for these professions and, in view of the high costs involved, this trend will unquestionably continue.

Business and Labor Organizations

Business and industry, being concerned with production and efficiency, are giving increasing attention and support to medical and health programs for their employees. These programs include not only the provision of healthful conditions of employment but also health instruction and the provision of medical services. In some cases these services are provided not only for the workers but also for the members of their families. Experience has convinced leaders of industry that health services pay big dividends in efficiency, in morale, and in productivity.

Labor unions and some fraternal organizations are also becoming increasingly interested in the health of their members and are supporting or participating in various types of health and welfare programs.

Insurance Companies

Life insurance companies spend enormous sums of money each year to support medical research and to provide health information, periodic health examinations to holders of certain types of policies, and nursing service to groups insured under industrial

[587]

contracts. This is effective public health work and the insurance companies can show that it represents a good investment for them. They make money by prolonging the lives of their policy holders and, naturally, the policy holders do not object.

Other insurance companies make a contribution in the health field by offering insurance which provides cash payments in case of illnesses or accidents which require medical and hospital care and result in loss of time from employment. Policies are also being offered with special provisions to cover in whole or in part the costs of medical and hospital care.

About 800 private insurance companies sell policies that provide at least partial protection against the costs of accidents, hospitalization, surgical treatment, and physicians' services in the hospital, office, or home. By the end of 1951 more than 91 million persons were covered by some type of hospital insurance; 73 million people had insurance against surgical expenses; and almost 36 million persons had medical-expense insurance. At the present rate of growth it will not be long until most people will be using some type of insurance to protect themselves against the financial hardships occasioned by serious accidents or illnessess.

Of special interest is the development by the hospitals of this country of the Blue Cross programs of hospital insurance. These are nonprofit enterprises, most of which are operated on a state-wide basis. The national organization represents merely an affiliation of the state plans for cooperation and exchange of information. Although Blue Cross had been well established for only about 15 years by the end of 1952, some 43 million persons were insured against the costs of hospitalization under these programs. The cost of and the benefits provided by these plans are not standardized, but in general for approximately a dollar and a half a month one obtains coverage of all or almost all the hospital costs of illness over a period of three or four weeks.

Another type of insurance still more recently developed but now rapidly expanding is called Blue Shield. This provides for the payment of physicians' services on an insurance basis. Some plans provide coverage only for surgical operations, others include all kinds of medical care. In some places Blue Cross and

Blue Shield are combined in a single policy. By the end of 1952 almost 28 million persons were insured against surgical expenses and 18 million against medical expenses under Blue Shield programs.

A Place for All

In the modern public health program, which has as its objective the prevention of disease, the prolongation of life, and the improvement of physical and mental health and efficiency, there is a place and a need for these many different types of health organizations. They can succeed, however, only if and when they have the intelligent interest, support, and participation of the citizens whom they are attempting to serve.

DISCUSSION SUGGESTIONS

1. Discuss the contributions that the philanthropic foundations have made to public health.
2. What are some of these foundations which operate on a national scale?
3. Discuss the role of voluntary health organizations, in distinction to official health agencies.
4. What are some of the major voluntary health organizations in this country and what service does each render?
5. Discuss the major professional organizations in the health field.
6. Discuss the reasons for the great increase in the use of hospitals.
7. How can the needs of communities for hospitals be determined? Are the hospitals in your community adequate to meet the need?
8. What contributions do pharmaceutical companies and pharmacists make to the medical and health services?
9. What can business and labor organizations accomplish in the field of health?
10. Discuss the role of insurance companies in the health program of the country.

REFERENCES AND READING SUGGESTIONS

1. Anderson, Odin W.: "National Family Survey of Medical Costs and Voluntary Health Insurance," Health Information Foundation, New York.
2. Faxon, N. W.: "The Hospital in Contemporary Life," Harvard University Press, Cambridge, Massachusetts, 1919.
3. Freeman, Lucy: "It's Your Hospital and Your Life," Public Affairs Pamphlets, New York, 1952.
4. Gunn, S. M., and P. S. Platt: "Voluntary Health Agencies, An Interpretive Study," National Health Council, New York, 1945.

5. Kandle, R. P.: "Who Should Do What in Public Health?" *American Journal of Public Health*, vol. 43, p. 1539, December, 1953.
6. Shepard, W. P., C. E. Smith, R. R. Beard, and L. B. Reynolds: "Essentials of Public Health," J. B. Lippincott Company, Philadelphia, 1952.
7. "Accident and Health Coverage in the United States," Health Insurance Council, New York, 1953.
8. "Voluntary Prepayment Plans," Council on Medical Service, American Medical Association, Chicago, 1950.
9. Reports and bulletins from the following organizations:

American Academy of Pediatrics, 636 Church Street, Evanston, Ill.
American Association for Health, Physical Education and Recreation, 1201 16th Street, N.W., Washington 6, D.C.
American Cancer Society, 47 Beaver Street, New York 4, N.Y.
American Dental Association, 222 E. Superior Street, Chicago, Ill.
American Hearing Society, 1537 35th Street N.W., Washington, D.C.
American Heart Association, 1790 Broadway, New York 19, N.Y.
American Hospital Association, 18 E. Division Street, Chicago 10, Ill.
American Medical Association, 535 N. Dearborn Street, Chicago 10, Ill.
American Nurses' Association, 1790 Broadway, New York 19, N.Y.
American Public Health Association, 1790 Broadway, New York 19, N.Y.
American Red Cross, 17th and D Streets N.W., Washington 7, D.C.
American School Health Association, 3335 Main Street, Buffalo 14, N.Y.
American Social Hygiene Association, 1790 Broadway, New York 19, N.Y.
Arthritis and Rheumatism Foundation, 23 W. 45th Street, New York, N.Y.
Child Study Association of America, 221 W. 57th Street, New York 19, N.Y.
Child Welfare League of America, 130 E. 22nd Street, New York 10, N.Y.
Metropolitan Life Insurance Company, 1 Madison Avenue, New York, N.Y.
National Committee for Mental Hygiene, 1790 Broadway, New York 19, N.Y.
National Education Association, 1201 16th Street N.W., Washington 6, D.C.
National Foundation for Infantile Paralysis, 120 Broadway, New York 5, N.Y.
National Health Council, 1790 Broadway, New York 19, N.Y.
National Safety Council, 20 N. Wacker Drive, Chicago 6, Ill.
National Society for Crippled Children and Adults, 10 S. LaSalle Street, Chicago 3, Ill.
National Society for the Prevention of Blindness, 1790 Broadway, New York 19, N.Y.
National Tuberculosis Association, 1790 Broadway, New York 19, N.Y.

Chapter XXX

HEALTH IN THE FUTURE

FURTHER progress in the improvement of health and in the reduction of illnesses and preventable deaths is clearly possible but it will be more difficult to attain than the brilliant achievements of the past. It will not be possible in the next half century, as it was in the past, by improved sanitation of drinking water and food supplies to save 50,000 lives a year from typhoid fever and 175,000, mostly of children, from diarrhea and enteritis; or (by immunization) to prevent 60,000 deaths a year from diphtheria; or even to reduce the deaths from tuberculosis by a quarter of a million a year. (See Table 29.)

In considering the possibilities of further improvement in health, we naturally think first of improved and expanded public health and medical services and of research to provide new methods for the prevention and treatment of disease. These are all essential elements in a program for better health. But much more is necessary. The public must be better informed on matters of personal and public health, and people everywhere, acting as individuals and as groups, must make better use of available information concerning the improvement of health and the prevention of accidents and of disease. Other factors too, such as housing and an income adequate to provide the essentials of healthful living, are in many instances more important than medical services for improved health.

[591]

TABLE 29

COMPARATIVE DEATH RATES, 1856–1865 AND 1951

(Per 100,000 population, in Massachusetts)

Cause of Death	1951	1856–1865	Decline, Per Cent
Infant mortality per 1,000 live births.............	21.9	174.4	87.4
Typhoid fever and paratyphoid.................	0.1	92.5	99.9
Diarrhea and enteritis........................	1.4	166.0	99.2
Diphtheria and croup.........................	0.2	86.1	99.8
Measles.....................................	0.1	17.1	99.4
Whooping cough..............................	0.1	23.8	99.6
Scarlet fever.................................	0.0	101.3	100.0
Smallpox....................................	0.0	11.0	100.0
Tuberculosis (all forms).......................	18.3	446.4	95.9
Pneumonia (all forms)........................	26.8	107.4	76.0

Housing

Poor health and poor housing cannot fail to be associated in the mind of any physician, nurse, or social worker who has been called upon to see patients in the slums or blighted areas of our cities. Associated, of course, with poor housing are other factors and conditions prejudicial to health: poverty, overcrowding, and ignorance and carelessness about nutrition, hygiene, sanitation, and other basic principles of personal health. Typhoid and paratyphoid fever have been reported to be twice as frequent in houses with outside toilets. The communicable diseases of childhood, as well as tuberculosis and pneumonia, are more prevalent in crowded than uncrowded houses. Accident rates are consistently higher in old dilapidated houses than in newer, well-maintained ones.

Recognizing the importance of housing to health, the American Public Health Association a few years ago set up a Committee on the Hygiene of Housing. This committee has published two reports which summarize the principles of healthful housing as follows:[1]

---

[1] "Basic Principles of Healthful Housing" (pamphlet), American Public Health Association, New York, 1946.

FUNDAMENTAL PHYSIOLOGICAL NEEDS

Maintenance of a thermal environment which will avoid undue heat loss from the human body

Maintenance of a thermal environment which will permit adequate heat loss from the human body

Provision of an atmosphere of reasonable chemical purity

Provision of adequate daylight illumination and avoidance of undue daylight glare

Provision for admission of direct sunlight

Provision of adequate artificial illumination and avoidance of glare

Protection against excessive noise

Provision of adequate space for exercise and for the play of children

FUNDAMENTAL PSYCHOLOGICAL NEEDS

Provision of adequate privacy for the individual

Provision of opportunities for normal family life

Provision of opportunities for normal community life

Provision of facilities which make possible the performance of the tasks of the household without undue physical and mental fatigue

Provision of facilities for maintenance of cleanliness of the dwelling and of the person

Provision of possibilities for esthetic satisfaction in the home and its surroundings

Concordance with prevailing social standards of the local community

PROTECTION AGAINST CONTAGION

Provision of a water supply of safe sanitary quality, available to the dwelling

Protection of the water supply system against pollution within the dwelling

Provision of toilet facilities of such a character as to minimize the danger of transmitting disease

Protection against sewage contamination of the interior surfaces of the dwelling

Avoidance of insanitary conditions in the vicinity of the dwelling

Exclusion from the dwelling of vermin which may play a part in the transmission of disease

Provision of facilities for keeping milk and food undecomposed

Provision of sufficient space in sleeping-rooms to minimize the danger of contact infection

PROTECTION AGAINST ACCIDENTS

Erection of the dwelling with such materials and methods of construction as to minimize danger of accidents due to collapse of any part of the structure

[593   ]

Control of conditions likely to cause fires or to promote their spread
Provision of adequate facilities for escape in case of fire
Protection against danger of electrical shocks and burns
Protection against gas poisonings
Protection against falls and other mechanical injuries in the home
Protection of the neighborhood against the hazards of automobile traffic

Research

Medical research has made possible the prevention or control of many of the age-old scourges of mankind—smallpox, typhoid fever, yellow fever, malaria, diphtheria, rickets, beriberi, cholera, typhus, and bubonic plague. It has made possible also the successful treatment of many other diseases that a generation ago were taking a heavy toll of life and health—diabetes, pernicious anemia, most types of pneumonia, syphilis, appendicitis. These far-reaching accomplishments mean for millions not only the difference between living and dying, but even more important, the difference between useful, happy living and unfruitful existing.

In spite of all this progress, however, the unknown in medicine still far exceeds the known. Medical science can neither prevent nor treat successfully the major causes of death today—heart disease, high blood pressure, cancer. It has not yet achieved the successful control of other diseases that greatly reduce our effectiveness and pleasure in living—arthritis or rheumatism, influenza, asthma, the common cold, various forms of mental illnesses. It does not yet know the basic cause of diabetes, how infantile paralysis is spread, or the physiological reasons for growing old.

The most difficult problems, in other words, remain to be solved. A scientific discovery or development which would make possible the prevention or cure of any one of the leading causes of illness would contribute more to the health of the people of this country than any amount of money expended on the building of hospitals or the extension of medical services. Clearly then, high priority in health planning for the future must be given to the provision of the funds necessary to train research workers and to provide able scholars and scientists with the time, facilities, and support for investigative work.

In the past most of the money for the support of medical research has come from private philanthropy. It is highly important that this be continued but all the funds needed cannot possibly be provided from this source. During the past few years the Federal Government and some states have been appropriating funds to support medical research in the universities and research institutes of the country.

In 1941 approximately $18,000,000 was provided for the support of medical research in this country. In 1951, a decade later, the corresponding amount was $181,000,000, of which 41 per cent was provided by the Federal Government, 33 per cent by industry, and 25 per cent from other services.[2]

This is a valuable beginning but the total appropriations for medical research are but a small fraction of the amount required for the care of patients ill with diseases which, with a little more knowledge, we could prevent or cure.

Extension of Public Health Services

A realization as to how much improvement in community and individual health results from an efficient and well-supported local health department can lead only to one conclusion; namely, that the extension of such services to the many areas of the country in which they do not now exist is one of the most urgent aspects of a future health program. The major responsibility for the developments of local health units should devolve upon the people to be served by them. But encouragement and financial aid when necessary should be given to local health departments by increased state and federal appropriations for this purpose.

Needs for Health Personnel and Facilities

Basic also to an improved and expanded health program is the need for more personnel and facilities. Specially trained and qualified public health personnel of all kinds—health officers, epidemiologists, public health engineers, public health nurses, etc.—are needed in increasing numbers. Federal appropriations

[2] *Science*, September 25, 1953.

are proposed to expand schools of public health and to provide scholarships for those in training.

More nurses, dentists, and physicians are also needed; just how many it is difficult to know. The increasing complexity of medical care is requiring more and better-qualified nurses. To supplement the services of professional nurses special training programs for practical nurses are being developed. These courses are 1 year in length, in comparison to the 3-year hospital course in nursing and the 4- or 5-year nursing courses offered by colleges and universities. The practical nurse is able under supervision to perform many of the nursing services required both in hospitals and in homes.

There is a national shortage also of dentists. In fact, there have never been nearly enough dentists to provide the dental services which are needed to keep the teeth of the people of this country in good condition. It is hoped that effective measures to prevent dental caries will reduce the amount of dental service required, but until that is accomplished provisions should be made to train more dentists.

As to physicians, the situation is less clear. This country has more physicians in relation to population than any other country in the world and the number of physicians is increasing at a greater rate than is the general population. In spite of this there are physician shortages in certain areas and in certain fields. This is due in part to the disruption of civilian medical service and medical training in wartime; in part to the increasing specialization and complexity of medical care; in part to new demands for physicians in special fields, such as industrial medicine, public health, research, and school health services; and in part to inefficient utilization and uneven distribution of these services. Some of the larger cities have more physicians than are needed, while certain rural areas are desperately in need of doctors.

The correction of the physician shortage problem probably will require, at least on a temporary basis, some increase in the number of doctors being trained. More important, however, are measures that will improve the distribution of physicians and increase the efficiency of the utilization of their services. This can be accomplished, in part at least, by the provision of strategically located and well-equipped hospitals and diagnostic centers in which physicians can work efficiently.

One of the reasons why many physicians prefer to practice in urban rather than rural communities is that they are not happy in situations where they do not have available the facilities for diagnosis and treatment upon which modern medical practice so largely depends. Such facilities must be provided by community hospitals and health centers if the best of medical care is to be made generally available. Surveys by the U.S. Public Health Service indicate that large areas of the country have no satisfactory general hospitals at all and that for the country as a whole the number of general hospital beds should be approximately doubled to meet the need. It is agreed that a hospital should be available within an hour's distance of any given home and that rural community health centers with emergency beds should be located even more conveniently. These hospitals and clinics should provide not only x-ray and laboratory facilities, with trained personnel to operate them, but also offices for the physicians who practice in the community.

Meeting the Costs of Medical Care

Widespread discussion concerning the costs of medical care has created the impression that these costs are excessively high. Yet government reports show that each year the American people spend more than twice as much for tobacco as they spend for the services of physicians and dentists. And it is estimated that annual expenditures for alcoholic beverages exceed the total expenditures for all medical care. Furthermore, the American people spend more than a third as much on advertised preparations for self-medication as they spend for all medical services combined. It would hardly seem unreasonable if we were to spend as much on the maintenance and improvement of health as we spend upon habits and practices which are at best unprofitable.

On the other hand, the occasional illness is extremely expensive. It may wreck the family finances. Most of these costs are

[597]

for hospitalization, nursing care, and other expenses incident to the illness rather than for medical service itself. Yet, these costs must be met. In fact, they usually are paid before physicians receive their fees. The important questions are whether the American people can pay for their medical care, and, if so, on what basis.

Analysis of national income and expenditures indicates that practically all except the very lowest income groups could pay for all the medical care that they need if they would give medical care a high priority in their expenditures, with preference over expenditures for alcoholic liquors, tobacco, automobiles, recreation, and savings. The major problem is not so much inability to pay for medical care as unwillingness to forego other expenditures.

Every owner of an automobile assumes a heavy risk for possible damage to the person or property of others, a risk which may exceed almost any possible expense for medical care. Responsible automobile owners, for the protection of themselves and of those whose property or persons might be injured by the cars they own, take out liability insurance. In some states automobile owners are required to carry such insurance.

Common sense says that this same principle could be applied to the financial risks incident to illness. The problem of providing for the cost of medical care can be solved for those with incomes by budgeting. For other essential services one expects to pay regularly; why not for medical service? Disability insurance can be carried as protection against the major hazards of prolonged illness and unemployment; regular medical and dental service can be provided without hardship either on a similar insurance basis or by budgeting or regularly saving for this purpose.

For those who wish to spread the financial risk of illness on an insurance basis, various plans are available. Commercial insurance companies, as well as the Blue Cross and Blue Shield organizations, offer various types of policies. Insurance of this sort is relatively new; yet by the end of 1952 more than half of the people of this country had some sort of insurance protection against the costs of accidents and illnesses.

[598]

The system of private medical practice, which has always existed in this country, is founded upon the free choice of physician by the patient and the payment of professional services on an individual fee basis. The amount of the fee usually depends upon the type of service rendered, the eminence of the physician, and the ability of the patient to pay. Most physicians care for many patients from whom they receive little or nothing in payment for their services, but they are able to do this because of the larger fees which they charge to those in good financial circumstances. In utilizing this sliding scale of fees, physicians have long followed a principle which more recently has been incorporated into our income tax laws.

This system of medical practice has given to the American people probably the best medical care found anywhere in the world. Yet it does not adequately meet the needs of all groups. During the past decade the problem of providing medical care for low-income groups has been receiving increasing attention. European countries have developed various types of plans to meet this problem. Some of these are on a compulsory insurance basis; others are supported out of tax funds and administered by the government. In certain of these countries a high quality of medical service has been maintained, but in others the service has been inferior and both the physicians and the public have suffered.

In the rural provinces of western Canada where it was impossible for physicians to earn a living in private practice, various communities have arranged to pay physicians out of public funds. In the United States also, various modifications of the system of private practice have grown up to meet special situations. Medical schools and the larger hospitals have long maintained free clinics for those unable to pay. In many localities relief funds can be used to provide necessary medical services. Certain industries have established their own medical departments to safeguard the health of and provide medical care for their employees. Most colleges and universities have developed excellent health services for their students. States operate public hospitals for patients with tuberculosis, mental illnesses, and contagious diseases; and health departments aid physicians in the provision of better care for mothers and infants and in the diagnosis and treatment of such diseases as pneumonia, diphtheria, syphilis, gonorrhea, and tetanus.

At the present time various studies and experiments are under way to determine the best way to provide low-income groups with medical services. Some are of the opinion that we should have compulsory sickness insurance, paid for in part by payroll deductions on a national basis and administered by the Federal Government. Others advocate voluntary insurance programs with special appropriations of governmental funds to provide medical care for those unable to pay the costs of insurance programs.

As a distinguished American physician said recently, "One of the worst mistakes that can be made about medical care is to look upon it as a commodity. It no more lends itself to being a commodity than does religion because it is on the very next shelf to religion in its closeness to the lives of human beings."

One of the considerations which is fundamental to the development of any sound program for the extension of medical service is that the service shall apply first to those conditions for which we have effective preventive and curative measures. If funds and facilities were unlimited, it might be justifiable to attempt to provide everything in the way of medical and hospital care for all people, but with limited funds the only intelligent basis upon which to proceed is to provide the essential services first and to postpone the expensive refinements and frills of medical care. Otherwise available funds will be dissipated so widely that little or nothing will be well done. Above all, it is essential that plans for the provision of medical care safeguard the quality of the service rendered. To fail to do so would be a catastrophe for both the public and the medical profession.

The late President Coffman of the University of Minnesota said that there are certain things in life for which we pay whether we have them or not. He was referring to education, but the same might well be said of medical care. If we fail to pay for it in dollars and cents, we will pay for it eventually in terms of inefficiency, illness, disability, and possibly even life itself.

Individual Responsibility for Health

Science is constantly making available more and more effective measures for the prevention and control of human illnesses and disabilities. Society utilizes some of this information to safeguard the health and welfare of the public. Much more, however, could be accomplished if the public were properly informed and sufficiently interested to insist upon aggressive health programs. This in turn requires constructive leadership of a type which college and university students have a special obligation to provide. The education and training which they have had place upon them the responsibility to provide the leadership upon which progress in a democratic society depends.

DISCUSSION SUGGESTIONS

1. What is the need for research and study of health and medical needs?
2. What are some of the major objectives of a health program?
3. What should be emphasized in a health program?
4. What are effective ways of solving health problems?
5. Discuss housing in relation to health.
6. How may health be related to economic status?
7. Discuss the advantages and disadvantages of government-administered compulsory sickness insurance.
8. Discuss the possibilities of voluntary hospital and medical care insurance.
9. Discuss the advantages and shortcomings of the system of private medical care which has been traditional in this country.
10. How can one arouse individual and community interest in health problems?

REFERENCES AND READING SUGGESTIONS

1. Dickinson, Frank G.: "The Cost and Quantity of Medical Care in the United States," *Bulletin* 66, American Medical Association, Chicago, 1948.
2. Dublin, Louis I.: "Health Progress, 1936–1945," Metropolitan Life Insurance Company, New York, 1948.
3. Hester, Harriet: "Antivivisection Threatens You," *Today's Health*, vol. 31, p. 18, January, 1953.
4. Heyman, D. M.: "The Health Issue: A Middle Course," *New York Times Magazine*, March 6, 1949.
5. Matthews, H. L.: "Report on Britain's Cradle-to-grave Plan," *New York Times Magazine*, January 9, 1949.
6. Meriam, L., and G. W. Bachman: "The Issue of Compulsory Health Insurance," Brookings Institution, Washington, D.C., 1948.
7. Mott, F. D., and M. I. Roemer: "Rural Health and Medical Care," McGraw-Hill Book Company, Inc., New York, 1948.

8. National Health Assembly: "America's Health: A Report to the Nation," Harper & Brothers, New York, 1949.

9. Rusk, Howard: "The Way to Better Medical Care," *New York Times Magazine*, June 29, 1947.

10. Simmons, J. S., ed.: "Public Health in the World Today," Harvard University Press, Cambridge, Mass., 1949.

11. Winslow, C.-E. A.: "The Cost of Illness and the Price of Health," Columbia University Press, New York, 1951.

12. Woodbury, C.: "How to Pay the Doctor," *Woman's Home Companion*, March, 1949.

13. "National Conference on Rural Health," *Journal of the American Medical Association*, vol. 139, pp. 928–941, April 2, 1949.

14. "Housing and Health," Milbank Memorial Fund, New York, 1951.

15. The President's Commission on the Health Needs of the Nation: "Building America's Health," Government Printing Office, Washington, D.C., 1953.

In Conclusion

If this book may be said to have any special theme or keynote it is "Be intelligent and responsible in matters of health," and practice:

THE ART OF LIVING

To touch the cup with eager lips and
taste, not drain it;
To woo and tempt and court a bliss—and
not attain it;
To fondle and caress a joy, yet hold it
lightly,
Lest it become necessity and cling too
tightly;
To watch the sun set in the West without
regretting;
To hail its advent in the East—the night
forgetting;
To smother care in happiness and grief in
laughter;
To hold the present close—not questioning
the hereafter;
To have enough to share—to know the joy
of giving;
To thrill with all the sweets of life—is
living.

—Anonymous.

APPENDIX A

Tables of Standard Weight

STANDARD WEIGHTS FOR MEN*

Age	5 Ft.	5 Ft, 1 In.	5 Ft, 2 In.	5 Ft, 3 In.	5 Ft, 4 In.	5 Ft, 5 In.	5 Ft, 6 In.	5 Ft, 7 In.	5 Ft, 8 In.	5 Ft, 9 In.	5 Ft, 10 In.	5 Ft, 11 In.	6 Ft.	6 Ft, 1 In.	6 Ft, 2 In.	6 Ft, 3 In.	6 Ft, 4 In.	6 Ft, 5 In.
16	109	111	114	117	120	124	128	132	136	140	144	149	154	159	164	169	174	179
17	111	113	116	119	122	126	130	134	138	142	146	151	156	161	166	171	176	181
18	113	115	118	121	124	128	132	136	140	144	148	153	158	163	168	173	178	183
19	115	117	120	123	126	130	134	138	142	146	150	155	160	165	170	175	180	185
20	117	119	122	125	128	132	136	140	144	148	152	156	161	166	171	176	181	186
21	118	120	123	126	130	134	138	141	145	149	153	157	162	167	172	177	182	187
22	119	121	124	127	131	135	139	142	146	150	154	158	163	168	173	178	183	188
23	120	122	125	128	132	136	140	143	147	151	155	159	164	169	175	180	185	190
24	121	123	126	129	133	137	141	144	148	152	156	160	165	171	177	182	187	192
25	122	124	126	129	133	137	141	145	149	153	157	162	167	173	179	184	189	194
26	123	125	127	130	134	138	142	146	150	154	158	163	168	174	180	186	191	196
27	124	126	128	131	134	138	142	146	150	154	158	163	169	175	181	187	192	197
28	125	127	129	132	135	139	143	147	151	155	159	164	170	176	182	188	193	198
29	126	128	130	133	136	140	144	148	152	156	160	165	171	177	183	189	194	199
30	126	128	130	133	136	140	144	148	152	156	161	166	172	178	184	190	196	201
31	127	129	131	134	137	141	145	149	153	157	162	167	173	179	185	191	197	202
32	127	129	131	134	137	141	145	149	154	158	163	168	174	180	186	192	198	203
33	127	129	131	134	137	141	145	149	154	159	164	169	175	181	187	193	199	204
34	128	130	132	135	138	142	146	150	155	160	165	170	176	182	188	194	200	206
35	128	130	132	135	138	142	146	150	155	160	165	170	176	182	189	195	201	207
36	129	131	133	136	139	143	147	151	156	161	166	171	177	183	190	196	202	208
37	129	131	133	136	140	144	148	152	157	162	167	172	178	184	191	197	203	209
38	130	132	134	137	140	144	148	152	157	162	167	173	179	185	192	198	204	210
39	130	132	134	137	140	144	148	152	157	162	167	173	179	185	192	199	205	211
40	131	133	135	138	141	145	149	153	158	163	168	174	180	186	193	200	206	212
41	131	133	135	138	141	145	149	153	158	163	168	174	180	186	193	200	207	213
42	132	134	136	139	142	146	150	154	159	164	169	175	181	187	194	201	208	214
43	132	134	136	139	142	146	150	154	159	164	169	175	181	187	194	201	208	214
44	133	135	137	140	143	147	151	155	160	165	170	176	182	188	195	202	209	215
45	133	135	137	140	143	147	151	155	160	165	170	176	182	188	195	202	209	215
46	134	136	138	141	144	148	152	156	161	166	171	177	183	189	196	203	210	216
47	134	136	138	141	144	148	152	156	161	166	171	177	183	190	197	204	211	217
48	134	136	138	141	144	148	152	156	161	166	171	177	183	190	197	204	211	217
49	134	136	138	141	144	148	152	156	161	166	171	177	183	190	197	204	211	217
50	134	136	138	141	144	148	152	156	161	166	171	177	183	190	197	204	211	217
51	135	137	139	142	145	149	153	157	162	167	172	178	184	191	198	204	212	218
52	135	137	139	142	145	149	153	157	162	167	172	178	184	191	198	205	212	218
53	135	137	139	142	145	149	153	157	162	167	172	178	184	191	198	205	212	218
54	135	137	139	142	145	149	153	158	163	168	173	178	184	191	198	205	212	219
55 and up	135	137	139	142	145	149	153	158	163	168	173	178	184	191	198	205	212	219

* Based on the records of 136,504 women and 221,819 men accepted by American and Canadian life insurance companies. Medico-Actuarial Investigation, Vol. I, The Association of Life Insurance Medical Directors and the Actuarial Society of America, New York, 1912.

STANDARD WEIGHTS FOR WOMEN*

Age	4 Ft. 8 In.	4 Ft. 9 In.	4 Ft. 10 In.	4 Ft. 11 In.	5 Ft.	5 Ft. 1 In.	5 Ft. 2 In.	5 Ft. 3 In.	5 Ft. 4 In.	5 Ft. 5 In.	5 Ft. 6 In.	5 Ft. 7 In.	5 Ft. 8 In.	5 Ft. 9 In.	5 Ft. 10 In.	5 Ft. 11 In.	6 Ft.
16	102	104	106	108	109	111	114	117	120	124	128	132	136	139	143	148	153
17	103	105	107	109	111	113	116	119	122	125	129	133	137	140	144	149	154
18	104	106	108	110	112	114	117	120	123	126	130	134	138	141	145	150	155
19	105	107	109	111	113	115	118	121	124	127	131	135	139	152	146	151	155
20	106	108	110	112	114	116	119	122	125	128	132	136	140	143	147	151	156
21	107	109	111	113	115	117	120	123	126	129	133	137	141	144	148	152	156
22	107	109	111	113	115	117	120	123	126	129	133	137	141	145	149	153	157
23	108	110	112	114	116	118	121	124	127	130	134	138	142	146	150	153	157
24	109	111	113	115	117	119	121	124	127	130	134	138	142	146	150	154	158
25	109	111	113	115	117	119	121	124	128	131	135	139	143	147	151	154	158
26	110	112	114	116	118	120	122	125	128	131	135	139	143	147	151	155	159
27	110	112	114	116	118	120	122	125	129	132	136	140	144	148	152	155	159
28	111	113	115	117	119	121	123	126	130	133	137	141	145	149	153	156	160
29	111	113	115	117	119	121	123	126	130	133	137	141	145	149	153	156	160
30	112	114	116	118	120	122	124	127	131	134	138	142	146	150	154	157	161
31	113	115	117	119	121	123	125	128	132	135	139	143	147	151	154	157	161
32	113	115	117	119	121	123	125	128	132	136	140	144	148	152	155	158	162
33	114	116	118	120	122	124	126	129	133	137	141	145	149	153	156	159	162
34	115	117	119	121	123	125	127	130	134	138	142	146	150	154	157	160	163
35	115	117	119	121	123	125	127	130	134	138	142	146	150	154	157	160	163
36	116	118	120	122	124	126	128	131	135	139	143	147	151	155	158	161	164
37	116	118	120	122	124	126	129	132	136	140	144	148	152	156	159	162	165
38	117	119	121	123	125	127	130	133	137	141	145	149	153	157	160	163	166
39	118	120	122	124	126	128	131	134	138	142	146	150	154	158	161	164	167
40	119	121	123	125	127	129	132	135	138	142	146	150	154	158	161	164	167
41	120	122	124	128	128	130	133	136	139	143	147	151	155	159	162	165	168
42	120	122	124	126	128	130	133	136	139	143	147	151	155	159	162	166	169
43	121	123	125	127	129	131	134	137	140	144	148	152	156	160	163	167	170
44	122	124	126	128	130	132	135	138	141	145	149	153	157	161	164	168	171
45	122	124	126	128	130	132	135	138	141	145	149	153	157	161	164	168	171
46	123	125	127	129	131	133	136	139	142	146	150	154	158	162	165	169	172
47	123	125	127	129	131	133	136	139	142	146	151	155	159	163	166	170	173
48	124	126	128	130	132	134	137	140	143	147	152	156	160	164	167	171	174
49	124	126	128	130	132	134	137	140	143	147	152	156	161	165	168	172	175
50	125	127	129	131	133	135	138	141	144	148	152	156	161	165	169	173	176
51	125	127	129	131	133	135	138	141	144	148	152	157	162	166	170	174	177
52	125	127	129	131	133	135	138	141	144	148	152	157	162	166	170	174	177
53	125	127	129	131	133	135	138	141	144	148	152	157	162	166	170	174	177
54	125	127	129	131	133	135	138	141	144	148	153	158	163	167	171	174	177
55 and up	125	127	129	131	133	135	138	141	144	148	153	158	163	167	171	174	177

* Based on the records of 136,504 women and 221,819 men accepted by American and Canadian life insurance companies. Medico-Actuarial Investigation, Vol. I, The Association of Life Insurance Medical Directors and the Actuarial Society of America, New York, 1912.

APPENDIX B

Food Values in Common Portions

This compact food composition table, for reference use in class work and meal planning, will enable nurses, clinicians, extension workers, and students to compare quickly the nutritive value of foods and to estimate the nutritive value of diets.

Data are given in quantities that can be readily adjusted to servings of different sizes. Values for prepared foods and food mixtures have been calculated from typical recipes. Values for cooked vegetables are without added fat.

Table 11, page 115, shows recommended amounts of key nutrients. It is adapted from the recommended daily allowances of the Food and Nutrition Board of the National Research Council.

The following abbreviations are used: gm. for gram; mg. for milligram; I.U. for International Unit; cal. for calories; Tr. for Trace. Ounce refers to weight; fluid ounce to measure.

NUTRIENTS IN HOUSEHOLD QUANTITIES OF FOODS[a]

Food and Approximate Measure or Common Weight	Water, per cent	Food Energy, cal.	Protein, gm.	Fat, gm.	Total Carbohydrate, gm.	Calcium, mg.	Iron, mg.	Vitamin A Value, I.U.	Thiamine, mg.	Riboflavin, mg.	Niacin Value, mg.	Ascorbic Acid, mg.
Milk and milk products												
Buttermilk, from skim milk, 1 cup	90	85	9	Tr.	12	288	.2	10	.09	.43	.3	3
Milk, cow:												
Fluid, whole, 1 cup	87	165	9	10	12	288	.2	390	.09	.42	.3	3
Fluid, nonfat (skim), 1 cup	90	85	9	Tr.	13	303	.2	10	.09	.44	.3	3
Evaporated (undiluted), 1 cup	74	345	18	20	25	612	.4	1,010	.12	.91	.5	3
Condensed (undiluted), 1 cup	27	980	25	26	168	835	.6	1,300	.16	1.19	.6	3
Dry, whole, 1 tablespoon	4	40	2	2	3	76	0	110	.02	.12	.1	1
Dry, nonfat solids, 1 tablespoon	4	30	3	Tr.	4	98	0	Tr.	.03	.15	.1	1
Milk, goat, fluid, 1 cup	87	165	8	10	11	315	.2	390	.10	.26	.7	2
Cheese, 1 ounce:												
Cheddar (1 in. cube)	37	115	7	9	1	206	.3	400	.01	.12	Tr.	0
Cheddar, processed	40	105	7	8	1	191	.3	370	Tr.	.12	Tr.	0
Cheese foods, Cheddar	43	90	6	7	2	162	.2	300	.01	.16	Tr.	0
Cottage, from skim milk	76	25	6	Tr.	1	27	.1	10	.01	.09	Tr.	0

Food												
Cream	51	105	3	10	1	19	.1	410	Tr.	.06	Tr.	0
Swiss	39	105	8	8	Tr.	262	.3	410	Tr.	.11	Tr.	0
Cream, 1 tablespoon:												
Light	72	30	Tr.	3	1	15	0	120	Tr.	.02	Tr.	Tr.
Heavy	59	50	Tr.	5	Tr.	12	0	220	Tr.	.02	Tr.	Tr.
Beverages, 1 cup:												
Chocolate (all milk)	80	240	8	12	26	260	.5	350	.08	.40	.3	2
Cocoa (all milk)	79	235	10	12	27	298	1.0	400	.10	.46	.5	3
Chocolate flavored milk	83	185	8	6	26	272	.2	230	.08	.40	.2	2
Malted milk	78	280	12	12	32	364	.8	680	.18	.56	—	3
Desserts:												
Blanc mange, 1 cup	76	275	9	10	39	290	.2	390	.08	.40	.2	2
Custard, baked, 1 cup	77	285	13	13	28	283	1.2	840	.11	.49	.2	1
Custard pudding, canned, strained (infant food, 1 ounce)	75	30	1	1	5	26	.1	60	Tr.	.04	Tr.	Tr.
Ice cream, plain:												
¼ of quart brick	62	165	3	10	17	100	.1	420	.03	.15	.1	1
8 fluid ounces	62	295	6	18	29	175	.1	740	.06	.27	.1	1
Fats, oils, related products												
Bacon, medium fat, broiled or fried, 2 slices	13	95	4	9	Tr.	4	.5	0	.08	.05	.8	0
Butter, 1 tablespoon	16	100	Tr.	11	Tr.	3	0	460[b]	Tr.	Tr.	Tr.	0
Fats, cooking (vegetable fats):												
1 cup	0	1,770	0	200	0	0	0	0	0	0	0	0
1 tablespoon	0	110	0	12	0	0	0	0	0	0	0	0
Lard, 1 tablespoon	0	125	0	14	0	0	0	0	0	0	0	0

[a] Adapted from the more comprehensive tables in "Composition of Foods—Raw, Processed, Prepared," Agriculture Handbook 8, U.S. Bureau of Human Nutrition and Home Economics, Washington, D.C., 1951.

[b] Year-round average.

NUTRIENTS IN HOUSEHOLD QUANTITIES OF FOODS (*Continued*)

Food and Approximate Measure or Common Weight	Water, per cent	Food Energy, cal.	Protein, gm.	Fat, gm.	Total Carbohydrate, gm.	Calcium, mg.	Iron, mg.	Vitamin A Value, I.U.	Thiamine, mg.	Riboflavin, mg.	Niacin Value, mg.	Ascorbic Acid, mg.
Margarine, 1 tablespoon	16	100	Tr.	11	Tr.	3	0	460c	0	0	0	0
Oils, salad or cooking, 1 tablespoon	0	125	0	14	0	0	0	0	0	0	0	0
Salad dressings, 1 tablespoon:												
French	40	60	Tr.	5	3	0	0	0	0	0	0	0
Home-cooked	68	30	1	2	3	15	.1	80	.01	.03	Tr.	Tr.
Mayonnaise	16	90	Tr.	10	Tr.	2	.1	30	Tr.	Tr.	0	0
Eggs												
Eggs, raw, medium:												
1 whole	74	75	6	6	Tr.	26	1.3	550	.05	.14	Tr.	0
1 white	88	15	3	0	Tr.	2	.1	0	0	.08	Tr.	0
1 yolk	49	60	3	5	Tr.	25	1.2	550	.05	.06	Tr.	0
Eggs, dried, whole, 1 cup	5	640	51	45	3	205	9.5	4,040	.36	1.14	.3	0
Meat, poultry, fish												
Beef, 3 ounces, without bone, cooked:												
Chuck	51	265	22	19	0	9	2.6	0	.04	.17	3.5	0
Hamburger	47	315	19	26	0	8	2.4	0	.07	.16	4.1	0
Sirloin	54	255	20	19	0	9	2.5	0	.06	.16	4.1	0
Beef, canned:												
Corned beef, medium fat, 3 ounces	59	180	22	10	0	17	3.7	0	.01	.20	2.9	0
Corned beef hash, 3 ounces	70	120	12	5	6	22	1.1	Tr.	.02	.11	2.4	0
Strained (infant food), 1 ounce	78	30	5	1	0	3	1.2	0	Tr.	.06	.9	0

Food												
Beef, dried, 2 ounces	48	115	19	4	0	11	2.9	0	.04	.18	2.2	0
Beef and vegetable stew, 1 cup	79	250	13	19	17	31	2.6	2,520	.12	.15	3.4	15
Chicken, canned, boned, 3 ounces	62	170	25	7	0	12	1.5	0	.03	.14	5.4	0
Chile con carne, canned (without beans), ⅓ cup	67	170	9	13	5	32	1.2	130	.01	.10	1.9	
Clams, raw, meat only, 4 ounces	80	90	15	2	4	109	7.9	120	.11	.20	1.8	
Cod, dried, 1 ounce	12	105	23	1	0	14	1.0	0	.02	.13	3.1	
Crab meat, canned or cooked, 3 ounces	77	90	14	2	1	38	.8	—	.04	.05	2.1	
Flounder, raw, 4 ounces	83	80	17	1	0	69	.9	—	.07	.06	1.9	
Haddock, fried, 1 fillet (4 by 3 by ½ in.)	67	160	19	6	7	18	.6	—	.04	.09	2.6	
Halibut, broiled, 1 steak (4 by 3 by ½ in.)	64	230	33	10	0	18	1.0	30	.08	.09	13.1	
Heart, beef, raw, 3 ounces	78	90	14	3	1	8	3.9	980	.50	.75	6.6	5
Kidneys, beef, raw, 3 ounces	75	120	13	7	1	8	6.7	0	.32	2.16	5.5	11
Lamb, leg roast, cooked, 3 ounces	56	230	20	16	0	9	2.6	0	.12	.21	4.4	0
Lamb, canned, strained (infant food), 1 ounce	79	30	4	1	0	5	.7	0	.01	.07	1.1	
Liver, beef, fried, 2 ounces	57	120	13	4	5	5	4.4	30,330	.15	2.25	8.4	0
Liver, canned, strained (infant food), 1 ounce	78	30	5	1	Tr.	7	2.0	5,440	.01	.61	1.8	18
Mackerel, canned, solids and liquid, 3 ounces	66	155	16	9	0	157	1.8	370	.05	.18	4.9	
Oysters, meat only, raw, 1 cup (13–19 medium size oysters, selects)	80	200	24	5	13	226	13.4	770	.35	.48	2.8	
Oyster stew, 1 cup with 6 to 8 oysters	80	245	17	13	14	262	7.0	820	.21	.46	1.6	
Pork loin or chops, cooked, 3 ounces without bone	50	285	20	22	0	9	2.6	0	.71	.20	4.3	0
Pork, cured ham, cooked, 3 ounces without bone	39	340	20	28	Tr.	9	2.5	0	.46	.18	3.5	0

ᶜ Based on the average vitamin A content of fortified margarine. Most margarines manufactured for use in the United States have 15,000 I.U. of vitamin A added per pound; minimum Federal specifications for fortified margarine require 9,000 I.U. per pound.

NUTRIENTS IN HOUSEHOLD QUANTITIES OF FOODS (Continued)

Food and Approximate Measure or Common Weight	Water, per cent	Food Energy, cal.	Protein, gm.	Fat, gm.	Total Carbohydrate, gm.	Calcium, mg.	Iron, mg.	Vitamin A Value, I.U.	Thiamine, mg.	Riboflavin, mg.	Niacin Value, mg.	Ascorbic Acid, mg.
Pork luncheon meat, canned, spiced, 2 ounces..	55	165	8	14	1	5	1.2	0	.18	.12	1.6	0
Salmon, canned, pink, 3 ounces..	70	120	17	5	0	159d	.7	60	.03	.16	6.8	0
Sardines, canned in oil, drained solids, 3 ounces..	57	180	22	9	1	328	2.3	190	.01	.15	4.1	0
Sausage:												
Bologna, 1 piece (1 by 1½ in diam.)..	62	465	31	34	8	19	4.6	0	.37	.40	5.7	0
Frankfurter, 1 cooked..	62	125	7	10	1	3	.6	0	.08	.09	1.3	0
Pork, bulk, canned, 4 ounces..	55	340	17	29	0	10	2.6	0	.23	.27	3.4	0
Scallops, raw, 4 ounces..	80	90	17	Tr.	4	29	2.0	0	.05	.11	1.6	
Shad, raw, 4 ounces..	70	190	21	11	0	—	.6	50	.17	.27	9.6	
Shrimp, canned, meat only, 3 ounces..	66	110	23	1	—	98	2.6		.01	.03	1.9	0
Soups, canned, ready-to-serve:												
Beef, 1 cup..	91	100	6	4	11	15	.5	—		.12	1.5	
Chicken, 1 cup..	94	75	4	2	10	20	.5	—	.02			
Chicken, strained (infant food), 1 ounce..	87	15	1	1	2	11	.1	70	Tr.	.03	.1	Tr.
Clam chowder, 1 cup..	91	85	5	2	12	36	3.6	0	.14	.33	5.7	0
Tongue, beef, raw, 4 ounces..	68	235	19	17	Tr.	10	3.2	0	.04	.10	10.9	0
Tuna fish, drained solids, 3 ounces..	60	170	25	7	0	7	1.2	70				
Veal cutlet, cooked, 3 ounces without bone..	60	185	24	9	0	10	3.0	0	.07e	.24e	5.2e	0

Mature beans and peas; nuts

Almonds, shelled, unblanched, 1 cup	5	850	26	77	28	361	6.2	0	.35	.95	6.5	Tr.
Beans, canned or cooked, 1 cup:												
Red kidney	76	230	15	1	42	102	4.9	0	.12	.12	2.0	0
Navy or other varieties with:												
Pork and tomato sauce	72	295	15	5	48	107	4.7	220	.13	.09	1.2	7
Pork and molasses	70	325	15	8	50	146	5.5	90	.13	.09	1.2	7
Beans, lima, dry, 1 cup	13	610	38	2	113	124	13.7	0	.88	.32	3.6	3
Brazil nuts, shelled, 1 cup	5	905	20	92	15	260	4.8	Tr.	1.21			
Coconut, dried, shredded (sweetened), 1 cup	3	345	2	24	33	27	2.2	0	Tr.	Tr.	Tr.	0
Cowpeas, dry, 1 cup	11	685	46	3	123	154	13.0	60	1.84	.32	4.5	3
Peanuts, roasted, shelled, 1 cup	3	805	39	64	34	107	2.7	0	.42	.19	23.3	0
Peanut butter, 1 tablespoon	2	90	4	8	3	12	.3	0	.02	.02	2.6	0
Peas, split, dry, 1 cup	10	690	49	2	123	66	10.2	740	1.53	.56	6.3	4
Pecans, 1 cup halves	3	750	10	79	14	80	2.6	50	.77	.12	1.0	2
Soybeans, dry, 1 cup	7	695	73	38	73	477	16.8	230	2.25	.65	4.9	Tr.
Walnuts, English, 1 cup halves	3	655	15	64	16	83	2.1	30	.48	.13	1.2	3
Vegetables												
Asparagus:												
Cooked, 1 cup cut spears	92	35	4	Tr.	6	33	1.8	1,820	.23	.30	2.1	40
Canned green, 6 spears, medium size	92	20	2	Tr.	3	18	1.8	770	.06	.08	.9	17
Canned bleached, 6 spears, medium size	92	20	2	Tr.	3	15	1.0	70	.05	.07	.8	17
Beans, lima, immature, cooked, 1 cup	75	150	8	1	29	46	2.7	460	.22	.14	1.8	24
Beans, snap, green, cooked, 1 cup	92	25	2	Tr.	6	45	.9	830	.09	.12	.6	18
Beets, cooked, diced, 1 cup	88	70	2	Tr.	16	35	1.2	30	.03	.07	.5	11
Broccoli, cooked, flower stalks, 1 cup	90	45	5	Tr.	8	195	2.0	5,100	.10	.22	1.2	111
Brussels sprouts, cooked, 1 cup	85	60	6	1	12	44	1.7	520	.05	.16	.6	61

[d] If bones are discarded, calcium content would be much lower. Bones equal about 2 per cent of total contents of can.

[e] Data assume cut to be prepared by braising or pot roasting. Use of proportionate quantity of drippings would add approximately 50 per cent more thiamine and niacin and 25 per cent more riboflavin.

[613]

NUTRIENTS IN HOUSEHOLD QUANTITIES OF FOODS (Continued)

Food and Approximate Measure or Common Weight	Water, per cent	Food Energy, cal.	Protein, gm.	Fat, gm.	Total Carbohydrate, gm.	Calcium, mg.	Iron, mg.	Vitamin A Value, I.U.	Thiamine, mg.	Riboflavin, mg.	Niacin Value, mg.	Ascorbic Acid, mg.
Cabbage, 1 cup:												
Raw, shredded	92	25	1	Tr.	5	46	.5	80	.06	.05	.3	50
Cooked	92	40	2	Tr.	9	78	.8	150	.08	.08	.5	53
Carrots:												
Raw, grated, 1 cup	88	45	1	Tr.	10	43	.9	13,200	.06	.06	.7	7
Cooked, diced, 1 cup	91	45	1	1	9	38	.9	18,130	.07	.07	.7	6
Canned, strained (infant food), 1 ounce	92	10	Tr.	0	2	7	.2	2,530	.01	.01	.1	1
Cauliflower, cooked, flower buds, 1 cup	92	30	3	Tr.	6	26	1.3	110	.07	.10	.6	34
Celery, 1 cup:												
Raw, diced	94	20	1	Tr.	4	50	.5	0	.05	.04	.4	7
Cooked, diced	94	25	2	Tr.	5	65	.6	0	.05	.04	.4	6
Collards, cooked, 1 cup	87	75	7	1	14	473	3.0	14,500	.15	.46	3.2	84
Corn, sweet:												
Cooked, 1 ear (5 in. long)	75	85	3	1	20	5	.6	390f	.11	.10	1.4	8
Canned, solids and liquid, 1 cup	80	170	5	1	41	10	1.3	520f	.07	.13	2.4	14
Cowpeas, immature seed, cooked, 1 cup	75	150	11	1	25	59	4.0	620f	.46	.13	1.3	32
Cucumbers, raw, 6 slices (1/8 in. thick, center section)	96	5	Tr.	0	1	5	.2g	0g	.02	.02	.1	4
Dandelion greens, cooked, 1 cup	86	80	5	1	16	337	5.6	27,310	.23	.22	1.3	29
Endive, raw, 1 pound	93	90	7	1	18	359	7.7	13,600	.30	.53	1.8	49
Kale, cooked, 1 cup	87	45	4	1	8	248	2.4	9,220	.08	.25	1.9	56
Lettuce, headed, raw, 2 large or 4 small leaves	95	5	1	Tr.	1	11	.2	270	.02	.04	.1	4

Mushrooms, canned, solids and liquid, 1 cup.	93	30	3	Tr.	9	17	2.0	0	.04	.60	4.8	
Mustard greens, cooked, 1 cup.	92	30	3	Tr.	6	308	4.1	10,050	.08	.25	1.0	63
Okra, cooked, 8 pods (3 in. long, ⅝ in. diam.).	90	30	2	Tr.	6	70	.6	630	.05	.05	.7	17
Onions, raw:												
Mature, 1 onion (2½ in. diam.).	88	50	2	Tr.	11	35	.6	60	.04	.04	.2	10
Young green, 6 small onions without tops.	88	25	Tr.	Tr.	5	68	.4	30	.02	.02	.1	12
Parsnips, cooked, 1 cup.	84	95	2	1	22	88	1.1	0	.09	.16	.3	19
Peas, green:												
Cooked, 1 cup.	82	110	8	1	19	35	3.0	1,150	.40	.22	3.7	24
Canned, strained (infant food), 1 ounce.	87	15	1	Tr.	2	5	.4	180	.03	.02	.3	2
Peppers, green, raw, 1 medium.	92	15	1	Tr.	4	7	.3	400	.02	.04	.2	77
Potatoes:												
Baked, 1 medium (2½ in. diam.).	74	95	2	Tr.	22	13	.8	20	.11	.05	1.4	17
Boiled in skin, 1 medium (2½ in. diam.).	78	120	3	Tr.	27	16	1.0	30	.14	.06	1.6	22
Boiled after peeling, 1 medium (2½ in. diam.).	78	105	3	Tr.	24	14	.9	20	.12	.04	1.3	17
French-fried, 8 pieces (2 by ½ by ½ in.).	20	155	2	8	21	12	.8	20	.07	.04	1.3	11
Potato chips, 10 medium (2 in. diam.).	3	110	1	7	10	6	.4	10	.04	.02	.6	2
Pumpkin, canned, 1 cup.	90	75	2	1	18	46	1.6	7,750	.04	.14	1.2	5
Radishes, raw, 4 small.	94	5	Tr.	0	1	7	.2	10	.01	Tr.	.1	
Rutabagas, cooked, cubed or sliced, 1 cup.	91	50	1	Tr.	12	85	.6	540	.08	.11	1.1	33
Sauerkraut, canned, drained solids, 1 cup.	91	30	2	Tr.	7	54	.8	60	.05	.10	.2	24
Soybean sprouts, raw, 1 cup.	86	50	7	1	6	51	1.1	190	.24	.21	.9	14

[f] Vitamin A based on yellow corn; white corn contains only a trace.

[g] Based on pared cucumber; unpared contains about 0.6 mg. of iron and 130 I.U. vitamin A.

NUTRIENTS IN HOUSEHOLD QUANTITIES OF FOODS (Continued)

Food and Approximate Measure or Common Weight	Water, per cent	Food Energy, cal.	Protein, gm.	Fat, gm.	Total Carbohydrate, gm.	Calcium, mg.	Iron, mg.	Vitamin A Value, I.U.	Thiamine, mg.	Riboflavin, mg.	Niacin Value, mg.	Ascorbic Acid, mg.
Spinach:												
Cooked, 1 cup	91	45	6	1	6	223^h	3.6	21,200	.14	.36	1.1	54
Canned, strained (infant food), 1 ounce	94	5	1	Tr.	1	22^h	.4	1,190	.01	.03	.1	2
Squash:												
Summer, cooked, diced, 1 cup	95	35	1	Tr.	8	32	.8	550	.08	.15	1.3	23
Winter, baked, mashed, 1 cup	86	95	4	1	23	49	1.6	12,690	.10	.31	1.2	14
Winter, canned, strained (infant food), 1 ounce	91	10	Tr.	Tr.	2	9	.1	560	.01	.02	.1	1
Sweetpotatoes, peeled, 1 sweetpotato:												
Baked (5 by 2-in.)	61	185	3	1	41	44	1.1	11,410^i	.12	.08	.9	28
Boiled (5 by 2½ in.)	69	250	4	1	57	62	1.4	15,780^i	.18	.11	1.3	41
Tomatoes:												
Raw, 1 medium (2 by 2½ in.)	94	30	2	Tr.	6	16	.9	1,640	.08	.06	.8	35
Canned or cooked, 1 cup	94	45	2	Tr.	9	27	1.5	2,540	.14	.08	1.7	40
Tomato juice, canned, 1 cup	94	50	2	Tr.	10	17	1.0	2,540	.12	.07	1.8	38
Turnips, cooked, diced, 1 cup	92	40	1	Tr.	9	62	.8	Tr.	.06	.09	.6	28
Turnip greens, cooked, 1 cup	90	45	4	1	8	376	3.5	15,370	.09	.59	1.0	87
Vegetables, mixed, canned, strained (infant food), 1 ounce	90	10	Tr.	0	2	9	.3	j	.01	.01	.1	1
Fruits												
Apples, raw, 1 medium (2½ in. diam.)	84	75	Tr.	1	20	8	.4	120	.05	.04	.2	6
Apple juice, fresh or canned, 1 cup	86	125	Tr.	0	34	15	1.2	90	.05	.07	Tr.	2
Apple betty, 1 cup	64	345	4	7	70	34	.2	370	.13	.09	1.1	3
Applesauce, canned, sweetened, 1 cup	80	185	1	Tr.	50	10	1.0	80	.05	.03	.1	3

Apricots:												
Raw, 3 apricots	85	55	1	Tr.	14	17	.5	2,990	.03	.05	.9	7
Canned in sirup, 4 medium halves and 2 tablespoons sirup	77	95	1	Tr.	26	12	.4	1,650	.02	.03	.4	5
Canned, strained (infant food), 1 ounce	83	15	Tr.	Tr.	4	6	.3	480	.01	.01	.1	1
Dried, cooked, unsweetened, fruit and liquid, 1 cup	75	240	5	Tr.	62	80	4.6	6,900	.01	.14	2.8	9
Avocados, raw, ½ peeled fruit (3½ by 3¼ in.)	65	280	2	30	6	11	.7	330	.07	.15	1.3	18
Bananas, raw, 1 medium (6 by 1½ in.)	75	90	1	Tr.	23	8	.6	430	.04	.05	.7	10
Blackberries, raw, 1 cup	85	80	2	1	18	46	1.3	280	.05	.06	.5	30
Blueberries, raw, 1 cup	83	85	1	1	21	22	1.1	400	.04	.03	.4	23
Cantaloups, raw, ½ melon (5 in. diam.)	94	35	1	Tr.	8	31	.7	6,190[k]	.09	.07	.9	59
Cherries, 1 cup pitted:												
Raw	83	65	1	1	16	19	.4	710	.05	.06	.4	9
Canned red sour	87	120	2	1	30	28	.8	1,840	.07	.04	.4	14
Cranberry sauce, sweetened, 1 cup	48	550	Tr.	1	142	22	.8	80	.06	.06	.3	5
Dates, "fresh" and dried, pitted and cut, 1 cup	20	505	4	1	134	128	3.7	100	.16	.17	3.9	0
Figs, raw, 3 small (1½ in. diam.)	78	90	2	Tr.	22	62	.7	90	.06	.06	.6	2
Figs, dried, 1 large (2 by 1 in.)	24	55	1	Tr.	14	39	.6	20	.03	.02	.4	0
Fruit cocktail, canned, solids and liquid, 1 cup	81	180	1	1	48	23	1.0	410	.03	.03	.9	5
Grapefruit, raw, 1 cup sections	89	75	1	Tr.	20	43	.4	20	.07	.04	.4	78
Grapefruit juice:												
Canned, unsweetened, 1 cup	89	90	1	Tr.	24	20	.7	20	.07	.04	.4	85
Frozen concentrate, 6-ounce can	58	295	4	1	77	63	2.4	60	.24	.13	1.4	272

[h] Calcium may not be usable because of presence of oxalic acid.
[i] If very pale varieties only were used, the vitamin A value would be very much lower.
[j] Vitamin A value ranges from 270 to 1,510 I.U. per ounce.
[k] Vitamin A based on deeply colored yellow varieties.

[617]

NUTRIENTS IN HOUSEHOLD QUANTITIES OF FOODS (Continued)

Food and Approximate Measure or Common Weight	Water, per cent	Food Energy, cal.	Protein, gm.	Fat, gm.	Total Carbohydrate, gm.	Calcium, mg.	Iron, mg.	Vitamin A Value, I.U.	Thiamine, mg.	Riboflavin, mg.	Niacin Value, mg.	Ascorbic Acid, mg.
Grapes, 1 cup:												
American type (slip skin)	82	85	2	2	18	20	.7	90	.07	.05	.3	5
European type (adherent skin)	82	100	1	1	26	26	.9	120	.09	.06	.4	6
Grape juice, bottled, 1 cup	81	170	1	0	46	25	.8	—	.09	.12	.6	Tr.
Lemon juice, fresh, 1 cup	91	60	1	Tr.	19	34	.2	0	.11	.01	.3	122
Lime juice, fresh, 1 cup	91	60	1	0	20	34	.2	0	.11	.01	.3	65
Oranges, 1 medium (3-in. diam.)	87	70	1	Tr.	17	51	.6	290	.12	.04	.4	77
Orange juice:												
Fresh, 1 cup	88	110	2	Tr.	27	47	.5	460	.19	.06	.6	122
Canned, unsweetened, 1 cup	88	110	2	Tr.	27	25	.7	240	.17	.04	.6	103
Frozen concentrate, 6-ounce can	58	300	5	1	75	69	2.0	670	.48	.11	1.5	285
Papayas, raw, cubed, 1 cup	89	70	1	Tr.	18	36	.5	3,190	.06	.07	.5	102
Peaches:												
Raw, 1 medium (2½ by 2-in. diam.)	87	45	1	Tr.	12	8	.6	880	.02	.05	.9	8
Canned in sirup, solids and liquid, 1 cup	81	175	1	Tr.	47	13	1.0	1,160	.02	.05	1.8	11
Canned (infant food), 1 ounce	83	15	Tr.	Tr.	4	2	.3	180	.01	.01	.2	1
Dried, cooked unsweetened, 1 cup (10–12 halves and 6 tablespoons liquid)	76	225	2	1	59	38	5.9	2,750	.01	.16	4.3	11
Pears:												
Raw, 1 pear (3 by 2½ in. diam.)	83	95	1	1	24	20	.5	30	.03	.06	.2	6
Canned in sirup, 2 medium size halves and 2 tablespoons sirup	81	80	Tr.	Tr.	22	9	.2	Tr.	.01	.02	.2	2
Canned (infant food), 1 ounce	86	15	Tr.	Tr.	4	3	.1	10	Tr.	.01	.1	Tr.

Persimmons, Japanese, raw, seedless kind, 1 persimmon (2¼ in. diam.)..	78	95	1	Tr.	24	7	.4	3,270	.06	.05	Tr.	13
Pineapple:												
Raw, diced, 1 cup..	85	75	1	Tr.	19	22	.4	180	.12	.04	.3	33
Canned in sirup, 2 small or 1 large slice and 2 tablespoons juice..	78	95	Tr.	Tr.	26	35	.7	100	.09	.02	.2	11
Pineapple juice, canned, 1 cup..	86	120	1	Tr.	32	37	1.2	200	.13	.04	.4	22
Plums, raw, 1 plum (2-in. diam.)..	86	30	Tr.	Tr.	7	10	.3	200	.04	.02	.3	3
Prunes, cooked, unsweetened, 1 cup (16–18 prunes and ⅓ cup liquid)..	65	310	3	1	82	62	4.5	2,210	.07	.20	2.0	2
Prune juice, canned, 1 cup..	80	170	1	0	46	60	4.3	—	.07	.19	1.0	2
Rasins, dried, 1 cup..	24	430	4	1	114	125	5.3	80	.24	.13	.8	Tr.
Raspberries, red, raw, 1 cup..	84	70	1	Tr.	17	49	1.1	160	.03	.03	.4	29
Rhubarb, cooked with sugar, 1 cup..	63	385	1	Tr.	98	112¹	1.1	70	.02	—	.2	17
Strawberries:												
Raw, 1 cup..	90	55	1	1	12	42	1.2	90	.04	.10	.4	89
Frozen, 3 ounces..	72	90	1	Tr.	23	19	.5	30	.02	.04	.2	35
Tangerines, 1 medium (2½ in. diam.)..	87	35	1	Tr.	9	27	.3	340	.06	.02	.2	25
Tangerine juice, canned, 1 cup..	89	95	2	1	23	47	.5	1,040	.15	.06	.6	64
Watermelons, ½ slice (¾ by 10 in.)..	92	45	1	Tr.	11	11	.3	950	.08	.08	.3	10
Grain products												
Barley, pearled, light, dry, 1 cup..	11	710	17	2	160	32	4.1	0	.25	.17	6.3	0
Biscuits, baking powder, enriched flour, 1 biscuit (2½ in. diam.)..	27	130	3	4	20	83	.7	0	.09	.08	.7	0
Bran flakes, 1 cup..	4	115	4	1	32	24	2.0	0	.19	.09	3.5	0
Breads, 1 slice:												
Boston brown, unenriched..	44	105	2	1	22	89	1.2	70	.04	.06	.7	0
Rye..	35	55	2	Tr.	12	17	.4	0	.04	.02	.4	0

¹ Calcium may not be usable because of presence of oxalic acid.

[619]

NUTRIENTS IN HOUSEHOLD QUANTITIES OF FOODS (Continued)

Food and Approximate Measure or Common Weight	Water, per cent	Food Energy, cal.	Protein, gm.	Fat, gm.	Total Carbohydrate, gm.	Calcium, mg.	Iron, mg.	Vitamin A Value, I.U.	Thiamine, mg.	Riboflavin, mg.	Niacin Value, mg.	Ascorbic Acid, mg.
White, unenriched, 4 per cent nonfat milk solids[m]	35	65	2	1	12	18	.1	0	.01	.02	.2	0
White, enriched, 4 per cent nonfat milk solids[m]	35	65	2	1	12	18	.4[n]	0	.06[n]	.04[n]	.5[n]	0
White, enriched, 6 per cent nonfat milk solids[m]	34	65	2	1	12	21	.4[n]	0	.06[n]	.04[n]	.5[n]	0
Whole wheat	37	55	2	1	11	22	.5	0	.07	.03	.7	0
Cakes:												
Angel food, 2-inch sector (1/12 of cake, 8 in. diam.)	32	110	3	Tr.	23	2	.1	0	Tr.	.05	.1	0
Doughnuts, cake-type, 1 doughnut	19	135	2	7	17	23	.2	40	.05	.04	.4	0
Foundation, 1 square (3 by 2 by 1¾ in.)	25	230	4	8	36	82	.3	100[o]	.02	.05	.2	0
Foundation, plain icing, 2 inch sector, layer cake (1/16 of cake, 10 in. diam.)	24	410	6	11	72	121	.5	150[o]	.03	.08	.2	0
Fruit cake, dark, 1 piece (2 by 2 by ½ in.)	23	105	2	4	17	29	.8	50[p]	.04	.04	.3	0
Gingerbread, 1 piece (2 by 2 by 2 in.)	30	180	2	7	28	63	1.4	50	.02	.05	.6	0
Plain cake and cupcakes, 1 cupcake (2¾ in. diam.)	27	130	3	3	23	62	.2	50[q]	.01	.03	.1	0
Sponge, 2-inch sector (1/12 of cake, 8 in. diam.)	32	115	3	2	22	11	.6	210	.02	.06	.1	0
Cereal foods, dry, precooked (infant food), 1 ounce	6	105	4	1	21	185	9.6	0	.34	.13	1.4[r]	0
Cookies, plain and assorted, 1 3-inch												

cooky	5	110	2	3	19	6	.2	0	.01	.01	.1	0
Corn bread or muffins made with enriched, degermed corn meal, 1 muffin (2¾ in. diam.)	49	105	3	2	18	67	.9	60[s]	.08	.11	.6	0
Corn flakes, 1 cup	4	95	2	Tr.	21	3	.3	0	.01	.02	.4	0
Corn grits, degermed, cooked, 1 cup:												
Unenriched	87	120	3	Tr.	27	2	.2	100[t]	.04	.01	.4	0
Enriched	87	120	3	Tr.	27	2	.7	100[t]	.11	.08	1.0	0
Crackers:												
Graham, 4 small or 2 medium	6	55	1	1	10	3	.3	0	.04	.02	.2	0
Soda, plain, 2 crackers (2½ in. diam.)	6	45	1	1	8	2	.1	0	.01	.01	.1	0
Farina, enriched, cooked, 1 cup	89	105	3	Tr.	22	7	.5	0	.10	.07	.4	0
Macaroni, cooked, 1 cup:												
Unenriched	61	210	7	1	42	13	.8	0	.03	.02	.7	0
Enriched	61	210	7	1	42	13	1.5	0	.24	.15	2.0	0
Muffins, made with enriched flour, 1 muffin (2¾ in. diam.)	37	135	4	4	20	99	.8	50	.09	.10	.7	0
Noodles, containing egg, unenriched, cooked, 1 cup	84	105	4	1	20	6	.6	60	.05	.03	.6	0
Oatmeal or rolled oats:												
Cooked, 1 cup	85	150	5	3	26	21	1.7	0	.22	.05	.4	0
Precooked (infant food), dry, 1 ounce	7	105	4	1	19	225	8.9	0	.36	.10	.7[u]	0

[m] When the amount of nonfat milk solids in commercial bread is unknown, use bread with 4 per cent nonfat milk solids.

[n] Iron, thiamine, riboflavin, and niacin are based on the minimum levels of enrichment specified in the standards of identity of breads proposed by the Federal Security Agency and published in the Federal Register, Aug. 3, 1943.

[o] If fat used is butter or fortified margarine, the vitamin A value would be 350 I.U. per square, and 520 I.U. per 2-inch sector, iced.

[p] If fat used is butter or fortified margarine, the vitamin A value would be 120 I.U.

[q] If fat used is butter or fortified margarine, the vitamin A value would be 150 I.U. per cupcake.

[r] Based on products ranging from 0.7 to 1.9 mg. per ounce. The niacin value of some products is as high as 6.5 mg.

[s] Based on recipe using white corn meal; if yellow corn meal is used, vitamin A value is 120 I.U.

[t] Vitamin A based on yellow corn grits; white corn grits contain only a trace.

[u] Based on products ranging from 0.4 to 1.2 mg. per ounce of cereal. The niacin value of some products is as high as 6.5 mg. per ounce.

NUTRIENTS IN HOUSEHOLD QUANTITIES OF FOODS (Continued)

Food and Approximate Measure or Common Weight	Water, per cent	Food Energy, cal.	Protein, gm.	Fat, gm.	Total Carbohydrate, gm.	Calcium, mg.	Iron, mg.	Vitamin A Value, I.U.	Thiamine, mg.	Riboflavin, mg.	Niacin Value, mg.	Ascorbic Acid, mg.
Pancakes, baked, wheat, with enriched flour, 1 cake (4-in. diam.)	55	60	2	2	7	43	.4	50	.05	.06	.3	Tr.
Pies, 4-inch sector (9-in. diam.):												
Apple	48	330	3	13	53	9	.5	220	.04	.02	.3	1
Custard	59	265	7	11	34	162	1.6	290	.07	.21	.4	0
Lemon meringue	47	300	4	12	45	24	.6	210	.04	.10	.2	1
Mince	43	340	3	9	62	22	3.0	10	.09	.05	.5	1
Pumpkin	59	265	5	12	34	70	1.0	2,480	.04	.15	.4	0
Pretzels, 5 small sticks	8	20	Tr.	Tr.	4	1	0	0	Tr.	Tr.	Tr.	0
Rice, cooked, 1 cup:												
Converted	72	205	4	Tr.	45	14	.5	0	.10	.02	1.9	0
White or milled	71	200	4	Tr.	44	13	.5	0	.02	.01	.7	0
Rice, puffed, 1 cup	4	55	1	Tr.	12	3	.3	0	.01	.01	.1	0
Rolls, plain, enriched, 1 roll (12 per pound)	29	120	3	2	21	21	.7^v	0	.09^v	.06^v	.8^v	0
Spaghetti, unenriched, cooked, 1 cup	61	220	7	1	44	13	.9	0	.03	.02	.7	0
Waffles, baked, with enriched flour, 1 waffle (4½ by 5⅝ by ½ in.)	40	215	7	8	28	144	1.4	270	.14	.20	1.0	0
Wheat flours:												
Whole, 1 cup stirred	12	400	16	2	85	49	4.0	0	.66	.14	5.2	0
All purpose or family flour:												
Unenriched, 1 cup sifted	12	400	12	1	84	18	.9	0	.07	.05	1.0	0
Enriched, 1 cup sifted	12	400	12	1	84	18	3.2^w	0	.48^w	.29^w	3.8^w	0
Wheat germ, 1 cup stirred	11	245	17	7	34	57	5.5	0	1.39	.54	3.1	0

Food												
Wheat, shredded, 1 large biscuit, 1 ounce.	6	100	3	1	23	13	1.0	0	.06	.03	1.3	0
Sugars, sweets												
Candy, 1 ounce:												
Caramels	7	120	1	3	22	36	.7	50	.01	.04	Tr.	Tr.
Chocolate, sweetened, milk	1	145	2	9	16	61	.6	40	.03	.11	.2	0
Fudge, plain	5	115	Tr.	3	23	14[x]	.1	60	Tr.	.02	Tr.	Tr.
Hard	1	110	0	0	28	0	0	0	0	0	0	0
Marshmallows	15	90	1	0	23	0	0	0	0	0	0	0
Chocolate sirup, 1 tablespoon	39	40	Tr.	Tr.	11	3[y]	.3	0	Tr.	.01	Tr.	1
Honey, strained or extracted, 1 tablespoon	20	60	Tr.	0	17	1	.2		Tr.	Tr.		
Jams, marmalades, preserves, 1 tablespoon	28	55	Tr.	Tr.	14	2	.1	Tr.		.01	Tr.	1
Molasses, cane, 1 tablespoon:												
Light	24	50	—	—	13[z]	33	.9	—	.01	.04	Tr.	
Blackstrap	24	45	—	—	11[z]	116	2.3	—	.02		.3	
Sirup, table blends, 1 tablespoon	25	55	0	0	15	9	.8	0	0	Tr.	Tr.	0
Sugar, 1 tablespoon:												
Granulated, cane or beet	Tr.	50	0	0	12	—	—	0	0	0	0	0
Brown	3	50	0	0	13	10[aa]	.4	0	0	0	0	0
Miscellaneous												
Beverages, carbonated, kola type, 1 cup.	88	105	—	—	28			0				

[623]

v Iron, thiamine, riboflavin, and niacin are based on the minimum levels of enrichment specified in the standards of identity of breads proposed by the Federal Security Agency and published in the Federal Register, Aug. 3, 1943.

w Iron, thiamine, riboflavin, and niacin are based on the minimum levels of enrichment specified in the standards of identity promulgated under the Food, Drug, and Cosmetic Act.

x The calcium contributed by chocolate may not be usable because of presence of oxalic acid; in that case the value would be 11 mg. per ounce.

y Calcium may not be usable because of presence of oxalic acid.

z Total sugars only.

aa Calcium is based on dark brown sugar; value would be lower for light brown sugar.

NUTRIENTS IN HOUSEHOLD QUANTITIES OF FOODS (Continued)

Food and Approximate Measure or Common Weight	Water, per cent	Food Energy, cal.	Protein, gm.	Fat, gm.	Total Carbohydrate, gm.	Calcium, mg.	Iron, mg.	Vitamin A Value, I.U.	Thiamine, mg.	Riboflavin, mg.	Niacin Value, mg.	Ascorbic Acid, mg.
Bouillon cubes, 1 cube	5	2	Tr.	Tr.	0	—	—	—	—	.07	1.0	0
Chocolate, unsweetened, 1 ounce	2	140	2	15	8	23[v]	1.2	20	.01	.06	.3	0
Gelatin dessert, plain, ready-to-serve, 1 cup	83	155	4	0	35	0	0	0	0	0	0	0
Olives, pickled "mammoth" size, 10 olives:												
Green	75	70	1	7	2	48	.9	160	Tr.	Tr.		
Ripe, Mission variety	72	105	1	12	1	48	.9	40	Tr.			
Pickles:												
Dill, cucumber, 1 large (4 in. long)	93	15	1	Tr.	3	34	1.6	420	Tr.	.09	.1	8
Sweet, cucumber or mixed, 1 pickle (2¾ in. long)	70	20	Tr.	Tr.	5	3	.3	20	0	Tr.	Tr.	1
Sherbet,[bb] ½ cup	68	120	1	0	29	48	0	0	.02	.07	0	0
Vinegar, 1 tablespoon	—	2	0	—	1	1	.1	—				
White sauce, medium, 1 cup	73	430	11	33	23	305	.3	1,350	.09	.41	.3	1
Yeast:												
Compressed, baker's, 1 ounce	71	25	3	Tr.	3	7	1.4	0	.13	.59	8.0	0
Dried brewer's, 1 tablespoon	7	20	3	Tr.	3	8	1.5	0	.78	.44	2.9	0

[v] Calcium may not be usable because of presence of oxalic acid.
[bb] Based on 6.8 pounds to the gallon, factory packed.

APPENDIX C

Personal Health Record

A continuous personal health record is exceedingly important for your own and your physician's future reference. Since this is to be a permanent record, check accuracy of "Personal and Family Health History" with parents and family physician. Upon completion of your health examinations request the physician for the information necessary to complete this record.

Name_____

PERSONAL AND FAMILY HEALTH HISTORY

Date of initial health examination_____

Father: If living, age_____Condition of health_____
                If dead, age at death_____Cause of death_____

Mother: If living, age_____Condition of health_____
                If dead, age at death_____Cause of death_____

Paternal
  grandfather: If living, age_____Condition of health_____
                If dead, age at death_____Cause of death_____

Paternal
  grandmother: If living, age_____Condition of health_____
                If dead, age at death_____Cause of death_____

Maternal
  grandfather: If living, age_____Condition of health_____
                If dead, age at death_____Cause of death_____

Maternal
  grandmother: If living, age_____Condition of health_____
                If dead, age at death_____Cause of death_____

Brothers: Living, ages_____Condition of health_____
                Dead, ages at death_____Cause of death_____

Sisters: Living, ages_____Condition of health_____
                Dead, ages at death_____Cause of death_____

Have any of the following diseases occurred among your relatives? If so, indicate what relatives.

Tuberculosis or consumption	Convulsions or epilepsy
Apoplexy or stroke	Nervous trouble
Mental trouble	Diabetes
Cancer	Tendency to bleed easily
Kidney trouble or Bright's disease	Hay fever
High blood pressure	Asthma
Heart disease	Hives
Sick headaches	Eczema

Indicate which of the following diseases you have had. If you have had a disease, write the age at which you had it after the name; if you have not had it, write "0"; if you are not certain write "?".

Scarlet fever	Measles	Syphilis
Diphtheria	Smallpox	Gonorrhea
Inflammatory rheumatism	Pneumonia	Whooping cough
St. Vitus's dance	Influenza	Malaria
Nervous breakdown	Tuberculosis	Chicken pox
Typhoid fever	Pleurisy	Heart disease

Other diseases:

Broken bones. If so, what?

Operations on nose or throat. If so, what?

Other operations?

IMMUNIZATION HISTORY

Have you been vaccinated against smallpox_____Age of first vaccination_____
Did it leave a scar_____Age of most recent vaccination_____.

Have you been vaccinated against diphtheria_____Age_____Did you have a Schick test before vaccination_____Result_____After vaccination_____Result_____Date of most recent Schick test_____Result_____.

Have you been vaccinated against tetanus_____Age_____.

Have you ever had a Mantoux test_____If so, when was the first one and what was the result_____If you have had more than one, when and what was the result of the most recent one_____.

Have you had any other vaccinations or inoculations_____If so, for what and when

_____

_____

_____

Summary of present symptoms or complaints.
(Date)

SUBSEQUENT EXAMINATIONS

Changes in personal or family health history since last examination.

1. (Date)

_____

2. (Date)

_____

3. (Date)

_____

4. (Date)

_____

5. (Date)

_____

6. (Date)

_____

7. (Date)

_____

8. (Date)

_____

9. (Date)

_____

10. (Date)

_____

PHYSICAL EXAMINATIONS

Dates.............									
Age................									
Height............									
Weight............									
Per cent of standard.									
Temperature.......									
Vision:									
Color vision.....									
Eye...............									
Ear...............									
Nose.............									
Throat...........									
Hearing..........									
Teeth............									
Hemoglobin.......									
Blood pressure:									
Systolic.........									
Diastolic........									
Pulse rate:									
Sitting..........									
After exercise....									
2 min. later......									
Heart:									
Condition of.....									
Lungs:									
Condition of.....									
Posture:									
A, B, C, D......									
Mantoux test......									
Schick test........									
Dick test..........									
Smallpox									
vaccination......									
Wassermann test...									
Urine examination.									
X-ray examinations.									
Special examina-									
tions...........									

Summary of Physical Findings and Health Advice.
First Examination:
(Date)

Subsequent Examinations.

1. (Date)

_____

2. (Date)

_____

3. (Date)

_____

4. (Date)

_____

5. (Date)

_____

6. (Date)

_____

7. (Date)

_____

8. (Date)

_____

9. (Date)

_____

10. (Date)

_____

APPENDIX D

Control of Communicable Diseases in Man

This section is from the official report of the American Public Health Association on the Control of Communicable Diseases in Man (8th edition, 1955). It is reprinted by the courtesy and with the permission of the American Public Health Association.

DEFINITIONS

(Technical meaning of terms used in the text)

1. *Animal host.* An animal other than man which under natural conditions harbors an infectious agent pathogenic for man.

2. *Carrier.* A carrier is a person who harbors a specific infectious agent in the absence of discernible clinical disease and serves as a potential source or reservoir of infection for man. The carrier state may occur with infections inapparent throughout their course (commonly known as healthy carriers), and also as a feature of incubation period, convalescence and post-convalescence of infections having a recognized clinical stage (commonly known as incubationary and convalescent carriers). Under either circumstance the carrier state may be short or long (temporary or chronic carriers). The same applies to animal carriers.

3. *Cleaning.* The removal from surfaces by scrubbing and washing, as with hot water, soap, and washing soda (Na_2CO_3) or other detergent, of infectious agents and organic matter on which and in which infectious agents may find favorable conditions for prolonging life and virulence.

4. *Communicable disease.* An illness due to an infectious agent or its toxic products which is transmitted directly or indirectly to a well person from an infected person or animal, or through the agency of an intermediate animal host, vector, or the inanimate environment. (This report also includes infestations by ectoparasites such as pediculosis, see 20, Infestation.)

5. *Communicable period.* The time or times during which the etiologic agent may be transferred directly or indirectly from an infected person to another person, or from an infected animal to man.

In diseases such as diphtheria and scarlet fever, in which mucous membranes are involved from the first entry of the pathogen, the period of communicability is from the date of first exposure to a source of infection, until the infecting microorganism is no longer disseminated from the involved mucous membranes; i.e., from before the prodromata until the termination of a carrier state, if such develops.

In diseases such as tuberculosis, syphilis, and gonorrhea, the communicable state may be at any time over a long and sometimes intermittent period when unhealed lesions of the disease permit the discharge of infectious agents from the surface of the skin or through any of the body orifices. In certain diseases communicability does not occur during the early incubation period or after full recovery; e.g., measles and chickenpox.

In diseases transmitted by arthropods, such as malaria and yellow fever, the periods of communicability are those during which the etiologic agent occurs in the blood or other tissues of the infected person in infective form and in sufficient numbers for vector infection; and similarly in the tissues of the arthropod.

6. *Contact.*   A contact is any person or animal known to have been in such association with an infected person or animal as to have had the opportunity of acquiring the infection. Contact may be immediate and intimate, involving touching or close approximation of sick and well; or remote or casual with no direct physical contact. Familial contacts are those living within a single household, and commonly distinguished from those arising through work, school or play.

7. *Contamination.*   The presence of a pathogenic agent on a body surface or on or in an inanimate article or substance.

8. *Disinfection.*   Killing of pathogenic agents outside the body by chemical or physical means directly applied.

Concurrent disinfection is the application of disinfection as soon as possible after the discharge of infectious material from the body of an infected person, or after the soiling of articles with such infectious discharges, all personal contact with such discharges or articles being prevented prior to such disinfection.

Terminal disinfection indicates the process of rendering the personal clothing and immediate physical environment of the patient free from the possibility of conveying the infection to others, after the patient has ceased to be a source of infection or isolation practices have been discontinued.

9. *Disinfestation.*   Any physical or chemical process serving to destroy undesired animal forms, especially arthropods or rodents, present upon the person, the clothing, or in the environment of an individual, or on domestic animals. (See Insecticide and Rodenticide infra.) This includes the processes commonly called "delousing" as applied to infestation with Pediculus humanus, the body louse.

10. *Education in personal cleanliness.*   This phrase includes the various means available to impress upon all members of the community, young and old, and especially when communicable disease is prevalent or during epidemics, by spoken and printed word, and by illustration and suggestion, the necessity of:

   a. Keeping the body clean by sufficiently frequent soap and water baths.

   b. Washing hands in soap and water immediately after voiding bowels or bladder and always before eating.

   c. Keeping hands and unclean articles, or articles that have been used for toilet purposes by others, away from the mouth, nose, eyes, ears, genitalia, and wounds.

   d. Avoiding the use of common or unclean eating, drinking, or toilet articles of any kind, such as cutlery and crockery, drinking cups, towels, handkerchiefs, combs, hairbrushes, and pipes.

[631   ]

e. Avoiding exposure of persons to spray from the nose and mouth, as in coughing, sneezing, laughing, or talking.

f. Washing hands thoroughly after handling the patient or his belongings and wearing a protective overall apron while in the sickroom.

11. *Epidemic.* An epidemic or outbreak is here defined as the occurrence in a community or region of a group of illnesses of similar nature, clearly in excess of normal expectancy, and derived from a common or propagated source. The number of cases indicating presence of an epidemic will vary according to the etiologic agent, size and type of population exposed, previous experience or lack of exposure to the disease, and time and place of occurrence; epidemicity is thus relative to usual frequency of the disease in the same area, among the specified population, at the same season of year. A single case of a communicable disease long absent, or first invasion by a disease never previously recognized in that area, is considered to meet these requirements, as dengue fever in Florida or American trypanosomiasis in Texas.

12. *Fumigation.* Any process by which the killing of animal forms, especially arthropods and rodents, is accomplished by the employment of gaseous agents. (See 21, Insecticide and 30, Rodenticide.)

13. *Immune person.* An immune person is one who possesses specific protective antibodies or cellular immunity as a result of previous infection or immunization, or is so conditioned by such previous specific experience as to respond adequately with production of antibodies sufficient in either instance to protect from illness following exposure to the etiologic agent of the disease. This applies also to animals. Immunity is relative; an ordinarily effective protection may be overwhelmed by an excessive dose of the infectious agent or an unusual portal of entry.

14. *Inapparent infection.* A person or animal has an inapparent infection (also known as latent or subclinical infection) when the infectious agent has so mild an effect that even though infection be present and is identifiable by laboratory means, it is likely to be undetected clinically.

15. *Incidence.* The number of cases of disease, of infection or other event occurring during a prescribed time period, in relation to the unit of population in which they occur (a dynamic measurement); thus the incidence of tuberculosis expressed as a rate is the number of new cases recognized and reported per 100,000 population per year.

16. *Incubation period.* The time interval between the infection of a susceptible person or animal and the appearance of signs or symptoms of the disease in question.

17. *Infected person.* Infected persons include patients or sick persons, persons with inapparent infection, and carriers. The same expression holds for animals, including arthropods.

18. *Infection.* The entry and development or multiplication of a particular pathogen in the body of man or animal. The presence of living infectious agents on exterior surfaces of the body or upon articles of human use, as apparel or toilet articles, is not infection but soiling of such surfaces and articles. The term "infection" should not be used to describe conditions of inanimate matter such as soil, water, sewage, milk, or food; the term "contamination" applies (see 7, Contamination).

19. *Infectious disease.* A disease of man or animal resulting from an infection.

20. *Infestation.* By infestation of persons and animals is meant the lodgment, development, and reproduction of arthropods on the surface of the body or in the clothing. Infested articles or premises are such as harbor or give shelter to animal forms, especially arthropods and rodents.

21. *Insecticide.* Any chemical substance used for the destruction of arthropods, whether applied as powder, liquid, atomized liquid, aerosol, or as a paint-spray with residual action. The term larvicide is generally used to designate insecticides applied specifically for destruction of immature stages of arthropods, imagocide and adulticide to mature and adult forms.

22. *Isolation.* The separation for the period of communicability of infected persons from other persons, in such places and under such conditions as will prevent the direct or indirect conveyance of the infectious agent from infected persons to other persons who are susceptible or who may spread the agent to others. This applies also to animals.

Strict isolation of the patient for the period of communicability is necessary in certain diseases, notably smallpox. However, isolation of the patient has but little effect in limiting the spread of many other diseases, for instance poliomyelitis.

When used in connection with such diseases as the common cold, influenza, chicken-pox, mumps, and the pneumonias, isolation is not to be understood, under ordinary circumstances, as a necessary or practicable procedure for official requirement or enforcement, but a modified practice to be instituted under the direction of the attending physician, and its duration to be generally, if not exclusively, at his discretion.

Other than for rare exceptions and under special circumstances, the placarding of premises has no place in public health practice as a means to enforce isolation.

23. *Patient or sick person.* A person suffering from a recognizable attack of a communicable disease.

24. *Prevalence.* The number of cases of disease, of infected persons, or of persons with some other attribute, present at a particular time and in relation to the size of the population from which drawn (a static measurement); thus the prevalence of tuberculosis is commonly expressed as the number of cases (all forms, old and new) existing at a designated time per 100,000 persons.

25. *Quarantine.* (1) Complete quarantine is the limitation of freedom of movement of such well persons or domestic animals as have been exposed to a communicable disease, for a period of time equal to the longest usual incubation period of the disease, in such manner as to prevent effective contact with those not so exposed.

(2) Modified quarantine is a selective, partial limitation of freedom of movement of persons or domestic animals, commonly on the basis of known or presumed differences in susceptibility, but sometimes because of danger of disease transmission. It may be designed to meet particular situations; examples are exclusion of children from school or exemption of immune persons from provisions required of susceptible persons, prohibition of contacts from acting as food handlers, or restriction of military populations to the post or to quarters.

(3) Surveillance is the practice of close supervision of contacts for purposes of prompt recognition of infection or illness without restricting their movements.

(4) Segregation is the separation for special consideration, control, or observation of some part of a group of persons or of domestic animals from the others, to facilitate the control of a communicable disease. Removal of susceptible children to homes of immune persons, or the establishment of a sanitary boundary to protect uninfected from infected portions of a population are examples.

26. *Repellent.* A chemical applied to the skin or clothing or other places to discourage arthropods from lighting on and attacking an individual who cannot be protected otherwise.

27. *Report of a disease.* Official report is notification of the occurrence of a com-

municable or other disease in man or animals; to the local health authority for diseases of man, to the livestock, sanitary or agriculture authority for diseases of animals, and in some instances, disease of both animal and man to the health authority. Report should include suspect cases of diseases of particular public health importance, ordinarily those requiring epidemiologic investigation or initiation of special control measures.

When a person is infected in one health jurisdiction and the case is reported from another, the authority receiving the report should notify the other jurisdiction involved, especially if the disease is such as to require examination of contacts for infection, and of food or water supplies as vehicles.

In addition to routine reporting of specified diseases, as determined by the needs of the particular health jurisdiction, special notification of all epidemics or outbreaks of disease, including those not in the list declared reportable, is regularly to be required (see 11, Epidemic).

28. *Reservoir of infection.* Reservoirs of infection are man, animals, plants, soil, or inanimate organic matter, in which an infectious agent lives and multiplies and depends primarily for survival, reproducing itself in such manner that it can be transmitted to man. Man himself is the most frequent reservoir of infectious agents pathogenic for man.

29. *Resistance.* The sum total of body mechanisms which interpose barriers to the progress of invasion of infectious agents.

    a. Immunity—Immunity is here defined as that resistance usually associated with possession of antibodies for a specific disease. Passive immunity is attained either naturally by maternal transfer, or artificially by inoculation of specific protective antibodies (convalescent or immune serum, or gamma globulin) and is of brief duration. Active immunity is attained either naturally by infection, with or without clinical manifestations, or artificially by inoculation of fractions or products of the infectious agent, or of the agent itself in killed, modified or variant form.

    b. Inherent insusceptibility—Inherent insusceptibility is an ability to resist disease independently of antibodies or specifically developed tissue response; it commonly rests in anatomic or physiologic characteristics of the host; it may be genetic or acquired; permanent or temporary; autarcesis.

30. *Rodenticide.* A chemical substance used for the destruction of rodents, generally through ingestion. (Compare 12, Fumigation.)

31. *Source of infection.* The thing, person, object or substance from which an infectious agent passes immediately to a host. Transfer is often direct from reservoir to host in which case the reservoir is also the source of infection (measles). The source may be at any point in the chain of transmission, as a vehicle, vector, intermediate animal host or fomite; thus, contaminated water (typhoid), an infective mosquito (yellow fever), beef (tapeworm infection), or a toy (diphtheria). In each instance cited the reservoir is an infected person. (Compare 28, Reservoir.)

32. *Susceptible.* A person or animal presumably not possessing resistance against a particular pathogenic agent and for that reason liable to contract a disease if exposed to such agent.

33. *Suspect.* A person whose medical history and symptoms suggest that he may have or be developing some communicable disease.

34. *Transmission of infection.* Modes of transmission are the mechanisms by which an infectious agent is transported from reservoir to susceptible human host. They are:

    a. Contact:

[634]

(1) Direct contact: Actual touching of the infected person or animal or other reservoir of infection, as in kissing, sexual intercourse or other contiguous personal association.

(2) Indirect contact: Touching of contaminated objects such as toys, handkerchiefs, soiled clothing, bedding, surgical instruments and dressings, with subsequent hand to mouth transfer; less commonly, transfer to abraded or intact skin or mucous membrane.

(3) Droplet spread: The projection on to the conjunctivae and the face or into the nose or mouth of the spray emanating from an infected person during sneezing, coughing, singing or talking. Such droplets usually travel not more than 3 feet from the source. Transmission by droplet infection is considered a form of contact infection, since it involves reasonably close association between two or more persons.

b. Vehicle: Water, food, milk, biological products to include serum and plasma, or any substance or article serving as an intermediate means by which the infectious agent is transported from a reservoir and introduced into a susceptible host through ingestion, through inoculation or by deposit on skin or mucous membrane.

c. Vector: Arthropods or other invertebrates which transmit infection by inoculation into or through the skin or mucous membrane by biting, or by deposit of infective materials on the skin or on food or other objects. The vector may be infected itself or may act only as a passive or mechanical carrier of the agent.

d. Air-borne:

(1) Droplet nuclei: The inhalation of the small residues which result from evaporation of droplets (see a 3 above) and remain suspended in air of enclosed spaces for relatively long periods of time. Droplet nuclei also may be created purposely by a variety of atomizing devices, or accidentally in the course of many laboratory procedures.

(2) Dust: The inhalation or settling on body surfaces of coarser particles which may arise from contaminated floors, clothes, bedding, or soil, and ordinarily remain suspended in the air for relatively short periods of time.

ACTINOMYCOSIS

1. *Identification.* A chronic suppurative or granulomatous process, most frequently localized in jaw, lungs or abdomen, and characterized by swellings, firm at first but later breaking down to form multiple draining sinuses. The course is long and recovery uncommon, with death usually from some intercurrent disease.

Naked eye or hand lens examination of materials from lesions or discharges usually show small "sulfur granules" which microscopic examination identifies as actual colonies of the fungus; diagnosis confirmed by anaerobic culture of the fungus.

2. *Etiologic agent.* Actinomyces bovis (Actinomyces israeli).

3. *Source and reservoir of infection.* The source of clinical infection is the oral cavity of man where the fungus maintains an inapparent infection around carious teeth and in tonsillar crypts; reservoir unknown.

4. *Mode of transmission.* From the site of inapparent infection in the mouth, the fungus may be swallowed, inhaled or introduced into jaw tissues by injury. Not known to be transmissible in nature from man to man or from animal to animal.

5. *Incubation period.* Unknown; probably weeks or months.

[635]

6. *Period of communicability.* Contamination of the environment as long as infection persists; a chronic disease.
7. *Susceptibility and resistance.* Natural susceptibility is low. No immunity follows attack.
8. *Occurrence.* An infrequent disease of man, occurring sporadically all over the world. All races, both sexes and all age groups may be infected; the ratio of males to females is approximately two to one, and most cases are between ages 15 and 35. Primarily a disease of cattle, swine, horses and other animals.
9. *Methods of control:*
   A. Preventive measures: Meat inspection of slaughtered animals with condemnation of infected parts is commonly required by law.
   B. Control of the infected individual, contacts and environment:
      1. Report to local health authority: Official report not ordinarily justifiable.
      2. Isolation: None.
      3. Concurrent disinfection: Of discharges and contaminated dressings.
      4. Terminal disinfection: Thorough cleaning.
      5. Quarantine: None.
      6. Immunization: None.
      7. Investigation of contacts and source of infection: Not profitable.
      8. Specific treatment: Prolonged administration of sulfonamides, penicillin, aureomycin or chloramphenicol.
   C. Epidemic measures: Not applicable, a sporadic disease.
   D. International measures: None.

ANCYLOSTOMIASIS

1. *Identification.* A chronic debilitating infection with nematodes commonly known as hookworms. A variety of vague symptoms occur, varying greatly according to degree of infection. The blood-sucking activity of the worms and a predisposing malnutrition lead to hypochromic microcytic anemia. Infected children may be retarded in mental and physical development. Death is infrequent either in acute or chronic stages, and then usually in association with other infection. Synonyms: Uncinariasis, hookworm disease.

   Hookworm infection is confirmed by finding the eggs in feces; species recognition is through microscopic examination of adult worms.
2. *Etiologic agent.* Necator americanus and Ancylostoma duodenale. Third-stage larvae pass from the skin via lymphatics and blood stream to the lungs, enter the alveoli, migrate up the trachea to the pharynx, are swallowed and reach the small intestine where they attach to the intestinal wall, develop to maturity and produce eggs.

   Infective larvae of cat and dog hookworm (Ancylostoma braziliense and A. caninum) cause a dermatitis in man called creeping eruption; the larvae are destroyed in the skin and do not otherwise affect man.
3. *Source and reservoir of infection.* The usual source of infection is soil contaminated with infective larvae. (Reservoir is feces of infected persons.)
4. *Mode of transmission.* Eggs in feces are deposited on the ground, hatch, larvae develop to the third stage (infective form) and penetrate the skin, usually the foot, in so doing characteristically producing a dermatitis (ground itch). Infection via the alimentary tract is also possible.

5. *Incubation period.* The first eggs appear in the feces about six weeks after infection. Symptoms may appear after a few weeks to many months or even years, depending on intensity of infection.

6. *Period of communicability.* Infected individuals are potential spreaders of infection as long as they remain infected and continue to pollute soil, often many years. Under favorable conditions, third-stage infective larvae remain alive in soil for several weeks.

7. *Susceptibility and resistance.* Susceptibility is universal but disease is less frequent among Negroes than whites. Some immunity develops with infection.

8. *Occurrence.* Widely endemic in those tropical and subtropical countries where disposal of feces is inadequate and soil, moisture, and temperature favor development of infective larvae. N. americanus is the prevailing species throughout tropical West Africa and southeastern United States; and A. duodenale in Mediterranean countries, including the Nile valley. Both forms occur in many parts of Asia, South America and the West Indies.

9. *Methods of control:*

    A. Preventive measures:

        1. Education as to dangers of soil pollution and methods of prevention.

        2. Prevention of soil pollution by installation of sanitary disposal systems for human discharges, especially sanitary privies in rural areas, and education of the public in the use of such facilities.

        3. Personal prophylaxis by cleanliness and the wearing of shoes.

    B. Control of the infected individual, contacts and environment:

        1. Report to local health authority: Official report not ordinarily justifiable.

        2. Isolation: None.

        3. Concurrent disinfection: Sanitary disposal of feces to prevent contamination of soil and water.

        4. Terminal disinfection: None.

        5. Quarantine: None.

        6. Immunization: None.

        7. Investigation of contacts and source of infection: Each patient and carrier is a potential or actual spreader of the disease. Examine all family contacts.

        8. Specific treatment: Tetrachlorethylene or hexylresorcinol; toxic reactions are infrequent and therapy can be repeated if necessary. The duration of communicability is shortened.

    C. Epidemic measures: Surveys for prevalence in highly endemic areas, public health education in sanitation of the environment and in personal hygiene, and provision of facilities for treatment.

    D. International measures: None.

ANTHRAX

1. *Identification.* An acute bacterial infection of animals and man; in man usually a disease of the skin. An initial papule and vesicle at the site of inoculation turns into an eschar, followed by hard edematous swelling of deeper and adjacent tissues. Pain in the early stages is unusual. If untreated, infection extends progressively to regional lymph nodes and blood stream and may result in overwhelming septicemia and death. Primary anthrax pneumonia and primary gastro-intestinal anthrax are rare. Untreated cutaneous anthrax has a fatality of

[637]

about 20%; other forms are highly fatal; appreciably lower rates with effective antibiotic therapy. Synonym: Malignant pustule.

Laboratory confirmation is by inoculation of mice with exudates from lesions or with blood or other tissues; also by direct demonstration of bacilli in lesions or discharges, and by culture.

2. *Etiologic agent.* Bacillus anthracis.
3. *Source and reservoir of infection.* The source of infection is the tissues of animals dying of the disease, or contaminated hair, wool and hides. The reservoir is any one of several species of herbivorous animals, cattle, sheep, goats, horses, and others.
4. *Mode of transmission.* Infection of skin is by common vehicles (fomites), hair, wool, hides, contaminated shaving brushes and other manufactured products, or by direct contact with infected tissues. Primary anthrax pneumonia when it occurs, presumably results from inhalation of spores. Gastro-intestinal anthrax results from ingestion of heavily contaminated meat; milk not involved. The disease spreads among herbivorous animals through contaminated soil or feed, and among omnivorous and carnivorous animals through contaminated meat, bone meal or other feed products. Flies may serve as mechanical carriers. Vultures have spread the infection from one area to another. Accidental infections occur among laboratory workers.
5. *Incubation period.* Within 7 days, usually less than 4.
6. *Period of communicability.* Rarely if ever transmitted from man to man, although discharges from lesions are infective. Contaminated articles and soil may remain infective for years.
7. *Susceptibility and resistance.* In comparison with animals man has a natural high resistance to the infection.
8. *Occurrence.* Infrequent and sporadic in man, primarily as an occupational hazard to veterinarians and agricultural workers handling animals, and to industrial workers processing hides, hair and wool. Endemic in some agricultural areas (Balkans); small localized epidemics may occur. Enzoötic in cattle, sheep and goats in most parts of the world.
9. *Methods of control:*
    A. Preventive measures:
    1. Animals suspected of having anthrax should be promptly isolated and treated; otherwise, destroyed.
    2. Post-mortem examination of animals dying of suspected anthrax should be made by a veterinarian, and with care not to contaminate soil or environment with blood or infected tissues. Carcasses should be disposed of by incineration or deep burial with quick lime.
    3. Immunization of exposed animals under direction of U.S. Department of Agriculture or comparable government authority in other nations.
    4. Control of effluents and trade wastes of rendering plants that may handle infected animals and of factories that manufacture products using potentially contaminated hair, wool or hides.
    5. Education of employees handling potentially contaminated vehicles in personal cleanliness and care of skin abrasions. Prompt medical care of all suspicious skin lesions to exclude anthrax.
    6. Dust control and proper ventilation in hazardous industries.

[638]

7. Thorough washing, disinfection or sterilization, when possible, of hair, wool or hides and bone meal or other feed of animal origin, prior to further processing.

8. Hides of animals infected with anthrax must not be sold, nor carcasses used as food.

B. Control of the infected individual, contacts and environment:

1. Report to local health authority: Case report obligatory in most states and countries. Report also to appropriate livestock, sanitary or agriculture authority.

2. Isolation: Until lesions are healed.

3. Concurrent disinfection: Of discharges from lesions and articles soiled therewith. Spores require steam sterilization under pressure, or burning.

4. Terminal disinfection: Thorough cleaning.

5. Quarantine: None.

6. Immunization: None. Vaccines used for animals are not applicable to man.

7. Investigation of contacts and source of infection: Search for history of exposure to infected animal product and trace to origin for discovery of disease in sporadic or epizootic form. If traced to a manufacturing plant, inspect for adequacy of preventive measures outlined in 9A above.

8. Specific treatment: Penicillin, also tetracycline antibiotics; supplementary sulfadiazine or anti-anthrax serum may be useful in severe cases.

C. Epidemic measures: Epidemics in man are rare. Trace source of infection and eliminate it. In animals, epizootics may be controlled by vaccination and treatment, removal of animals from contaminated pastures, and sterilization of feed products of animal origin.

D. International measures: Sterilization of imported bone meal before use as animal feed. Sterilization of hair for use in shaving brushes; regulation of processing of imported hair, wool, hides to minimize the hazard to man.

ASCARIASIS

1. *Identification.* A common chronic intestinal infection with a round worm. Symptoms are variable and often vague or absent; heavy infection may give digestive disturbances, abdominal pain, exaggerated reflexes, restlessness, and disturbed sleep. Live worms passed in the stools or vomited are frequently the first sign of infection. Ordinarily a mild infection, but complications may be serious and occasional deaths among children in tropical countries are related to this cause.

Identification of eggs in feces is the usual method of diagnosis.

2. *Etiologic agent.* Ascaris lumbricoides, the large intestinal round worm of man. After ingestion, embryonated eggs hatch in the intestinal canal, larvae penetrate the wall, and reach the lungs by way of lymphatic and circulatory systems. Most larvae reaching the lungs pass into air passages, ascend bronchi, are swallowed and eventually reach the small intestine where they grow to maturity.

3. *Source and reservoir of infection.* Infective eggs from human feces deposited in and about houses where facilities for sanitary disposal of human excreta are lacking or not used.

4. *Mode of transmission.* By direct or indirect transmission of the embryonated eggs from soil or other contaminated material to the mouth; embryonation requires about a month. Salads and other foods eaten raw are vehicles. Contaminated soil may be carried long distances on feet or footwear into houses and conveyances.

[639]

5. *Incubation period.* The worms reach maturity about 2 months after ingestion.
6. *Period of communicability.* As long as mature fertilized female worms live in the intestine. Each worm produces about 20,000 eggs a day, permitting a high content of eggs in feces even when infection is light.
7. *Susceptibility and resistance.* Susceptibility is general. Relative resistance may develop from repeated infections.
8. *Occurrence.* A world-wide and common infection, but more frequent in moist tropical countries where prevalence may exceed 50% of a population. Children of preschool and early school age tend to be more frequently and more heavily infected than older children and adults. Area of major prevalence in the United States is lower Appalachian plateau, eastern Tennessee and surrounding areas.
9. *Methods of control:*
   A. Preventive measures:
      1. Provision of adequate facilities for proper disposal of feces and prevention of soil contamination in areas immediately adjacent to houses, particularly in play areas of children.
      2. In rural areas, privies should be so constructed as to obviate dissemination of ascarid eggs through overflow, drainage or similar circumstance.
      3. Education of all members of the family, particularly children, to use toilet facilities.
      4. Encouragement of satisfactory hygienic habits on the part of children, especially the practice of washing the hands before handling food, and after defecating.
   B. Control of the infected individual, contacts and environment:
      1. Report to local health authority: Official report not ordinarily justifiable.
      2. Isolation: None.
      3. Concurrent disinfection: Sanitary disposal of feces.
      4. Terminal disinfection: None.
      5. Quarantine: None.
      6. Immunization: None.
      7. Investigation of contacts and source of infection: Individual and environmental sources of infection should be sought, particularly in the persons and premises of the family.
      8. Specific treatment: Hexylresorcinol: the drug is mildly caustic and capsules must not be chewed.
   C. Epidemic measures: Surveys for prevalence in highly endemic areas, public health education in sanitation of the environment and in personal hygiene, and provision of facilities for treatment.
   D. International measures: None.

BRUCELLOSIS

1. *Identification.* A general infection with acute or insidious onset, characterized by continued, intermittent or irregular fever of variable duration, headache, weakness, profuse sweating, chills or chilliness, and generalized aching. The disease may last for several days, many months or occasionally for several years. Recovery is usual but disability is often pronounced. Fatality rate about 2% or less; higher for B. melitensis than other varieties. Synonym: Undulant fever.
   Laboratory diagnosis is by isolation of the infectious agent from blood, bone

marrow or other tissue, or from discharges of the patient. The agglutination test is a valuable aid.

2. *Etiologic agent.* Brucella melitensis; Brucella abortus; Brucella suis.

3. *Source and reservoir of infection.* The sources of infection are tissues, blood, urine, milk, and especially placentas, vaginal discharges and aborted fetuses of infected animals. Reservoirs of infection are cattle, swine, sheep and goats.

4. *Mode of transmission.* By contact with infected animals, animal tissues or secretions, and by ingestion of milk and dairy products from infected animals. Airborne infection may occur in laboratories.

5. *Incubation period.* Highly variable and difficult to ascertain: onset is insidious and date of infection usually not established; usually 14 to 30 days, occasionally 3 months.

6. *Period of communicability.* Rarely communicable from man to man; the infecting microorganism may be discharged in urine and other excretions for long periods.

7. *Susceptibility and resistance.* Susceptibility is variable, as indicated by wide differences in severity and duration of clinical illness, lesser susceptibility of children to manifest disease, and frequency of mild and inapparent infections. Duration of acquired immunity is uncertain.

8. *Occurrence.* World-wide, especially Mediterranean countries of Europe and North and South America. Males more often affected than females because of occupational hazards. Sporadic cases and outbreaks occur among consumers of unpasteurized milk or milk products from cows and goats. More prevalent than present reports indicate because of diagnostic difficulties; in the United States less than 4,000 cases reported annually, with actual number estimated in excess of 10,000.

9. *Methods of control.* Ultimate control in man rests in the elimination of the disease among domestic animals.

  A. Preventive measures:

    1. Education of farmers and workers in slaughterhouses, packing plants and butcher shops as to the nature of the disease and the danger of handling carcasses or products of infected animals.

    2. Search for infection among livestock by the agglutination reaction and elimination of infected animals from herds by segregation or slaughter. The control of infection among swine usually requires slaughter of the drove.

    3. Pasteurization of milk and dairy products from cows, sheep or goats. Boiling milk is practicable when pasteurization is not possible.

    4. Vaccination of calves; sometimes adult animals.

    5. Care in handling and disposal of discharges and fetus from an aborted animal. Disinfection of areas contaminated.

    6. Meat inspection and condemning of infected carcasses of pork and pork products; not a useful procedure for cattle.

  B. Control of the infected individual, contacts and environment:

    1. Report to local health authority: Case report obligatory in most states and countries.

    2. Isolation: None.

    3. Concurrent disinfection: Of body discharges.

    4. Terminal disinfection: None.

    5. Quarantine: None.

6. Immunization: None.
7. Investigation of contacts and source of infection: Trace infection to the common or individual source, usually infected domestic goats, swine, or cattle, or unpasteurized milk or dairy products from cows and goats.
8. Specific treatment: The tetracycline antibiotics usually produce prompt subsidence of fever and symptoms within several days. The relapse rate is high. More satisfactory results are obtained with a combination of aureomycin and dihydrostreptomycin with or without the addition of a sulfonamide. Treatment should be continued for at least 3 weeks.

C. Epidemic measures: Search for common source of infection, usually unpasteurized milk or milk products from an infected herd. Stop distribution or provide pasteurization.
D. International measures: Control of domestic animals in international trade and transport.

CAT SCRATCH FEVER

1. *Identification.* A benign infection marked by appearance within 3 to 5 days of a red or purple inflammatory lesion of the skin at the site of cat bite or trauma; resembles a furuncle and may become crusted or pustular. Two to 3 weeks after injury, with limits of 4 days to more than a month, one or more regional lymph nodes becomes enlarged but usually solitary with overlying skin inflamed. Some patients have an evanescent rash. Symptoms of malaise, headache, anorexia and occasionally chills become more pronounced and temperature may rise to 102°–104° F., persisting for days and weeks until rupture of suppurating lymph node. The process then subsides, healing is rapid and recovery usual. Instances of a fatal meningoencephalitis have been described. Some patients have neither cutaneous lesion nor suppurating lymph node. Synonym: Benign inoculation lymphoreticulosis.

   A skin test and complement fixation with psittacosis–granuloma venereum group antigen are aids in diagnosis. Confirmation is by inoculation of monkeys with material from local lesions or discharges from suppurating lymph nodes.
2. *Etiologic agent.* Unknown; a virus closely related to the psittacosis–lymphogranuloma venereum group has been isolated from lesions.
3. *Source and reservoir of infection.* Probably several animals, usually with inapparent infection, of which the domestic cat is best known.
4. *Mode of transmission.* Commonly by bite, scratch or lick of a cat, exposure to other animals including birds, or bite of an insect. Frequent absence of such exposure suggests other modes of transmission, as through minor trauma after thorn scratch, or puncture by splinters of wood, spicules of bone or porcupine quill.
5. *Incubation period.* Several days; 2 to 8 days in instances of definite trauma.
6. *Period of communicability.* Unknown for reservoir host or for man; in man presumably for duration of open lesions; not known to be communicable from man to man.
7. *Susceptibility and resistance.* Unknown.
8. *Occurrence.* Apparently universal; reported from nearly every country in Europe, from South Africa, the United States and Canada, and several countries in South America. Commonly sporadic with occasional family or community outbreaks. Seasonal variation not determined; sex distribution equal; approximately one-

third of patients are aged less than 10 years; more than one-half are under 20 years.

9. *Methods of control:*

    A. Preventive measures:

        1. A disease first recognized in 1950. No defined preventive measures, other than avoidance of cats.

    B. Control of the infected individual, contacts and environment:

        1. Report to local health authority: Official report not ordinarily justifiable.

        2. Isolation: None.

        3. Concurrent disinfection: Of discharges from cutaneous lesions or lymph nodes.

        4. Terminal disinfection: None.

        5. Quarantine: None.

        6. Immunization: None.

        7. Investigation of contacts and source of infection: Examination of family contacts for common exposure and search for cats as possible reservoirs.

        8. Specific treatment: None; chloramphenicol and tetracycline antibiotics are stated to shorten the course.

    C. Epidemic measures: None.

    D. International measures: None.

CHANCROID

1. *Identification.* An acute, localized, self-limiting autoinoculable infectious disease characterized clinically by necrotizing ulcerations at the site of inoculation. Genital lesions frequently are accompanied by painful inflammatory swelling and suppuration of regional lymph nodes. Extragenital lesions of umbilicus, tongue, lip, breast, chin and bulbar conjunctiva are on record. Synonyms: Ulcus molle, chancre mou, soft chancre and soft sore.

    Microscopic examination of stained exudate from edges of lesion, bacteriologic culture of pus from buboes, intradermal skin test, autoinoculation and biopsy are diagnostic aids.

2. *Etiologic agent.* Hemophilus ducreyi, Ducrey bacillus.

3. *Source and reservoir of infection.* Patients with discharges from open lesions and pus from buboes; suggestive evidence that women are occasionally carriers.

4. *Mode of transmission.* Predominantly venereal except for rare instances of professionally acquired lesions on hands of doctors and nurses; also accidental inoculation of children. Indirect transmission is rare. Prostitution, indiscriminate sexual promiscuity and uncleanliness are important factors favoring transmission.

5. *Incubation period.* 3 to 5 days, occasionally longer; if abrasions of mucous membrane are present, as short as 24 hours.

6. *Period of communicability.* As long as the etiologic agent persists in the original lesion or discharging regional lymph nodes; usually parallels healing and in most instances a matter of weeks.

7. *Susceptibility and resistance.* Susceptibility is general; no evidence of natural or acquired immunity.

8. *Occurrence.* No particular differences in incidence according to age, race or sex except as determined by sexual habits. Geographically widespread and a relatively frequent disease. Incidence in military forces is sometimes higher than for syphilis.

9. Methods of control:

  A. Preventive measures:

    1. Except for specific reference to chancroid as such, and those measures specific for syphilis, the preventive measures are those of syphilis.

  B. Control of the infected individual, contacts and environment:

    1. Report to local health authority: Case report obligatory in many states and countries. With the decline in syphilis, reporting of chancroid assumes importance as a better index of sexual promiscuity.

    2. Isolation: None; avoid sexual or other personal contact until lesions are healed.

    3. Concurrent disinfection: None; ordinary personal cleanliness.

    4. Terminal disinfection: None.

    5. Quarantine: None.

    6. Immunization: None.

    7. Investigation of contacts and source of infection: Search for sexual contact of the period 2 weeks before lesions appeared and since signs and symptoms became evident.

    8. Specific treatment: Sulfonamides (sulfanilamide, sulfathiazole or sulfadiazine); tetracycline antibiotics (aureomycin) and chloramphenicol only in sulfonamide-resistance because of potentially masking syphilis.

  C. Epidemic measures: Non-declining levels of occurrence or any increase in incidence are indication for increased vigilance and more rigid application of measures outlined in 9A and 9B.

  D. International measures: See Syphilis.

CHICKENPOX

1. *Identification.* An acute infectious disease of sudden onset with slight fever, mild constitutional symptoms and an eruption which is maculopapular for a few hours, vesicular for 3 to 4 days, and leaves a granular scab. Lesions tend to be more abundant on covered than on exposed parts of the body; may appear on scalp, and mucous membrane of upper respiratory tract; commonly occur in successive crops with several stages of maturity present at the same time; may be so few as to escape observation. Essentially nonfatal; such deaths as occur are almost invariably the result of septic complications. Synonym: Varicella.

    Laboratory tests for identification of variola virus are sometimes necessary to distinguish chickenpox from smallpox.

2. *Etiologic agent.* The virus of chickenpox; whether an independent virus or identical with that of herpes zoster remains controversial.

3. *Source and reservoir of infection.* Lesions of the skin and respiratory tract of infected persons.

4. *Mode of transmission.* From person to person by direct contact or droplet spread; indirectly through articles freshly soiled by discharges from the skin and mucous membranes of infected persons. One of the most readily communicable of diseases, especially in the early stages of the eruption.

5. *Incubation period.* 2 to 3 weeks; commonly 13 to 17 days.

6. *Period of communicability.* Probably not more than one day before nor more than 6 days after the appearance of the first crop of vesicles.

APPENDIX D

7. *Susceptibility and resistance.* Susceptibility is universal among those not previously attacked; ordinarily a more severe disease of adults than of children. An attack confers long immunity; second attacks are rare.
8. *Occurrence.* Nearly universal. In metropolitan communities probably 70 per cent of persons have had the disease by 15 years of age. Not uncommon in early infancy. Winter is the season of greatest prevalence in temperate zones.
9. *Methods of control:*
   A. Preventive measures:
      1. The chief public health importance of this disease is that cases thought to be chickenpox in persons over 15 years, or of any age during an epidemic of small-pox, should be viewed with suspicion and investigated to eliminate possibility of smallpox.
   B. Control of the infected individual, contacts and environment:
      1. Report to local health authority: Official report is not ordinarily justifiable. Case report of chickenpox in adults may be required where smallpox is infrequent.
      2. Isolation: Exclusion from school for the period of communicability, and avoidance of contact with non-immune persons.
      3. Concurrent disinfection: Articles soiled by discharges from the nose and throat and from lesions.
      4. Terminal disinfection: None.
      5. Quarantine: None.
      6. Immunization: None.
      7. Investigation of contacts and source of infection: Of no importance.
      8. Specific treatment: None.
   C. Epidemic measures: No procedures in common use can be relied upon as a means of effective control of the disease or of epidemics.
   D. International measures: None.

CHOLERA

1. *Identification.* A serious acute intestinal infection characterized by sudden onset, vomiting, profuse watery diarrhea, rapid dehydration and collapse. Severity differs greatly from place to place and within epidemics; mild cases show only diarrhea. Death may occur within 24 hours. Epidemics have a fatality from 10 to 80%.

   Cholera vibrios can be cultivated from feces; if abundant, can be recognized on direct smear.
2. *Etiologic agent.* Vibrio cholerae, cholera vibrio.
3. *Source and reservoir of infection.* Feces and vomitus of patients, feces of persons in-cubating the disease and of convalescents.
4. *Mode of transmission.* Fecal contamination of water; of foods by soiled hands, utensils, or flies. Contact carriers do not play a significant role in spread of the infection.
5. *Incubation period.* From a few hours to 5 days, usually 3 days.
6. *Period of communicability.* While cholera vibrios are present in feces, usually 7 to 14 days after onset.
7. *Susceptibility and resistance.* Susceptibility is general, although natural resistance

[645]

varies. Clinical attack confers temporary immunity which may afford some protection for several years. Immunity artificially induced by vaccines is of variable degree and uncertain duration.

8. *Occurrence.* Endemic in parts of India and certain adjacent areas of Southeast Asia. From these centers, spreads along lines of communication, from time to time reaching remote countries and causing widespread epidemics. Absent from Europe and Western Hemisphere for many years although has invaded repeatedly.

9. *Methods of control:*
   A. Preventive measures:
   1. Sanitary disposal of human feces.
   2. Protection and purification of public water supplies and construction of safe private supplies.
   3. Boiling of milk and pasteurization of milk and dairy products.
   4. Sanitary supervision of processing, preparation, and serving of foods, especially those that are moist and eaten raw; special attention to provision and use of hand-washing facilities.
   5. Fly control, control of fly breeding and protection of foods against fly contamination by screening.
   6. Education of public in habits of personal cleanliness, especially washing hands before eating and after defecation.
   7. Active immunization with cholera vaccine of persons subject to unusual risk.
   B. Control of the infected individual, contacts and environment:
   1. Report to local health authority: Case report universally required by international regulation.
   2. Isolation: Of patient in hospital or screened room during communicable period.
   3. Concurrent disinfection: Prompt and thorough disinfection of feces and vomitus, and of articles used by patient. Practice by attendants of scrupulous cleanliness, disinfection of hands each time after handling or touching articles contaminated by feces, avoidance of eating or drinking in room of patient in order to avoid infection; entering kitchen prohibited.
   4. Terminal disinfection: Thorough cleaning.
   5. Quarantine: Surveillance of contacts for 5 days from last exposure and longer if feces contain cholera vibrio.
   6. Immunization: No passive immunization. Inoculation of contacts with cholera vaccine to protect against subsequent or continued exposure.
   7. Investigation of contacts and source of infection: Search for unreported cases and carriers. Investigate possible infection from polluted drinking water or from contaminated uncooked foods.
   8. Specific treatment: None. Replacement of fluid and electrolyte and other measures for shock are paramount.
   C. Epidemic measures:
   1. Boiling of water used for drinking, toilet purposes, or washing dishes or food containers, unless water supply is adequately treated as by chlorination.
   2. Inspection service for early detection of infected persons; provision of temporary and ad hoc facilities for isolation of patients and suspects; identification and isolation of carriers desirable but usually impracticable; detention in suitable camps for 5 days, of those desirous of leaving for another locality.

3. Immediate administration of cholera vaccine to exposed population groups, despite questionable value on existing evidence.
4. Careful supervision of food and drink. After cooking or boiling should be protected against contamination, as by flies and human handling.
5. Control of flies, by limiting fly breeding, by use of appropriate insecticides and by screening kitchens and eating places.

D. International measures:

1. Telegraphic notification of WHO and of adjacent countries by governments of the existence of an epidemic of cholera.
2. Measures applicable to ships, aircraft and land transport arriving from cholera areas are specified in International Sanitary Regulations (WHO Techn. Rept. Ser. No. 41, Geneva, 1951).
3. International travellers: Most countries within endemic areas, particularly Southeast Asia, require immunization for entry; many others for travellers returning from those countries. International cholera immunization certificate is valid from 6 days until 6 months after the first injection of vaccine, or in the event of revaccination within such period of 6 months, on the date of that revaccination.

COCCIDIOIDOMYCOSIS

1. *Identification.*
   A. Primary infection: May be entirely asymptomatic or resemble an acute febrile influenzal illness, with fever, chills, cough, and pleural pain. About one-fifth of clinically recognized cases (an estimated 5% of all primary infections) develop erythema nodosum (valley fever); or more rarely erythema multiforme, a complication most frequent in white females and rarest in Negro males. Primary infection may (1) heal completely without detectable residuals, (2) leave radiographic fibrosis or calcification of pulmonary lesions, (3) leave a persistent thin-walled cavity, or (4) and most rarely, progress to the disseminated form of the disease, comparable to progressive primary tuberculosis.
   The fungus may be found in sputum by direct examination or by culture. Reaction to skin test with coccidioidin appears within two days to three weeks after onset; precipitin and complement fixation tests are usually positive at an early date.
   B. Coccidioidal granuloma: A progressive, highly fatal granulomatous disease characterized by lung lesions and single or multiple abscesses throughout the body, especially in subcutaneous tissues, skin, bone, peritoneum, testes, thyroid and central nervous system. Coccidioidal meningitis resembles tuberculous meningitis.
   The fungus can be demonstrated in sputum and in materials from lesions by microscopic examination or by culture.
   A granulomatous disease, sometimes referred to as paracoccidioidal granuloma, has no relationship to coccidioidomycosis.

2. *Etiologic agent.* Coccidioides immitis.
3. *Source and reservoir of infection.* Source is soil contaminated with spores of the fungus. Reservoir of infection is unknown.
4. *Mode of transmission.* Inhalation of spores in dust and dry vegetation, and in

[647]

laboratories inhalation of spores from cultures. Infection through open wounds is a possible but infrequent route. Not directly transmissible in nature from man to man.

5. *Incubation period.* Ten days to three weeks in primary infection. Coccidioidal granuloma develops insidiously, not necessarily preceded by symptoms of primary pulmonary infection.

6. *Period of communicability.* Contamination of environment as long as open lesions remain.

7. *Susceptibility and resistance.* Susceptibility to primary infection is general; high incidence of positive coccidioidin reactors in endemic areas; recovery apparently is followed by solid immunity. Susceptibility to coccidioidal granuloma is highest in dark skinned adult males and lowest in young white females.

8. *Occurrence.* Primary infections are extremely common in scattered, highly endemic areas; in the United States from California to West Texas, and in South America several areas having similar climate and terrain. Affects all ages, both sexes, and all races. Infection most frequent in summer, especially after wind and dust storms. Coccidioidal granuloma has the geographic distribution of Valley fever. More than half of cases occur between 15 and 35 years of age; males are infected five times as frequently as females; and dark-skinned individuals ten times more than others.

9. *Methods of control:*
   A. Preventive measures:
      1. In endemic areas, planting of grass, oiling and other dust-control measures. Individuals from non-endemic areas should not be recruited to dusty occupations such as road-building.
   B. Control of the infected individual, contacts and environment:
      1. Report to local health authority: Case report of coccidioidal granuloma in selected endemic areas (USA); in many countries not a reportable disease.
      2. Isolation: None.
      3. Concurrent disinfection: Of discharges and soiled articles.
      4. Terminal disinfection: Thorough cleaning.
      5. Quarantine: None.
      6. Immunization: None.
      7. Investigation of contacts and source of infection: Not profitable.
      8. Specific treatment: None.
   C. Epidemic measures: Epidemics occur only when groups of susceptibles are infected by air-borne spores. Dust control measures should be instituted where practicable.
   D. International measures: None.

COLORADO TICK FEVER, VIRAL

1. *Identification.* An acute febrile, erythematous disease without macular rash, usually with brief remission followed by a second bout of fever, each of two or three days duration; no reported deaths.

   Specific serological tests using mouse adapted virus are used in laboratory confirmation of diagnosis.

   Clinical course, symptomatology and leukocyte response are almost identical with dengue; to be differentiated from Rocky Mountain Spotted Fever.

2. *Etiologic agent.* The virus of Colorado tick fever.

3. *Source and reservoir of infection.* Source of infection is vector ticks, usually Dermacentor andersoni, and the blood of infected persons. An animal reservoir other than man probably exists but has not been demonstrated.

4. *Mode of transmission.* Ticks presumably acquire infection through feeding on infected animals during period of viremia and after suitable extrinsic incubation transmit to man by feeding. Transovarian transmission by infected ticks has been demonstrated.

5. *Incubation period.* Usually 4 to 5 days.

6. *Period of communicability.* Not directly communicable in nature from man to man. Virus is present in man during febrile course, from 1 to 10 days after onset.

7. *Susceptibility and resistance.* Susceptibility apparently universal. Second attacks are unknown; experimental reinfection unsuccessful.

8 *Occurrence.* Known area of occurrence limited to United States: Oregon, Utah, Idaho, Wyoming, Montana and Colorado; a similar virus isolated from Dermacentor variabilis Long Island, New York, but disease in man not recognized. Predominantly a disease of adults; seasonal incidence corresponds to greatest tick activity; sporadic and endemic distribution; an uncommon disease even in affected areas.

9. *Methods of control:*
   A. Preventive measures:
      1. Control of ticks; see Rocky Mountain Spotted Fever, 9 A1 and 2.
      2. No available vaccine.
   B. Control of the infected individual, contacts and environment:
      1. Report to local health authority: In endemic areas (USA); in most states and countries not a reportable disease.
      2. Isolation: None.
      3. Concurrent disinfection: All ticks on patient should be destroyed.
      4. Terminal disinfection: None.
      5. Quarantine: None.
      6. Immunization: None.
      7. Investigation of contacts and source of infection: Identification of ticks and tick infested areas.
      8. Specific treatment: None.
   C. Epidemic measures: Not applicable.
   D. International measures: None.

COMMON COLD

1. *Identification.* An acute catarrhal infection of the upper respiratory tract characterized by coryza, lacrimation, irritated nasopharynx, chilliness and malaise lasting 2 to 7 days. Probably never fatal; importance rests in days of disability and in predisposing to more serious respiratory tract infections. Fever is uncommon, particularly in infants and adults. Complications of catarrhal sinusitis, otitis media, laryngitis, tracheitis or bronchitis are frequent.

   No confirmatory laboratory tests; leucocyte count and distribution are normal.

2. *Etiologic agent.* The infection has been transmitted experimentally to chimpanzees and man by a filter-passing agent, presumably a virus. Cultivation and characterization not achieved; existence of more than one type undetermined. Role of

bacteria in the usual case is uncertain; pyogenic bacteria of respiratory tract (pneumococci, streptococci, H. influenzae) may cause suppurative complications.

3. *Source and reservoir of infection.* Discharges from nose and mouth of patients.

4. *Mode of transmission.* Usual transmission is by direct contact or by droplet spread; indirectly by handkerchiefs, eating utensils or other articles freshly soiled by discharges of the infected person.

5. *Incubation period.* Between 12 and 72 hours, usually 24 hours.

6. *Period of communicability.* Nasal washings taken 24 hours before to 5 days after onset of symptoms transmit infection experimentally to man.

7. *Susceptibility and resistance.* Susceptibility is universal. Inapparent and abortive attacks occur; frequency undetermined. Epidemiological evidence suggests limited and transient immunity; no immunity demonstrated in volunteers reinoculated after 3 weeks. No artificial immunization.

8. *Occurrence.* World-wide distribution; endemic and epidemic. In temperate zones, incidence rises during winter months. Most persons, except in small isolated communities, have 1 to 6 colds yearly. Incidence highest in children under 5 years; gradual decline with increasing age. For unknown reasons, after childhood rates are higher for females than males. No racial selectivity.

9. *Methods of control:*
   A. Preventive measures:
      1. Education in the niceties of personal hygiene as in covering the mouth when coughing and sneezing and disposal of nose and mouth secretions.
   B. Control of the infected individual, contacts and environment:
      1. Report to local health authority: Official report not ordinarily justifiable.
      2. Isolation: On first recognition of a common cold the infected person should avoid direct and indirect exposure of others, particularly little children, feeble or aged persons, or persons suffering from other illness. Such modified isolation as can be accomplished by rest in bed during the acute stage is advised.
      3. Concurrent disinfection: Of eating and drinking utensils; disposal of nose and mouth discharges, preferably by collecting on soft paper and burning.
      4. Terminal disinfection: Airing and sunning of room and bedding.
      5. Quarantine: None.
      6. Immunization: None.
      7. Investigation of source of infection: Unprofitable.
      8. Specific treatment: None. Indiscriminate use of antibiotics for uncomplicated colds or mild sore throat is to be discouraged. These valuable therapeutic agents should be reserved for complications such as pneumonia, tracheobronchitis, otitis, and sinusitis.
   C. Epidemic measures: Effective measures for the control of epidemics are not known. Isolation precautions may be helpful in institutions but procedures such as ultraviolet irradiation, aerosols and dust control have not been effective.
   D. International measures: None.

CONJUNCTIVITIS, ACUTE INFECTIOUS

1. *Identification.* The disease begins with lacrimation, irritation, and vascular injection of the palpebral and bulbar conjunctivae of one or both eyes, followed by edema of the lids, a mucopurulent exudate, photophobia and pain; in severe

cases, ecchymoses of the bulbar conjunctiva and transient phlyctenules on the cornea. A non-fatal disease with usual clinical course of 2–3 weeks; many patients have no more than vascular injection and slight exudate for a few days. Synonyms: Sore eyes, pink eye.

Confirmation by bacteriologic culture, or microscopic examination of smears of exudate.

Other forms of acute conjunctivitis are to be differentiated: acute conjunctivitis of the newborn to include gonorrheal ophthalmia, ophthalmia neonatorum and babies' sore eyes of the first 21 days of life, trachoma and keratoconjunctivitis.

2. *Etiologic agent.* Haemophilus aegyptius (Koch-Weeks bacillus) appears to be the most important; Haemophilus influenzae, Moraxella lacunatus, staphylococci, streptococci, and pneumococci may produce the disease.

3. *Source and reservoir of infection.* Discharges from the conjunctiva or upper respiratory tract of infected persons, possibly including chronic carriers with subacute infections.

4. *Mode of transmission.* Contact with infected individuals through contaminated fingers, clothing or other fomites. In some areas may be mechanically transmitted by eye-gnats or flies, but importance as a vector undetermined and probably differs from area to area.

5. *Incubation period.* Usually 24 to 72 hours.

6. *Period of communicability.* During the course of active infection.

7. *Susceptibility and resistance.* Children under 5 are most susceptible and the incidence decreases with age. Acquired immunity does not follow attack.

8. *Occurrence.* Wide-spread throughout the world, particularly in warmer climates; frequently epidemic. In the United States, infection with H. aegyptius is largely confined to rural areas of southernmost states, Georgia to California, primarily during summer and early autumn months; in those areas an important cause of absenteeism from school. Infection with other organisms occurs throughout the United States, often associated with acute respiratory infection during cold seasons.

9. *Methods of control:*
    A. Preventive measures:
        1. Report to local health authority: Obligatory report of epidemics; no case report.
        2. Isolation: Children should not attend school during the acute stage.
        3. Concurrent disinfection: Of discharges and soiled articles.
        4. Terminal disinfection: Thorough cleaning.
        5. Quarantine: None.
        6. Immunization: None.
        7. Investigation of contacts and source of infection: Usually not profitable.
        8. Specific treatment: Application of an appropriate antibiotic such as aureomycin, terramycin, streptomycin or penicillin, the latter primarily for the less common streptococcal and pneumococcal infection; or a chemotherapeutic agent such as $\frac{1}{4}$% solution of zinc sulphate; usually results in shortened course and period of communicability.
    B. Epidemic measures:
        1. Adequate and intensive treatment of patients.

[651]

2. In areas where insects are suspected of mechanically transmitting infection, measures to prevent access of eye-gnats or flies to eyes of sick and well persons.
3. Insect control, depending on the suspected vector.

C. International measures: None.

DENGUE

1. *Identification.* An acute febrile infection of sharp onset, occasionally with two paroxysms of short duration; fever of about five days and rarely more than seven, intense headache, joint and muscle pains, and eruption. Eruption usually appears 3 to 4 days after onset of fever, either musculo-papular or scarlatiniform; petechiae may appear on feet, legs, axillae, or palate on last day of fever or shortly thereafter. Leucopenia is usual with an absolute decrease of segmented neutrophiles and a marked increase of nonsegmented forms. Case fatality is exceedingly low. Synonym: Breakbone fever.

   Laboratory tests contributing to identification include hemagglutination, complement fixation, or neutralization with specific type of virus.

2. *Etiologic agent.* The viruses of dengue fever; at least two immunologically distinct types have been identified.

3. *Source and reservoir of infection.* The immediate source of infection is an infected vector mosquito. Reservoir unknown; may be man, mosquito or possibly an animal.

4. *Mode of transmission.* By the bite of mosquitoes, Aëdes aegypti, Aëdes albopictus, or one of the Aëdes scutellaris complex, infected by biting a patient.

5. *Incubation period.* Three to 15 days, commonly 5 or 6 days.

6. *Period of communicability.* Not directly communicable in nature from man to man; for the mosquito, from the day before onset to the 5th day of disease. The mosquito becomes infective from 8–11 days after the blood meal and remains so for life.

7. *Susceptibility and resistance.* Susceptibility is apparently universal. Homologous immunity to either type of virus is of long duration; heterologous immunity, though present, is brief and may permit mild febrile illness without rash.

8. *Occurrence.* Endemic areas are limited to parts of the world where mosquito vectors survive in large numbers throughout the year; also may depend on continued immigration of susceptibles such as occurs during war and on distant military posts. Islands of the south-west Pacific, Indo-China, Indonesia, India, and northern Australia are areas commonly involved. Imported epidemics can occur wherever the vectors are present.

9. *Methods of control:*

A. Preventive measures:
   1. Measures directed toward elimination of vector mosquitoes, and where practicable their breeding places.
   2. Screening of rooms.
   3. Use of mosquito repellents.

B. Control of the infected individual, contacts and environment:
   1. Report to local health authority: Obligatory report of epidemics; no case report.
   2. Isolation: Patient should be kept in screened room for 5 days after onset, or in quarters treated with insecticide with residual effect, such as DDT.

[652]

3. Concurrent disinfection: None.
4. Terminal disinfection: None.
5. Quarantine: None.
6. Immunization: None.
7. Investigation of contacts and source of infection: Place of residence of patient during fortnight previous to onset. Search for unreported or undiagnosed cases. Determine density of Aëdes mosquitoes in vicinity and search for breeding places.
8. Specific treatment: None.

C. Epidemic measures:
  1. Community survey for breeding places of vector mosquitoes, and their elimination.
  2. Search for and destruction of Aëdes mosquitoes in places of human habitation.
  3. Use of mosquito repellents by persons exposed through occupation or necessity to bites of vector mosquitoes.

D. International measures:
  1. Enforcement of provisions of international agreements designed to prevent mosquito transfer by public conveyances (ships, airplanes, land transport) from areas of prevalence to areas free of the disease.

DIARRHEA OF THE NEWBORN, EPIDEMIC

A variety of diseases of children aged less than 2 years, having diarrhea and usually fever as the common clinical manifestations are grouped under the general term of infantile enteritis. Two broad classes are recognized. The larger and generally more serious group includes specific infections that result in primary infectious enteritis. Some are due to known pathogenic agents such as Salmonella and Shigella; some are associated with serologically recognizable types of Escherichia coli or a number of other common bacteria; and others may be caused by filtrable viruses. The second class includes various forms of secondary enteritis associated with parenteral infection. The several kinds of primary enteritis can not be distinguished accurately by clinical methods. A number are seen principally among older infants; any one may attack the newborn.

A form of acute enteritis of the newborn has characteristics sufficiently distinctive to be recognized individually; as an epidemiologic entity by reason of its practical limitation to outbreaks among infants housed in hospital nurseries, and as a clinical entity by manifestations which set it apart from the usual infantile diarrhea. It is probably not an etiologic entity. This is the condition now presented as epidemic diarrhea of the newborn.

1. *Identification.* An acute communicable disease characterized by severe diarrhea with watery feces containing little or no mucus and no blood, by dehydration. and commonly acidosis. Signs other than of enteric infection are lacking in uncomplicated cases; the temperature is normal or only slightly elevated except with severe dehydration or with pneumonia or other complication. The disorder spreads rapidly from infant to infant in a nursery for the newborn and ordinarily has a high case fatality, with variation from 0 to 40%.

Stool culture serves to identify specific infection with known pathogenic bacteria but is of no help in viral infections. Post-mortem examination shows remarkably few changes and none pathognomonic of the disorder.

[653]

2. *Etiologic agent.* Still doubtful, but probably more than one infectious agent is responsible. Some outbreaks have been attributed to a filtrable virus; others are associated with the presence in the intestine of serologically recognizable types of E. coli, 0–111, 0–55 and others.

3. *Source and reservoir of infection.* Unknown; presumably feces of infected persons. The specific types of E. coli appear to be present only in the feces of patients and of close contacts.

4. *Mode of transmission.* Direct or indirect person to person transfer. Faults in aseptic nursing technic are a principal factor in many outbreaks, as with milk formulas and rubber nipples. In epidemics associated with specific types of E. coli, the whole of the patient's environment is contaminated and the organism can be demonstrated on bed clothing and in dust of the ward, suggesting airborne transmission and other indirect avenues of spread. Nurses and doctors rarely may act as healthy carriers.

5. *Incubation period.* Unknown; estimates are from 2 to 21 days, most frequently 6 to 7 days.

6. *Period of communicability.* Readily communicable among newborn infants as long as symptoms are present or a carrier state persists.

7. *Susceptibility and resistance.* Restricted in general to infants under one month of age, most frequently those 8 to 9 days old. Premature infants are more susceptible and have a decidedly higher fatality. Older infants and adults seem to be less susceptible; most other bacterial and viral diseases producing diarrhea in the newborn also affect adults. No known means to induce immunity artificially.

8. *Occurrence.* Frequent in North America and Europe, and probably more widespread than reports from other countries indicate. Primarily a disease of hospitals caring for newborn infants in nurseries. No definite seasonal incidence.

9. *Methods of control.* Current practice is empirical, with principal dependence on general measures for limiting spread of infection and for conduct of a clean nursery.

   A. Preventive measures:

      1. A hospital nursery for the newborn or premature should accommodate no more than 12 infants; should not communicate directly with other nurseries; have at least 24 square feet of floor space per infant; and provide mechanically controlled running hot and cold water for hand washing. A "suspect" nursery should be provided to which infants can be transferred on the slightest suspicion of illness. Infants with established illness should be transferred to a separate isolation nursery or to the pediatric service. Because of the ease with which the infection spreads, once introduced into a nursery, the increasing practice of keeping each baby with its mother has much to recommend it.

      2. Individual equipment, kept at the bassinet, should be provided each infant; no common bathing or dressing tables and no bassinet stands for holding or transporting more than one infant at a time.

      3. No nurse to care for more than 12 infants and their equipment, such care to be given at the bedside.

      4. Feeding formulas including glucose water should be prepared aseptically, placed in clean bottles with clean nipples attached and covered with a cap. The entire product should be subjected to terminal heating, either by steam under pressure (15 lbs. at 250° F. for 5 minutes, or 6 lbs. at 230° F. for 10

minutes) or by flowing steam, 212° F. for 30 minutes; then refrigerated with nipple caps left on bottles until feeding time. Periodic bacteriological sampling of heated formulas is recommended; coliform organisms should be absent and the total plate count should not exceed 10 organisms per ml.

5. Normal newborn infants should not be kept in the same nursery with sick infants or older children. An infant born outside the hospital or to a mother who has diarrheal or respiratory illness should not be admitted to the nursery for well infants except after isolation for at least four days, preferably with stool examination for potential pathogens. Nurses caring for patients should have no association with nurseries for normal newborn or premature infants; nurses engaged in the milk kitchen should not attend the infants' toilet; control of visitors to minimize spread of infection; laundry procedures to assure absence of pathogenic organisms from finished product as returned to nursery.

6. Systematic daily record of number and consistency of stools for each infant.

B. Control of the infected individual, contacts and environment:

1. Report to local health authority: Obligatory report of epidemics; no individual case report. Two or more concurrent cases in a nursery are to be interpreted as an epidemic.

2. Isolation: Of infected infant, also suspects.

3. Concurrent disinfection: Of all discharges and articles soiled therewith.

4. Terminal disinfection: Thorough cleaning of nursery and equipment.

5. Quarantine: Complete quarantine of all newborn contacts.

6. Immunization: None.

7. Investigation of contacts and source of infection: See 9C2.

8. Specific treatment: The tetracycline antibiotics, chloramphenicol or sulfadiazine in illnesses due to coliform group.

C. Epidemic measures:

1. Permit no new admissions to the contaminated hospital nursery; suspend maternity service unless uninfected nurseries with separate personnel and facilities are available. Exposed babies in the contaminated nursery should be cared for by separate medical and nursing personnel skilled in care of communicable disease; observe contacts for at least 2 weeks after last case leaves the nursery; promptly remove each new case to isolation. Maternity service may be resumed after discharge of all contact babies and mothers and thorough cleaning. Put into practice recommendations of 9A so far as feasible in the emergency.

2. Epidemiologic investigation: (a) Assure adequate treatment of missed cases by follow-up examination of all infants discharged from hospital during 2 weeks preceding first recognized case; (b) examine mothers and maternity service personnel for early signs of illness; (c) bacteriologic examination of feces of all sick and exposed babies, mothers and maternity service personnel to detect missed cases and carriers due to a known pathogen; (d) survey hospital for sanitary hazards; (e) investigate preparation of feeding formulas for adequacy of sterilization and refrigeration; bacteriologic examination of solutions and sugars used in formulas and their storage; bacteriologic examination of rubber nipples and bottle caps; (f) inquiry into technic of aseptic nursing of infants, of changing diapers, and of laundering diapers and other clothing.

D. International measures: None.

[655]

DIPHTHERIA

1. *Identification.* An acute febrile infection, generally of tonsils, throat, and nose, marked by a patch or patches of grayish membrane from which the diphtheria bacillus is readily cultured. Occasionally, and especially in adults, there is only slight inflammation with little or no membrane. Nasal diphtheria is commonly marked by one-sided nasal discharge and excoriated nares. Non-respiratory forms include infection of skin and wound surfaces; rarely the vagina. Case fatality is variable; in some epidemics 10–12%, commonly 2–5%.

   Diagnosis is by clinical symptoms with confirmation by bacteriologic examination of discharges. Failure to demonstrate the bacillus in suspected diphtheria is not a valid reason for withholding specific treatment.

2. *Etiologic agent.* Corynebacterium diphtheria, the Klebs-Loeffler bacillus.

3. *Source and reservoir of infection.* Discharges and secretions from mucous surfaces of nose, pharynx and nasopharynx of infected persons, and from skin and other lesions.

4. *Mode of transmission.* Contact with a patient or carrier or with articles soiled with discharges of such persons. Milk has served as a vehicle.

5. *Incubation period.* Usually 2 to 5 days, occasionally longer.

6. *Period of communicability.* Variable, until virulent bacilli have disappeared from secretions and lesions; usually 2 weeks or less, seldom more than 4 weeks.

7. *Susceptibility and resistance.* Infants born of immune mothers are relatively immune, a passive protection in most instances lost by the 6th month; in North America, probably not more than half of mothers are immune. Recovery from an attack of the disease is usually but not necessarily followed by persisting immunity. Immunity is often acquired through unrecognized infection. Passive temporary immunity of 10 days to 3 weeks and active immunity of prolonged duration can be induced artificially.

8. *Occurrence.* Endemic and epidemic; a disease of autumn and winter months. In communities where active immunization has been neglected, approximately one-fourth of cases and one-half of deaths occur in children under 5 years of age. In communities where childhood immunization has been adequate but reinforcing doses of toxoid were not continued, age distribution tends towards older persons. Clinical disease is more common in temperate zones than in the tropics, although infection rates are often much the same. Relatively, the tropics have more inapparent infection, less faucial diphtheria and more diphtheria of the skin.

9. *Methods of control:*
   A. Preventive measures:
      1. The only effectual control of diphtheria is through active immunization on a population basis. All children should be inoculated with diphtheria toxoid. The following procedure is recommended: at 2 to 6 months of age 2 adequate doses of diphtheria precipitated toxoid alone or combined with tetanus toxoid, 4 to 8 weeks between doses; or 3 doses of combined pertussis vaccine and diphtheria toxoid (with or without added tetanus toxoid) administered at 3 to 5 week intervals; or 3 doses of fluid toxoid. Whether with toxoid alone or combined, the basic course of inoculations must be reinforced by at least one recall or "booster" dose within 3–12 months. Reinforcing doses are essential

[656]

in pre-school life, desirable on entrance to school, and elective through school life and early adulthood. Where protection has been neglected in infancy, the program should be carried through as soon as the opportunity arises.

2. Adults subject to unusual risk such as physicians, teachers, nurses, nurse maids, orderlies and other hospital personnel, should receive diphtheria toxoid. It is desirable to identify susceptibles by a Schick test (0.1 ml intradermally containing 0.001 of stabilized nonphenolized toxin). In order to serve as an adequate control of the Schick test and to reduce the hazard of severe local and constitutional reactions, an intradermal toxoid reaction test (0.1 cc of 1:100 dilution fluid toxoid in saline solution) is recommended. Schick positive non-reactors to the control may be given toxoid in the usual dosage; Schick positive reactors should be given small doses of suitably diluted purified toxoid containing a minimal amount of alum.

3. Pasteurization of milk supply.

4. Educational measures to inform the public and particularly the parents of little children of the hazards of diphtheria and the necessity and advantages of active immunization.

B. Control of the infected individual, contacts and environment:

1. Report to local health authority: Case report obligatory in most states and countries.

2. Isolation: Until two cultures from throat and two from nose taken not less than 24 hours apart fail to show diphtheria bacilli. Local or general application of antibiotic or chemotherapeutic agents invalidates the usefulness of bacteriological examination. Isolation may be terminated if the microorganism reported present is proved avirulent. Where termination of case by culture is impracticable, isolation may end with fair safety 14 days after onset. Where practicable, a virulence test should be made if throat cultures are reported positive 3 weeks or more after onset.

3. Concurrent disinfection: Of all articles in contact with patient, and all articles soiled by discharges of patient.

4. Terminal disinfection: Thorough airing and sunning of the sick room, with cleaning.

5. Quarantine: All intimate contacts, especially young children, should be kept under surveillance if found to be carriers or suffering from nasal discharge or sore throat. Adult contacts whose occupation involves handling of food or close association with children should be excluded from these occupations until shown not to be carriers by bacteriological examination.

6. Immunization: Child contacts less than 10 years of age, intimately exposed and not previously immunized with toxoid, may be given a prophylactic dose of antitoxin, 10,000 units, and at the same time a first dose of toxoid. Daily examination by a physician is advised for older children and adults, with such further active immunization as may be indicated. Groups of persons, as in institutions, barracks, or in closely congested quarters should have immediate Schick test, with toxoid reaction test, followed by combined active and passive immunization of Schick positives; passive immunization has hazard of serum sensitivity.

7. Investigation of contacts and source of infection: Search for unreported and atypical cases, carriers, and contaminated milk.

[657]

8. Specific treatment: If diphtheria is suspected, antitoxin should be given without awaiting bacteriological confirmation. The earlier antitoxin is given the more effective it is; 20,000 to 80,000 units depending upon duration of symptoms, area of involvement, and severity of the disease; and in a single dose after completion of sensitivity tests. Intramuscular administration usually suffices; in severe infection antitoxin both intravenously and intramuscularly is indicated. Bed rest is essential to minimize the hazard of cardiac and other complications. Sulfonamides are of no value. Penicillin may be used in conjunction with antitoxin but is *not* a substitute for antitoxin. Diphtheria antitoxin cannot be relied upon to shorten materially the period of communicability; penicillin does. Penicillin soaked compresses (500 units per cc) are of value in cutaneous diphtheria; also erythromycin and bacitracin.

C. Epidemic measures:
 1. Immediate intensification of efforts to provide artificial immunization by diphtheria toxoid to the largest possible numbers of the population affected, with first and greatest emphasis upon protection of infants and preschool children.

D. International measures:
 1. Active immunization of susceptible travelers, especially infants and young children.
 2. Epidemiological intelligence service.

DYSENTERY, AMEBIC

1. *Identification.* Amebic infection has a wide range of clinical manifestations. The primary site is the colon; infection may be asymptomatic, or with mild symptoms that include abdominal discomfort and diarrhea alternating with constipation, or a chronic diarrhea with mucus and some blood, or an acute dysentery with profuse blood and mucus, usually with little pus. Amebiasis is only occasionally a direct cause of death. Infection may spread by the blood stream or by direct extension, producing amebic hepatitis, abscess of liver, lung or brain, or ulceration of skin. Synonym: Amebiasis.

 Definitive diagnosis is through identifying trophozoites or cysts of Endamoeba histolytica in the feces, or trophozoites in smears or sections from lesions.

 Differential diagnosis includes shigellosis, appendicitis, and ulcerative colitis. Other intestinal protozoa are associated with diarrhea in man. Balantidiasis, caused by the ciliate protozoan Balantidium coli usually produces abdominal discomfort and a watery or mucoid diarrhea; sometimes severe ulceration of the colon similar to amebic dysentery. Giardia lamblia, an intestinal flagellate inhabiting the duodenum, is often associated with epigastric discomfort and mucoid diarrhea (giardiasis); both may exist concomitantly with E. histolytica.

2. *Etiologic agent.* Endamoeba histolytica.

3. *Source and reservoir of infection.* Cysts from feces of infected persons, usually chronic or asymptomatic cases. Acute infections are of little menace because of fragility of trophozoites.

4. *Mode of transmission.* Contaminated vegetables, especially those commonly served raw, cold and moist; contaminated water; flies; soiled hands of infected food handlers.

[658]

5. *Incubation period.* From 5 days in severe infections to several months in subacute and chronic cases; commonly 3 to 4 weeks.
6. *Period of communicability.* During intestinal infection, which may be years if unrecognized and untreated.
7. *Susceptibility and resistance.* Susceptibility to infection is general; relatively few persons harboring the organism develop recognized symptoms; acute cases tend to become chronic. Immunity to reinfection is not recognized in man. No artificial immunity.
8. *Occurrence.* Distribution is world wide. Prevalence of infection is 50% or more in some unsanitated areas, especially in populations of moist tropics and in mental institutions; low (1–5%) in well sanitated cities. Foreigners entering tropical regions are particularly liable to acute dysenteric attack.
9. *Methods of control:*
   A. Preventive measures:
      1. Sanitary disposal of human feces.
      2. Protection of public water supplies against fecal contamination, and boiling drinking water where necessary. Chlorination of water supplies as generally practiced is inadequate for destruction of cysts; sand filtration removes nearly all cysts, diatomaceous earth filters completely. Avoidance of cross-connections between public and private auxiliary water and of back-flow connections in plumbing systems. Small quantities of water, as in Lyster bags and canteens, are best protected by tablets of tetraglycine hydroperiodide (globaline).
      3. Supervision of general cleanliness, personal health, and sanitary practices of persons preparing and serving food in public eating places, especially moist foods eaten raw. Pre-employment examination of food handlers is of value in institutions and military units; routine periodic examination is valueless.
      4. Chloramelamine has had extended trial in military practice in treatment of potentially contaminated fruits and vegetables.
      5. Fly control and protection of foods against fly contamination by screening or other appropriate measure.
      6. Instruction of convalescents and of the general public in personal hygiene, particularly as to sanitary disposal of feces, and hand washing after defecation and before preparing or eating food.
   B. Control of the infected individual, contacts and environment:
      1. Report to local health authority: In selected endemic areas; in many states and countries not a reportable disease.
      2. Isolation: None. Exclusion of patient from food preparation, processing, and serving.
      3. Concurrent disinfection: Sanitary disposal of feces. Hand washing after defecation.
      4. Terminal disinfection: Cleaning.
      5. Quarantine: None.
      6. Immunization: None.
      7. Investigation of contacts and source of infection: Microscopic examination of feces of members of household, and of other suspected contacts, supplemented by search for direct contamination of water and foods by human feces.
      8. Specific treatment: Acute amebic dysentery: Any one of the tetracycline antibiotics; relapse rate (about 5%) is reduced by combining with other anti-

amebic drugs. Emetine hydrochloride will relieve symptoms, but will usually not eliminate the intestinal infection; should be accompanied or followed by carbarsone, chiniofon, vioform or diodoquin. Some patients with ulceration of lower colon and rectum may require retention enemas of carbarsone or chiniofon.

Chronic or symptomless intestinal infections usually respond to antibiotic therapy, or to a single course of carbarsone, chiniofon, vioform or diodoquin. Emetine is not indicated.

Amebic hepatitis and liver abscess; chloroquin or emetine hydrochloride. If abscess requires drainage, precede by chloroquin or emetine to limit infection, even if parasite is not found in feces.

Repeated fecal examination at intervals up to six months is necessary to assure that pathogenic amebae have been eliminated.

C. Epidemic measures: Any grouping of several cases from a single area requires prompt epidemiologic investigation to determine source of infection and mode of transmission. If a common vehicle is indicated, such as water or food, take appropriate measures to correct the situation. Food handlers should be investigated, and if found infected, removed from duty. If the epidemiologic evidence points to person-to-person transmission, the emphasis is on sanitary disposal of feces, personal cleanliness and fly control.

D. International measures: None.

DYSENTERY, BACILLARY

1. *Identification.* An acute bacterial infection characterized by diarrhea, fever, tenesmus and in severe cases blood and mucus in stool. Many mild undiagnosed cases have only transient diarrhea or are without intestinal symptoms. Severe infections are most frequent in infants, in elderly debilitated persons and in persons infected with Shiga bacillus; under other circumstances, the disease is rarely fatal. Synonym: Shigellosis.

   Bacteriological diagnosis is by isolation of dysentery bacilli from feces or rectal swabs.

2. *Etiologic agent.* Various species of genus Shigella (dysentery bacilli), Sonne, Flexner, Shiga and others.

3 *Source and reservoir of infection.* Feces of infected persons. Many inapparent, mild and unrecognized infections.

4. *Mode of transmission.* By eating contaminated foods, or drinking contaminated water or milk, and by hand-to-mouth transfer of contaminated material; by flies; by objects soiled with feces of a patient or carrier.

5. *Incubation period.* One to 7 days, usually less than 4.

6. *Period of communicability.* During acute infection and until microorganism is absent from feces, usually within a few weeks even without specific therapy; with some strains of shigella a few individuals become carriers for a year or two, rarely longer.

7. *Susceptibility and resistance.* Susceptibility is general but disease is more common and more severe in children than in adults. A relative and transitory strain-specific immunity follows recovery.

8. *Occurrence.* More common in United States than generally recognized; a high proportion of unreported diarrheas are dysentery. In England, Sonne infection is

responsible for 90% of recognized cases; in United States, the distribution of Flexner and Sonne strain is nearly equal. Shiga infection is rare in United States and Europe. Institutional outbreaks are frequent, with spread apparently by direct contact with unrecognized cases, or indirectly through nursing procedures and sometimes by food. In many parts of world, especially the Orient, tropics and subtropics, dysentery is a common and serious infection, occurring at all ages and causing many deaths, particularly in small children.

9 *Methods of control:*

A. Preventive measures:

1. Sanitary disposal of human feces.
2. Sanitary supervision of processing, preparation and serving of all foods, particularly those moist and eaten raw; special attention to provision and use of hand washing facilities.
3. Boiling of milk or pasteurization of milk and dairy products.
4. Persons suffering from diarrhea should be excluded from handling food for public consumption, and from handling family food supply if possible.
5. Fly control and control of fly breeding; screening to protect foods against fly contamination.
6. Protection and purification of public water supplies and construction of safe private supplies.
7. Reduction of infant mortality in areas with high rates usually depends upon prevention of intestinal infection. Attention to the hygiene of breast feeding, scrupulous cleanliness in preparation, handling and refrigeration of food for children, boiling of milk for infant feeding, and continuous supervision of diet will contribute much to this aim. All infantile diarrhea should be regarded as bacillary dysentery until proved otherwise by bacteriologic examination of feces.

B. Control of the infected individual, contacts and environment:

1. Report to local health authority: Case report obligatory in most states and countries. Recognition and report of epidemics especially in schools and institutions has more than usual importance.
2. Isolation: During acute illness. Rigid personal precautions by attendants. Surveillance during carrier state, which is usually temporary, and prohibition from food handling.
3. Concurrent disinfection: Of feces and of articles soiled therewith. In communities with a modern and adequate sewage disposal system, feces can be disposed of directly into sewer without preliminary disinfection.
4. Terminal disinfection: Cleaning.
5. Quarantine: Contacts should not be employed as food handlers during period of contact nor before repeated negative feces cultures are obtained.
6. Immunization: No known satisfactory method.
7. Investigation of contacts and source of infection: Search for unrecognized mild cases and convalescent carriers among contacts. For sporadic cases, such investigation is time consuming and gives meagre results.
8. Specific treatment: The tetracycline antibiotics (aureomycin, terramycin), chloramphenicol and streptomycin give rapid relief of symptoms, with marked reduction in numbers of bacilli in from 24–48 hours and elimination regularly within several days. Streptomycin orally is also effective, especially when com-

bined with sulfadiazine. Sulfadiazine may be used alone when antibiotics are not available.

C. Epidemic measures:
1. Groups of cases of acute diarrheal disorder should always be reported to local health authority at once, even in absence of exact identification of the disease.
2. Investigation of food, water, and milk supplies, general sanitation, and search for recognized mild cases and carriers.
3. Reduction in incidence may be expected from prophylactic administration of chemotherapeutic and antibiotic agents (see 9B8), given orally under medical supervision to groups of persons exposed temporarily to high risk of infection.

D. International measures: None.

ENCEPHALITIS, ARTHROPOD-BORNE VIRAL

1. *Identification.* A group of acute inflammatory diseases of short duration, involving parts of the brain, spinal cord and meninges. Several viruses produce clinical reaction, with variation in severity and rate of progress. Mild cases may resemble non-paralytic poliomyelitis. Severe infections usually have acute onset, high fever, meningeal signs, stupor, disorientation, coma, spasticity, tremors, convulsions occasionally in infants and spastic but rarely flaccid paralysis. The Russian type frequently leads to paralysis and atrophy of shoulder girdle. Fatality ranges from 5 to 60%, that of Japanese B and Eastern equine types being highest. Permanent sequelae are rare except in infants; no parkinsonism. Mild leucocytosis is usual; leucocytes in spinal fluid from 50 to 200, occasionally 1,000 or more in infants.

Specific identification is by demonstrated rise in antibody between early and late serum specimens; by neutralization and complement fixation, for some types by hemagglutination inhibition. Virus may be isolated from brain of fatal cases: histopathology not specific for individual viruses.

These diseases require differentiation from encephalitic and nonparalytic forms of poliomyelitis, rabies, mumps, meningoencephalitis, lymphocytic choriomenginitis, herpes encephalitis, post-vaccinal or postinfection encephalitis, bacterial, protozoal, leptospiral and fungal meningitides or encephalitides; also the von Economo type of encephalitis (encephalitis lethargica) of unknown etiology, a disease of frequent occurrence in the years just before and after 1920 but now rarely reported.

2. *Etiologic agent.* Each form of the disease is caused by a specific virus—Eastern equine, Western equine, St. Louis, Venezuelan equine, Japanese B, Murray Valley, Russian Spring-Summer, West Nile and others. Some are interrelated immunologically.

3. *Source and reservoir of infection.* Wild and domestic birds are the principal reservoir for mosquito infection in the United States; although serving as hosts, horses are not important, nor is man for types found in United States; rodents in Russian type.

4. *Mode of transmission.* By the bite of mosquitoes, except for Russian Spring-Summer type which is tick-borne. In western and central United States and in Canada, Culex tarsalis is believed the principal vector; C. tritaeniorhynchus in the Far East; Culiseta melanura strongly suspect in eastern United States. Genus and species elsewhere are undetermined.

5. *Incubation period.* Usually 5 to 15 days.

6. *Period of communicability.* Probably not communicable from man to man. Virus not demonstrable in blood of man after onset of disease except in Venezuelan and Russian types.

7. *Susceptibility and resistance.* Susceptibility to clinical disease usually highest in infancy and old age; inapparent or undiagnosed infection more common at other ages. Infection of any degree apparently results in homologous immunity but not to other types. In several Far Eastern areas most adults are immune through mild infection, and susceptibles are mainly children.

8. *Occurrence.* Eastern and Western equine and St. Louis types are recognized human infections in United States and Canada, in some Central and South American countries one or other or both, and also the Venezuelan equine type. Japanese B type is present in Japan, Korea, China, Malaya, and a number of Pacific islands. Murray Valley type of Australia is probably the originally described Australian X disease. Russian Spring-Summer type occurs in both European and Siberian Russia. West Nile is prevalent in parts of northeast Africa, the Middle East and India. Other types of virus have been reported from United States and elsewhere, but pathogenicity for man is ill defined. A disease of summer and early fall, commonly limited to areas and years of high sustained temperature and many mosquitoes; has persisted for successive years in hot, irrigated western valley regions of the United States; irregularly epidemic in dry farming areas of midwest, southwest, and east. Highest rates in rural and suburban districts.

9. *Methods of control:*

   A. Preventive measures:

      1. Destruction of larvae and elimination of breeding places of known or suspected vector mosquitoes.

      2. Killing mosquitoes by space spraying of human habitations.

      3. Screening of sleeping and living quarters; when disease is present, use mosquito bed-nets.

      4. Avoid exposure to mosquitoes during hours of biting, or use repellents.

      5. Education of the public as to mode of spread and control.

      6. Immunization of persons at great risk (laboratory workers and others) with formalinized vaccines; not recommended for general use.

      7. Passive protection of accidentally exposed laboratory workers, by human or animal immune serum.

   B. Control of the infected individual, contacts and environment:

      1. Report to local health authority: Case report obligatory in most states of the United States and in some other countries.

      2. Isolation: None. Virus not usually found in blood, secretions, or discharges during clinical manifestations.

      3. Concurrent disinfection: None.

      4. Terminal disinfection: None.

      5. Quarantine: None.

      6. Immunization: Of contacts, none.

      7. Investigation of contacts and source of infection: Search for missed cases and presence of vector mosquitoes; primarily a community problem.

      8. Specific treatment: None.

   C. Epidemic measures: Identification of cases among horses and recognition of other

human cases in the community is of epidemiological value to indicate frequency of
infection and areas involved.

D. International measures: Insecticide spray of airplanes from recognized areas of
prevalence.

ENTEROBIASIS

1. *Identification.* An exceedingly common non-fatal intestinal infection which usually
produces no symptoms. If severe, may cause pruritus ani, with disturbed sleep
and irritability, and local irritation from scratching. A variety of severe manifestations including appendicitis and salpingitis have been described, but their relationship is indefinite. Synonyms: Pinworm or threadworm infection.

Diagnosis is by swabbing a cellophane tipped applicator over the perianal
region and examining microscopically for eggs; the swab is best obtained in the
morning before bathing or defecation.

2. *Etiologic agent.* Enterobius vermicularis, an intestinal round worm infecting only
man. Eggs are infective within a few hours after leaving the gastrointestinal
tract. After ingestion, eggs hatch in the stomach and small intestine; young
worms mature in lower small intestine, cecum and upper portions of colon.
Gravid worms migrate to the rectum to discharge eggs on perianal skin; may
migrate up genital tract of females and enter peritoneal cavity.

3. *Source and reservoir of infection.* Clothing and bedding soiled with feces containing
eggs; contaminated food. Reservoir of infection is infected persons, particularly
children.

4. *Mode of transmission.* Infective eggs may be transferred by hand from anal region to
mouth of the same host, and indirectly to same host or new hosts through contamination of food and other objects. Dust-borne infection by inhalation is
possible in contaminated households.

5. *Incubation period.* The life cycle requires about two months. Infections ordinarily
build up from successive reinfections and are not noticed for several months.

6. *Period of communicability.* Infected persons are potential spreaders of infection as
long as they harbor the parasites.

7. *Susceptibility and resistance.* Susceptibility is universal. Differences in incidence
and intensity of infection are due to differences in frequency of exposure. No
apparent resistance to repeated infections.

8. *Occurrence.* Distribution is world-wide. An estimated 20 percent of the general
population of the United States are infected. Prevalence is highest in children of
school age, next highest in those of preschool age, and lowest in adults except
for mothers of infected children, who commonly have a high rate. Infection is
characteristically familial. Crowding is an important factor; incidence often high
in institutions.

9. *Methods of control:*
   A. Preventive measures:
      1. Maintenance of clean facilities for defecation.
      2. Insistence upon practice of personal hygiene of the toilet, particularly the
      washing of hands after defecation and always before eating or preparing food.
      3. Reduction of overcrowding in living accommodations; adequate provision of
      toilets and privies.

[664]

4. Bathing with sufficient frequency to keep the body clean; use of clean underclothing, night clothes and bed sheets at frequent intervals.

5. Habits of nail biting and scratching bare anal area should be discouraged.

B. Control of the infected individual, contacts and environment:

1. Report to local health authority: Official report not ordinarily justifiable. School authorities should be advised of school outbreaks.

2. Isolation: None.

3. Concurrent disinfection: Sanitary disposal of feces and washing of hands in soap and water after defecating and before eating. Change bed linen and underwear of infected person daily and boil to kill eggs.

4. Terminal disinfection: None.

5. Quarantine: None.

6. Immunization: None.

7. Investigation of contacts and source of infection: Each infected individual is a source of infection. All members in an infected family or institution should be examined.

8. Specific treatment: Medicinal gentian violet by mouth is the usual therapy. The tetracyclines and particularly terramycin recently have been reported as preferred. All members of a household should be treated simultaneously.

C. Epidemic measures: Outbreaks in schools and insitutions require strict hygienic measures and cleanliness. Toilet seats should be washed daily with disinfectant. Control measures should include facilities for treatment.

D. International measures: None.

FILARIASIS*

1. *Identification.* A nematode infection with early acute manifestations of fever, lymphadenitis, retrograde lymphangitis of extremities, orchitis, epididymitis, funiculitis and abscess. These are primarily allergic reactions, but secondary bacterial infection may occur and end in the occasionally recorded death. After prolonged or repeated infection, obstruction to lymph flow often leads to hydrocele and elephantiasis of limbs, genitalia or breasts, or to chyluria. Female worms give birth to larvae, microfilariae, which in the absence of lymphatic obstruction, reach the blood stream. Many infected persons have no clinical manifestations but do have circulating microfilariae; many persons with clinical manifestations do not have circulating microfilariae. A nocturnal periodicity of microfilariae in the peripheral blood (10 p.m.–2 a.m.) occurs in all endemic areas except in those Pacific Islands where Aëdes mosquitoes are the vectors.

Microfilariae are best detected in blood specimens taken at optimum time of day, and examined in thick-film preparation, or in stained sediment of laked blood. Skin test is non-specific and experimental.

Other filarial infections within an endemic area require differentiation, such as loaiasis (Loa loa) in central West Africa.

2. *Etiologic agents.* Nematode worms, Wuchereia bancrofti and W. malayi.

3. *Source and reservoir of infection.* Source is a mosquito; reservoir is blood of an infected person bearing microfilariae.

4. *Mode of transmission.* By bite of mosquitoes harboring infective larvae. W. bancrofti is transmitted in nature by many species, the most important Culex

* Sometimes called elephantiasis.

[665]

fatigans, C. pipiens, Aëdes polynesiensis (pseudoscutellaris), and several species of Anopheles. W. malayi is transmitted by several species of Mansonia and Anopheles. The microfilariae penetrate the stomach wall of the mosquito, lodge in thoracic muscles, develop into infective larvae, migrate to the proboscis, and are transmitted to the new host as the infected mosquito bites.

5. *Incubation period.* Allergic manifestations may appear as early as 3 months after infection. Microfilariae do not appear in the blood until at least 9 months.

6. *Period of communicability.* In man, as long as microfilariae are present in the blood, which may be years. In the mosquito, from at least 10 days after infective feed until all infective larvae have been discharged or mosquito dies.

7. *Susceptibility and resistance.* All persons are probably susceptible. Repeated infection apparently occurs in endemic regions. Acquired immunity is unknown.

8. *Occurrence.* W. Bancrofti is endemic in the West Indies, coastal Central America, northern and eastern South America, Central and Northern Africa, a few small areas of southern Europe, Arabia, Madagascar, India, Southeast Asia, China, Korea, Japan, northern Australia, and most of the Pacific Islands. W. malayi is endemic only in southeast Asia, India, central China and a few islands of Indonesia. Local foci of high prevalence are often surrounded by non-endemic areas. High prevalence depends upon a large reservoir of infection and abundant vector breeding.

9. *Methods of control:*

    A. Preventive measures:

        1. Anti-mosquito measures. Determine by dissection the vector or vectors in each locality; study times and places of feeding and locate breeding places. Attack adult mosquitoes by residual spraying of buildings with an acceptable insecticide, DDT or other, screening of houses, use of bednets, and insect repellents; larvae by eliminating small breeding places and treating others with larvicides. Each local situation requires individual study.

        2. Education of the public concerning mode of transmission, and methods of mosquito control.

    B. Control of infected individual, contacts and environment:

        1. Report to local health authority: In selected endemic regions; in most countries not a reportable disease. Reporting of cases with demonstrated microfilariae provides data on potential transmission. Cases of elephantiasis without microfilariae in the blood should not be reported as filariasis, but are usefully recorded in estimating prevalence or in planning control programs.

        2. Isolation: Not practicable. So far as possible patients with microfilariae in blood should be protected from mosquito bites as a means of reducing transmission.

        3. Concurrent disinfection: None.

        4. Terminal disinfection: None.

        5. Quarantine: None.

        6. Immunization: None.

        7. Investigation of source of infection: Only as a part of a general community effort.

        8. Specific treatment: Diethylcarbamazine (hetrazan) results in rapid disappearance of most or all microfilariae from the blood, but may not kill or even sterilize the adult female worm; microfilariae reappear in most cases after several

[666]

months. Sodium thiacetarsamide (Caparsolate sodium) causes slow disappearance of microfilariae during treatment without subsequent increase over a 2-year period. Action of this compound apparently is against adult worms rather than microfilariae.

C. Epidemic measures: The first essential in a program of control in areas of high endemicity is an appraisal of the local situation, particularly the bionomics of mosquito vectors, prevalence and incidence of disease, and environmental factors responsible for transmission. Vector control is the fundamental approach. Even partial control by anti-mosquito measures may reduce incidence of new infections and restrict the endemic focus. Measurable results are slow because of the long incubation period. Mass treatment of known infected persons by chemotherapy contributes materially.

D. International measures: Coordinated programs entered into by neighboring countries where the disease is endemic with the purpose of limiting migration of infected persons across international boundaries, and instituting treatment and other control measures near such boundaries.

FOOD INTOXICATIONS AND INFECTIONS

Food poisoning is a generic term for disease of man characterized by gastro-enteritis of abrupt evolution, acquired through food, having a characteristic grouping of cases, and arising either from intoxication or infection. Numerous organic and inorganic substances act as agents of intoxication, and a number of microorganisms as infectious agents. The interest here is in intoxications of bacterial origin, and in infections due to salmonella.

Food poisoning is distinguished from food-borne infection. The effects of food poisoning are promptly evident and the amount of the particular food ingested has a relation to severity, suggesting the importance of preformed elements. Food-borne infection with a number of intestinal pathogens, with streptococci and with the agents of diphtheria, tuberculosis and undulant fever, follows a usual incubation for the particular disease, and clinical course and manifestations are not as a rule materially altered by the circumstance of food serving as the vehicle of infection.

A. STAPHYLOCOCCUS INTOXICATION

1. *Identification.* A poisoning (not infection) of abrupt and sometimes violent onset with severe nausea, vomiting and prostration; sometimes severe diarrhea. Deaths are exceedingly rare. Diagnosis is usually on the basis of grouping of cases and short interval between eating food and onset of symptoms.

   Isolation of large numbers of staphylococci from suspected food permits presumptive diagnosis. Demonstration of ability of the organism to produce enterotoxin is essential for confirmation.

2. *Etiologic agent.* Toxin (enterotoxin) of certain strains of staphylococci. Toxin is stable at boiling temperature; staphylococci multiply in food, producing toxin which causes poisoning.

3. *Source and reservoir of infection.* (Not an infection but a poisoning.) Source of contamination not known in most instances; believed to be of human origin.

4. *Mode of transmission.* Most common vehicle is custard-filled pastry; processed meats, especially ham, responsible for some outbreaks; milk from cows with specifically infected udders.

[667]

5. *Incubation period.* Interval between taking food and onset is one-half hour to 4 hours, usually 2 to 4.
6. *Period of communicability.* Not applicable.
7. *Susceptibility and resistance.* Most persons susceptible, though individual reaction is variable.
8. *Occurrence.* Widespread and a relatively frequent disease; the principal cause of acute food poisoning in the United States.
9. *Methods of control:*
   A. Preventive measures:
      1. Prompt refrigeration of sliced and chopped meats and of custards and cream fillings, to avoid multiplication of staphylococci accidentally introduced; filling of pastries with custard immediately before sale, or adequate heat treatment of finished product. Avoid improper care of leftover foods.
      2. Some health departments have forbidden sale of custard-filled products during summer months.
      3. Temporary exclusion from food handling of persons suffering from pyogenic skin infections, especially those of hands.
      4. Education of food handlers in strict attention to sanitation, including refrigeration, hand-washing and danger of working with skin infections.
   B. Control of the infected individual, contacts and environment:
      1. Report to local health authority: Obligatory report of epidemics; suspect or confirmed cases with evidence of grouping or association with others in time and place.
      2. Isolation: None.
      3. Concurrent disinfection: None.
      4. Terminal disinfection: None.
      5. Quarantine: None.
      6. Immunization: None.
      7. Investigation of contacts and source of infection: Search for food contaminated with staphylococci, and for food handlers showing pyogenic skin infections or sore throat.
      8. Specific treatment: None.
   C. Epidemic measures:
      1. Search for food contaminated with staphylococci and for food handlers with skin infections or sore throat.
      2. Destruction of any remainder of contaminated food after samples have been taken for laboratory examination.
   D. International measures: None.

B. Botulinus Intoxication (Botulism)

1. *Identification.* A highly fatal afebrile poisoning (not infection) characterized by headache, weakness, constipation, a lack of gastrointestinal symptoms, oculomotor or other paralyses. Death is by cardiac or respiratory paralysis; in about two-thirds of patients, and usually within 3 to 7 days. Symptoms develop according to amount of toxin ingested in relation to body weight.

   Biologic and toxicologic tests may confirm presence of bacterium or its toxin in suspected food or stomach contents.
2. *Etiologic agent.* Toxins produced by Clostridium botulinum or Cl. parabotulinum

[668]

APPENDIX D

(botulinus bacilli). Most outbreaks are due to toxin from type A or B organisms; a few from type E. Toxin is produced in improperly processed food only under anaerobic conditions and particularly in non-acid foods. Toxin is easily destroyed by boiling but spores require higher temperatures.

3. *Source and reservoir of infection.* Not an infection but a poisoning. The immediate source is food containing botulinus toxin. The reservoir of botulinus bacillus is soil and the intestinal tract of animals. Toxin is formed by anaerobic growth of spores in food.
4. *Mode of transmission.* By ingestion of food containing botulinus toxin, usually eaten uncooked from jars or cans inadequately processed during canning. Most poisonings in the United States are due to home canned vegetables; in Europe most cases due to sausages or other smoked or preserved meat.
5. *Incubation period.* Symptoms usually appear within 18 hours after eating food containing toxin, possibly longer, the interval being determined by amount of contaminated food taken and content of botulinus toxin.
6. *Period of communicability.* Not applicable.
7. *Susceptibility and resistance.* Susceptibility is general.
8. *Occurrence.* Sporadic and grouped cases occur in all countries and always in relation to some perishable food product which has been so kept or preserved as to permit botulinus bacilli to develop.
9. *Methods of control:*
   A. Preventive measures:
      1. Governmental control by regulation and inspection of commercial processing of canned and preserved foods.
      2. Education of housewives and others concerned with home canning of foods, in essentials of safe processing, as to time, pressure and temperature factors.
      3. Education in value of boiling home canned green and leafy vegetables before serving; also thorough cooking of sausage and other meat and fish products.
   B. Control of the affected (poisoned) individual, contacts and environment:
      1. Report to local health authority: Case report obligatory in most states and countries. Includes suspect and confirmed cases.
      2. Isolation: None.
      3. Concurrent disinfection: None.
      4. Terminal disinfection: None.
      5. Quarantine: None.
      6. Immunization: Polyvalent botulinus antitoxin of appropriate type, if available, should be given to all who have eaten suspected food.
      7. Investigation of contacts and source of infection: Search for contaminated food. Study of food habits and recent food history of persons attacked.
      8. Specific treatment: Intramuscular administration of botulinus antitoxin.
   C. Epidemic measures:
      1. Suspicion or recognition of a case of botulism should immediately raise question of a group outbreak. Single sporadic cases are uncommon.
      2. Immediate search for persons who shared suspected food, for persons who may have eaten comparable food from same source, and for any remaining food from same source that may be similarly contaminated, such food if found to be destroyed after samples have been taken for laboratory examination. Search for limberneck in chickens.
   D. International measures: None.

C. Salmonella Infection

1. *Identification.* Salmonellosis includes a variety of clinical syndromes. The most common is an acute gastro-enteritis with diarrhea and abdominal cramps, to which attention is here limited. Fever, nausea and vomiting are frequently present. Deaths are uncommon but somewhat more frequent than for staphylococcal food poisoning.

   Microorganism may be recovered from feces or from site of a localized infection during acute illness; progressively more difficult during convalescence.

2. *Etiologic agent.* Numerous species of genus Salmonella of the group pathogenic for animals and occasionally for man, and excluding primarily human pathogens (see typhoid and paratyphoid fevers). Among the more common in United States are S. typhimurium, S. choleraesuis, S. newport, S. oranienburg, S. montevideo, S. panama and S. anatum; much variation from country to country; total serological types involved in food poisoning approach one hundred.

3. *Source and reservoir of infection.* Feces of patients and convalescent carriers, especially mild and unrecognized infections. Feces of domestic fowl, household pets, rodents and domestic animals; eggs of ducks, less commonly of chickens.

4. *Mode of transmission.* Epidemics are usually traced to (1) improperly prepared food, especially meat pies and roast fowl; (2) insufficiently cooked foods containing dried hen eggs, or duck eggs; (3) unpasteurized milk or dairy products; (4) pastries contaminated by rodent feces, possibly through medium of cockroaches; (5) food prepared by infected food handler. Sporadic cases probably originate through direct contact with infected person or animal.

5. *Incubation period.* In epidemics, 6 to 48 hours, usually about 12 hours. Not known for sporadic cases, but believed to be from 1 to 7 days.

6. *Period of communicability.* Throughout infection. Extremely variable, usually three days to three weeks and as long as carrier state persists.

7. *Susceptibility and resistance.* Susceptibility general; apparently bears important relationship to size of infecting dose. No active or passive artificial immunization. Some species-specific immunity of brief duration probably follows recovery.

8. *Occurrence.* World-wide and a common disease. Usually recognized in its epidemic form by groupings of cases among individuals having a common food supply. In such circumstances, a high proportion of individuals develop clinical symptoms. Sporadic cases tend to include more instances of mild unrecognized infection than of clinically evident disease.

9. *Methods of control:*
   A. Preventive measures:
   1. Thorough cooking of all foodstuffs derived from animal sources. Particular attention to preparation of fowl, egg products and meat dishes.
   2. Protection of prepared food against rodent or insect contamination.
   3. Refrigeration of prepared food during storage.
   4. Attempts to control salmonella infection among domestic animals.
   5. Meat and poultry inspection with adequate supervision of abattoir hygiene.
   B. Control of the infected individual, contacts and environment:
   1. Report to local health authority: Obligatory report of epidemics; suspect or confirmed cases with evidence of grouping or association with others in time and place.

2. Isolation: Exclusion of infected persons from food handling and occupations involving care of young children until negative feces cultures have been obtained.

3. Concurrent disinfection: Of feces and of articles soiled therewith. In communities with modern and adequate sewage disposal systems, feces can be disposed of directly into sewer without preliminary disinfection.

4. Terminal disinfection: Cleaning.

5. Quarantine: Family contacts should not be employed as food handlers during period of contact nor before repeated negative feces cultures have been obtained.

6. Immunization: None.

7. Investigation of contacts and source of infection: Search for unrecognized mild cases and convalescent carriers among contacts.

8. Specific treatment: None; chloramphenicol and the tetracyclines serve irregularly.

C. Epidemic measures:

1. Intensive search for case or carrier who is source of infection.

2. Search for food which may have served as a vehicle of spread and attempt to determine method of contamination.

3. Destruction of any remainder of suspected food after samples have been taken for laboratory examination.

D. International measures: An International Salmonella Center in Copenhagen, Denmark, and national salmonella centers in various countries (e.g., Communicable Disease Center, Atlanta, U.S.A.) facilitate proper identification of the various salmonella types. These centers provide uniformity of method and are essential to proper epidemiologic investigation of salmonellosis.

GONOCOCCAL INFECTION

Acute and chronic urethritis, vulvovaginitis of children and ophthalmia of the newborn and of adults are inflammatory conditions of man caused in common by gonococci. The maintenance of all depends upon the continued presence of gonorrhea in a population; together they constitute an epidemiologic entity and similar principles of control apply to the group. Clinically indistinguishable infections of the same anatomic structures are caused by a number of other infectious agents. This presentation relates specifically to gonococcal disease but the final paragraph under identification of each of the three gonococcal conditions gives the general characteristics of these other infections. They occur frequently and methods of control are often ill defined.

A. Gonococcal Urethritis (Gonorrhea)

1. *Identification.* A more or less self-limited infectious disease of venereal origin initiated by the gonococcus, an organism having affinity for columnar and transitional epithelium. The disease is thereby limited to areas where such tissues are found. Accordingly, gonorrhea in the male and female differs in course, in seriousness and in ease of identification. In males, a thick yellow purulent discharge of the anterior urethra usually appears 3 to 9 days after effective exposure; infection may extend to the posterior urethra and after varying intervals result in epididymitis, prostatitis, arthritis, and endocarditis. In females, the disorder is in three stages: a few days after exposure, an initial urethritis or

[671]

cervicitis, often so mild as to pass unnoticed; a stage of pelvic invasion, usually accompanying the first, second, or later menstrual period after infection, with mild or severe symptoms of salpingitis or pelvic peritonitis; the third stage is that of residua and often chronic infection. Death from gonorrhea is rare, but early and late manifestations, especially complications, are commonly and seriously incapacitating.

Bacteriologic culture is requisite to diagnosis of gonorrhea in the female, and desirable in gonorrhea of the male.

Widespread and frequent non-gonococcal urethritis, possibly also of sexual origin, seriously complicates the clinical diagnosis of gonorrhea in the male. In some countries the incidence exceeds that of gonorrhea and the condition is reportable; notoriously resistant to treatment, with many deficiencies in knowledge of etiology, communicability, clinical course and control; may be initiated by a number of infectious agents.

2. *Etiologic agent.* Neisseria gonorrhoeae, the gonococcus.

3. *Source and reservoir of infection.* Exudate from mucous membranes of infected persons. Man is the only reservoir.

4. *Mode of transmission.* Almost wholly by sexual intercourse, even in children; occasionally, in the newborn from ophthalmic infection acquired during birth; and in institutions for children, by careless and indiscriminate use of rectal thermometers.

5 *Incubation period.* Usually 3 to 9 days, sometimes 14.

6. *Period of communicability.* For months or years unless interrupted by specific therapy, which ends communicability within hours or days.

7. *Susceptibility and resistance.* Susceptibility is general. Spontaneous recovery is usual in the absence of reinfection. Acquired immunity not demonstrated; one attack does not protect against subsequent infection.

8. *Occurrence.* Worldwide and a common disease, particularly among persons of lower economic status; affects both sexes and practically all ages, especially the age groups of greatest sexual activity. The decline in frequency of gonorrhea has not kept pace with that of syphilis; lack of accurate diagnosis and incomplete reporting preclude reliable estimates of incidence.

9. *Methods of control:*

A. Preventive measures:

1. Except for measures applying specifically to gonorrhea, primarily the use of chemo prophylactic agents in the eyes of the newborn and special attention (abortive treatment) to female contacts of male patients, the preventive measures are those of syphilis.

B. Control of the infected individual, contacts and environment:

1. Report to local health authority: Case report is required in many states and countries.

2. Isolation: None; antibiotics promptly render discharges noninfectious. Refrain from sexual intercourse with untreated previous sexual partners to avoid reinfection.

3. Concurrent disinfection: None; care in disposal of discharges from lesions and articles soiled therewith.

4. Terminal disinfection: None.

5. Quarantine: None.

6. Immunization: None.
7. Investigation of contacts and source of infection: Interview of patients and tracing of contacts are the fundamental features of a program for control. Trained interviewers obtain the best results. Female contacts of male patients with gonorrhea should be treated at once, on epidemiologic grounds only, because of delays and difficulties in diagnosis and the practical fact that sexual exposure continues despite advice to the contrary. Include all sexual contacts of ten days prior to onset; also examine serologically for syphilis.
8. Specific treatment: Procaine penicillin or bicillin in one intramuscular injection on clinical, laboratory or epidemiological grounds; smaller doses for prophylaxis.
C. Epidemic measures: Intensification of routine procedures, especially therapy on epidemiologic grounds.
D. International measures: (See Syphilis).

B. Gonococcal Vulvovaginitis of Children

1. *Identification.* An inflammatory reaction of the urogenital tract of prepubescent females, characterized by redness and swelling of mucous membrane and mucopurulent discharge of varying degree; in severe infections, excoriation of labia and thighs and extension to urethra and bladder. A self-limited disease in that more than three-fourths of patients recover spontaneously within 3 to 6 months; a carrier state sometimes persists.

   Diagnosis is established by bacteriologic culture of exudates; examination of stained smears is unreliable.

   Gonococcal vulvovaginitis is to be differentiated from acute vulvovaginitis due to a variety of other infectious agents. In the United States, the gonococcus is responsible for only a small proportion (about 25%) of all cases. Clinical manifestations are usually indistinguishable and recognition is by bacteriological means. Outbreaks of non-gonococcal proctitis and vulvovaginitis occur in institutions for children.
2. *Etiologic agent.* Neisseria gonorrhoeae, gonococcus.
3. *Source and reservoir of infection.* Exudates from infected persons; infrequently, contaminated moist articles. The existence of transient inapparent gonococcus infection among children has been proven.
4. *Mode of transmission.* Intimate direct contact with adult patients in the home, willing and unwilling sexual contact, and insertion of contaminated instruments and foreign bodies in vagina and rectum.
5. *Incubation period.* Usually 3 to 9 days.
6. *Period of communicability.* While discharges persist, usually 3–6 months; communicability may continue after clinical manifestations cease.
7. *Susceptibility and resistance.* Susceptibility is related to type of epithelium lining vagina; until puberty: columnar or transitional epithelium, changes at puberty to stratified squamous type, not attacked by gonococci. Susceptibility general among female children; the frequency of spontaneous recovery is proof of a developing resistance. One attack does not protect against subsequent infection.
8. *Occurrence.* Extent not known but presumably widespread, particularly in families of lower social and economic levels where standards of personal, sexual, and general hygiene are low. Epidemics are most frequent in institutions for children.

9. *Methods of control:*

  A. Preventive measures:

    1. Fundamentally dependent on control of gonorrhea (see above): general measures are those of syphilis.

    2. Proper supervision of institutions for children, with rigid enforcement of hygienic principles and realization that sex education must begin earlier in life than commonly believed.

  B. Control of the infected individual, contacts and environment:

    1. Report to local health authority: Case report is required in most states and countries.

    2. Isolation: For the first 24 hours after administration of antibiotics

    3. Concurrent disinfection: None; care in disposal of discharges from lesions and articles soiled therewith.

    4. Terminal disinfection: None.

    5. Quarantine: None.

    6. Immunization: None.

    7. Investigation of contacts and source of infection: The proven importance of sexual transmission among children calls for trained interviewers to elicit history of sexual contact among playmates, family members and older males within the family group and outside. Histories are unreliable; therefore search for gonorrhea among persons in environment of child.

    8. Specific treatment: Penicillin in a single repository dose.

  C. Epidemic measures:

    1. Prompt search for source of infection within the institution or group affected and measures to protect pre-adolescent and younger girl children.

    2. Education of those in charge of children as to causes of outbreaks, sources and development of disease, with special emphasis upon personal cleanliness of children. The importance of probable sexual transmission should be emphasized.

  D. International measures: None.

C. Gonococcal Ophthalmia Neonatorum

1. *Identification.* Acute redness and swelling of the conjunctiva of one or both eyes, with mucopurulent or purulent discharge in which gonococci are identifiable by microscopic and cultural methods.

    Gonococcal ophthalmia neonatorum is but one of a number of acute inflammatory conditions of the eye or of the conjunctiva occurring within the first 3 weeks of life, and collectively known as ophthalmia neonatorum, acute conjunctivitis of the newborn, and babies' sore eyes of the first 21 days of life. Differentiation within the group is by bacteriologic means; clinical distinction is indefinite. The gonococcus is the most important but not necessarily the most frequent among infecting agents, which include meningococci, hemophilic bacilli, a virus (inclusion blenorrhea) and others. All purulent inflammation of the conjunctiva of the newborn is to be regarded as gonococcal until proved otherwise.

2. *Etiologic agent.* Neisseria gonorrhoeae, gonococcus.

3. *Source and reservoir of infection.* Infected maternal birth canal.

4. *Mode of transmission.* Contact during childbirth.

[674]

5. *Incubation period.* Usually 36 to 48 hours.

6. *Period of communicability.* During the course of the disease and until discharges from infected mucous membrane have ceased.

7. *Susceptibility and resistance.* Susceptibility is general. Immunity to subsequent gonococcal infection does not follow attack.

8. *Occurrence.* Varies widely according to observance or neglect of prophylactic use of a solution of silver nitrate or equivalent preparation in the eyes of the newborn by attendants at delivery. Infrequent where care of the newborn is adequate; globalwise, the disease is still an important cause of blindness.

9. *Methods of control:*

    A. Preventive measures:

        1. Specific protection by diagnosis and treatment of gonorrhea in prenatal period and instillation of silver nitrate or equivalent preparation at birth.

        2. Depends fundamentally on control of gonorrhea (see above); general preventive measures are those of syphilis.

    B. Control of the infected individual, contacts and environment:

        1. Report to local health authority: Case report is required in most states and countries.

        2. Isolation: For the first 24 hours after administration of antibiotic.

        3. Concurrent disinfection: None; care in disposal of conjunctival discharges and articles soiled therewith.

        4. Terminal disinfection: None.

        5. Quarantine: None.

        6. Immunization: None.

        7. Investigation of contacts and source of infection: Examination and treatment of mother and her consort.

        8. Specific treatment: Parenteral penicillin.

    C. Epidemic measures: None; a sporadic disease.

    D. International measures: None.

HEMORRHAGIC FEVER

1. *Identification.* An acute infectious disease characterized by fever of three to six days duration, conjunctival injection, prostration, anorexia, vomiting, hemorrhagic manifestations which begin about the third day and are an outstanding clinical feature, proteinuria about the fourth day and hypotension about the fifth; renal abnormalities continue for several weeks. About one-fourth of cases show an alarming hypotension and the majority of deaths (fatality about 6%) occur during shock. Increased fragility and permeability of capillaries are among the basic physiologic abnormalities of the disease, and contribute materially to the severe manifestations late in the first week. Convalescence is usually rapid during the third week but some loss of ability of the kidney to concentrate urine may persist for a month or so. Synonyms: Epidemic hemorrhagic fever, hemorrhagic nephroso-nephritis.

    Specific laboratory diagnostic tests are not available; clinical laboratory findings such as proteinuria, leucocytosis, thrombocytopenia and elevated nonprotein nitrogen assist in establishing the diagnosis.

    This disease is not to be confused with a number of other clinically similar

[675   ]

acute infectious hemorrhagic fevers (Crimean, Omsk, Bukovinan and Uzbeki-
stan) which occur in the U.S.S.R., are of viral etiology and transmitted by ticks.

2. *Etiologic agent.* Relatively little known; Berkefeld and Seitz filtrates of infectious
   human materials induce hemorrhagic fever in experimentally inoculated volunteers. The agent has not been established in laboratory animals.

3. *Source and reservoir of infection.* Assumed to be maintained in nature by a cycle involving some terrestrial arthropod and some rodent, with man only an accidental
   victim.

4. *Mode of transmission.* Unknown. Epidemiologic observations in Korea suggest an
   analogy to scrub typhus and implicate a non-flying arthropod vector of limited
   mobility; trombiculid mites are a likely suggestion.

5. *Incubation period.* Usually 12 to 16 days but varying from 9 to 35.

6. *Period of communicability.* Not communicable from man to man.

7. *Susceptibility and resistance.* Newcomers to endemic areas are uniformly susceptible
   but indigenous populations probably have some acquired resistance. Mild or
   inapparent infections are suspected but remain unproved in the absence of
   specific diagnostic tests. Second attacks have not been observed.

8. *Occurrence.* The disease was encountered in Korea in the vicinity of the 38th parallel
   among United Nations troops in 1951. Earlier Russian experience in Manchuria
   and Siberia along the Amur River and its tributaries indicates that women and
   children acquire the malady, as well as men. Two seasonal outbreaks, in May and
   June and in October and November, account for most cases; a few occur throughout the year. The majority are isolated events but outbreaks involving 5 to 20
   persons within a small unit are observed, with all infections apparently acquired
   at the same time and place.

9. *Methods of control:*
   A. Preventive measures: Lacking adequate information of etiologic agent and mode
      of transmission, preventive measures are those of diseases with an arthropod
      vector and a rodent host; in Korea since the summer of 1952 essentially as for
      scrub typhus.
   B. Control of the infected individual, contacts and environment:
      1. Report to local health authority: In selected endemic areas; in most countries
         not a reportable disease.
      2. Isolation: None.
      3. Concurrent disinfection: None.
      4. Terminal disinfection: None.
      5. Quarantine: None.
      6. Immunization: None.
      7. Investigation of source of infection: None.
      8. Specific treatment: None.
   C. Epidemic measures: Since outbreaks apparently result from simultaneous infec-
      tion of groups, control measures are not applicable to the episode. For measures in
      an endemic area, see 9A, and Scrub Typhus.
   D. International measures: None.

HEPATITIS, INFECTIOUS

1. *Identification.* An acute infection characterized by a prodromal period with constitutional manifestations, and a second phase commonly associated with

[676]

jaundice and symptoms referable to liver damage. Prodromal symptoms include fever, anorexia, nausea with or without vomiting, fatigue, lassitude, headache, and abdominal discomfort. Leucopenia is usual. Fever subsides after a few days, bile may be detected in the urine, and clinically recognizable jaundice appears. The second phase is of variable duration, with occasional chronic impairment of liver function and possible cirrhosis. Convalescence may be prolonged. Severity varies greatly, from mild infection without jaundice and recognizable only by liver function test, to the rare fulminating and usually fatal acute yellow atrophy of the liver. Most infections are benign; in epidemics the fatality rarely exceeds 0.5% and commonly is nearer 0.2%. Synonyms: Epidemic hepatitis, epidemic jaundice, catarrhal jaundice.

No specific laboratory tests are available.

2. *Etiologic agent.* The virus of infectious hepatitis.
3. *Source and reservoir of infection.* Feces and blood from infected persons. Presence of virus in discharges of nose and throat is poorly established; commonly assumed on epidemiological behavior of the disease.
4. *Mode of transmission.* Probably through intimate person-to-person contact via the intestinal-oral route, with respiratory spread secondary; transmitted by transfusion of whole blood, blood serum, or plasma from infected persons, and by accidental contamination of syringes or needles with traces of blood from such persons; transmissible to human volunteers by ingestion or parenteral inoculation of blood or filtered fecal suspensions from patients in the acute phase. Epidemics have been related to contaminated water, food, and milk.
5. *Incubation period.* Long and variable, from 10 to 40 days, commonly 25 days.
6. *Period of communicability.* Unknown; virus demonstrated in blood before clinically recognized disease; evidence of a fecal carrier state of at least 5 to 15 months. Clinically experience suggests most communicable from a few days before to a few days after onset, usually not exceeding 7 days.
7. *Susceptibility and resistance.* Susceptibility is general. Degree and duration of immunity after attack unknown but probably life-long; second attacks are infrequent. No known animal other than man is susceptible.
8. *Occurrence.* Worldwide, sporadically and in epidemics, with outbreaks most common in institutions, in rural areas, and in military forces during wars. Incidence in rural areas is decidedly higher than in cities. Most common among children and young adults, less with advancing years. Incidence highest in autumn and early winter in temperate zones.
9. *Methods of control:*
   A. Preventive measures:
      1. Good community sanitation and personal hygiene, with particular emphasis on sanitary disposal of feces and respiratory discharges.
      2. Proper technical procedure to prevent transmission by blood or blood products from an infected donor or through use of improperly sterilized syringes and needles (see Serum Hepatitis).
   B. Control of the infected individual, contacts and environment:
      1. Report to local health authority: In selected endemic areas (U.S.A.); in most states and countries not a reportable disease.
      2. Isolation: During first week of illness.
      3. Concurrent disinfection: Feces, and nose and throat secretions.

[677]

4. Terminal disinfection: None.
5. Quarantine: None.
6. Immunization: Immune serum globulin, 0.01 mlgm. per pound of body weight intramuscularly and promptly after exposure, gives passive protection even as late as 6 days before onset of disease and lasting 6 to 8 weeks.
7. Investigation of contacts and source of infection: Search for missed cases and surveillance of contacts.
8. Specific treatment: None.

C. Epidemic measures:
1. Epidemiologic investigation to determine possible transmission by food, water, blood or blood products.
2. Special efforts to improve sanitary and hygienic practices in the community, with the object of reducing fecal contamination of foods and water and carelessness in disposal of nose and mouth discharges.
3. Focal concentrations of disease in schools and institutions of limited populations may suggest mass prophylaxis with immune serum globulin.

D. International measures: None.

HEPATITIS, SERUM

1. *Identification.* Clinically indistinguishable from infectious hepatitis. The chief differences are in longer incubation period of serum hepatitis; that serum hepatitis is not known to be transmitted in nature from man to man, and higher case fatality varying from 6 to 12%. The relationship between the diseases is not completely understood, although the evidence suggests that each is caused by an independent virus. Synonym: Homologous serum jaundice.

   Absence of naturally occurring infection among associates and history of infection by blood products 2 to 6 months previously, are essential to differentiation from infectious hepatitis.

2. *Etiologic agent.* The virus of serum hepatitis.

3. *Source and reservoir of infection.* Blood or blood products from an infected person.

4. *Mode of transmission.* By parenteral (intravenous, intramuscular, or subcutaneous) inoculation of infected human blood, plasma, serum or thrombin; or by administration of prophylactic or therapeutic agents with syringes and needles contaminated with traces of blood from infected persons. Immune serum globulin and albumin, although blood derivatives, do not transmit the disease.

5. *Incubation period.* Estimated at 2 to 6 months, usually 12 to 14 weeks.

6. *Period of communicability.* Virus demonstrated in blood of experimentally inoculated volunteers long before onset of symptoms. How long harbored after infection is unknown; blood donors have infected recipients in each of three successive years. Some persons are carriers without experiencing a clinically recognized attack.

7. *Susceptibility and resistance.* Susceptibility is high, as measured by manifest disease relatively low in children and progressively higher for adults.

8. *Occurrence.* Worldwide in distribution, wherever appropriate circumstances exist for transmission. Incidence among recipients of pooled blood products varies from 2 to 15%, and of known icterogenic plasma as high as 60%.

[678]

9. *Methods of control:*
   A. Preventive measures:
      1. Limiting administration of whole blood, and particularly pooled blood serum or plasma, to patients or others with clear indication of therapeutic usefulness or necessity. Pooling increases the likelihood that blood products will contain the infectious agent. Use of blood substitutes free of virus, such as human albumin or dextran, where feasible. Donor recruitment programs should rigidly exclude persons with a past history of hepatitis.
      2. Thorough heat sterilization of syringes and needles, and of stylets for finger-puncture. A fresh sterile syringe and needle or stylet is essential for each patient; traces of blood from previous use contaminate these instruments.
      3. No available technical method of treatment assures destruction of serum hepatitis virus in infected blood and blood derivatives. Ultraviolet light irradiation, as now practiced, is ineffective. Recent evidence suggests storage for 6 months as a practical procedure.
   B. Control of infected individual, contacts and environment:
      1. Report to local health authority: In selected endemic areas (U.S.A.); in most states and countries not a reportable disease.
      2. Isolation: None. Not known to be communicable except by injection.
      3. Concurrent disinfection: Of equipment contaminated with blood.
      4. Terminal disinfection: None.
      5. Quarantine: None.
      6. Immunization: None. Immune serum globulin of no value.
      7. Investigation of contacts and source of infection: Search for groupings of cases among others who have attended in common a clinic or hospital where parenteral therapy is much employed, as a clinic for diabetes or syphilis.
      8. Specific treatment: None.
   C. Epidemic measures: Surveys in areas of high incidence of persons receiving blood or blood products, to determine incidence and to control technics associated with parenteral injections.
   D. International measures: None.

HERPANGINA

1. *Identification.* An acute infection characterized by sudden onset with fever and small vesicular lesions of the pharynx which promptly ulcerate and cause moderate discomfort. The illness lasts 3–5 days, with occasional relapse of fever one week later; no deaths.

   Definitive diagnosis is established during acute illness by recovery of the etiologic agent from lesions, from stool specimens well into convalescence and by neutralizing and complement fixing antibody response.

   Clinically, herpangina is to be distinguished from herpetic stomatitis which has larger, deeper and more painful lesions commonly located in the front of the mouth.

2. *Etiologic agent.* At least six distinct immunologic types of Coxsackie virus, Group A.

3. *Source and reservoir of infection.* Pharyngeal (nose and throat) discharges and feces of infected persons, frequently in the absence of clinically recognized attack.

[679]

4. *Mode of transmission.* Direct contact with infected persons, and by droplet spread. Contaminated flies have been found, but with no reliable evidence of spread by insects, water, food or sewage.

5. *Incubation period.* Usually 3 to 5 days.

6. *Period of communicability.* During the acute stage of illness and perhaps longer, since the virus persists in stools for several weeks.

7. *Susceptibility and resistance.* Susceptibility to infection is general. Immunity is acquired by infection, clinical and inapparent; duration unknown. Second attacks occur with Group A virus of different immunological type.

8. *Occurrence.* Throughout the world, both sporadically and in epidemics; highly prevalent and with greatest incidence in summer and early autumn. A common communicable disease of children under 10 years, but adult cases are relatively frequent.

9. *Methods of control:*

   A. Preventive measures: None.

   B. Control of the infected individual, contacts and environment:
   1. Report to local health authority: Obligatory report of epidemics; no case report.
   2. Isolation: None.
   3. Concurrent disinfection: Of nose and throat discharges, feces, and articles soiled therewith.
   4. Terminal disinfection: None.
   5. Quarantine: None.
   6. Active immunization: None.
   7. Investigation of source of infection: Of no practical value.
   8. Specific treatment: None.

   C. Epidemic measures:
   1. General notice to physicians of the prevalence or increased incidence of the disease, description of usual characteristics of onset and necessity for differential diagnosis, especially from poliomyelitis.
   3. Isolation in bed of all children with fever, pending diagnosis.

   D. International measures: None.

HISTOPLASMOSIS

1. *Identification.* Most infections are asymptomatic, with evidence of past infection limited to a positive skin test to histoplasmin, sometimes associated with calcified pulmonary lesions. A generalized highly fatal form of the disease is rare, and is characterized by enlargement of the liver, spleen and lymph nodes, ulcerations of mouth, nose, pharynx and larynx, and lung lesions. Gastro-intestinal lesions are not infrequent. Recent studies of outbreaks in groups exposed in closed areas, such as a cave, storm cellar or silo, indicate that infection may result in symptoms of general malaise, weakness, fever, chest pains and nonproductive cough; recovery is the rule.

In the rare generalized infection, the fungus is frequently seen within monocytes by microscopic examination of stained blood. Culture of blood, sternal bone marrow or exudates from ulcers confirms the diagnosis.

[680]

2. *Etiologic agent.* Histoplasma capsulatum, a fungus.

3. *Source and reservoir of infection.* Man is apparently infected from his environment. The fungus has been isolated from soils in areas where infection exists in man or animals; also from dogs, cats, rats, skunks, opossums and foxes.

4. *Mode of transmission.* Presumably through inhalation of air-borne spores; possibly by ingestion of spores on contaminated food or other articles.

5. *Incubation period.* In the few reported epidemics, symptoms appeared within 5 to 18 days after exposure.

6. *Period of communicability.* Probably for duration of active lesions; direct transmission from man to man not established.

7. *Susceptibility and resistance.* Susceptibility is general. Inapparent infections are extremely common in endemic areas; resulting immunity is likely, but not established.

8. *Occurrence.* Reported from widely scattered areas of North, Central and South America, Europe, Africa, Hawaii, Java and the Philippines. The disease occurs in all age groups but is more common in infants and in adults over 40 years; males outnumber females, especially at ages over ten years where the ratio is 7 to 1. Histoplasmin hypersensitivity, indicating antecedent infection, is highly prevalent in the central regions of the United States as compared with Rocky Mountain and coastal areas. No differences between sexes; the proportion of positive reactors increases from childhood to 30 years of age. Racial differences not discerned.

9. *Methods of control:*

   A. Preventive measures: None.

   B. Control of the infected individual, contacts and environment:

      1. Report to local health authority: In selected endemic areas (U.S.A.); in many states and countries not a reportable disease. Reporting limited to systemic disease.

      2. Isolation: None.

      3. Concurrent disinfection: Discharges from skin lesions and necrotic lymph nodes, sputum and articles soiled therewith.

      4. Terminal disinfection: None.

      5. Quarantine: None.

      6. Immunization: None.

      7. Investigation of contacts and source of infection: Household contacts of patients with systemic disease for evidence of infection.

      8. Specific treatment: None.

   C. Epidemic measures: The occurrence of grouped cases of acute pulmonary infection in an endemic area, particularly with a history of exposure to dust in a closed space, should arouse suspicion of primary histoplasmosis. Suspected sources such as barns, silos, caves, and basements should be investigated.

   D. International measures: None.

IMPETIGO CONTAGIOSA

1. *Identification.* A purulent dermatitis, characterized initially by vesicular lesions which later become crusted seropurulent plaques, commonly of the face and

[681]

hands, but sometimes widely over the body: a disfiguring and offensive disease but rarely serious.

2. *Etiologic agent.* Probably streptococci, with staphylococci secondarily. Crater-like ulcers of the corium commonly indicate mixed infection with hemolytic strepto-coccus and staphylococcus aureus.

3. *Source and reservoir of infection.* Lesions on the skin of an infected person; possibly discharges from the nose and throat.

4. *Mode of transmission.* By direct contact with moist discharges of skin lesions, or in-direct contact with articles recently soiled by discharges. Infection may be readily inoculated from place to place on the patient's body by scratching. Some evidence of airborne transmission through dust in hospital wards for children.

5. *Incubation period.* Usually within 5 days, often 2.

6. *Period of communicability.* While lesions remain unhealed.

7. *Susceptibility and resistance.* Susceptibility general, especially among children and debilitated persons.

8. *Occurrence.* Common among children, especially in warm weather. Occurs sporad-ically and as small epidemics in nurseries for infants, institutions for children, and summer camps. Likely to spread rapidly where measures of personal hygiene are neglected and where other skin lesions lead to scratching; association with scabies and pediculosis is common.

9. *Methods of control:*

   A. Preventive measures:

      1. Personal cleanliness, particularly avoidance of common use of toilet articles by children.

      2. Prompt treatment of the first case in a group of children will abbreviate the period of communicability and prevent extension of lesions to new sites and to other children.

      3. Prompt treatment of parasitic infections of the skin.

   B. Control of the infected individual, contacts and environment:

      1. Report to local health authority: Obligatory report of epidemics, especially in institutions, schools, hospitals and among groups of children; no individual case report.

      2. Isolation: Prevent contact with other children or debilitated persons until pustules are healed.

      3. Concurrent disinfection: Of dressings and moist discharges from the patient; sterilization of underclothes and towels before laundering; avoid reinfection from contaminated washcloths, combs, and other toilet articles.

      4. Terminal disinfection: Thorough cleaning of towels, hair brushes, combs and other toilet articles.

      5. Quarantine: None.

      6. Immunization: None.

      7. Investigation of contacts and source of infection: In family cases, of little profit; see 9C.

      8. Specific treatment: Adequate treatment will materially shorten the period of communicability. Remove crusts with bacitracin ointment or 5% ammoniated mercury ointment; continue either with ointment or 5% ammoniated mercury in calamine lotion; 3% aureomycin ointment is also effective. Parenteral

penicillin (aqueous soluble) for severe spreading infections but never penicillin locally; aureomycin if penicillin resistant.

C. Epidemic measures: Child contacts should be kept under surveillance; search for skin infections among attendants of infants; persons with skin lesions should be restricted from contact with newborn babies.

D. International measures: None.

INFLUENZA

1. *Identification.* An acute, highly communicable group of diseases, characterized by abrupt onset with fever lasting 1 to 6 days, chills or chilliness, aches and pains in the back and limbs, and prostration. Respiratory symptoms include coryza, sore throat and cough. Recognition is ordinarily on the basis of symptoms and the presence of an epidemic. Sporadic cases are difficult to identify. Usually a self limited disease with recovery in 48–72 hours; influenza derives its importance from the complications that follow, especially pneumonia in those debilitated by old age, by other disease, or in young infants.

   Laboratory confirmation is by recovery of virus from throat washings or by demonstration of a significant rise in antibiotics against a specific influenza virus in serums obtained during acute and convalescent stages of the disease.

2. *Etiologic agent.* Two types of influenza virus, Influenza A and Influenza B are long recognized; a third, Influenza C, is more recently identified. Types A and B include numerous serologically distinct strains. One strain tends to be replaced from epidemic to epidemic by another of slightly different nature, the first disappearing; hence the importance of continued epidemiologic and serologic studies.

3. *Source and reservoir of infection.* Discharges from the mouth and nose of infected persons.

4. *Mode of transmission.* By direct contact, through droplet infection, or by articles freshly soiled with discharges of the nose and throat of infected persons; possibly air-borne.

5. *Incubation period.* Short, usually 24 to 72 hours.

6. *Period of communicability.* Probably limited to one week after onset.

7. *Susceptibility and resistance.* Susceptibility is close to universal but of varying degree, as evidenced by frequent inapparent and atypical infections during epidemics. After early infancy, presence of serum antibody is a result of infection. For a population, antibody content for different types of virus, and varieties within types is a reflection of the experience of that population; for individuals it tends to broaden with age and to exist in varying degree and extent. Immunity after attack may persist for several years against homologous or closely related strains, but freedom from disease is often short because of the variety of influenza viruses and of other microbial agents capable of inducing the influenzal syndrome.

8. *Occurrence.* Variable, in pandemics, local epidemics and as sporadic cases, the latter commonly unrecognized. Epidemics may affect up to half a population within 4 to 6 weeks; attack rates ordinarily vary from less than 5 to 20–30%. The last serious pandemic of influenza, representing a world wide distribution of the

[683]

infectious agent, was in 1918; those since then have been mild and of relatively little consequence. In temperate zones epidemics tend to occur in winter, in the tropics irregularly. The disease shows a cyclic tendency, with influenza A appearing in epidemic form at shorter intervals than does influenza B. One serologic type of virus is usually obtained from patients of the same epidemic, but presence of two types is known.

9. *Methods of control:*

  A. Preventive measures:

    1. Education of the public as to sanitary hazards from spitting, sneezing and coughing in the close presence of other persons with stress that the viruses of influenza are in discharges from the upper respiratory tract. Avoid use of common towels, glasses, eating utensils, or toilet articles and encourage use of disposable paper handkerchiefs and napkins.

    2. Active immunization with currently available vaccines achieves a substantial reduction in incidence of influenza, provided the prevailing strain of virus matches closely the antigenic components of the vaccine used. Opinion differs on duration of protection but immunization oftener than once a year appears unnecessary. Major shifts in antigenic structure of influenza virus occur and discount the effectiveness of general immunization programs.

      Inoculation of vaccine during an epidemic is valueless; the disease spreads rapidly and protection does not follow until seven days. For practical effect, must be practiced in advance of an anticipated epidemic; international control measures under D2 and D3 below are designed to this purpose and are also applicable within a country.

      General inoculation of whole populations is not feasible, but experimental use of influenza vaccines under controlled conditions is increasingly practiced for selected groups; in general not including children because of reactions that follow.

  B. Control of the infected individual, contacts and environment:

    1. Report to local health authority: Obligatory report of epidemics resembling influenza; no individual case report. Confirmation of the epidemic disease as influenza should be sought promptly through laboratory procedures.

    2. Isolation: During the acute illness; not as an official requirement but as directed by the attending physician.

    3. Concurrent disinfection: Discharges from the nose and throat of the patient.

    4. Terminal disinfection: None.

    5. Quarantine: None.

    6. Immunization: Of contacts, none.

    7. Investigation of contacts and source of infection: Of no practical value.

    8. Specific treatment: None. Sulfonamides and antibiotics do not affect the uncomplicated disease; should be employed if pulmonary complications arise.

  C. Epidemic measures:

    1. To minimize severity and to protect the patient from secondary infections thus reducing mortality, patients should go to bed at the beginning of an attack and not return to work without the approval of a physician.

    2. The aggregation of large numbers of persons is to be discouraged. The closing of schools is not effective in checking spread.

    3. Crowding of beds in hospitals and institutions to accommodate increased

numbers of patients and other inmates is especially to be avoided. Increased spacing between beds in wards and dormitories reduces risk of attack and of pneumonia.

4. Continued dissemination of current information on extent and nature of the epidemic to local health authorities by state or national health agencies.

D. International measures:

1. Prompt notification to WHO of epidemics within a country, especially those involving institutional, military or other considerable groups.

2. Identification of virus type in such situations through prompt dispatch of the necessary blood samples or throat washings to one of the official influenza virus detection centers which now number close to 60, and are widely distributed in many countries. The World Influenza Center is in London.

3. Continuing epidemiologic studies by official health agencies and exchange of information in order to establish broad movements of epidemic influenza, to facilitate early recognition of outbreaks within a country, and to identify the prevailing type and strain.

LEPROSY

1. *Identification.* A chronic communicable disease characterized by lesions of the skin— infiltration, macules, plaques, papules and nodules—and by involvement of peripheral nerves with consequent anesthesia, muscle weakness and paralysis, and trophic changes in skin, muscle and bone. In lepromatous (cutaneous) leprosy, the mucous membranes of the upper respiratory tract are also usually invaded. Progress of the disease is slow but ultimate fatality is high.

Demonstration of acid-fast bacilli in suspected lesions is confirmatory in lepromatous cases; bacilli may be rare or not demonstrable in tuberculoid (maculo-anesthetic) lesions and diagnosis depends primarily upon presence of anesthesia in areas served by affected nerves.

2. *Etiologic agent.* Mycobacterium leprae, leprosy bacillus.

3. *Source and reservoir of infection.* Discharges from lesions of infected persons.

4. *Mode of transmission.* Not definitely known; the bacillus probably gains entrance through skin or mucous membrane of the upper respiratory tract.

5. *Incubation period.* Prolonged, undetermined, from one to several years.

6. *Period of communicability.* Commences when lesions become open and discharge leprosy bacilli; continues until healing, communicability being shortened by adequate chemotherapy. Patients with demonstrable acid-fast bacilli in smears from skin or mucous membrane are potentially open cases even if demonstrable ulceration is not present.

7. *Susceptibility and resistance.* No racial immunity. More frequent in persons exposed in early life; the lesser incidence among adults is seemingly dependent on differences in opportunity for infection.

8. *Occurrence.* Mostly in the tropics and subtropics. Prevalence rates of 5 per 1,000 or higher are found only in the tropics. A few countries with temperate climates have estimated rates of 1:1,000, including China, Japan and Korea. China and India have about one-half of the estimated world total of 3–4,000,000 cases. In Europe, low endemicity in Greece, Portugal, Spain; residual foci only in several other countries. Endemic but decreasing in Hawaii, present at a low level in

Canal Zone, Puerto Rico and Virgin Islands, and in continental United States, chiefly limited to Gulf Coast areas of Florida, Louisiana and Texas.

9. *Methods of control:*

A. Preventive measures:

1. In endemic areas leprosy is usually contracted in childhood but may be acquired in adult life. Infants should be separated from leprous parents at birth; educational efforts should stress greater risk when exposure is early in life. The exaggerated fear of leprosy and belief in its high communicability should be discounted.

B. Control of the infected individual, contacts and environment:

1. Report to local health authority: Case report obligatory in most states and countries and desirable in all.

2. Isolation: In endemic areas, patients with demonstrable leprosy bacilli in smears from the lesions should be isolated in hospitals or colonies and treated until bacteriologically negative for at least six months. The next best procedure is institutional treatment until ulcerative lesions are healed followed by home isolation with medical supervision. In many countries of high endemicity only clinic supervision is practicable. In areas where the disease is not indigenous, home isolation is sufficient. Patients discharged from institutions should be examined periodically, the suggested interval being six months.

3. Concurrent disinfection: Discharges of lesions and articles soiled therewith.

4. Terminal disinfection: Thorough cleaning of living premises of patient.

5. Quarantine: None.

6. Immunization: None.

7. Investigation of contacts and source of infection: Should be undertaken in cases of apparently recent origin; the long and uncertain period of incubation makes discovery of the source of infection difficult. Periodic examination of contacts for secondary cases.

8. Specific treatment: Sulfones (promin, diasone and D.D.S., di-amino-diphenyl sulfone), the preferred therapeutic agents, are continued for long periods. Promin is administered intravenously, diasone orally, with slowly increased doses. Initial small oral doses of D.D.S. are slowly increased to tolerance. Streptomycin probably has value equal to sulfones and may be substituted when sulfone therapy fails or is not tolerated. Isoniazid and a number of other drugs are under evaluation. Penicillin is of value only for control of secondary infection.

C. Epidemic measures: In areas giving evidence of spread of infection (high endemicity or those uncommon situations justifying epidemic characterization) provision of facilities for bacteriological diagnosis, treatment clinics, case finding to include examination of family contacts of known cases every six months, separation of children of leprous parents from birth and repatriation of immigrants developing the disease within five years of arrival; also the usual measures of reporting and isolation.

D. International measures:

1. Exercise of the recognized international rights of governments to refuse entry of immigrants who are found to have leprosy is usual and desirable.

2. Reciprocal measures between governments at authorized points of entry of immigrants to prevent introduction or spread of the disease.

LEPTOSPIROSIS

1. *Identification.* An acute systemic infection characterized by fever, chills, severe malaise and muscular aches, headache, vomiting, stiff neck, injection of conjunctivae, and infrequently jaundice, renal insufficiency, hemolytic anemia, and hemorrhage in skin and mucous membranes. Leucocytosis is common, pleocytosis of spinal fluid frequent. The acute illness lasts from one to three weeks; relapses may occur. Case fatality is low; in severe cases with jaundice and kidney damage, formerly considered the common manifestations of the disease, may reach 20% or more, being greater with advancing age. Synonyms: Weil's disease, canicola fever, swineherd disease, mud fever, hemorrhagic jaundice.

2. *Etiologic agent.* Many species of the genus Leptospira; L. icterohemorrhagiae, L. canicola and a member of the sero-group autumnalis have been recovered from human cases in the United States; and in addition serologic evidence of human infection with members of the serogroup pomona, bataviae and grippotyphosa; others are probable. At present at least 21 serogroups containing 35 serotypes are recognized.

3. *Source and reservoir of infection.* The source is urine of chronically infected animals and possibly infected tissues. Reservoirs include cattle, dogs and swine, rats and other wild rodents.

4. *Mode of transmission.* Contact with water contaminated with urine of infected animals, as in swimming or accidental immersion; direct contact with infected animals. Infection presumably results from penetration of abraded skin or mucous membrane, or possibly from ingestion.

5. *Incubation period.* Four to 19 days, usually 10 days.

6. *Period of communicability.* Communicability from man to man is negligible; urine of patients infrequently contains leptospira.

7. *Susceptibility and resistance.* Susceptibility of man is general. Demonstrable antibodies are generally present in serum up to one year; may persist for many years.

8. *Occurrence.* Outbreaks among swimmers exposed to contaminated waters are reported with increasing frequency. An occupational hazard to veterinarians, animal husbandmen, abattoir workers, fish workers, and those who live or work in rat infested premises. Distribution of reservoirs of infection and of one or another species of leptospira is probably world wide.

9. *Methods of control:*

   A. Preventive measures:

      1. Protection with boots and gloves of workers exposed to hazard of infection.

      2. Avoidance of swimming in potentially contaminated waters.

      3. Rodent control in human habitations, agricultural and recreational.

      4. Segregation of domestic animals and prevention of contamination of human living and working areas by urine of infected animals.

   B. Control of the infected individual, contacts and environment:

      1. Report to local health authority: Obligatory case report in many states and countries.

      2. Isolation: None.

      3. Concurrent disinfection: None.

      4. Terminal disinfection: None.

      5. Quarantine: None.

6. Immunization: None of established value.
7. Investigation of contacts and source of infection: Search for exposure to infected animals or swimming in contaminated waters.
8. Specific treatment: Penicillin, streptomycin, and the broad spectrum antibiotics are leptospirocidal in vitro, but not yet of demonstrated value in human infections.

C. Epidemic measures: Search for source of infection, such as a swimming pool; eliminate contamination, or prohibit further use.
D. International measures: None.

LYMPHOGRANULOMA VENEREUM

1. *Identification.* A venereally acquired virus infection of lymph channels and lymph nodes manifesting itself in a variety of ways: bubo formations, ulcerations, elephantiasis of genitalia, and rectal stricture. The disease sometimes begins with a small painless evanescent erosion, papule, or herpetiform lesion, followed shortly by acute, subacute or chronic adenitis and periadenitis, usually with multiple foci of suppuration and with grooved adherent skin of a purplish hue; more commonly the bubo is the first manifestation. Constitutional symptoms during lymphatic progression include fever, chills, headache, vague abdominal aches, joint pains and anorexia. Spontaneous regression of buboes does not indicate recovery; the course is often long, disability is great, and death occasionally follows pyogenic complications. Synonyms: Lymphogranuloma inguinale, climatic bubo, poradenitis, and lymphopathia venereum.

Diagnosis is aided by skin test with Frei antigen or by demonstration of complement fixing antibodies against lymphogranuloma venereum-psittacosis group of viruses; neither test is conclusive.

2. *Etiologic agent.* The virus of lymphogranuloma venereum, immunologically related to virus of psittacosis.
3. *Source and reservoir of infection.* Lesions of rectum and urethra and sinuses and ulcerations of infected persons.
4. *Mode of transmission.* Through direct contact during sexual intercourse; by indirect contact with articles contaminated by infectious exudates, especially infections of children.
5. *Incubation period.* 5 to 21 days from primary lesion, usually 7 to 12; if inguinal bubo is first manifestation, 10 to 30 days, sometimes several months.
6. *Period of communicability.* Variable, from weeks to years, during presence of active lesions.
7. *Susceptibility and resistance.* Susceptibility seemingly is general. Immunity does not follow attack; no artificial immunity.
8. *Occurrence.* A commoner disease than ordinarily believed; widespread throughout the world, especially tropical and subtropical areas. Endemic in southern United States, particularly among Negroes. Age incidence is that of greatest sexual activity, with the disease most frequent among the sexually promiscuous. Sex differences are not pronounced and all races are affected.
9. *Methods of control:*
A. Preventive measures:
1. Except for specific information relating to lymphogranuloma venereum, preventive measures are those for the venereal diseases.
B. Control of the infected individual, contacts and environment:

[688]

1. Report to local health authority: In selected endemic areas (U.S.A. some states); in most states and countries not a reportable disease.
2. Isolation: None; avoid sexual and other intimate contact until lesions are healed.
3. Concurrent disinfection: None; care in disposal of dicharges from lesions and of articles soiled therewith.
4. Terminal disinfection: None.
5. Quarantine: None.
6. Immunization: None.
7. Investigation of contacts and source of infection: Search for sexual contacts exposed prior and subsequent to appearance of disease.
8. Specific treatment: Varies with stage of the disease; aureomycin in the bubo phase, with sulfadiazine moderately successful; for proctitis and other ulcerative lesions, tetracycline antibiotics (aureomycin, terramycin), chloramphenicol or sulfadiazine, administered for 30 days or more after discharges subside.

C. Epidemic measures: Intensification of preventive and control activities.
D. International measures: See Syphilis.

MALARIA

1. *Identification.* A severe systemic disease, acute and often chronic, commonly beginning with a brief and indefinite illness shortly followed by a characteristic shaking chill with rapidly rising temperature, usually accompanied by headache and nausea and ending with profuse sweating; after an interval free of fever, the cycle of chills, fever and sweating is repeated. As the disease progresses the paroxysms tend to occur daily, every other day or every third day, depending on species and strain of etiologic agent. The duration of untreated primary attack varies from a week to a month or longer. Relapses are common and may occur at irregular intervals for several years. Fatality in untreated cases varies from less than 1% to 10% or even higher, depending on character of the parasite and degree of host resistance. In treated cases the rate may be 0.1% and rarely exceeds 0.5%. Clinical diagnosis depends upon development of the characteristic recurrent chills and fever, enlargement of the spleen and secondary anemia, often with palpable spleen and mild icterus.

Laboratory confirmation should always be sought through demonstration of malaria parasites in blood films by microscopic examination. Repeated examinations may be necessary; the thick film method is most likely to reveal the parasite; often not demonstrable in films from patients recently or actively under treatment.

2. *Etiologic agent.* Plasmodium vivax for tertian malaria, P. malariae for quartan malaria, P. falciparum for falciparum malaria and P. ovale for the rare ovale malaria.

3. *Source and reservoir of infection.* The immediate source is an infected mosquito. Man is the only known reservoir.

4. *Mode of transmission.* Certain species of Anopheles ingest human blood containing plasmodia in the gametocyte stage and act as definitive hosts. The parasite develops into sporozoites in from 8 to 35 days depending on species of parasite and temperature to which the insect is exposed. Sporozoites lodge in the salivary glands and are injected into man as the insect thereafter takes a blood meal. In the susceptible host, gametocytes usually appear in the blood within 3 to 14

days, according to species of parasite. Malaria may be transmitted also by injection or transfusion of blood of infected persons or by use of contaminated hypodermic syringes, as by drug addicts.

5. *Incubation period.* Average 12 days for P. falciparum, 13 to 15 days for P. vivax, and 28 to 30 days for P. malariae. With some strains of P. vivax, primary attack may be delayed for 8 to 10 months, the period of latency being known as protracted incubation period. With infection by blood transfusion, incubation may be much shorter.

6. *Period of communicability.* As long as infective gametocytes circulate in the blood, varies with species and strain of parasite and with response to therapy. May extend indefinitely in quartan malaria, from 1 to 3 years in vivax, and rarely more than 1 year in falciparum. The infected mosquito remains infective for life; only the female takes blood meals.

7. *Susceptibility and resistance.* Susceptibility is universal; the degree of susceptibility is sometimes lessened by previous infection. A high degree of tolerance to the effects of infection may develop in highly endemic primitive communities where nightly exposure to infective anophelines is continuous over many years.

8. *Occurrence.* Highly infrequent in the United States and in several other countries where malaria was a health problem a decade ago. Even in the tropics, Ceylon and Venezuela among other countries have now greatly reduced the incidence of malaria by modern control measures. The disease is still a major cause of ill health in many parts of tropical and subtropical Africa, Asia, and the Southwest Pacific.

9. *Methods of control:*
   A. Preventive measures:
      1. Application of residual insecticide (such as DDT, benzene hexachloride or dieldrin) in suitable formula and dosage at appropriate intervals on the inside walls of dwellings and on other surfaces upon which vector anophelines habitually rest will generally result in effective malaria control. Usually entire communities are included in a spraying project and the latter is routinely carried forward year after year until malaria ceases to be endemic.
      2. Where residual insecticide is not available, nightly spraying of living and sleeping quarters with a liquid or an aerosol preparation of pyrethrum is useful.
      3. In endemic areas, living and sleeping quarters should be screened and bed nets used.
      4. Insect repellents (such as dimethylphthalate or 2-ethylhexane-diol, 1, 3, commonly called "612") applied to uncovered skin or impregnated in the clothing of persons exposed to bites of vector anophelines are useful.
      5. Sanitary improvements, such as filling and draining, to eliminate breeding places of vector anophelines should not be neglected. Larvicides (such as oil and Paris green) are now not commonly used where residual spraying is effective but may have usefulness under special conditions.
      6. Regular use of suppressive drugs in highly malarious areas has special value (see 9B8).
      7. Effective treatment of acute and chronic cases is an important adjunct to malaria control.
      8. Malaria control projects often profit from health education that teaches modern drug treatment and suppression, and practical measures of prevention.

[690   ]

B. Control of the infected individual, contacts and environment:

1. Report to local health authority: Obligatory case report, in non-endemic areas and in areas where the disease has been brought under control, desirably limited to authenticated cases (USA).

2. Isolation: None; patients desirably are protected at night by screens or bed nets in areas where vector anophelines are present.

3. Concurrent disinfection: A single concurrent residual spraying of the neighborhood may be useful, if a primary or relapsing case occurs in an area not under control, previously free from the disease and where potential vectors are active.

4. Terminal disinfection: None.

5. Quarantine: None.

6. Immunization: None.

7. Investigation of contacts and source of infection: Determine history of previous infection or of exposure to infection by anophelines or otherwise.

8. Specific treatment: (a) Acute cases in non-immune subjects: Chloroquine diphosphate or sulphate immediately, six hours later, and on each of next two days; or amodiaquine dihydrochloride dihydrate, immediately, and daily for next two days. (b) Acute cases, emergency treatment: Quinine hydrobromide or dihydrochloride, well diluted in normal saline, administered intravenously and slowly, and repeated after six hours if necessary; or mepacrine methane sulphonate intramuscularly, repeated after six hours if necessary. (c) Acute cases in semi-immune subjects: Chloroquine diphosphate or sulphate in a single dose; or amodiaquine dihydrochloride dihydrate, in a single dose.

Suppression: Chloroquine diphosphate or sulphate, 300 mgm. of base once weekly or 100 mgm. daily; or amodiaquine dihydrochloride dihydrate, 400 mgm. of base once weekly; or proguanil monohydrochloride, 100 mgm. daily, or for semi-immune subjects, 300 mgm. once weekly; or pyrimethamine, 25 mgm. once weekly.

Prevention of relapse: Primaquine diphosphate, 15 mgm. of base daily for 14 days; for those leaving endemic areas should be given at time suppressive drugs are discontinued. In acute attacks, should be given concurrently with standard chloroquine or amodiquine treatment.

C. Epidemic measures: A field survey to determine nature and extent of the hyperendemic or epidemic situation is the point of departure. Intensify residual spraying, treatment of acute cases, and use of suppressive drugs. Sometimes the breeding places of anophelines responsible for an epidemic can be eliminated.

D. International measures:

1. Routine disinsectization of aircraft coming from malarial areas. Special disinsectization of aircraft, ships and other vehicles not possessing a valid disinsectization certificate, prior to arrival in areas freed from anophelines generally or from certain species.

2. So far as practicable, rigid anti-mosquito sanitation should be maintained within the mosquito flight range of all ports and airports.

MEASLES

1. *Identification.* An acute highly communicable viral disease with a prodromal stage characterized by catarrhal symptoms and Koplik spots on the buccal mucous

membranes. A morbilliform rash appears on the third or fourth day affecting face, body and extremities, and sometimes ending in branny desquamation. Leukopenia is usual. Death from uncomplicated measles is rare; usually a result of secondary pneumonia, in children under 2 years old and the aggregate is less than 1 per 1,000 cases of measles. Synonyms: Rubeola, morbilli.

Virus and serological identification of measles is not practicable.

2. *Etiologic agent.* The virus of measles.

3. *Source and reservoir of infection.* Secretions of nose and throat of infected persons.

4. *Mode of transmission.* By droplet spread or direct contact with an infected person; indirectly through articles freshly soiled with secretions of nose and throat. One of the most readily transmitted of communicable diseases; in some instances probably airborne.

5. *Incubation period.* About 10 days from exposure to initial fever; 13 to 15 days until rash appears; uncommonly longer or shorter. Late inoculation in attempted passive protection may extend incubation to 21 days.

6. *Period of communicability.* During the period of catarrhal symptoms; usually about 9 days, from 4 days before to 5 days after rash appears.

7. *Susceptibility and resistance.* Practically all persons are susceptible; permanent acquired immunity is usual after attack. Babies born of mothers who have had the disease are ordinarily immune for the first few months of life.

8. *Occurrence.* Common in childhood; probably 80 to 90% of persons surviving to age 20 years have had measles; a few persons go through life without an attack. Endemic and relatively mild in large metropolitan communities, attaining epidemic proportions about every other year. In smaller communities, and in rural areas outbreaks tend to be wider spaced and somewhat more severe. In areas previously free, or in isolated settlements with long intervals between outbreaks, measles often affects large proportions of the population and fatality is much increased. Prevalent in all seasons except summer, but primarily spring.

9. *Methods of control:*

A. Preventive measures:

1. Education as to special danger of exposing young children to those exhibiting any fever or acute catarrhal symptoms, particularly during years and seasons of epidemic measles.

2. Encouragement by health departments and by private physicians of administration of immune serum globulin (gamma globulin) to infants and children under 3 years of age in families where measles occurs. This product carries no hazard of serum hepatitis.

B. Control of the infected individual, contacts, and environment:

1. Report to local health authority: Case report is compulsory in some jurisdictions, optional in others. Early reporting may secure better isolation and adequate care for the underprivileged child and provide opportunity for passive protection of contacts.

2. Isolation: Commonly 7 days from rash to protect the patient against added infection and to limit transfer of measles to susceptible contacts, especially those under 3 years of age.

3. Concurrent disinfection: All articles soiled with secretions of nose and throat.

4. Terminal disinfection: Thorough cleaning.

5. Quarantine: Impractical and of no value in large communities. Exclusion of

exposed susceptible school children and teachers from school and from all public gatherings until 14 days from last exposure may be justifiable in sparsely settled rural areas. If date of single exposure is reasonably certain, an exposed susceptible child may be allowed to attend school for the first 7 days of incubation. Quarantine of institutions, wards or dormitories for young children exposed to measles is of value; strict segregation of infants if measles occurs in an institution.

6. Immunization: Administration of gamma globulin, or serum of convalescent patients or of healthy adults who have had measles, to an exposed person within 3 days after first exposure to a known case of measles, will avert the attack in most instances, and almost certainly modify it. Such passive immunity has a maximum duration of 4 weeks. Given between 4 and 6 days after first exposure, there is reasonable chance of modifying severity of attack and the patient probably will acquire the usual lasting immunity to measles; given after the sixth day, little effect is expected. Dosage of gamma globulin, 0.1 cc. per pound of body weight, of convalescent or normal human serum, 20–30 cc. intramuscularly.

7. Investigation of contacts and source of infection: Search for exposed susceptible children under 3 years of age is profitable. Carriers are not known to occur.

8. Specific treatment: None. Complications should be treated with an appropriate antibiotic or with sulfadiazine.

C. Epidemic measures:

1. Daily examination of exposed children and known susceptible adult contacts, with record of body temperature. Susceptible persons exhibiting a rise of temperature of 0.5° C (0.9° F) or more should be isolated promptly pending diagnosis.

2. Schools should not be closed or classes discontinued; daily observation of children by physician or nurse should be provided and sick children promptly removed.

3. Administration of gamma globulin to all susceptibles has value in institutional outbreaks, in checking spread of infection and in reducing fatality; accept no new admissions and exclude visitors under 16 years of age, whether the measles outbreak is in the institution or in the community. Removal of patients during the pre-eruptive period may prevent an outbreak.

D. International measures: None.

MENINGITIS, MENINGOCOCCAL

1. *Identification.* An acute bacterial infection characterized by sudden onset with fever, intense headache, nausea and often vomiting, signs of meningeal irritation, and frequently a petechial rash. With modern chemotherapy a case fatality of 5–10% is usual, supplanting the former 40–50%; much variation under both endemic and epidemic conditions. Delirium and coma may appear early; occasional fulminating cases (Waterhouse-Friderichsen syndrome) exhibit signs of collapse and shock from onset. Meningococcemia without extension to the meninges is not uncommon and should be suspected in cases of otherwise unexplained acute febrile illness, particularly if associated with skin eruption and high leucocytosis. Synonyms: Cerebrospinal fever, meningococcemia.

[693]

Meningococci can usually be cultivated from the blood, the spinal fluid and the nasopharynx. Smears from petechiae may reveal the infectious agent.

2. *Etiologic agent.* Neisseria meningitidis (N. intracellularis), Meningococcus.
3. *Source and reservoir of infection.* Discharges from nose and throat of patients or carriers. Carrier prevalence of 25% or more may exist without occurrence of cases. During epidemic periods more than half of a military organization may be healthy carriers of the strain of meningococcus responsible for the epidemic.
4. *Mode of transmission.* By contact with infected persons, direct and by droplet spread. Indirect transmission through contact with articles freshly soiled with discharges from the respiratory tract of infected persons has little significance because the meningococcus is especially susceptible to chilling and drying.
5. *Incubation period.* Varies from 2 to 10 days, usually 7 days.
6. *Period of communicability.* Until meningococci are no longer present in discharges from nose and mouth of patients. Meningococci usually disappear from the nasopharynx within 24 hours after administration of appropriate chemotherapeutic or antibiotic agent.
7. *Susceptibility and resistance.* Susceptibility to the clinical disease is slight as evidenced by the low ratio of cases to carriers. Younger age groups are more susceptible, but the disease may occur at all ages. Type, degree and duration of immunity after attack are unknown; no generally accepted methods for inducing immunity artificially.
8. *Occurrence.* Endemic and epidemic; no limits in geographic distribution, but primarily a disease of temperate climates. Sporadic cases occur throughout the year in both urban and rural areas, with greatest incidence during winter and spring. The disease exhibits high incidence at irregular intervals, with epidemic waves usually lasting 2 to 3 years.
9. *Methods of control:*
   A. Preventive measures:
      1. Education as to personal cleanliness and necessity of avoiding direct contact and droplet infection.
      2. Prevention of overcrowding in living quarters, public transportation, working places and especially in barracks, camps and ships.
   B. Control of the infected individual, contacts and environment:
      1. Report to local health authority: Obligatory case report in most states and countries.
      2. Isolation: Until recovery from acute illness.
      3. Concurrent disinfection: Of discharges from the nose and throat or articles soiled therewith.
      4. Terminal disinfection: Cleaning.
      5. Quarantine: No complete quarantine; surveillance is profitable.
      6. Immunization: None.
      7. Investigation of contacts and source of infection: Impracticable.
      8. Specific treatment: Sulfadiazine by mouth in an initial loading dose and smaller amounts thereafter; if vomiting is severe, solution of sodium sulfadiazine intravenously after proper hydration. Penicillin in large doses or the tetracyclines may be used in addition.
   C. Epidemic measures:
      1. Increase the separation of individuals and the ventilation of living and sleeping

quarters for such groups of people as are especially exposed to infection because of occupation or some necessity of living condition.

2. If a community—civil, industrial, or military—is suffering unusual risk of infection and the general administration of chemoprophylaxis to exposed persons under medical supervision is practicable, sulfadiazine will lower markedly the carrier rate and limit the spread of the disease (0.5 gm. twice daily for children, 1 gm. twice daily for adults, both for 4 days).

D. International measures: None.

MONILIASIS

1. *Identification.* The clinical reaction to this fungus infection varies according to location of lesions, allergic state of the patient, and other factors. Common manifestations are thrush, vaginitis or vulvovaginitis, skin lesions of various kinds, bronchopulmonary disease, meningitis and rare generalized infection. Skin and local infections are benign; systemic infections highly fatal. Synonyms: Candidiasis, thrush.

   Identification is difficult and depends upon repeated microscopic demonstration of budding and mycelial forms in direct smears of lesions; fungi may be found in sputum from patients with tuberculosis, other lung infections or tumors.

2. *Etiologic agent.* Candida albicans (Monilia albicans).

3. *Source and reservoir of infection.* Skin and gastrointestinal tract of apparently normal persons.

4. *Mode of transmission.* Probably from auto-inoculation; rarely transmitted from man to man.

5. *Incubation period.* Unknown.

6. *Period of communicability.* Unknown.

7. *Susceptibility and resistance.* Inapparent infections are common. Most adults are hypersensitive to the fungus and possess antibodies. Second attacks are common; clinical manifestations are likely to follow general or local lowering of resistance. Infections of fingers is associated with maceration through long exposure to water (bartenders, housewives). Skin lesions are common in obese people with excessive perspiration in frictional folds, in diabetics and in lactating women. Thrush occurs in debilitated infants, and in older people with ill-fitting dentures. The fungus is frequently found in patients receiving wide spectrum antibiotic therapy.

8. *Occurrence.* World-wide and sporadic. Clinical infection of adults is more frequent than of children, excluding infants. More common in females than in males.

9. *Methods of control:*

   A. Preventive measures: None.

   B. Control of the infected individual, contacts and environment:

      1. Report to local health authority: Official report ordinarily not justifiable.
      2. Isolation: None.
      3. Concurrent disinfection: None.
      4. Terminal disinfection: None.
      5. Quarantine: None.
      6. Immunization: None.
      7. Investigation of contacts and source of infection: Not profitable.

[695   ]

8. Specific treatment: None. Infections developing during antibiotic therapy sometimes disappear when medication is discontinued.

C. Epidemic measures: Not applicable.

D. International measures: None.

MONONUCLEOSIS, INFECTIOUS

1. *Identification.* An acute infection with irregular clinical manifestations usually accompanied by characteristic lymphocytosis and heterophile antibodies in the blood. Three common clinical entities have been described having one or both characteristics: (1) Glandular fever (Pfeiffer)—enlargement of lymphatic glands and spleen without throat manifestations; common in children; (2) Infectious mononucleosis—continued fever with absent or inconsequential glandular swelling or throat symptoms; common in young adults; (3) Monocytic angina—a characteristic involvement of throat structures with or without lymphatic gland involvement; common in older children and young adults. A rash of variable morphology is an irregular occurrence and jaundice and meningoencephalitis are sometimes seen. The disease rarely ends fatally.

Laboratory aids to diagnosis are through examination of blood smears and test for heterophile antibodies. Serologic tests for syphilis may be temporarily positive.

2. *Etiologic agent.* Unknown.

3. *Source of infection.* Unknown.

4. *Mode of transmission.* Unknown.

5. *Incubation period.* Unknown; seemingly varies from 4 to 14 or more days.

6. *Period of communicability.* Undetermined.

7. *Susceptibility and resistance.* Susceptibility apparently general, but incidence greatest among children and young adults. Mild unrecognized cases probably occur. The degree of immunity conferred by an attack is undetermined.

8. *Occurrence.* Reported from many parts of the world, particularly Continental Europe, Great Britain, Australia and the United States. Observed as isolated cases and in epidemics and probably much more prevalent and more widely distributed than indicated by reported cases. Epidemics are most frequently recognized in schools and institutions for children; cases are commonly reported among medical students, nurses and hospital personnel.

9. *Methods of control:*

A. Preventive measures: None.

B. Control of the infected individual, contacts and environment:

1. Report to local health authority: Obligatory report of epidemics; no individual case report.
2. Isolation: None.
3. Concurrent disinfection: Of articles soiled with nose and throat discharges.
4. Terminal disinfection: None.
5. Quarantine: None.
6. Immunization: None.
7. Investigation of contacts and source of infection: For the individual case, of little value.
8. Specific treatment: None.

[696   ]

C. Epidemic measures: Field investigation of epidemics should be undertaken with the hope of adding to knowledge of the disease.

D. International measures: None.

MUMPS

1. *Identification.* An acute viral infection of sudden onset characterized by fever and by swelling and tenderness of one or more of the salivary glands, usually of the parotid, sometimes of the sublingual or submaxillary glands. Involvement of ovaries and testicles is more frequent in persons past puberty; involvement of the central nervous system is not infrequent early or late in the course of the disease. Orchitis and meningoencephalitis due to mumps virus may occur without involvement of a salivary gland. Death from mumps is exceedingly rare. Synonym: Infectious parotitis.

Hemagglutination and complement fixation tests are of value in recognizing atypical forms of infection. The virus may be found in the saliva, blood and cerebrospinal fluid.

2. *Etiologic agent.* The virus of mumps.

3. *Source and reservoir of infection.* Saliva of infected persons.

4. *Mode of transmission.* By droplet spread and by direct contact with an infected person or with articles freshly soiled with the saliva of such persons.

5. *Incubation period.* From 12 to 26 days, commonly 18 days.

6. *Period of communicability.* From about 6 days before distinctive symptoms and persisting as much as 9 days thereafter, but no longer than swelling of a salivary gland. Susceptibles may contract the disease through exposure to persons with inapparent infection.

7. *Susceptibility and resistance.* Susceptibility believed to be general. Second attacks are uncommon; immunity generally held to be life-long; develops after inapparent as well as clinical attack. An allergic tuberculin-like response occurs when inactivated virus is injected intradermally in persons previously infected.

8. *Occurrence.* Clinical disease is less frequent than with other common communicable diseases of childhood such as measles and chickenpox; many inapparent infections. Winter and spring are seasons of greatest prevalence; sporadic and epidemic except in large cities, where it is endemic. Outbreaks occur more frequently and are more serious in aggregations of young people, especially military.

9. *Methods of control:*

A. Preventive measures: None.

B. Control of the infected individual, contacts and environment:

1. Report to local health authority: Official report not ordinarily justifiable.

2. Isolation: Until swelling of salivary glands has subsided.

3. Concurrent disinfection: Of eating and drinking utensils; of articles soiled with secretions of nose and throat.

4. Terminal disinfection: None.

5. Quarantine: None.

6. Immunization: None.

7. Investigation of contacts and source of infection: Search for unreported or recent cases among associates in school or family.

8. Specific treatment: None.

[697]

C. Epidemic measures: No procedures in common use can be relied upon as a means of effective control of the disease or of epidemics. Active immunization by vaccines is experimental.

D. International measures: None.

PARATYPHOID FEVER

1. *Identification.* A generalized bacterial infection with continued fever and involvement of lymphoid tissues of intestines, enlargement of spleen, sometimes rose spots on trunk, usually diarrhea. Many mild infections give no more than a transient diarrhea. Fatality is much less than for typhoid fever.

   Paratyphoid bacilli may be found in feces, blood, and urine.

2. *Etiologic agent.* Salmonella paratyphi, S. schottmuelleri, S. hirschfeldi, Paratyphoid bacilli, A, B, and C.

3. *Source and reservoir of infection.* Feces and urine of patients or carriers, with temporary carriers often in frequent epidemics.

4. *Mode of transmission.* Direct or indirect contact with patient or carrier. Vehicles of indirect spread are food, especially milk, milk products and shellfish, usually contaminated by hands of a carrier or missed case. Under some conditions, flies are vectors. Few outbreaks are related to water supplies. Most large outbreaks in England in recent years have been associated with synthetic cream.

5. *Incubation period.* One to 10 days; somewhat longer for paratyphoid A than for B and C.

6. *Period of communicability.* As long as paratyphoid bacilli appear in excreta; usually from appearance of prodromal symptoms, throughout illness and for varying periods after recovery.

7. *Susceptibility and resistance.* Susceptibility is general. Permanent immunity usually follows recovery. The degree of resistance conferred by typhoid vaccine is uncertain.

8. *Occurrence.* Incidence in United States has fallen with that of typhoid fever. Occurs sporadically or in limited outbreaks due to contact or to contaminated food, milk or water. Probably more common than reports suggest due to large number of unrecognized infections. Paratyphoid A infection is rare in United States, but common in Europe; paratyphoid B is common in the United States, often as a transient diarrhea of undetermined etiology; both are still frequent in countries where sanitation is defective. Paratyphoid C infection is extremely rare in United States but common in Eastern Europe and Asia.

9. *Methods of control:*
   A. Preventive measures:
      1. The preventive measures applicable to paratyphoid fever are those listed under Typhoid Fever.
   B. Control of the infected individual, contacts and environment:
      1. Report to local health authority: Obligatory case report in most states and countries, both suspect and confirmed infections.
      2. Items 2–8 of Typhoid Fever, also apply to paratyphoid fever. Therapeutic results from chloramphenicol are not striking.
   C. Epidemic measures:
      1. The procedures are those of typhoid fever.
   D. International measures: Inoculation of international travellers with triple ty-

phoid vaccine (TAB, typhoid, paratyphoid A, paratyphoid B) is advisable for travel in all areas except the United States, Canada, Great Britain and Northwest Europe, if not protected through previous attack.

PEDICULOSIS

1. *Identification.* Infestation with adult lice, larvae or nits, of the scalp, of the hairy parts of the body, or of clothing, especially along the seams of inner surfaces. Synonym: Lousiness.
2. *Infesting agents.* Pediculus humanus, head louse or body louse, and Phthirus pubis, crab louse.
3. *Source of infestation.* Infested persons or their personal belongings, particularly body clothing; infested beds.
4. *Mode of transmission.* Direct contact with an infested person and indirectly by contact with clothing and headgear of such persons.
5. *Incubation period.* Under optimum conditions, the eggs hatch in a week, and sexual maturity is reached in approximately 2 weeks.
6. *Period of communicability.* While lice remain alive on the infested person or in his clothing, and until eggs (nits) in hair and clothing have been destroyed.
7. *Susceptibility and resistance.* Any person may become lousy under suitable conditions of exposure. Repeated infestations often result in dermal hypersensitivity.
8. *Occurrence.* Cosmopolitan. The head louse is common in outbreaks among school children.
9. *Methods of control:*
   A. Preventive measures:
      1. Direct inspection of the heads and, when necessary, of the body and clothing where lousiness is found in groups of children or adults, particularly of children in schools, institutions and camp groups.
      2. Education in the value of using hot water and soap to maintain cleanliness, and laundering of clothing to destroy nits and lice.
      3. Provision of residual insecticide for freeing persons and clothing of lice. (See 9B8.)
   B. Control of the infested individual, contacts and environment:
      1. Report to local health authority: Official report not ordinarily justifiable; school authorities should be informed.
      2. Isolation: Not necessary after application of effective insecticide.
      3. Concurrent disinfestation: Of other members of family or associated group.
      4. Terminal disinfestation: None.
      5. Quarantine: None.
      6. Immunization: Does not apply.
      7. Investigation of contacts and source of infestation: Examination of household and other close personal contacts.
      8. Specific treatment: 10% DDT dusting powder for body and head lice; dust clothing, particularly along seams, and hairs; cover head with towel or cap for several hours; comb hair with fine tooth comb; repeat dusting in one week without washing hair or clothing in the interim. For crab lice, dust hairy parts of body and bathe after 12 to 24 hours; repeat treatment in one week; continue treatment at weekly intervals until lice or nits are no longer present. In parts of Korea and Egypt lice are known to have become DDT-resistant; gamma

isomer of benzene hexachloride (lindane) may then be substituted as a dusting powder.

C. Epidemic measures: Mass treatment as recommended in 9B8.

D. International measures: None.

PEMPHIGUS NEONATORUM

1. *Identification.* An acute vesicular or bullous eruption of the skin of newborn infants, particularly in nurseries. Onset is commonly between the 4th and 10th day of life as vesicles or bullae, usually first seen on the lower abdomen but spreading to the skin of any part of the body. Vesicles rupture, thin crusts form, and new lesions develop, tending to spread peripherally and often coalescing. Constitutional symptoms are unusual but if lesions are widespread, fever, diarrhea and a complicating pneumonia, meningitis or bacteremia may occur. Death sometimes follows. Synonym: Impetigo of the newborn.

2. *Etiologic agent.* Probably staphylococci, in frequent association with streptococci.

3. *Source and reservoir of infection.* Infected infants, attendants or visitors.

4. *Mode of transmission.* By direct contact with the skin of infected infants or with articles freshly contaminated with discharges from lesions; also by contact with other individuals whose skin is infected or contaminated with the infectious agents.

5. *Incubation period.* 2 to 5 days.

6. *Period of communicability.* Until the lesions have healed; usually about 1 or 2 weeks.

7. *Susceptibility and resistance.* Susceptibility of newborn infants is general. Immunity does not follow an attack.

8. *Occurrence.* Chiefly in nurseries for the newborn, particularly in association with laxness in nursing technics and much handling of infants. Incidence highest in countries such as the United States, where percentage of deliveries in hospitals is high and newborn infants are housed in nurseries. Occurs in all seasons of the year.

9. *Methods of control:*

   A. Preventive measures: Cleanliness is the most important preventive measure. The infant should be handled as little as possible. Excess vernix should be wiped gently from the scalp and face, and no water or oil bath given until ready for discharge. Examination by physicians should be at a minimum. Infants should be weighed not more than twice a week and temperature taken not oftener than once a day. Nurses and attendants should wash their hands with soap and water after diapering and before feeding an infant; those with infections of the skin should be excluded from care of infants. Visitors should not be permitted in nurseries. Scrupulous attention must be given to aseptic precautions, and to bedding, furnishings, gowns and masks of attendants.

   B. Control of the infected individual, contacts and environment:

   1. Report to local health authority: Obligatory report of epidemics; no individual case report. Any case in a hospital or other nursery is to be interpreted as a potential epidemic. Willful attempt to delay control measures by labelling cases as dermatitis or folliculitis is a common source of trouble.

   2. Isolation: Prompt isolation of infected infants.

   3. Concurrent disinfection: Collect and burn dressings; launder separately bedding and clothing of patients.

[700]

4. Terminal disinfection: Wash nursery, cribs and other furniture with soap and water after all infants have been discharged; instruments and basins boiled, and mattresses sterilized.

5. Quarantine: Of all exposed newborn infants.

6. Immunization: None.

7. Investigation of contacts and source of infection: Examine nurses and attendants for presence of skin lesions.

8. Specific treatment: Ammoniated mercury ointment or gentian violet solution or penicillin ointment. If lesions are widespread, use penicillin intramuscularly. ACTH or cortisone gives temporary relief in severe cases.

C. Epidemic measures:

1. If an outbreak (more than 1 case) occurs in a nursery, isolate all patients and quarantine contacts until all have been discharged. Permit no new admissions to quarantined nursery.

2. Exclude nurses and attendants with skin infections.

3. Investigate adequacy of nursing procedures; emphasize cleanliness and personal hygiene.

4. Nursing staffs of isolation and quarantined nurseries should not work in nurseries housing normal newborn infants.

D. International measures: None.

PERTUSSIS

1. *Identification.* An acute bacterial infection involving trachea, bronchi and bronchioles, and characterized by a typical cough, usually of one to two months duration. The initial catarrhal stage has an insidious onset with irritating cough, which gradually becomes paroxysmal, usually within one to two weeks. Paroxysms are characterized by a repeated series of violent coughs, each series having many coughs without intervening inhalation and followed by characteristic crowing or high pitched inspiratory whoop; frequently ends with vomiting of clear, tenacious mucus. Young infants and adults often do not have the typical paroxysm. An absolute lymphocytosis is usually present. The overall case fatality is low, less than 0.5%, but approximately 85% of deaths and 15% of cases are among children aged less than 2 years. Synonym: Whooping cough.

The etiologic agent is readily recovered during catarrhal and early paroxysmal stages by nasopharyngeal swab. Bacteriological characteristics differentiate infections with Hemophilus parapertussis which is immunologically distinct from H. pertussis.

2. *Etiologic agent.* Hemophilus pertussis. Pertussis bacillus.

3. *Source and reservoir of infection.* Discharges from the laryngeal and bronchial mucous membranes of infected persons.

4. *Mode of transmission.* By direct contact with an infected person, by droplet spread or indirectly by contact with articles freshly soiled with discharges of such persons.

5. *Incubation period.* Commonly 7 days, almost uniformly within 10 days, and not exceeding 21 days.

6. *Period of communicability.* Particularly communicable in early catarrhal stage before paroxysmal cough confirms provisional clinical diagnosis. After paroxysms are established communicability gradually decreases and becomes negligible for

ordinary non-familial contacts in about 3 weeks even though spasmodic cough with whoop may persist. For control purposes, the communicable stage is considered to extend from 7 days after exposure to 3 weeks after onset of typical paroxysms.

7. *Susceptibility and resistance.* Susceptibility is general; no good evidence of temporary passive immunity in young infants born of immune mothers. Pertussis is predominantly a childhood disease, the incidence being highest under seven years of age and mortality highest in infants, particularly those under six months. One attack confers a definite and prolonged immunity but second attacks occasionally occur, particularly in exposed adults. Fatality is higher in females than males at all ages. Both active and passive artificial immunity may be induced by appropriate means.

8. *Occurrence.* A frequent and common disease among children everywhere regardless of race, climate, or geographic location. In large communities the incidence is generally higher in late winter and early spring; in smaller communities the seasonal incidence is variable.

9. *Methods of control:*
   A. Preventive measures:
      1. General immunization of all susceptible pre-school children is an effective procedure for control of pertussis. Plain or alum adjuvant vaccines may be used either alone or in combination with diphtheria and tetanus toxoids. Three doses of an alum adjuvant vaccine mixed with diphtheria and generally tetanus toxoid, administered at four-week intervals, beginning at 2–6 months of age, is commonly and effectively used in the U. S. A. for simultaneous immunization against all three diseases. In general, routine immunization can be started at 3–4 months of age. The need for subsequent reinforcing doses of pertussis vaccine is not definitely established but when primary immunization is properly carried out in infancy, a single reinforcing dose is generally advised at 1–2 and again at 4–5 years of age; in addition, under circumstances of known direct exposure through familial contact. Infants living in institutions and in households with other susceptible children, particularly during the months when pertussis is prevalent in the community, should have active immunization started by the time they are 2 months of age.
      2. Educational measures to inform the public and particularly parents of infants of the dangers of pertussis and of the advantages of immunization in infancy.
   B. Control of the infected individual, contacts and environment:
      1. Report to local health authority: Case report obligatory in most states and countries.
      2. Isolation: Separation of the patient from susceptible children and exclusion of the patient from school and public places for the recognized period of communicability. Isolation of children over 2 years of age is often impracticable; even for those under 2, should not be insisted upon at the expense of fresh air in the open if weather permits.
      3. Concurrent disinfection: Discharges from the nose and throat articles soiled therewith.
      4. Terminal disinfection: Thorough cleaning.
      5. Quarantine: Limited to exclusion of non-immune children from school and public gatherings for 14 days after last exposure to a household or similar case;

may be omitted if exposed non-immune children are seen by a physician or nurse on arrival at school each day for 14 days after last exposure. Particularly important to protect children under 3 years against contact with known or suspected whooping cough.

6. Immunization: Brief and relative passive immunity may be conveyed to young children by administration of appropriate amounts of hyperimmune or convalescent serum. The risk of homologous serum jaundice from use of human serum must be kept in mind. Artificial active immunization after effective exposure is of no proven value.

7. Investigation of contacts and source of infection: Carriers in the exact sense of the term are not known; search for missed and atypical cases among contacts.

8. Specific treatment: None; convalescent serum, serum from immunized donors, and similar agents appear to help when given early in severe cases. The tetracyclines and probably chloramphenicol tend to abort the infection, but not the symptoms, although minor amelioration may follow.

C. Epidemic measures: A search for unrecognized and unreported cases is of value to protect young children from exposure and to assure adequate medical care for those exposed, especially infants. The comparatively high mortality in young infants justifies intensive effort toward their protection.

D. International measures:
  1. Active immunization of susceptible infants and young children travelling to other countries.

PLAGUE

1. *Identification.* A severe and highly fatal disease, characterized by rapid clinical course with high fever, progressive heart failure and nervous symptoms such as loss of coordinating power over voluntary muscles, delirium or coma. Conjunctival injection is common, skin hemorrhages or pustular eruptions may occur. Three clinical forms are recognized: a) The bubonic type is most common; acutely inflamed and painful swellings of lymph nodes draining the site of original inoculation. The infection often progresses to septicemia with localization in any part of the body. Secondary terminal pneumonia is an important complication; b) Primary septicemia plague is rare and probably represents a form of bubonic plague in which the bubo is obscure; c) Primary pneumonic plague is ordinarily uncommon but occurs in localized and sometimes devastating outbreaks among closely associated groups during epidemics of bubonic plague. Bubonic plague has a fatality of 25 to 50% or greater when untreated, primary pneumonic and septicemic forms are usually fatal. Modern methods of therapy reduce these rates, especially for bubonic plague.

Diagnosis is confirmed by demonstrating the infectious agent in fluid aspirated from buboes, in blood, or in sputum in severe or pneumonic forms.

2. *Etiologic agent.* Pasteurella pestis, plague bacillus.

3. *Source and reservoir of infection.* The source of bubonic infection is the flea; in pneumonic plague, exhaled droplets and sputum of patients. The reservoir of plague, and the source of flea infection, is a large series of wild rodents infected in nature in many parts of the world (sylvatic plague or wild rodent plague). The infection is apt to pass over to domestic rodents in large cities, particularly in seaports (urban plague).

[703]

4. *Mode of transmission.* Bubonic plague results from the bite of the infected rat flea, Xenopsylla cheopis and certain other species. Pneumonic plague is spread by person-to-person contact from patients with primary pneumonic plague or from patients with bubonic plague who develop terminal plague pneumonia. Accidental infections may occur among laboratory workers.

5. *Incubation period.* From 2 to 6 days in bubonic plague; 3–4 days in pneumonic plague; may be shorter, rarely longer.

6. *Period of communicability.* Bubonic plague is not directly communicable from person to person except through terminal plague pneumonia. Fleas remain infective for life, days or weeks, or may clear themselves of the infection. Pneumonic plague may become intensely communicable under climatic or social conditions which lead to overcrowding in unsanitary dwellings.

7. *Susceptibility and resistance.* Susceptibility is general. Occasionally bubonic infection may remain localized and of short duration, pestis minor. Immunity after recovery is temporary and relative. Active immunization with a vaccine of killed bacteria may confer considerable protection for some months when administered in 2 or 3 doses at weekly intervals; repeated stimulating injections are necessary for continued protection. Vaccines prepared with living avirulent strains may confer satisfactory immunity in one dose, repeated once yearly.

8. *Occurrence.* Sylvatic plague exists in the western third of the United States and in large areas in South America, in Central and South Africa, and in the Near East with the center in Iranian Kurdistan. The foci in southeast Russia and in Central Asia are possibly quiescent. The human disease in the United States is confined to rare instances of exposure to wild rodents. Urban plague has been largely controlled throughout most of the world but rural bubonic plague of rat origin continues as a serious health problem in some countries, particularly India, Burma, Indonesia (Java) and China. The threat of re-established urban plague thus continues.

9. *Methods of control:*
   A. Preventive measures:
      1. Periodic surveys in endemic and in potential epidemic areas to determine the prevalence of rats and rat fleas; suppression of rats by poisoning or trapping in urban areas. Continuing inspection and survey of wild rodents and their ectoparasites in areas of sylvatic plague. In areas where plague is present or threatening, systematic search for evidence of infection in rodents and their fleas by pooling methods.
      2. Rat-proofing of buildings and reduction of breeding places and harborages, particularly on docks and in warehouses.
      3. Rat control on ships by rat-proofing or periodic fumigation, combined when necessary with destruction of rats and their fleas in vessels and cargoes arriving from plague localities.
   B. Control of the infected individual, contacts and environment:
      1. Report to local health authority: Case report of suspect and confirmed cases universally required by international regulation.
      2. Isolation: Hospitalize all patients if practical; reasonable aseptic precautions for patients with bubonic plague, and strict isolation for primary pneumonic plague or patients developing plague pneumonia.
      3. Concurrent disinfection: Sputum and purulent discharges, and articles soiled therewith; urine and feces of patients.

4. Terminal disinfection: Thorough cleaning; bodies of persons dying of plague should be handled with strict aseptic precautions.

5. Quarantine: Contacts of bubonic plague, disinfestation with insecticide powder such as 5–10% DDT in talc or pyrophyllite and surveillance for 6 days; contacts of pneumonic plague, quarantine for 6 days with close surveillance for developing illness; dust with insecticide powder.

6. Immunization: None; the management of contacts is by chemoprophylaxis. For all contacts of pneumonic plague, sulfadiazine, 3 gms daily for 6 days; and similarly for contacts of bubonic plague if risk is judged appreciable.

7. Investigation of contacts and source of infection: Search for infected rodents and fleas or exposure to preceding cases of plague pneumonia or pneumonic plague.

   Focal attack on fleas should precede anti-rat measures, using an appropriate insecticide powder with residual effect such as 10 per cent DDT in talc or pyrophyllite. Dust rat runs and rat harborages in known or suspected focal areas. Disinfect by dusting or insecticide spray the houses, outhouses and household furnishings in the same areas. Dust the persons and clothing of immediate contacts and all other residents in the immediate vicinity. Supplemental suppression of rat populations by poisoning or trapping then follows.

8. Specific treatment: Streptomycin and the broad spectrum antibiotics are highly effective for all forms of plague when used early, results good even in pneumonic plague if therapy is begun within 24 hours of onset, poor later. Recurrence of fever during streptomycin therapy may indicate secondary pneumonia caused by gram positive cocci; in such cases, penicillin should be used with continued streptomycin; penicillin not effective against plague itself. Sulfadiazine should be used if antibiotics are not available; frequently used to continue treatment begun with antibiotics. These drugs are also effective in protection of contacts, sulfadiazine being most used.

C. Epidemic measures:

1. Investigate all deaths, with autopsy and laboratory examinations when indicated. Develop case-finding facilities. Establish the best possible provision for diagnosis and treatment. Alert all existing medical facilities toward immediate reporting and toward utilization of diagnostic and therapy services. Provide adequate laboratory services, and supplies of antibiotics.

2. Institute intensive flea control in expanding circles from known focal areas.

3. Supplemental rat destruction within affected areas.

4. Prophylactic administration of appropriate antibiotics or sulfadiazine to all medical, nursing and public health personnel exposed to risk; surveillance to detect disease in its earliest stages.

5. Personal protection of field workers aginst fleas by weekly dusting of underclothing with insecticide powder or daily use of insect repellents.

D. International measures:

1. Telegraphic notification of WHO and adjacent countries by governments of the existence of an epidemic of plague.

2. Measures applicable to ships, aircraft and land transport arriving from plague areas are specified in International Sanitary Regulations (WHO Techn. Rep. Ser. No. 41, Geneva, 1951).

3. All ships should be periodically deratized, or be permanently kept in such condition that rat populations are reduced to a minimum.

[705]

4. Rat-proofing of buildings of ports and airports; application of appropriate insecticide with residual effect every 6 months; deratization with effective rodenticide.

5. International travellers: No country requires immunization against plague as a requisite for entry. Because of the short duration of protection, the recommendation in the face of an existing epidemic or anticipated unusual exposure, is for immunization on arrival.

PLEURODYNIA

1. *Identification.* An acute infectious disease characterized by sudden onset of severe paroxysmal pain commonly localized at the costodiaphragmatic border and accompanied by intermittent fever, headache, anorexia, and malaise. Duration one to three days; remissions frequent. A nonfatal illness usually recognized in localized epidemics. Synonyms: Epidemic pleurodynia, Bornholm disease, epidemic myalgia, Devil's grippe.

   Since Coxsackie group B viruses have been repeatedly implicated as causative agents, diagnosis may be aided by isolation from feces and by demonstrating a rise in titer of type-specific neutralizing antibodies in blood serums of early and late illness. Differential count of blood leucocytes is usually normal.

2. *Etiologic agent.* Various Coxsackie Group B viruses have been implicated. Immunologically distinct Types 1 and 3 have repeatedly been associated with the illness, and other types may occur.

3. *Source and reservoir of infection.* Coxsackie group B viruses types 1 and 3 frequently have been found in feces and also in throat discharges of persons ill with epidemic pleurodynia. These viruses have been found less frequently in well persons in an epidemic area; occasionally, in persons with illnesses not typical of pleurodynia.

4. *Mode of transmission.* Probably contact with an infected person or with articles freshly soiled with infective material. Group B viruses have been found in sewage, on flies and mosquitoes; the relation to production of human disease is not clear.

5. *Incubation period.* 3 to 5 days is usual.

6. *Period of communicability.* Unknown, but certainly during the acute stage of the disease.

7. *Susceptibility and resistance.* Susceptibility is likely general, and presumably a type-specific immunity results from infection.

8. *Occurrence.* The disease is not common, usually occurs in epidemics, with outbreaks reported in Europe, England, Australia, New Zealand, and North America. A summer and early autumn disease, occurring in all age groups but most commonly manifest in children and young adults. Multiple cases frequently occur in a household.

9. *Methods of control:*

   A. Preventive measures: None.

   B. Control of the infected individual, contacts, and environment:

      1. Report to local health authority: Obligatory report of epidemics; no individual case report.

      2. Isolation: None.

[706]

3. Concurrent disinfection: Prompt and safe disposal of nose and throat discharges and of feces. Articles soiled therewith should be disinfected.
4. Terminal disinfection: None.
5. Quarantine: None.
6. Active immunization: None.
7. Investigation of contacts and source of infection: Of no practical value.
8. Specific treatment: None.

C. Epidemic measures:
1. General notice to physicians of the epidemic occurrence of the disease and the necessity for differential diagnosis of illness which might mistakenly be considered a medical or surgical emergency.

D. International measures: None.

THE PNEUMONIAS

A. Pneumococcal—Acute Lobar Pneumonia

1. *Identification.* An acute bacterial infection characterized by sudden onset with chill followed by fever, often pain in the chest, usually a productive cough, dyspnea, and leucocytosis. Roentgen-ray examination may disclose pulmonary lesions prior to other evidence of consolidation. Not infrequently pneumococcal pneumonia is bronchial rather than lobar, especially in children, with vomiting and convulsions often the first manifestations. Pneumococcal pneumonia remains an important cause of death, generally among acute infections. Case fatality is greatly reduced by antibiotic and chemotherapy; rates formerly were 20–40% for hospital patients, but now are ordinarily a small fraction of those figures; much variation according to serologic type of pneumococcus and age of patient, being highest among infants and the aged.

Laboratory confirmation is by bacteriological examination of sputum or discharges of the respiratory tract. A rise in antibody titer between acute-phase and convalescent-phase serums is useful in problem cases, and culture of the blood in severe infections.

2. *Etiologic agent.* Diplococcus pneumoniae. Pneumococci Types I to XXXII account for about 95% of cases; the remainder are due to rarely recognized types.

3. *Source and reservoir of infection.* Respiratory tract secretions of patients and carriers. Pneumococci may be found in the upper respiratory tract of healthy members of most communities throughout the world.

4. *Mode of transmission.* By droplet spread, by direct contact with patients or carriers, or indirectly through articles freshly soiled with discharges of nose and throat of such persons. Transmission by air-borne particles may be possible but has not been established as important. Person-to-person transmission of the pneumococcus is common, but secondary cases in contacts and attendants are infrequent.

5. *Incubation period.* Not well determined; believed to be 1 to 3 days.

6. *Period of communicability.* Unknown; presumably until the discharges of mouth and nose no longer carry the infectious agent in appreciable numbers or in virulent form. Penicillin will eliminate the pneumococcus from most patients within 3 days.

7. *Susceptibility and resistance.* Resistance is generally high but may be lowered by wet, cold, and exposure, and apparently under certain conditions by physical

[707]

and mental fatigue and by alcoholism. Inapparent infection is common, particularly with Type 3 pneumococci and strains of higher types. Immunity to the homologous type of pneumococcus usually follows an attack, may last for months or years, and is highly specific. Active immunization against specific types is possible but rarely practical.

8. *Occurrence.* Common; affecting a large proportion of the population at one time or other between adolescence and old age. No race or color and neither sex is exempt from the disease. More prevalent in industrial cities and lower economic groups. Occurs in all climates and seasons, most often in winter and spring in temperate zones, and in regions where cold, windy, changeable, and inclement weather prevails. Usually sporadic in the United States, but epidemics occur in institutions and in barracks; persistent occurrence of epidemics has been described in South African mines. A rising incidence is commonly associated with influenza epidemics.

9. *Methods of control:*
   A. Preventive measures:
      1. Whenever practicable and particularly in institutions, barracks, and on shipboard, crowding in living and sleeping places should be avoided. General resistance should be conserved by good food, fresh air, sufficient sleep, temperance in the use of alcoholic beverages, and other hygienic measures.
      2. Chemoprophylaxis with sulfonamide or antibiotic drugs is feasible for closed population groups in time of epidemics, but has not been adequately evaluated.
      3. Active immunization with bacterial vaccines or polysaccharides of prevailing types of pneumococci may be effective for the control of epidemics in limited populations such as mine workers and military units.
   B. Control of the infected individual, contacts, and environment:
      1. Report to local health authority: Obligatory report of epidemics; no individual case report. Reported deaths are a better index of frequency of the disease.
      2. Isolation: None.
      3. Concurrent disinfection: Of discharges from nose and throat.
      4. Terminal disinfection: Thorough cleaning and airing.
      5. Quarantine: None.
      6. Immunization: None.
      7. Investigation of contacts and source of infection: Of no practical value.
      8. Specific treatment: Penicillin intramuscularly; recent reports indicate that oral penicillin G is effective. The tetracycline antibiotics produce comparable results, in event of penicillin sensitivity or delayed response to penicillin. Sulfonamide drugs and erythromycin are usually effective.
   C. Epidemic measures:
      1. Applicable only in outbreaks in institutions or in other limited or closed population groups. General hygienic measures may be supported by immunization against prevailing types of pneumococci or by chemoprophylaxis with sulfonamides or antibiotics.
   D. International measures: None.

B. BACTERIAL PNEUMONIA, OTHER THAN PNEUMOCOCCAL

1. *Identification.* An acute febrile disease with pulmonary involvement evidenced by symptoms, physical signs, or Roentgen-ray examination. Often occurs in associa-

tion with other infections of the respiratory tract, particularly epidemic influenza. Case fatality with adequate treatment is low but appreciable, and variable according to infectious agent and age of the patient.

Appropriate bacteriologic examination of sputum, nasopharyngeal swabs and blood aid materially in diagnosis.

2. *Etiologic agents.* Various pathogenic bacteria of the mouth, nose, and throat, as Streptococcus pyogenes or Group A hemolytic streptococci, Staphylococcus aureus, Klebsiella pneumoniae (Friedlander's bacillus) and Hemophilus influenzae.

3. *Source and reservoir of infection.* Discharges from mouth and nose of patients and carriers.

4. *Mode of transmission.* By droplet spread, by direct contact with patient or carrier or indirectly through articles freshly soiled with discharges of nose or throat of such persons.

5. *Incubation period.* Variable, usually short, 1 to 3 days.

6. *Period of communicability.* Unknown; probably while the infectious agent is present in discharges of nose and throat of patients. For many of the agents involved, antibiotic therapy greatly decreases the period of communicability.

7. *Susceptibility and resistance.* Susceptibility appears to be low grade; highest in infants and young children, and in the aged. Immunity varies with the infecting organism and is probably minimal except for type-specific immunity to Group A streptococci. Immunization procedures are not feasible.

8. *Occurrence.* Worldwide in distribution and a frequent disease in infancy and old age, and in winter months in temperate climates. No racial selectivity. Usually sporadic, but epidemics occur in association with influenza, measles or other respiratory infection.

9. *Methods of control:*
   A. Preventive measures:
      1. Good personal hygiene; avoid crowding in institutions and hospitals.
      2. Immunization against influenza and chemoprophylaxis of streptococcal infections may be applied to limited or general populations.
   B. Control of the infected individual, contacts, and environment:
      1. Report to local health authority: Obligatory report of epidemics; no individual case report. Identification of a preceding respiratory infection is of public health significance.
      2. Isolation: None.
      3. Concurrent disinfection: Of discharges from mouth and nose and of articles soiled therewith.
      4. Terminal disinfection: Thorough cleaning and airing.
      5. Quarantine: None.
      6. Immunization: None.
      7. Investigation of contacts and source of infection: Of no practical value.
      8. Specific treatment: Streptococcal: Same as pneumococcal pneumonia. Staphylococcal: Procaine penicillin; if organism proves resistant, tetracycline antibiotics as in pneumococcal pneumonia; sensitivity tests with the organism isolated may aid in selecting the most suitable antibiotic. H. influenzae: The tetracyclines or chloramphenicol are all effective; combined sulfadiazine-streptomycin is also used. K. pneumoniae: (Friedlander's) Streptomycin initially, then the tetracyclines or chloramphenicol after the acute phase.

[709   ]

C. Epidemic measures:

    1. Applicable only in outbreaks in institutions or in other limited or closed population groups when associated with influenza, measles or other respiratory infection. Active immunization against influenza and passive immunization of infants and children against measles may be employed. Chemoprophylaxis may be effective but has not been adequately evaluated.

D. International measures: None.

C. Primary Atypical Pneumonia (Virus Pneumonia)

1. *Indentification.* An acute respiratory infection characterized by gradual and insidious onset, constitutional symptoms of chilliness, feverishness, headache, malaise and fatigue, and respiratory symptoms of cough and sputum. Physical signs in the lungs are initially minimal but develop later. Early patchy infiltration demonstrable by roentgenographic examination of chest, is often more extensive than clinical findings suggest. Count and distribution of leucocytes usually normal. Duration of illness averages about a week and complications are infrequent; case fatality is about 1 per 1,000.

    Development of cold hemagglutinins during convalescence or of agglutinins for streptococcus MG, or both, confirms diagnosis in one-half to two-thirds of cases.

    Differentiation required from psittacosis, influenza, Q fever, and a number of other infections with similar clinical reaction.

2. *Etiologic agent.* Most cases apparently due to a virus or viruses, not yet isolated or characterized or given specific name.

3. *Source and reservoir of infection.* Probably discharges from mouth and nose of patients, and of persons with mild, unrecognized infections.

4. *Mode of transmission.* By intimate contact with a patient or with articles freshly soiled with discharges of nose and throat of such person.

5. *Incubation period.* Believed to be 7 to 21 days, commonly 12.

6. *Period of communicability.* Unknown; presumably during late incubation and throughout febrile illness.

7. *Susceptibility and resistance.* The low incidence in general populations and low attack rate among contacts suggest a relatively high resistance. Most infected persons suffer no more than mild respiratory illness with no pneumonia. Degree and duration of immunity after attack are unknown; second attacks are rare. No available immunization.

8. *Occurrence.* World-wide distribution, as a sporadic, endemic, and occasionally epidemic disease especially in institutions and military populations. No reliable attack rates for civilian populations; rates of 10 per 1000 per annum are recorded among military populations. Incidence greatest during winter months in temperate zones, with much variation from year to year and in different geographic areas. No selectivity for race or sex. Occurs at all ages, but recognized disease is more frequent among adolescents and young adults.

9. *Methods of control:*

    A. Preventive measures:

        1. When possible, crowding in living and sleeping quarters should be avoided, especially in institutions, in barracks, and on shipboard. General resistance should be maintained by adequate food, sufficient sleep, fresh air, and good personal hygiene.

[**710**   ]

B. Control of the infected individual, contacts, and environment:
  1. Report to local health authority: Obligatory report of epidemics; no individual case report.
  2. Isolation: None.
  3. Concurrent disinfection: Of discharges from nose and throat.
  4. Terminal disinfection: Thorough cleaning and airing.
  5. Quarantine: None.
  6. Immunization: None.
  7. Investigation of contacts and source of infection: Of no practical value.
  8. Specific treatment: Beneficial results in individual cases have been reported through use of tetracycline antibiotics. Symptomatic and supportive treatment is effective in most instances.
C. Epidemic measures:
  No certainly effective measures for control are available. Isolation precautions in epidemic situations may be helpful.
D. International measures: None.

POLIOMYELITIS

1. *Identification.* An acute illness, usually febrile, varying in early symptomatology, but usually with headache and almost always a characteristic stiffness of neck and spine and tightness of hamstring muscles, often justifying an examination of spinal fluid. In about half such cases a lower neurone paralysis develops within the first few days of illness, with a marked tendency for spontaneous improvement after reaching its height. If the patient is first seen after the acute stage has passed, diagnosis depends upon detection of a flaccid paralysis irregularly involving various muscles or muscle groups. Presumptive diagnosis in nonparalytic cases depends upon detection of clinical manifestations compatible with the illness and demonstration of moderate increase in cells or protein in the spinal fluid. A form of illness presumptively poliomyelitis (abortive) but with only vague symptoms and without signs referable to the central nervous system, occurs during epidemics. Many inapparent infections. Fatality rates vary from 4 to 15%, for bulbar poliomyelitis from 5 to 60%. Synonym: Infantile paralysis.

   Virus may be isolated from feces or throat secretions; rising titer of antibodies to one type of virus can be demonstrated by complement fixation or neutralization test; microscopic and chemical examination of spinal fluid.
2. *Etiologic agent.* Poliomyelitis viruses, Types 1, 2 and 3, readily distinguished immunologically although having minor, common antigenic components.
3. *Source of infection.* Pharyngeal secretions and feces of infected persons, frequently those not suffering from clinically recognizable disease. Carriers are common.
4. *Mode of transmission.* By direct contact and droplet spread through close association with infected persons. Milk has been a vehicle in a few outbreaks. Flies and sewage have been found contaminated with virus, but no reliable evidence incriminates insects, water, food other than milk, or sewage in transmission of the infection.
5. *Incubation period.* From 7 to 21 days, commonly 12.
6. *Period of communicability.* Greatest communicability is apparently in late incubation and first few days of acute illness, virus usually being present in throat and feces; persists in feces for 3 to 6 weeks or more.

[711]

7. *Susceptibility and resistance.* Susceptibility to infection is general, but few develop paralytic disease. Type specific immunity is acquired by infection, whether clinically apparent or inapparent, and probably is of long duration; second attacks are rare and may be due to infection by virus of another type. Infants born of immune mothers possess passive immunity, also to be acquired through injection of gamma globulin or specific immune serum.

8. *Occurrence.* Infection prevails throughout most of the world; occurs both sporadically and in epidemics at irregular intervals, with the highest incidence in summer and early fall. Paralytic disease is more frequent in temperate zones. Wide variations in incidence occur from year to year and region to region. Even during epidemics the incidence of paralytic cases in large cities has rarely exceeded 100 per 100,000 population. Outbreaks in smaller communities tend to reach this level more frequently, and occasionally to be much higher. In the United States an annual reported incidence of 10 paralytic cases per 100,000 population has been normal expectancy; 18 to 37 in last 5 years. Children from one to 16 years of age are more frequently attacked than adults. In several countries, including the United States, older children and young adults constitute a higher proportion of reported cases than formerly.

9. *Methods of control:*
    A. Preventive measures: None other than those of 9B.
    B. Control of the infected individual, contacts and environment:
       1. Report to local health authority: Obligatory case report in most states and countries. Individual cases should be specified as paralytic or nonparalytic.
       2. Isolation: For one week from date of onset, or for the duration of fever if longer.
       3. Concurrent disinfection: Of throat discharges and feces and of articles soiled therewith.
       4. Terminal disinfection: None.
       5. Quarantine: Of doubtful value. Modified quarantine restricting intimate contacts for 7 to 21 days may be desirable in some circumstances.
       6. Immunization: Gamma globulin may be administered to family contacts and other intimate child contacts; no experimental data to determine dosage or effectiveness after infection has occurred.
       7. Investigation of contacts and source of infection: Thorough search for sick persons, especially children, to locate unrecognized and unreported cases.
       8. Specific treatment: None; attention to prevention and management of paralysis.
    C. Epidemic measures:
       1. General notice to physicians of prevalence or increased incidence of the disease, description of usual character of onset and necessity for diagnosis and medical care, particularly for bed rest of patient.
       2. Isolation in bed of all children with fever, pending diagnosis.
       3. Education in such technics of bedside nursing as will prevent transmission of infectious discharges from patients isolated at home.
       4. Protection of children so far as practicable against unnecessary close contact with other persons, especially with other family groups or outsiders during epidemic prevalence of the disease. Urban schools should not be closed nor opening delayed, but intensive or competitive athletic programs should be postponed. Rural schools, particularly where buses are used to gather children

[712]

from sparsely populated areas, and boarding schools which draw children from areas free of the disease and at a distance, should not be opened until the epidemic is clearly declining.

5. Postponement of elective nose or throat operations.

6. Avoidance by children of excessive physical strain as in violent exercise during an epidemic or with known exposure.

7. Postponement of inoculation of any precipitated type antigen of children over 6 months of age if the slightly increased risk of poliomyelitis is considered greater than risk of disease for which immunization is intended.

8. Avoidance of unnecessary travel and visiting, especially of children, during high prevalence of infection.

9. If available, passive immunization with gamma globulin of all children of the most susceptible ages in a limited community may be practiced where weekly number of cases is increasing rapidly and investigation suggests total rate will be unusually high. Under current conditions partial protection is afforded for 5 to 8 weeks by 0.14 cc gamma globulin per pound (0.31 per kilo) body weight. Results of such a program are too limited to recommend it as a general public health measure. Vaccines for active immunization are in experimental use.

D. International measures: Telegraphic notification of epidemics by national health authorities to WHO.

PSITTACOSIS

1. *Identification.* An acute generalized viral infection having an onset with fever and headache; early pneumonic involvement; cough initially absent or non-productive, later usually present and productive; sputum light yellow and extremely viscous; anorexia extreme; constipation the rule; pulse usually slow in relation to temperature; great prostration; delirium common; relapses not uncommon. Fatality is from 5 to 40% for reported cases; mild atypical infections not infrequent. Normal or slightly increased numbers of leucocytes early, leucopenia later. Synonym: Ornithosis.

   Laboratory diagnosis during first week of illness is by intracerebral or intraperitoneal inoculation of mice with sputum or blood, sputum if obtainable being more uniformly infectious than blood; repeated trials are often necessary. A rise in titer of complement fixing antibodies may be demonstrated through examination of early and late serum specimens from patients; serums from lymphogranuloma venereum infection also react.

2. *Etiologic agent.* The viruses of psittacosis or ornithosis, antigenically related to that of lymphogranuloma venereum.

3. *Source and reservoir of infection.* Infected parrots, parakeets, love birds, canaries, pigeons, ducks, turkeys, chickens and other birds. Apparently healthy birds occasionally transmit infection through virus in cloacal discharges. Sputum from infected persons is an occasional source. Mammalian hosts, calves and sheep, are now also suspect.

4. *Mode of transmission.* Contact with infected birds or their recent surroundings, chiefly household pets but also infected pigeons in cities; occasionally through a human infection. Virus may be airborne; laboratory infection frequent.

5. *Incubation period.* In human infections, 6 to 15 days.

[713   ]

6. *Period of communicability.* During acute severe illness, especially when coughing. Birds characteristically have latent infection but at irregular intervals appear sick and shed virus in large quantities.

7. *Susceptibility and resistance.* All ages susceptible, but more severe among older adults; one attack usually confers immunity.

8. *Occurrence.* Usually in sudden familial outbreaks among persons exposed to sick or apparently healthy birds. Deaths mainly confined to persons older than 30 years. An occupational infection in pet shops and aviaries.

9. *Methods of control:*
   A. Preventive measures:
      1. Strict regulation of import or traffic in birds of parrot family based on quarantine and laboratory examination.
      2. Quarantine of pet shops known to have harbored infected birds, until thoroughly cleaned.
      3. Education of community in the danger of making house pets of birds of the parrot family, particularly birds recently imported or with likely history of contact with sick birds.
   B. Control of the infected individual, contacts and environment:
      1. Report to local health authority: Obligatory case report in most states and countries.
      2. Isolation: Important during febrile acute stages. Nurses caring for patients with a cough should wear adequate gauze masks.
      3. Concurrent disinfection: Of all discharges.
      4. Terminal disinfection: Thorough wet cleaning and exposure to sunlight.
      5. Quarantine: Buildings having housed birds should not be used by humans until thoroughly cleaned and disinfected.
      6. Immunization: None.
      7. Investigation of contacts and source of infection: Trace source of suspect birds. Infected birds should be killed and bodies immersed in 2 per cent cresol. While feathers are wet, spleen, liver and kidneys should be aseptically removed, frozen in sterile container, and sent to nearest available laboratory. Carcasses should be burned after autopsy.
      8. Specific treatment: The tetracycline antibiotics (aureomycin and terramycin) and chloramphenicol continued several days after temperature becomes normal.
   C. Epidemic measures: See 9B7.
   D. International measures: Reciprocal respect for national regulations designed to control importation of psittacine birds by land, water, or air.

Q FEVER

1. *Identification.* Q fever is characterized by sudden onset, chilly sensations, headache, weakness, malaise, severe sweats, and considerable variation in severity and duration. Pneumonia, similar to that of atypical pneumonia, occurs in the majority of cases as well as mild cough, scanty expectoration, chest pain, minimal physical findings, and little or no upper respiratory involvement. Chronic general infections have been reported. Case fatality before introduction of specific therapy was not more than 1%; it is now negligible.

Laboratory diagnosis is by complement fixation reaction through demonstration of rise in antibody titer between acute and convalescent specimens; by agglutination test; or by recovery of the causative organism from blood of the patient, readily accomplished but hazardous to laboratory workers.

2. *Etiologic agent.* Rickettsia burneti (Coxiella burneti).

3. *Source and reservoir of infection.* Milk of infected domestic animals and dust laden air of barns and pens; carcasses of infected mammals, bodies of patients dead of the disease, and contaminated wool, straw and laundry have caused outbreaks. Ticks, wild animals (bandicoots), cattle, sheep and goats serve as natural reservoirs.

4. *Mode of transmission.* Commonly by air-borne dissemination of rickettsiae; drinking infected milk may be responsible for some cases (commercial pasteurization reduces but may not eliminate viable R. burneti in milk); also direct contact with infected meat.

5. *Incubation period.* Usually 2 to 3 weeks.

6. *Period of communicability.* Communicability from man to man has not been demonstrated.

7. *Susceptibility and resistance.* Susceptibility is general. An attack confers immunity of unknown duration. Vaccination increases resistance.

8. *Occurrence.* Reported from all continents except South America. Endemic in California where infection exists enzootically in animals raised for meat and milk; has occurred in explosive epidemics in a number of areas in United States, among workers in diagnostic laboratories, stock yards, meat packing and rendering plants and wool processing factories. The largest outbreaks were among troops of World War II in Italy and Greece.

9. *Methods of control:*

A. Preventive measures:

    1. Immunization with inactivated vaccine prepared from R. burneti infected yolk sac appears so useful in protecting laboratory workers that it should be considered for others in hazardous occupations.

    2. Pasteurization preferably above 145° F., or boiling of milk from cows, goats and sheep.

B. Control of the infected individual, contacts, and environment:

    1. Report to local health authority: Obligatory case report in most states and countries.

    2. Isolation: None.

    3. Concurrent disinfection: Of sputum and blood, and articles freshly soiled therewith.

    4. Terminal disinfection: None.

    5. Quarantine: None.

    6. Immunization: None, for contacts.

    7. Investigation of contacts and source of infection: Search for history of contact with cattle, sheep and goats, consuming raw milk and direct or indirect association with a laboratory handling R. burneti.

    8. Specific treatment: The tetracycline antibiotics or chloramphenicol, administered orally and continued for several days after afebrile; reinstitute if relapse occurs.

C. Epidemic measures: Individual outbreaks are generally of short duration; control measures are essentially limited to observation of exposed persons and therapy for

[715]

those ill. In hyperendemic situations immunization should be considered for persons at greatest risk.

D. International measures: Control of importation of domestic animals.

RABIES

1. *Identification.* An invariably fatal acute encephalitis that begins with a sense of apprehension, headache, fever, malaise and indefinite sensory changes often referred to the point of inoculation. The disease progresses to paresis or paralysis; spasm of muscles of deglutition on attempt to drink. Delirium and convulsions follow, ending in death from respiratory paralysis. Duration from onset to death varies from 2 to 6 days. Synonym: Hydrophobia.

   Verification of diagnosis depends upon demonstration of Negri bodies in nerve cells of the brain or upon animal inoculation.

2. *Etiologic agent.* The virus of rabies.

3. *Source and reservoir of infection.* The source of infection is the saliva of rabid animals. Reservoirs include any of a large group of wild and domestic canidae, including the dog, fox, coyote, wolf, and also cat, skunk, raccoon, opossum and other biting mammals. Vampire and fruit eating bats are infected in South and Central America; infection of insectivorous bats recently recognized in eastern United States.

4. *Mode of transmission.* The bite of a rabid animal or on rare occasions contact of saliva of such animals with a scratch or other break in the skin.

5. *Incubation period.* Usually 2 to 6 weeks or longer; depends on extent of laceration, site of wound in relation to richness of nerve supply, and length of nerve path to brain.

6. *Period of communicability.* In the dog, for 3 to 5 days before onset of clinical symptoms and through the clinical course of the disease; rarely communicated from man to man.

7. *Susceptibility and resistance.* Susceptibility general among mammals. Natural immunity is unknown in man or among animals subject to rabies. Prophylactic antirabic treatment of infected humans ordinarily will prevent the disease if begun soon after injury and if the wound does not extensively involve the distribution of the facial nerve. Antirabic vaccination leads to artificial active immunity in dogs.

8. *Occurrence.* Uncommon in man; primarily a disease of animals. Occurs throughout the world except in Australia, New Zealand, Hawaii and other Pacific Islands, some of the West Indies, Great Britain and the Scandinavian peninsula. Urban rabies is a problem of dogs and occasionally other pets, sylvatic or rural rabies primarily of wild biting animals, with sporadic infection of dogs and domestic livestock.

9. *Methods of control:*
   A. Preventive measures:
   1. Detention and observation for 10 days of dogs and other animals suspected of rabies or having bitten a person. Rabid animals have a change in behavior excitability or paralysis, and death occurs within 10 days.
   2. Immediate destruction or 6 months detention of dogs or cats bitten by known rabid animals.

[716]

3. Emphasis on preventive vaccination of dogs; all owned dogs in congested areas should be kept on leash when not within homes of owners. Ownerless dogs should be destroyed by public authority.

4. Education of the public and especially of dog owners and police in handling suspected rabid dogs or those that have bitten a person. Such dogs should be confined for 10 days and observed for symptoms of rabies; should not be killed until rabies is established clinically; the intact head should then be submitted for laboratory examination.

5. Cooperative programs with wild life and conservation authorities toward reduction of foxes and other reservoir animals in areas of sylvatic rabies.

B. Control of the infected individual, contacts and environment:

1. Report to local health authority: Obligatory case report required in most states and countries.

2. Isolation: None; immediate attendants should be warned of the hazard of inoculation through saliva of patient.

3. Concurrent disinfection: Of saliva and articles soiled therewith.

4. Terminal disinfection: None.

5. Quarantine: None.

6. Immunization: Human anti-rabies vaccination is based on the following principles:

    a. When apprehended, observe animal for 10 days. Give vaccine during this 10 day period to persons with severe bites on head or hands, especially with known rabies in the area. Give vaccine if laboratory diagnosis of rabies is established in the animal. In less severe bites, give vaccine if animal develops clinical rabies or dies during observation, whether or not laboratory diagnosis is established.

    b. If animal is not apprehended, vaccine should be administered when rabies is known to be present in the area. If vaccine is administered, 14 consecutive daily doses are usual. In severe exposures, vaccine should be continued for 21 days. Due to recognized occurrence of post-vaccinal paralysis, vaccine should not be given unless the skin is broken. Chances that rabies will develop must carefully be weighed against the small but finite chance of paralysis. For persons who have previously received anti-rabic vaccine, particularly within one year, consideration should be given to reducing the schedule of inoculations. An anti-rabies serum is in course of experimental development; may be useful in severe exposures in conjunction with vaccination.

7. Investigation of contacts and source of infection: Search for rabid animal and for persons and other animals bitten.

8. Specific treatment: For clinical rabies, none. Wounds caused by bite or scratch of an animal with rabies or suspected rabies are thoroughly cleaned and irrigated with a solution of tincture of green soap, or other antiseptic detergents; corrosive agents such as fuming nitric acid are not recommended.

C. Epidemic measures:

1. Establishment of area control under authority of state laws, regulations and local ordinances, in cooperation with appropriate wildlife, conservation and livestock sanitary authorities.

2. Strict enforcement of regulations requiring leashing of owned dogs, and of

collection, detention and destruction of ownerless, stray or unvaccinated dogs found off owner's premises.

3. Intensive program for vaccination of owned dogs with an objective of protecting 75% of resident dogs in the area involved.

4. Education of the public in the necessity of complying with restrictions on dogs, of vaccinating dogs, of seeking immediate medical attention if bitten by a dog, of confining and observing animals that inflict bites, of prompt reporting to the police of dogs manifesting strange behavior, and of reporting rabies in dogs and dog bites to the local health authority.

D. International measures: Strict compliance by common carriers and by travellers with national laws and regulations that institute quarantine or require vaccination of dogs intended for introduction into rabies-free areas.

RAT-BITE FEVER

Two diseases are included under the general term of rat-bite fever; one, also known as Sodoku, is caused by Spirillum minus; the other, also known as Haverhill fever, is caused by Streptobacillus moniliformis. The first disease has priority in recognition and description. Because of similarity in clinical and epidemiological behavior, and because Streptobacillus moniliformis infection is more common in the United States, only the latter disease is presented in detail. The essential variations manifested by Spirillum minus infection are noted under that disease.

A. SPIRILLUM MINUS INFECTION

1. A sporadic rat-bite fever, sodoku, is caused by *Spirillum* minus (Spirocheta morsus muris). It is less frequently observed in the United States than Streptobacillus moniliformis infection, but in Japan and the Far East is reported to be the common form. The incidence of rat-bite fever appears to be greater there than in western countries, although the data are inadequate. The fatality rate is approximately 10%. Clinically, Spirillum minus infection differs from streptobacillus infection in the usual absence of arthritic symptoms, and a more plaque-like rash. The incubation period is generally longer, one to 3 weeks, and usually more than 7 days. Laboratory methods are essential for differentiation of the two diseases.

B. STREPTOBACILLUS MONILIFORMIS INFECTION

1. *Identification.* Usually a history of rat bite within 10 days; primary edematous lesion; swelling of regional lymph nodes; sharp febrile paroxysms often alternating with afebrile intervals, and accompanied by a morbilliform and petechial rash, polyarthritis, and leucocytosis. Ulceration of the primary lesion may occur; also regional lymphadenitis. Fatality may reach 10% in untreated cases.

Bacteriologic examination of primary lesion, lymph nodes, blood and joint fluids, or serum test by specific agglutination, or mouse inoculation. Caution should be exercised lest the experimental mouse or rat be already naturally infected.

2. *Etiologic agent.* Streptobacillus moniliformis (Streptothrix muris rattis, Haverhillia multiformis, Actinomyces muris).

3. *Source and reservoir of infection.* An infected rat, rarely other rodents (squirrel, weasel). Sporadic cases without reference to bite have been recorded.

[718]

4. *Mode of transmission.* By the bite of an infected animal; animal blood escapes from the injured or diseased buccal mucosa into the wound, or the conjunctival secretion of the rat may contaminate the wound. Blood from an experimental laboratory animal may infect man. Localized epidemics may occur from contaminated milk or milk products (Haverhill fever); the means of contamination is not known, whether through infection of cows by rat bite, or direct contamination of milk by rats.

5. *Incubation period.* Three to 10 days, rarely longer.

6. *Communicability.* Not known to be transmitted from man to man.

7. *Susceptibility and resistance.* No data for man.

8. *Occurrence.* Distribution is world-wide. Uncommon in North and South America and in most European countries; case reports show this to be the usual form of rat-bite fever in the United States.

9. *Methods of control:*
   A. Preventive measures:
      1. Reduction of rat population. Rat proofing of dwellings.
      2. Pasteurization of milk may help in preventing Haverhill fever.
   B. Control of the infected individual, contacts, and environment:
      1. Report to local health authority. Obligatory report of epidemics; no individual case report.
      2. Isolation: None.
      3. Concurrent disinfection: None.
      4. Terminal disinfection: None.
      5. Quarantine: None.
      6. Immunization: None.
      7. Investigation of contacts and source of infection: Not practicable.
      8. Specific treatment: Penicillin; tetracycline antibiotics may be substituted. Treatment should be continued for seven to 10 days.
   C. Epidemic measures: Grouped cases presenting the typical symptoms require search for epidemiologic evidence of a relation to milk supply.
   D. International measures: None.

RELAPSING FEVER

Two disease entities, having minor clinical variations and distinguishable principally by differences in mode of transmission and geographic distribution, are known as relapsing fever. One is louse-borne, the other tick-borne.

A. Louse-borne Relapsing Fever

1. *Identification.* An epidemic spirochetal disease with short febrile paroxysms lasting 2 or 3 days, alternating with afebrile periods of 3 or 4 days and resulting in 2 to 10 relapses, more commonly the lesser number; each attack terminates by crisis and the average duration of the disease is 13 to 16 days. Transitory petechial-like rashes are common during the initial fever. Case fatality ranges between 2 and 10%.

Diagnosis is through demonstrating the infectious agent in darkfield preparations of fresh blood, stained thick blood films, or by intraperitoneal inoculation of white rats with 15 to 25 cc of blood taken during the pyrexial period and before crisis.

[719]

2. *Etiologic agent.* Borrelia recurrentis, a spirochete. Numerous specific names have been given to morphologically identical but biologically different spirochetes isolated from cases of relapsing fever in widely separated endemic areas.

3. *Source and reservoir of infection.* Blood of infected persons. Interepidemic reservoir is unknown.

4. *Mode of transmission.* By crushing an infected louse, Pediculus humanus, into the bite-wound or into an abrasion of the skin.

5. *Incubation period.* Up to 12 days, average 7 days.

6. *Period of communicability.* Not communicable from man to man. The louse becomes infective 4 to 5 days after ingestion of blood from an infected person and remains so for life (20–40 days).

7. *Susceptibility and resistance.* Susceptibility is general. The duration of immunity after clinical attack is unknown but probably does not exceed two years.

8. *Occurrence.* In limited localities in Europe and among peoples of Asia, North and South Africa, and Central America who are louse infested. Epidemics are commonly incidental to war and famine or other situations where malnourished, over-crowded populations with poor personal hygiene favor multiplication and wide dissemination of the vector. Not reported in the United States for many years.

9. *Methods of control:*
   A. Preventive measures:
      1. Routine application of insecticide with residual effect, such as DDT or a number of other compounds, at appropriate intervals to populations living under conditions favoring the development of lousiness.
      2. Individual prophylaxis through application of insecticide, DDT or equivalent, at appropriate intervals to clothing as dusting powder or by impregnation.
      3. Improvement of living conditions with provision for frequent bathing and washing of clothing.
   B. Control of the infected individual, contacts, and environment:
      1. Report to local health authority: Case report universally required by international regulation.
      2. Isolation: After proper chemical delousing of patient, clothing and bedroom. and of patient's household contacts, isolation is not required.
      3. Concurrent disinfection: None.
      4. Terminal disinfection: Careful terminal application of insecticides to body and clothing where death occurs before this has been done.
      5. Quarantine: Exposed lousy susceptibles are quarantined for 15 days or may be released after application of insecticide with residual effect, for example DDT.
      6. Immunization: None.
      7. Investigation of contacts and source of infection: For the individual case, unprofitable; a community effort (see 9C).
      8. Specific treatment: Penicillin G in adequate dosage; tetracyclines and chloramphenicol are also effective. Patients with central nervous system involvement, particularly with inadequate dosage, will likely experience relapse. Arsenical therapy, neo-arsphenamine and mapharsen, is widely used.
   C. Epidemic measures:
      1. The most important measure for the rapid control of relapsing fever, where reporting has been good and the number of cases small, is application of insecti-

[720]

cides with residual effect to contacts of all reported cases. Where infection is known to be widespread, systematic application of residual insecticide to all persons in the community is indicated; 2–5% DDT in an inert powder, talc or pyrophyllite for dusting.
  D. International measures:
   1. Telegraphic notification of WHO and of adjacent countries, by governments, of the existence of an epidemic of relapsing fever. An internationally quarantinable disease.
   2. Measures applicable to ships, aircraft and land transport arriving from relapsing fever areas are specified in International Sanitary Regulations (WHO Techn. Rep. Ser. No. 41, Geneva, 1951).

B. TICK-BORNE RELAPSING FEVER

1. *Identification.* Regularly an endemic disease with a clinical course similar to that of louse-borne infection, except that relapses are more frequent, averaging 6 or 7; deaths are rare. A satisfactory history of tick bite is unlikely and evidence of bite is seldom found.
      Diagnosis is by demonstrating the infectious agent in thick smears of blood at time of febrile attack, or from blood of mice, rats or monkeys inoculated with patient's blood at that time.
2. *Etiologic agent.* Borrelia duttoni, a spirochete. Numerous specific names have been given to morphologically identical but biologically different spirochetes isolated from cases of relapsing fever in widely separated endemic areas.
3. *Source and reservoir of infection.* Infected wild rodents or ticks.
4. *Mode of transmission.* Man is infected by the bite or coxal fluid of an infected tick, principally one of five species of the genus Ornithodoros; in the United States O. turicata and O. hermsi; O. rudis and O. talaje are vectors in Central and South America; O. moubata in tropical Africa; and O. tholozani in Near East, Middle East, and Far East. Transovarian infection occurs in ticks.
5. *Incubation period.* Three to 6 days, but may be as short as 2 days or as long as 12.
6. *Period of communicability.* Not communicable from man to man. Ticks can live for years without feeding and remain infective.
7. *Susceptibility and resistance.* Susceptibility is general. The duration of immunity after recovery is indefinite, but probably not more than 2 years.
8. *Occurrence.* Widespread throughout tropical Africa. Foci have been observed in Spain, North Africa, Arabia, Iran, India, and parts of Central Asia as well as in North and South America. In the United States human cases of tick-borne relapsing fever have been found in limited localities of 13 western states.
9. *Methods of control:*
  A. Preventive measures:
   1. Avoidance of tick-infested caves, camp sites, shacks, and ground areas. Exposed persons should use tick repellent on exposed areas of skin, such as dimethylphthalate, indalone, Rutgers 612, or a number of other compounds now under investigation. Clothing may be impregnated with repellent by sprayers or by dipping. Lindane can be used as a residual spray in buildings. The habits of argasid ticks differ from those of Ixodidae and consequently pose a different problem in prevention. Ticks of this genus attack, rapidly engorge. and promptly leave the body of the host.

B. Control of the infected individual, contacts, and environment:
   1. Report to local health authority: In selected endemic areas (U.S.A.); in many countries not a reportable disease.
   2. Isolation: None.
   3. Concurrent disinfection: None.
   4. Terminal disinfection: None.
   5. Quarantine: None.
   6. Immunization: None.
   7. Investigation of contacts and source of infection: Important.
   8. Specific treatment: See treatment of louse-borne relapsing fever.
C. Epidemic measures: Reduction of tick population in living quarters by periodic dusting with insecticides.
D. International measures: None.

RHEUMATIC FEVER

1. *Identification.* Rheumatic fever appears as an occasional sequella of group A hemolytic streptococcal upper respiratory infection, and sometimes in the absence of such recognized prior infection. The main clinical manifestations are migratory polyarthritis, carditis, chorea, subcutaneous nodules and erythema marginatum. Fever, rapid pulse, non-traumatic epistaxis, abdominal and precordial pain, pallor, anorexia, weight loss, a fast sedimentation rate, leuocytosis and electrocardiographic changes are a second group of findings of lesser diagnostic significance. With a history of previous attack, combinations of the above suggest recurrence of rheumatic fever. Mild and inapparent infections occur, their relative frequency unknown; definite and even severe right heart disease develops in absence of evident acute rheumatic fever. A leading cause of death among children of the United States, aged 6 to 10 years; case fatality is appreciable, commonly 3–5% in endemic areas. Synonym: Acute articular rheumatism.

   Bacteriologic or serologic (chiefly antistreptolysin O) evidence of a preceding group A streptococcal infection adds diagnostic weight to suggestive symptoms.

2. *Etiologic agent.* Unknown. Attacks are usually precipitated by group A streptococcal respiratory infections, frequently unrecognized or so mild as to have had no medical attention.

3. *Source and reservoir of infection.* Unknown.

4. *Mode of transmission.* Unknown.

5. *Incubation period.* Not applicable. Symptoms appear about 2–3 weeks after a recognized group A streptococcal infection.

6. *Period of communicability.* Not known to be communicable; the preceding streptococcal infection which may precipitate rheumatic fever is communicable but usually has subsided by the time rheumatic fever develops.

7. *Susceptibility and resistance.* All age groups are susceptible; the greatest incidence is in children from 6 to 12 years of age. The disease has a natural tendency to recur; no evidence that immunity develops.

8. *Occurrence.* A frequent disease in temperate zones throughout the world; in the United States most prevalent in Rocky Mountain region, New England, and North and Central Atlantic states; lowest in the South and Southwest. Seasonal incidence is that of streptococcal infections, in the United States a peak during spring months and a low point during summer and early autumn. Reliable data

on frequency in tropical areas are not available; the impression of a lesser prevalence than in temperate zones is not always supported. Predilection for race or sex has not been defined. For unknown reasons, incidence and mortality of rheumatic fever are declining.

9. *Methods of control:*

   A. Preventive measures:

   1. No practical measures of prevention except those for Group A streptococcal infections (see Scarlet Fever).

   B. Control of the infected individual, contacts and environment:

   1. Report to local health authority: In selected endemic areas (U.S.A.): in many states and countries not a reportable disease, Class 3B. Areas of high incidence will profit materially by encouraging individual case report over prescribed periods sufficient to acquire epidemiological data necessary for improved methods of control.

   2. Isolation: None.

   3. Concurrent disinfection: None.

   4. Terminal disinfection: None.

   5. Quarantine: None.

   6. Immunization: None.

   7. Investigation of contacts and source of infection: None.

   8. Specific treatment: Individuals known to have had rheumatic fever or convalescent from that disease should receive chemoprophylaxis until age 18 years, and past that age for a period of 5 years from last attack. Either a sulfonamide drug or penicillin may be employed, given orally throughout the year. Prior to prophylaxis, proper treatment should be instituted to free the patient of Group A streptococci (see Scarlet Fever).

   Salicylates are the method of choice in management of the acute phase, preferably acetylsalicylic acid, also sodium salicylate, continued for duration of active disease. Patients must be protected from intercurrent infection, particularly with group A hemolytic streptococci.

   C. Epidemic measures: Epidemics of rheumatic fever occur only in association with epidemics of Group A streptococcal infections. Proper therapy of the streptococcal infection (see Scarlet Fever) will prevent the subsequent development of rheumatic fever and thus prevent about half of the cases of rheumatic fever.

   D. International measures: None.

RICKETTSIALPOX

1. *Identification.* Rickettsialpox is characterized by an initial lesion, chills, fever, varicelliform rash, and a mild to severe course; even before specific therapy, case fatality was less than 1%. The initial lesion appears as a firm red papule about a week in advance of fever, most commonly on the covered parts of the body, the papule becomes vesicular, then covered by a scab and after about 3 weeks leaves a small pigmented scar. Fever, often preceded by chills, is remittent with peaks of 39.5° C. (103° F.) to 40.5° C. (105° F.), usually lasting less than one week. Headache, muscular pain, and general malaise are frequent. The secondary rash is manifest 3 to 4 days after onset of fever; has no characteristic distribution but seldom occurs on palms or soles; progresses through papular and papulovesicular stages, lasting usually less than one week and leaving no scars; local lymphade-

[723]

nopathy occurs in the region of the initial lesion, but splenomegaly or generalized lymph node enlargement is uncommon.

Specific diagnosis is by complement fixation test, positive between the second and third week of the disease. Sera from patients with rickettsialpox give Weil-Felix reactions with proteus OX antigens below the level regarded as significant in other rickettsial diseases.

2. *Etiologic agent.* Rickettsia akari, a member of the spotted fever group of rickettsiae.
3. *Source and reservoir of infection.* Infected house mice (Mus musculus musculus).
4. *Mode of transmission.* From mouse to mouse and probably from mouse to man by a rodent mite, Allodermanyssus sanguineus.
5. *Incubation period.* Probably 10 to 24 days.
6. *Period of communicability.* Not communicable from man to man. Duration of infectivity of mouse for mite, and mite for mouse or man are unknown.
7. *Susceptibility and resistance.* Susceptibility appears general. Duration of immunity after attack is unknown.
8. *Occurrence.* Approximately 150 cases occur annually in New York City, principally among inhabitants of apartment houses where the mouse, mite and rickettsia maintain a natural cycle of infection. A few cases have been recognized in Boston, Hartford, and Philadelphia; occurrence in other areas is probable.
9. *Methods of control:*
   A. Preventive measures:
      1. Rodent and mite control by elimination of mice and mouse harborages, including proper care and firing of incinerators in dwellings, and application of residual miticides (aldrine and others) to infested areas. Commercial vaccine not available and not currently needed.
   B. Control of the infected individual, contacts and environment:
      1. Report to local health authority: In selected endemic areas (U.S.A.); in most states and countries not a reportable disease, Class 3B.
      2. Isolation: None.
      3. Concurrent disinfection: None.
      4. Terminal disinfection: None.
      5. Quarantine: None.
      6. Immunization: None.
      7. Investigation of contacts and source of infection: Search for infested mice in dwelling and, if feasible, undertake isolation of rickettsiae from rodents and mites.
      8. Specific treatment: The tetracycline antibiotics and chloramphenicol are equally effective.
   C. Epidemic measures: When groups of cases occur in the same or adjacent dwellings the preventive measures listed under 9A should be applied. Other inhabitants should be observed and promptly treated if the disease develops.
   D. International measures: None.

RINGWORM

Ringworm is a general term applied to mycotic infections of keratinized areas of the body (hair, skin and nails). Various genera and species of a group of fungi known collectively as the dermatophytes are causative agents. For convenience in presentation, the dermatomycoses are subdivided according to sites of infection as follows: Tinea capitis (ringworm of the scalp), tinea corporis (ringworm of the body), tinea pedis (athlete's foot) and tinea unguium (ringworm of the nails). Synonyms: Favus, Jockey-Itch, Athlete's Foot, The Dermatomycoses).

A. RINGWORM OF SCALP (TINEA CAPITIS)

1. *Identification.* Infection begins as a small papule and spreads peripherally, leaving scaly patches of alopecia (baldness). Infected hairs become brittle and break off easily. Occasionally boggy, raised and suppurative lesions develop, called kerions. Examination of the scalp under Wood light for fluorescence is helpful in certain ringworm infections.

   Microscopic examination of hairs, cleared with sodium hydroxide solution, shows spores within the hair (endothrix type) or surrounding it (ectothrix type). The fungus should be cultured for genus and species identification.

   Favus of the scalp is a variety of tinea capitis, caused by Trichophyton schoenleini and characterized by formation of small, yellowish, cup-like crusts or scutulae giving the appearance of being stuck on to the scalp. Affected hairs do not break off but become gray and lusterless, eventually fall out and leave baldness which may be permanent. Microscopic examination of the hair in sodium hydroxide shows no spores, but the interior of the hair is filled with long branching mycelial filaments and characteristic air spaces.

   Tinea capitis is distinguished easily from piedra, a fungus infection of the hair occurring in South America and some countries of Southeast Asia, an infection characterized by hard "gritty" nodules in the hair shafts.

2. *Etiologic agent.* Various species of Microsporum and Trichophyton. Identification of genus and species is important epidemiologically and for estimation of prognosis.

3. *Source and reservoir of infection.* Sources are such materials as barber clippers, toilet articles or clothing contaminated with infected hair. Reservoirs are scalp lesions of man or lesions of infected animals, especially dogs, cats and cattle.

4. *Mode of transmission.* Direct contact with sources or reservoirs of infection.

5. *Incubation period.* 10 to 14 days.

6. *Period of communicability.* As long as infected lesions are present, and as long as viable spores are present on contaminated materials.

7. *Susceptibility and resistance.* Children before the age of puberty are notoriously susceptible to Microsporum infections and most adults are resistant. All ages are subject to Trichophyton infections but children are more susceptible. No immunity is developed.

8. *Occurrence.* Ringworm of the scalp caused by Microsporum audouini is widespread in the United States, particularly in urban areas. M. canis infection occurs both in rural and urban areas wherever infected cats and dogs are present. Trichophyton mentagrophytes and T. verrucosum (faviforme) infections are common in rural areas in association with infected cattle and horses. T. tonsurans infections are epidemic in urban areas in Southwestern United States and Mexico. Incidence in children is higher than adults, males are infected more frequently than females; significant differences in race have not been noted. Infection of animals is more common in damp cold seasons, especially when confined to barns, and incidence of human infection with animal transmitted strains is thus higher in colder weather.

[725]

9. *Methods of control:*
  A. Preventive measures: In epidemic areas young children should be surveyed by Wood light before entering school. The public, especially parents, should be warned of the dangers of acquiring infection from other infected children as well as from dogs, cats and other animals. Effective control of animal ringworm.
  B. Control of the infected individual, contacts and environment:
    1. Report to local health authority: Obligatory report of epidemics; no individual case report. School outbreaks should be reported to school authorities.
    2. Isolation: Impractical. The patient should be under a regulated regime of treatment with periodic visits to physician or clinic. Hair should be covered with a cap which can be sterilized frequently.
    3. Concurrent disinfection: Contaminated caps should be boiled after each use.
    4. Terminal disinfection: None.
    5. Quarantine: Not practicable.
    6. Immunization: None.
    7. Investigation of contacts and source of infection: Household contacts, and pets and farm animals, for evidence of infection.
    8. Specific treatment: Ointments containing salicylanilid, copper undecylenate or any one of a variety of similar compounds. Epilation by Roentgen-ray is instituted if progress is not satisfactory. Examine weekly and take cultures to assure recovery is complete.
  C. Epidemic measures: Epidemics in a school or institution require special measures such as education of children and parents, and enlistment of services of doctors and nurses for diagnosis. Follow-up surveys are important.
  D. International measures: Examination of scalps of immigrants coming from areas of high prevalence of favus or T. tonsurans or T. violaceum infections. Infected persons should be detained, placed under treatment and entry deferred until free of the disease; a procedure not to be loosely applied to all ringworm infection.

B. Ringworm of Body (Tinea Corporis)

1. *Identification.* Cutaneous infections other than of the scalp, bearded areas and feet, characteristically appearing as flat spreading ring-shaped lesions. The periphery is reddish, vesicular or pustular, and may be dry and scaly or moist and crusted. As lesions progress peripherally, the central area often clears and skin appears normal.

   Scrapings from the advancing margins, cleared in sodium hydroxide and examined microscopically, show segmented branching filaments.
2. *Etiologic agent.* Epidermophyton floccosum and various species of Microsporum and Trichophyton.
3. *Source and reservoir of infection.* Sources are contaminated floors, shower stalls, benches and similar articles; reservoir is skin lesions of man.
4. *Mode of transmission.* Direct contact with sources of infection.
5. *Incubation period.* 10 to 14 days.
6. *Period of communicability.* As long as viable spores are present on contaminated materials.
7. *Susceptibility and resistance.* Susceptibility is general. Clinical manifestations are

[726   ]

commonly exaggerated under conditions of friction and excessive perspiration, as in axillary and inguinal regions.

8. *Occurrence.* World-wide and relatively frequent. Males are infected more than females. All ages are susceptible and racial differences are immaterial.

9. *Methods of control:*

A. Preventive measures: Adequate sterilization of towels and general cleanliness in showers and dressing rooms of gymnasium, especially repeated washing of benches. A fungicidal agent such as cresol should be used for disinfection.

B. Control of the infected individual, contacts and environment:

1. Report to local health authority: Obligatory report of epidemics; no individual case report. Case report to school authority of infections of children, involving exposed parts of the body is desirable.

2. Isolation: Infected children should be excluded from gymnasiums, swimming pools and activities likely to lead to exposure of others.

3. Concurrent disinfection: Of clothing in contact with infected parts of the body.

4. Terminal disinfection: None.

5. Quarantine: None.

6. Immunization: None.

7. Investigation of contacts and source of infection: Examination of school and household contacts, and of household pets and farm animals.

8. Specific treatment: Thorough bathing with soap and water, removal of scabs and crusts, and application of any of a number of ointments containing salicylic acid or one of the higher fatty acids (propionic acid, undecylenic acid).

C. Epidemic measures: Education of children and of parents concerning the nature of the infection, its mode of spread and necessity of maintaining good body hygiene.

D. International measures: None.

C. Ringworm of Foot (Tinea Pedis)

1. *Identification.* Scaling or cracking of the skin, especially between the toes, or blisters containing a thin watery fluid are so characteristic that most laymen recognize "athlete's foot." In severe cases, vesicular lesions appear on various parts of the body, especially the hands. These dermatophytids do not contain the fungus and represent an allergic reaction to fungus products.

Microscopic examination of sodium hydroxide-treated scrapings from lesions between the toes reveals segmented branching filaments.

2. *Etiologic agent.* Epidermophyton floccosum and various species of Macrosporum and Trichophyton.

3. *Source and reservoir of infection.* Sources of infection are infected persons or contamined floors, shower stalls and other articles used by them. Reservoir is skin lesions of infected persons.

4. *Mode of transmission.* Direct contact with sources or reservoirs of infection.

5. *Incubation period.* Approximately 10 to 14 days.

6. *Period of communicability.* As long as infected lesions are present and as long as viable spores are present on contaminated materials.

7. *Susceptibility and resistance.* Susceptibility is variable and infection may be inapparent. Second attack is frequent.

8. *Occurrence.* World-wide and a common disease. Adults more often affected than children; males more than females. No differences in racial susceptibility. Infections are more prevalent in hot weather.

9. *Methods of control:*

   A. Preventive measures:

      1. As for tinea corporis above.
      2. Maintenance of strict personal hygiene, with special care in drying areas between toes after bathing.

   B. Control of the infected individual, contacts and environment:

      1. Report to local health authority: Official report not ordinarily justifiable. School outbreaks should be reported to school authorities.
      2. Isolation: None.
      3. Concurrent disinfection: Socks from heavily infected individuals should be boiled to prevent reinfection. Shoes should be placed in a box and subjected to formaldehyde for several hours, followed by airing to prevent irritation of skin from residual formalin.
      4. Terminal disinfection: None.
      5. Quarantine: None.
      6. Immunization: None.
      7. Investigation of contacts and source of infection: None.
      8. Specific treatment: Ointments, as recommended for tinea corporis, may be used. Exposure of feet to air through wearing sandals is often beneficial.

   C. Epidemic measures: Thorough cleaning and washing down of gymnasiums, showers, and similar sources of infection. Education of the public concerning the nature of the infection and its mode of spread.

   D. International measures: None.

D. RINGWORM OF NAILS (TINEA UNGUIUM)

1. *Identification.* A chronic infection involving one or more nails of the hand or foot. The nail gradually thickens, becomes discolored and brittle, and an accumulation of caseous-appearing material forms beneath the nail.

   Microscopic examination of sodium hydroxide preparations of the nail and of detritus beneath the nail show segmented branching mycelial filaments. The diagnosis should be confirmed by culture.

2. *Etiologic agent.* Epidermophyton floccosum and various species of trichophyton.

3. *Source and reservoir of infection.* Source is presumably direct extension from infections of foot, possibly contaminated floors and shower stalls; reservoir is skin or nail lesions of infected persons.

4. *Mode of transmission.* Unknown.

5. *Incubation period.* Unknown.

6. *Period of communicability.* As long as infected lesions are present.

7. *Susceptibility and resistance.* Unknown; injury to nail predisposes to infection.

8. *Occurrence.* Common. Adult males more frequently infected than females. No seasonal or racial differences.

9. *Methods of control:*

   A. Preventive measures: The measures described above for prevention of tinea pedis.

   B. Control of the infected individual, contacts and environment:

      1. Report to local health authority: Official report not ordinarily justifiable.

2. Items 2 through 7, see tinea pedis above.

8. Specific treatment: Scrape off as much of affected nail as possible. Apply ointments or other medication of types described for tinea pedis. Repeat frequently until nail appears normal.

C. Epidemic measures: Not applicable.

ROCKY MOUNTAIN SPOTTED FEVER, TICK-BORNE

1. *Identification.* This prototype of the diseases caused by the spotted fever group of rickettsiae is an infectious endangiitis characterized by sudden onset of fever, ordinarily persisting for two weeks, headache, conjunctival injection, and a maculopapular rash. The rash appears on the extremities about the third day and spreads rapidly to most of the body, including palms and soles, before becoming petechial. Case fatality is about 20% in absence of specific therapy; death is uncommon with prompt treatment.

The Weil-Felix reaction with Proteus OX-19 and usually with OX-2 becomes positive late in the second week; complement fixation tests using specific rickettsial antigen a few days later.

2. *Etiologic agent.* Rickettsia rickettsii.

3. *Source and reservoir of infection.* Infected ticks. In eastern and southern United States the common vector is the dog tick, Dermacentor variabilis; in northwestern United States, the wood tick, Dermacentor andersoni; in southwestern United States occasionally the Lone Star tick, Amblyomma americanum. In Brazil, Amblyomma cajennense is the common vector. The rabbit tick Haemaphysalis leporis palustris is infected in nature but does not bite man. The infection is passed from generation to generation in ticks and probably is maintained by infected and non-infected larvae feeding upon susceptible wild rodents.

4. *Mode of transmission.* Ordinarily by bite of infected tick but contamination of skin with crushed infected tick tissues or feces may lead to infection in man.

5. *Incubation period.* From 3 to about 10 days.

6. *Period of communicability.* Not directly communicable in nature from man to man.

7. *Susceptibility and resistance.* Susceptibility is general. One attack confers immunity which may or may not be permanent. Suitable vaccines induce immunity artificially.

8. *Occurrence.* Throughout most of the United States during spring and summer but most prevalent in Rocky Mountain and Middle Atlantic seaboard states. In western United States, adult males are most affected while in the East children are more frequently attacked; infection rates are related to opportunity for contact with infected ticks, and mortality rates increase with age. Infection also occurs in western Canada, western and central Mexico, Colombia and Brazil. Although limited to the Western Hemisphere, the disease is closely related to tick-borne rickettsial infections of other continents.

9. *Methods of control:*

A. Preventive measures:

1. Personal prophylaxis by avoiding tick-infested areas when feasible, by careful removal of ticks from the person as promptly as possible without crushing and with protection of the hands when removing ticks from animals. Some of the newer insect repellents (n-n-butyl-acetanilide) are of value against ticks.

[729]

2. Measures for reducing tick populations are generally impractical. Clearing the land, reducing small wild mammal populations, stray dog control and removing ticks from livestock by dipping may help. In selected areas direct application of appropriate insecticides effects excellent control of some tick vectors. DDT is used; newer preparations to include lindane, aldrin and others are undergoing field trial.

3. Vaccines containing killed R. rickettsii lessen the chance of infection and lower case fatality. Since advent of specific therapy, vaccination is generally limited to persons at high risk. Reinforcing doses at yearly intervals are necessary to maintain protection.

B. Control of the infected individual, contacts, and environment:

1. Report to local health authority: In selected endemic areas (U.S.A.); in many countries not a reportable disease.

2. Isolation: None.

3. Concurrent disinfection: All ticks on patients should be destroyed.

4. Terminal disinfection: None.

5. Quarantine: None.

6. Immunization: Of case contacts, unnecessary.

7. Investigation of contacts and source of infection: Not profitable except as a community measure; see 9C.

8. Specific treatment: The tetracycline antibiotics or chloramphenicol in daily oral doses until patient is afebrile (usually 3 days) and for one or two additional days.

C. Epidemic measures: In hyperendemic areas particular attention should be paid to identification of infected ticks and infested areas, and to recommendations in 9A1, 2.

D. International measures: None.

RUBELLA

1. *Identification.* A mild febrile infection with a rash of variable character, sometimes resembling that of measles, sometimes that of scarlet fever, and sometimes an admixture of both; few or no constitutional symptoms but almost always enlargement of the post-auricular, sub-occipital or post-cervical group of lymph nodes; occasionally others. Mild catarrhal symptoms may be present; absence of Koplik spots differentiates the disease from measles. Infection without a rash has been produced experimentally. Leukopenia is usual during fever. Synonym: German measles.

Roseola infantum (exanthem subitum) is to be distinguished from rubella by clinical and epidemiologic differences, notably the onset of rash after subsidence of fever and predilection for infants rather than older children and adults.

2. *Etiologic agent.* The virus of rubella.

3. *Source and reservoir of infection.* Nasopharyngeal secretions of infected persons; viremia shortly before and after onset of symptoms.

4. *Mode of transmission.* By droplet spread or direct contact with patient, or by indirect contact with articles freshly soiled with discharges from nose or throat. Airborne transmission also occurs.

5. *Incubation period.* From 14 to 21 days; usually 18 days.

6. *Period of communicability.* For at least 4 days after onset of catarrhal symptoms

and probably not much longer, the exact period being undetermined. Highly communicable.

7. *Susceptibility and resistance.* Susceptibility is general among young children. An attack usually confers permanent immunity.

8. *Occurrence.* Epidemic in expression, mostly in childhood, but with more adult patients than in measles; more prevalent in winter and spring than in other seasons. World wide in distribution and a common communicable disease.

9. *Methods of control.* Efforts to control rubella are prompted by the hazard of congenital defects in offspring of women who acquire the disease during pregnancy. The extent of the risk is indefinite, but approximately 10–20% of living infants born after maternal rubella during the first trimester of pregnancy have anomalies.

A. Preventive measures:

1. No attempt should be made to protect female children in good health against exposure to the disease before puberty.

B. Control of the infected individual, contacts and environment:

1. Report to local health authority: Obligatory report of epidemics; case report ordinarily serves no useful purpose; may be required specifically where contacts include susceptible women in first 4 months of pregnancy.

2. Isolation: None, except where contacts include a woman in early pregnancy; then under direction of the attending physician for 5 days after onset.

3. Concurrent disinfection: None.

4. Terminal disinfection: None.

5. Quarantine: None.

6. Immunization: Immune serum globulin (gamma globulin) appears to have some value in passive protection against rubella; results conflicting. Until evidence to the contrary and because of the serious risk to offspring, may be administered to adult female contacts with no definite history of rubella and exposure within the first 4 months of pregnancy; other non-immune family contacts may be included.

7. Investigation of contacts and source of infection: Of no practical value except to clarify possible confusion with scarlet fever; and to identify adult female contacts in the first 4 months of pregnancy.

8. Specific treatment: None.

C. Epidemic measures: No procedures in common use can be relied upon as a means of effective control of the disease or of epidemics.

D. International measures: None.

SCABIES

1. *Identification.* An infection of the skin caused by the itch mite and characterized by itching, by burrows which appear as slightly elevated grayish white lines and house the mite with eggs, and by papules and vesicles. The latter often become pustular from secondary infection by scratching. Lesions are most prominent in folds of the skin such as finger webs, elbow creases, armpits, between the thighs, and under the breasts of women; no fatality. Synonym: The itch.

The itch mite is identified by hand lens in scrapings from the burrows, the eggs microscopically.

[731]

2. *Etiologic agent.* Sarcoptes scabiei, the itch mite.
3. *Source and reservoir of infection.* Persons harboring the itch mite.
4. *Mode of transmission.* Transfer of young female mite by direct contact with the skin of infected persons; to a limited extent, by underclothing and linen recently used by infected individuals.
5. *Incubation period.* Until itch mites and eggs are destroyed, a period that varies from 1 to 2 weeks depending on treatment used.
6. *Period of communicability.* Until itch mites and eggs are destroyed, a period that varies from 1 to 2 weeks depending on treatment used.
7. *Susceptibility and resistance.* Anyone may become infected or reinfected. Initial infection results in sensitization accompanied by a rather marked tissue reaction and followed by a decreased susceptibility to reinfection.
8. *Occurrence.* Widespread and independent of climate, sex, or race. Commonly associated with overcrowding, body uncleanliness, neglect and lack of soap and water. Single infections in a family, without spread to others of the group, are uncommon. Epidemics occur characteristically in barracks, camps, and institutions.
9. *Methods of control:*
   A. Preventive measures:
   1. Cleanliness of body, underclothing and bed covering. Attention to proper laundering of linen.
   B. Control of the infected individual, contacts and environment:
   1. Report to local health authority: Official report not ordinarily justifiable; presence in schools should be reported to school authorities.
   2. Isolation: Children should be excluded from school until adequately treated. Infected persons should be denied common recreation and bathing facilities.
   3. Concurrent disinfection: Proper laundering of underwear and personal linen.
   4. Terminal disinfection: Unnecessary if effective treatment has been carried out.
   5. Quarantine: None.
   6. Immunization: None.
   7. Investigation of contacts and source of infection: Search for unreported or unrecognized cases in companions or in other members of the household.
   8. Specific treatment: (a) Benzyl benzoate; a 25% emulsion is applied with a 2 inch brush to the entire body, with special attention to areas with many lesions. A second application is made within 24 hours, and at 48 hours a bath is taken. (b) Hexachlorocyclohexane (Kwell); a 1% ointment is rubbed into the skin avoiding the eyes. A second application may be necessary. The drug is toxic in high concentration or if used repeatedly. (c) Sulfur; a 5% sulfur ointment is applied to the skin and repeated in 24 and 48 hours. The same underwear should be worn during this period. After another 24 hours a bath is taken.
   C. Epidemic measures:
   1. Segregation of infected individuals.
   2. Provision of convenient facilities for prompt treatment of the infection.
   3. Encouragement of bodily cleanliness and use of clean underclothes and bedding by people living in crowded quarters.
   D. International measures: None.

[732]

SCHISTOSOMIASIS

1. *Identification.* A blood-fluke (trematode) disease in which the adult male and female worms live in veins of the host (mainly mesenteric, portal and pelvic) and deposit eggs which produce minute granulomata and scars in organs in which they lodge. Early manifestations are remittent fever, giant urticaria, abdominal discomfort, right upper quadrant tenderness, and eosinophilia which may reach 85%; accompanied or soon followed by blood in feces or urine. Late manifestations are cirrhosis of liver with ascites and splenomegaly, or severe chronic cystitis or other pelvic manifestations. Eggs may be deposited in spinal cord or brain with resulting neurological manifestations. Death is uncommon except from complications, but more frequent for S. japonicum than for other species. Synonym: Bilharziasis.

    Definitive diagnosis is by finding the characteristic eggs in feces or urine; light infections require special concentration methods or rectal biopsy.

2. *Etiologic agents.* Schistosoma mansoni, S. haematobium and S. japonicum.

    The larvae of certain other schistosomes of birds and rodents may penetrate the human skin causing a dermatitis known as "swimmer's itch." These schistosomes do not become mature in man.

3. *Source and reservoir of infection.* Immediate source is snails infected with larval forms. Reservoir is usually persons harboring the infection. Pigs, cattle, water buffalo and dogs, also field mice and wild rats, are animal hosts of S. japonicum.

4. *Mode of transmission.* The eggs of S. haematobium leave the body mainly with the urine; those of S. mansoni and S. japonicum with the feces. The egg hatches in water and the liberated larva or miracidium enters a suitable fresh water snail host. Free swimming larvae, cercariae, emerge from the snail after several weeks and penetrate the human skin, usually while the person is swimming or wading; they enter the blood stream, are carried to blood vessels of the liver, develop to maturity, and then migrate to veins of the abdominal cavity. Adults of S. mansoni and S. japonicum usually remain in mesenteric veins; those of S. haematobium usually migrate through anastomoses into the pelvic veins. Eggs are deposited in venules and, by necrosis of tissue, escape into the lumen of bowel or bladder, but may lodge in other organs.

5. *Incubation period.* Systemic manifestations usually begin when the worms are reaching maturity, about 4 to 6 weeks after infection. Eggs usually are found in feces or urine a week or two after onset of symptoms.

6. *Period of communicability.* As long as eggs are discharged in urine or feces of infected persons which may be 25 years or longer. Infected snails may give off cercariae for several months.

7. *Susceptibility and resistance.* Susceptibility is general; whether or not resistance develops as a result of infection is controversial.

8. *Occurrence.* S. mansoni occurs in the West Indies, northeastern and eastern South America, the Arabian peninsula, and Africa. S. haematobium occurs in Africa, in parts of the Middle East and in Bombay State, India. S. japonicum occurs in the Orient (Japan, China, Formosa, Philippines, Celebes). No species is indigenous to continental North America. In some endemic areas more than half of the population is infected.

"Swimmer's itch" is prevalent among bathers in lakes in many parts of the world including North America; also in certain coastal sea water beaches.

9. *Methods of control:*
  A. Preventive measures:
  1. Disposal of feces and urine so that eggs will not reach bodies of fresh water containing snail intermediate host.
  2. Treatment of snail breeding places with molluscacides, and other methods of snail destruction.
  3. Provision of water for drinking, bathing and washing clothes from sources free from cercariae.
  4. Provision of cercaria-repellent or cercaria-proof clothing for persons required to enter contaminated water.
  5. Education of people in endemic areas regarding mode of transmission and methods of protection.
  6. Mass treatment of infected persons in endemic areas may help to reduce transmission but in the past has not materially reduced incidence.
  B. Control of the infected individual, contacts and environment:
  1. Report to local health authority: In selected endemic areas; in many countries not a reportable disease.
  2. Isolation: None.
  3. Concurrent disinfection: Disposal of feces and urine.
  4. Terminal disinfection: None.
  5. Quarantine: None.
  6. Immunization: None.
  7. Investigation of contacts and sources of infection: Examine contacts for infection from a common source. The search for the source is a community effort, see 9C.
  8. Specific treatment: For S. mansoni and S. haematobium, fuadin intramuscularly. For S. haematobium (nilodin, miracil dihydrochloride) is efficacious in light infections, less so in heavy infections; disagreeable side effects but no serious toxicity. For S. japonicum, tartar emetic intravenously; toxic side effects occur.
  C. Epidemic measures: In areas of high incidence, or in endemic areas where non-indigenous groups such as military forces become infected, snail breeding places should be carefully determined and treated with molluscacides; entering infected water should be prohibited. Clean water should be provided, population should be examined for infection, and infected persons treated.
  D. International measures: None.

SCRUB TYPHUS

1. *Identification.* A rickettsial disease transmitted by trombiculid mites and characterized by a primary lesion and a rash late in the first week of fever. The primary lesion, usually on a protected area of skin and representing the site of attachment of the infected mite, precedes the acute febrile onset by several days. Headache, conjunctival injection and lymphadenopathy accompany the fever. A dull red maculopapular eruption appears on the trunk, extends to the extremities, and disappears in a few days. Cough and roentgenographic evidence of pneumonitis are common. In the absence of specific antibiotic therapy, fever lasts for 14 days.

[734]

Case fatality in untreated cases varies with locality (1 to 40%) and is regularly higher in older age groups. Synonyms: Tsutsugamushi disease, mite-borne typhus.

Isolation of the etiologic agent in mice, and specific complement fixation tests supplement the Weil-Felix reaction (Proteus OXK) in laboratory diagnosis of the disease.

2. *Etiologic agent.* Rickettsia tsutsugamushi.

3. *Source of infection.* Infected larval mites of Trombicula akamushi and related species which vary with locality. The nymphs and adults do not feed on vertebrate hosts. The agent is passed from generation to generation in mites; also maintained by a mite—wild-rodent—mite cycle.

4. *Mode of transmission.* By the bite of infected mites.

5. *Incubation period.* Usually 10 to 12 days but varies from 6 to 21.

6. *Period of communicability.* Not communicable from man to man.

7. *Susceptibility and resistance.* Susceptibility is general. An attack confers prolonged immunity against the homologous strain of R. tsutsugamushi but only transient immunity against heterologous strains. Heterologous infection within a few months results in mild disease but such infection after a year produces the typical illness. Second and even third attacks of naturally acquired scrub typhus are not uncommon in persons who spend their lives in endemic areas. Inactivated vaccine is useless as an immunizing agent.

8. *Occurrence.* Scrub typhus occurs in eastern and southeastern Asia, northern Australia, the Indian subcontinent and adjacent islands. It is a place disease acquired by man in one of the innumerable small sharply delimited "typhus islands" where the rickettsiae, the vector and the rodent reservoir exist simultaneously. Occupational habits greatly influence sex distribution, but with few exceptions the disease is restricted to adult workers who frequent scrub or overgrown terrain. In the Pescadores Islands children are more often attacked because infected rodents and mites inhabit rock walls around gardens of homes. Epidemics occur when susceptibles are brought into endemic areas, a repeated observation among troops of World War II; in certain regiments and battalions 20 to 50% of men were infected within weeks or months.

9. *Methods of control:*

A. Preventive measures:

1. The aim is to prevent contact with infected mites, to eliminate mites and rodents from particular sites and to promote resistance to the disease.

2. Personal prophylaxis against the mite vector is by use of clothes and blankets impregnated with miticidal chemicals, together with application of mite repellents to exposed skin surfaces.

3. In military practice selected camp sites are cleared of vegetation by stripping with a bulldozer, the vegetation destroyed by burning, the area sprayed with residual miticidal chemicals (effective for several weeks or a month) and rodent control measures instituted.

4. Attempts to render man insusceptible to scrub typhus are generally impractical. That result can be attained in special instances by chemoprophylaxis with chloramphenicol, or immunization by a combined procedure of infection with living unattenuated vaccine and suppression of clinical disease by chemoprophylaxis.

B. Control of the infected individual, contacts and environment:

1. Report to local health authority: In selected endemic areas, with clear distinction from endemic and epidemic typhus; in many countries not a reportable disease.
2. Isolation: None.
3. Concurrent disinfection: None.
4. Terminal disinfection: None.
5. Quarantine: None.
6. Immunization: None.
7. Investigation of contacts and source of infection: None.
8. Specific treatment: One of the tetracycline antibiotics of chloramphenicol orally in a loading dose followed by divided doses daily until patient is afebrile (average 30 hours). If treatment is instituted within the first three days a second course should be given about the 8th day after onset to prevent relapse.

C. Epidemic measures:

1. Rigorously employed procedures described in 9A2 and 9A3 for all persons of the affected area.
2. Daily observation for fever and appearance of primary lesion of all persons at risk; institute treatment promptly at first indication of illness.
3. Consider use of chemoprophylaxis for key personnel in area; combined live vaccine–chemoprophylaxis may be considered prior to entering areas of known risk.

D. International measures: None.

SMALLPOX

1. *Identification.* An exanthematous disease characterized by sudden onset with fever, chills, headache, severe backache and prostration, continuing for 3 to 4 days. The temperature then falls and a rash appears which passes through stages of macule, papule, vesicle and pustule, forms crusts and finally scabs which fall off at about the end of the third week. The eruption is usually symmetrical and general, more profuse on prominences, extensor surfaces and surfaces exposed to irritation than on protected surfaces, flexures and depressions. Most abundant and earliest on the face, next on forearms, wrists and hands, and favoring the limbs, especially distally, more than the trunk. More abundant on shoulders and chest than on loins or abdomen, but lesions may be so few as to be overlooked.

Smallpox varies from a mild disease (variola minor) with a fatality under one per cent to a severe condition (classical smallpox, variola major) with about 30 per cent fatality; in recent years the disease has kept closely to these extremes, breeding true to type as regards severity. An uncommon fulminating form, hemorrhagic smallpox, is characterized by purpura, hemorrhages into the skin, and death within 3 to 4 days, usually before the typical rash appears. The mild type, variola minor or alastrim, has mild prodromal symptoms, a discrete and scanty rash and a more rapid progression of lesions. Previous vaccination commonly leads to modification of both the mild and classical forms of the disease, in timing and maturation of rash, and in other clinical features.

Laboratory confirmation can be had within 24 hours through demonstration of specific antigen in vesicular and pustular fluid from cutaneous lesions by com-

[736]

plement-fixation with rabbit antivaccinal serum; or within a few days through isolation of smallpox virus from chick embryos inoculated with such materials.

2. *Etiologic agent.* The virus of smallpox.

3. *Source and reservoir of infection.* Lesions of skin and mucous membrane and respiratory discharges of patients.

4. *Mode of transmission.* By contact with persons sick with the disease. Contact need not be intimate; aerial transmission may occur over short distances within closed spaces. Also spread by articles or persons freshly contaminated by respiratory discharges or by lesions of the skin and mucous membranes of the sick; scabs remain infectious for variable periods.

5. *Incubation period.* Seven to 16 days, commonly 12 days. A good working value in epidemiological investigations is 10 days from rash to onset of second illness, or 14 days from rash to rash, the latter being the more useful in field practice.

6. *Period of communicability.* From first symptoms to disappearance of all scabs and crusts, a period of about 2 to 3 weeks. Most communicable in the early stages of the disease.

7. *Susceptibility and resistance.* Susceptibility is universal, although exposure of a susceptible person does not always result in the disease. Permanent immunity usually follows recovery; second attacks are rare. Immunity acquired by vaccination gradually diminishes; it may be completely effective for less than 2 years or for more than 20 years.

8. *Occurrence.* Distributions within countries of the world range from sporadic to endemic to epidemic, varying widely according to immunity status of a population and frequency of imported infection. Incidence is greatest in winter and least in summer. The disease is still a serious problem in parts of Asia, Africa and South America.

9. *Methods of control:*
   A. Preventive measures:
   1. Vaccination at about the third month of age, revaccination on entering school, and of all persons facing unusual exposure, as in travel to endemic regions or presence of smallpox. Revaccination under conditions of sustained high risk may be practiced at intervals as short as every six months, as with troops in military operations.
   2. Measures to assure available supplies of potent glycerinated smallpox vaccine maintained below freezing up to the hour of vaccination, to include time in transit or shipment. Dried calf lymph vaccine is available for use under special conditions, mainly tropical.
   3. To avoid complications, insertion of vaccine should be over a small area of skin, not over one-eighth inch in any direction, and preferably by the multiple pressure method (acupuncture). If the scratch method is employed, care should be taken to avoid drawing blood. The site should be kept dry and cool without the use of shields or dressings. The deltoid area of the arm is the preferred site; leg vaccination should be avoided. Primary vaccination should be about the third month of age, provided the child has no eczema or other contraindication; patients with eczema should not come in contact with recently vaccinated persons. Vaccination during the warmer months is preferably avoided.

   Revaccination with a fully potent vaccine, of persons immunized more than ten years previously, gives at least 50% of vaccinoid (accelerated) reactions.

The site of revaccination should be carefully observed and the reaction recorded twice, on the 3rd and 9th days after vaccination, to determine whether the maximum diameter of redness occurred under three days (immediate or early reaction, formerly called immune reaction), or after 7 days (vaccinia), or intermediate between the two (vaccinoid reaction). The common result is either an immediate or accelerated reaction. The accelerated reaction indicates persisting protection; the immediate reaction, if marked by a firm indurated papule at the site of revaccination, probably does. Errors in interpretation of the early reaction are frequent; inactive vaccine sometimes gives the same response, trauma also confuses and sometimes secondary infection. If in doubt, revaccinate; with no reaction, always revaccinate.

B. Control of the infected individual, contacts and environment:

1. Report to local health authority: Case report universally required by international regulation.
2. Isolation: Hospital isolation in screened wards or rooms until all scabs and crusts have disappeared.
3. Concurrent disinfection: Oral and nasal discharges to be deposited in a paper bag or other suitable container and burned. All articles associated with the patient to be sterilized by high pressure steam or by boiling.
4. Terminal disinfection: Thorough cleaning of sick room and furniture; sterilization of mattress, pillow and bedding.
5. Quarantine: All persons living or working on the same premises as the person who develops smallpox should be considered contacts, and quarantined until vaccinated with a fully potent vaccine or for 16 days from last exposure. If vaccination was within 48 hours of first exposure, surveillance may be substituted with daily medical observation until height of reaction has passed; sometimes the requirement of surveillance is 16 days. Any rise of temperature calls for prompt isolation until smallpox can be excluded.
6. Immunization: Prompt vaccination of contacts with a potent vaccine.
7. Investigation of contacts and source of infection: The immediately prior case should be sought assiduously. Adults with chickenpox or patients with hemorrhagic or pustular lesions of the skin, particularly those associated in time or place with known smallpox, need careful review for errors in diagnosis.
8. Specific treatment: None.

C. Epidemic measures:

1. Hospital care of patients and suspects until no longer communicable.
2. Careful listing of all contacts and rigorous enforcement of quarantine until protected by successful vaccination; surveillance for 16 days from last exposure.
3. Immediate publicity by all available methods, giving a simple, clear and frank statement of the situation and urging all individuals in the area to be vaccinated. Provide potent vaccine to physicians and hospitals; establish vaccination clinics for those without a private physician.
4. Mass immunization of whole populations of a community or larger area is an emergency measure to be used when smallpox has entered a community, given evidence of material spread, and obviously is out of control.

D. International measures:

1. Telegraphic notification of WHO and adjacent countries by governments of the existence of an epidemic of smallpox.

2. Measures applicable to ships, aircraft and land transport arriving from small-pox areas are specified in International Sanitary Regulations (WHO Techn. Rept. Ser. No. 41, Geneva, 1951).

3. International travellers: Evidence of a previous attack of smallpox or of recent vaccination is a widely enforced requirement for entrance to or departure from a country. The validity of an international certificate of vaccination against smallpox extends for a period of 3 years beginning 8 days after the date of a successful primary vaccination, or in the event of a revaccination, on the date of that revaccination.

STREPTOCOCCAL INFECTIONS, HEMOLYTIC

Group A hemolytic streptococci cause a wide variety of conditions differentiated clinically according to portal of entry and tissue of localization of the infectious agent, and presence or absence of a scarlatinal rash. The more important conditions are:

A. Scarlet fever and streptococcal sore throat (tonsillitis-pharyngitis).

B. Erysipelas.

C. Puerperal infection.

Streptococcal infections, other than those just mentioned but caused by the same strains of Group A streptococci, include: cellulitis, lymphadenitis, mastoiditis, osteo-myelitis, otitis media, peritonitis, septicemia, and various skin and wound infections. Those characterized by purulent exudates are most likely to spread infection, but others such as septicemia are also important because of frequent association with upper respira-tory streptococcal carrier states. Insofar as these clinical categories are caused by Group A streptococci, they are different manifestations of the same infectious agent, and there-fore should be treated together in their epidemiologic relationships. They constitute an epidemiologic entity, and similar principles of control hold generally for the group.

A. SCARLET FEVER AND STREPTOCOCCAL SORE THROAT (STREPTOCOCCAL TONSILLITIS, STREPTOCOCCAL NASOPHARYNGITIS)

1. *Identification.* Scarlet fever is ordinarily streptococcal sore throat in which the in-fectious agent is capable of producing erythrogenic toxin and the patient has relatively no antitoxic immunity. If the organism is not a good toxin producer, or if the patient is immune to the toxin, the rash does not occur and streptococcal sore throat results. The distinguishing characteristics are fever, sore throat, exudative tonsillitis or pharyngitis, tender cervical adenopathy, leucocytosis, enanthem, strawberry tongue and rash (exanthem). Infection and edema of the pharynx involve the faucial pillars and soft palate, often extending to the hard palate; petechiae are sometimes seen against the background of diffuse redness. Tonsils, if present, often show the exudate of acute follicular tonsillitis. The rash is usually a fine erythema, commonly punctate, blanching on pressure and ap-pearing most often on the neck, chest, in the folds of the axilla, elbow and groin and on the inner aspects of the thighs. Typically the rash does not involve the face except in Negroes, but there is flushing of the cheeks and circumoral pallor. Pyrexia, nausea, and vomiting accompany severe infections. The desquamation of convalescence is seen at the tips of the fingers and toes and less often over wide areas of the trunk and limbs, including palms and soles. Scarlet fever occasion-ally occurs in patients with other types of streptococcal infections, such as in-fected wounds. Severity of the disease has been decreasing in the United States

[739   ]

for unknown reasons, fatality is low, about one death for each 300–400 reported cases. Fatality rates in some parts of the world are 3–5%.

Streptococcal sore throat is scarlet fever infection without a rash. The manifestations of this clinical entity are similar to scarlet fever, except that toxic manifestations including rash do not occur, nor does desquamation follow.

Laboratory diagnostic aids include demonstration of a typable Group A streptococcus as the predominant organism in cultures of the throat, and a rise in serum antibody titer (antistreptolysin O, antistreptokinase) from acute to convalescent phase of the illness.

2. *Etiologic agent.* Streptococcus pyogenes, Group A streptococci, of at least 40 serologically distinct types which vary greatly in geographic and time distributions. Two immunologically different types (A and B) of erythrogenic toxin have been demonstrated.

3. *Source and reservoir of infection.* Discharges from nose, throat or purulent complications of acutely ill or convalescent patients or carriers, or objects contaminated with such discharges. Nasal carriers are particularly liable to contaminate their environment.

4. *Mode of transmission.* Transmission is by direct contact with patient or carrier, or by indirect contact through objects handled, or by droplet spread whereby streptococci are inhaled; casual contact rarely leads to infection. Streptococci reach the air via contaminated floor dust, lint from bedclothing, personal clothing, handkerchiefs, or occasionally in droplet nuclei discharged by coughing or sneezing; the importance of air-borne transmission and contamination of the environment in spread of infection has not been clearly established. Explosive outbreaks may follow the ingestion of contaminated milk or other food.

5. *Incubation period.* Short, usually 2 to 5 days.

6. *Period of communicability.* In uncomplicated cases, during incubation and clinical illness, approximately 10 days. Thereafter in untreated patients, communicability decreases progressively, becoming negligible in 2–3 weeks although the carrier state may persist for months. Persons with untreated complications resulting in purulent discharges may spread infection for weeks or months. Adequate treatment with penicillin will eliminate probability of transmission from patients or carriers within 24 hours.

7. *Susceptibility and resistance.* Susceptibility is general, although many persons develop either antitoxic or type-specific antibacterial immunity, or both, through inapparent infection. Antibacterial immunity develops only against the type of Group A streptococcus which induces the patient's disease or inapparent infection, and lasts at least several years. Second attacks of streptococcal sore throat, due to a different type of streptococcus, are not uncommon. The frequency of inapparent infection is unknown, but undoubtedly is related to the prevalence of streptococci, and possibly to the type of streptococcus.

Immunity against erythrogenic toxin, and hence to rash, develops within a week of the onset of scarlet fever and is usually permanent. Second attacks of scarlet fever are rare but may occur because of the two immunological forms of toxin.

Both active and passive immunization against erythrogenic toxin are possible but not practical. Neither active nor passive immunization against the streptococcus itself can be accomplished satisfactorily at the present time.

[740]

APPENDIX D

8. *Occurrence.* Clinical disease is most common in temperate zones, less common in semi-tropical areas and rare in tropical climates. Inapparent infections are as common or more common in the tropics than in temperate zones.

In the United States, epidemiological behavior may be endemic, epidemic, or sporadic. Epidemic occurrence is more frequent in certain geographic areas, such as New England, the Great Lakes region and the Rocky Mountain area. Apart from food-borne epidemics, which may occur in any season, the highest incidence is during late winter and spring; generally in the 5–9 year age group; no sex or racial susceptibilities have been defined. Scarlet fever has followed a similar pattern in central Europe, the Scandinavian countries and Spain during the past two decades.

9. *Methods of control:*
   A. Preventive measures:
      1. Provision for throat cultures, with isolation of hemolytic streptococci and identification of serologic group and type.
      2. Emphasis on the fact that absence of rash does not decrease the danger of streptococcal infection.
      3. Boiling or pasteurization of milk.
      4. Exclusion of infected persons from handling milk or other food likely to be contaminated.
      5. Milk from any cow with evidence of mastitis should be excluded from sale or use.
      6. Chemoprophylaxis with oral sulfonamide drugs (0.5 to 1.0 gram per day) or penicillin (200,000 to 250,000 units twice a day on an empty stomach) for persons in whom recurrent streptococcal infection provides a special risk, such as individuals who have had rheumatic fever or chorea within 5 years or are under 18 years of age.
   B. Control of the infected individual, contacts, and environment:
      Control of streptococcal infections depends on preventing the dissemination of Group A streptococci and their implantation in the tissues of susceptible subjects.
      1. Report to local health authority: Case report of scarlet fever required in most states and countries. Notification of streptococcal sore throat is inaccurate and of limited value in control because of difficulty in diagnosis and differentiation from non-bacterial exudative tonsillitis and pharyngitis; recommended that reporting be limited to epidemics.
      2. Isolation: In order of preference, in a single room, cubicle or small ward; in uncomplicated cases until clinical recovery or not less than 7 days from onset. Isolation may be terminated after 24 hours treatment with penicillin, provided therapy is continued for 7–10 days.
      3. Concurrent disinfection: Of purulent discharges and all articles soiled therewith.
      4. Terminal disinfection: Thorough cleaning; sunning or other treatment of blankets.
      5. Quarantine: None.
      6. Immunization: None.
      7. Investigation of contacts and source of infection: Not indicated in sporadic cases.
      8. Specific treatment: Penicillin, either procaine penicillin intramuscularly or bicillin or aqueous penicillin. Penicillin G by mouth may be effective, continued

for 10 days. Therapy should be started early and continued for six or seven days if rheumatic fever is to be prevented. The tetracycline antibiotics lead to rapid improvement and decreased incidence of rheumatic fever. Sulfonamide drugs are not recommended; scarlet fever antitoxin and pooled convalescent human serum are rarely used.

C. Epidemic measures:

1. Determine source and manner of spread, as person-to-person, by milk, or food-borne. Outbreaks can often be traced to an individual or animal with a persistent streptococcal infection through identification of the serologic type of streptococcus.

2. With limited population groups or under special circumstances, penicillin prophylaxis may be given to intimate and household contacts, to those known to have been exposed to contaminated milk or other food, or to the entire population group (see 9A6). In the latter circumstance, sulfonamide drugs should not be administered for prolonged periods because of likelihood that resistant strains of streptococci will develop.

3. Prompt investigation of any group of cases as to possibility of contaminated milk with exclusion of suspected milk supply from sale or use until pasteurized. Contamination of milk or food can occasionally or under special circumstances be determined by culture.

D. International measures: None.

B. ERYSIPELAS

1. *Identification.* An acute infection characterized by fever, constitutional symptoms, leucocytosis, and a red, tender, edematous, spreading lesion of the skin, having a well-marked, raised border. The central point of origin tends to clear as the periphery extends. Face and legs are common sites. Recurrences are frequent. The disease may be especially severe, with bacteremia, in patients suffering from debilitating disease.

Group A streptococci may be isolated from the margin of the skin lesion, the nose and throat, and occasionally from the blood. Erysipelas due to Group A streptococci is to be distinguished from erysipeloid, caused by Erysipelothrix rhusiopathiae, a localized cutaneous infection primarily an occupational disease of persons handling meat, fish, poultry and shellfish.

2. *Etiologic agent.* Streptococcus pyogenes, Group A streptococci, of at least 40 types. No specific strain or type has been shown to cause erysipelas.

3. *Source and reservoir of infection.* Persons infected with Group A streptococci, with the source either respiratory discharges of the same individual or of exogenous origin.

4. *Mode of transmission.* Transmission is by direct contact with patient or carrier, by indirect contact through objects handled, or by droplet spread whereby streptococci are inhaled. Streptococci reach the air through contaminated floor dust, lint from bedclothing, personal clothing, handkerchiefs, or occasionally in droplet nuclei discharged by coughing or sneezing. The importance of air-borne transmission has not been established. Erysipelas may be associated epidemiologically with other forms of Group A streptococcal infection.

5. *Incubation period.* Unknown; probably not more than 2 days.

6. *Period of communicability.* Unknown; presumably until clinical recovery, about 10 days in untreated patients. Adequate treatment with penicillin will eliminate probability of transmission from patients or carriers within 24 hours.

7. *Susceptibility and resistance.* Susceptibility is greatest in infants, in older persons and in the debilitated. One attack appears to predispose to subsequent attacks; recurrences may be due to streptococcal infection or to hypersensitivity. Whether or not type-specific immunity occurs is unknown. No available immunization procedures.

8. *Occurrence.* Geographic and seasonal distributions are similar to scarlet fever and streptococcal sore throat. Common after 20 years of age with highest attack rates at 40–60 years, occurs frequently in infants. No clear predilection for sex or race has been defined. Occurrence is sporadic, even during epidemics of streptococcal infection.

9. *Methods of control:*

    A. Preventive measures:

        1. Personal cleanliness and avoidance of transferring the infectious agent to the broken skin.

        2. Chemoprophylaxis with oral sulfonamide drugs or penicillin as for scarlet fever and streptococcal sore throat.

        3. Recurrence of erysipelas may be prevented by administration of oral sulfonamide drugs or penicillin during and after convalescence, to be continued for months or years depending on the individual situation.

    B. Control of the infected individual, contacts and environment:

        1. Report to local health authority: Obligatory report of epidemics; no individual case report.

        2. Isolation: During period of communicability; patients are a potential danger to young infants and to surgical and obstetrical patients. Isolation may be terminated after 24 hours treatment with penicillin, provided therapy is continued for 7–10 days.

        3. Concurrent disinfection: Of dressings and discharges from lesions.

        4. Terminal disinfection: Thorough cleaning; sunning or other treatment of blankets.

        5. Quarantine: None.

        6. Immunization: None.

        7. Investigation of contacts and source of infection: None.

        8. Specific treatment: Penicillin; procaine penicillin is preferred but oral penicillin G has been used; continue for 7 to 10 days. The tetracycline antibiotics or sulfonamide drugs may be substituted if patient is sensitive to penicillin.

    C. Epidemic measures: Erysipelas is now rarely epidemic in the western world. In the event of an outbreak in a limited population group, institution or hospital, prophylactic administration of penicillin or sulfonamide drugs, as outlined under scarlet fever and streptococcal sore throat.

    D. International measures: None.

C. Streptococcal Puerperal Fever (Puerperal Septicemia)

1. *Identification.* An acute infection, usually febrile, accompanied by local and general symptoms and signs of bacterial invasion of the genital tract and sometimes of the blood of the postpartum or postabortum patient.

[743]

The causative agent can be recovered by bacterial culture of vaginal discharges, cervix and blood and identified by bacteriologic and serologic methods.

A goodly proportion of puerperal infections are of other origin than hemolytic streptococci. They are to be differentiated by appropriate bacteriological means, for they are clinically similar. The infecting microorganisms include a variety of bacterial agents, nonhemolytic streptococci, anaerobic streptococci, Staphylococcus aureus, Escherichia coli, Clostridium welchii, Bacteroides sp., and others. Group A streptococci are of primary importance in postpartum infection; the anaerobic organisms, colon bacilli and staphylococci in postabortum infections. Treatment is by appropriate antibiotics. Epidemiologic characteristics and methods of control now described for Group A streptococcal infections apply equally to the others.

2. *Etiologic agent.* Streptococcus pyogenes, Group A hemolytic streptococci; hemolytic streptococci of Groups B, C, D, and G. Mixed infections with other bacteria are common.

3. *Source and reservoir of infection.* From an external source or from the respiratory tract, intestinal tract, genital tract, or skin of the patient. In postpartum infections due to Group A streptococci, the organism comes from an attendant in about half of cases, from a familial contact in about one-fifth, and from the patient's respiratory tract in the remainder. In postabortum infections, the organism most frequently comes from the patient herself due to faulty or inadequate aseptic technic.

4. *Mode of transmission.* Direct transfer of infectious agent to uterus may be accomplished by hands or by instruments used in examinations before, during or following parturition or abortion; transfer of organisms to the genital tract from nose and throat of a carrier or infected attendant, or from the patient's respiratory tract, intestinal tract or skin, is usually by the hands; indirectly as for other streptococcal and wound infections.

5. *Incubation period.* One to three days, rarely longer.

6. *Period of communicability.* During persistence of infectious discharges from genital tract of the patient. Infectiousness of the patient herself, in the case of Group A streptococcal infection, will become negligible after 24–48 hours of adequate penicillin therapy. In institutional outbreaks contamination of the environment may be extensive and persistent for days or weeks.

7. *Susceptibility and resistance.* Susceptibility is general. The birth process and the abortion procedure increase the opportunity for implantation of pathogenic bacteria.

8. *Occurrence.* World wide in distribution but reliable morbidity data are not available. In the United States, mortality has declined more than 80% in the past 15 years, and case fatality has dropped precipitously since the advent of antibiotic drugs; greater for white than non-white races. Similar changes have occurred throughout the western world. Now is chiefly a sporadic disease, although epidemics may occur in institutions where aseptic technics are faulty.

9. *Methods of control:*

A. Preventive measures:

    1. Maintenance of high standards of prenatal care and extension of such services to all segments of the population.

2. Strict asepsis in obstetrical procedures with special attention to possible contamination from mouth and nose of attendants as well as by hands and instruments.

3. Protection of patient during labor and postpartum from attendants, visitors and other patients with respiratory or skin infection.

4. Bacteriologic search for carriers among attendants, physicians, nurses, and nursemaids.

5. Prophylactic use of antibiotic drugs in patients undergoing difficult deliveries or sustaining complications that predispose to infection, such as premature rupture of membranes, severe lacerations or retained products of conception.

6. Education of women in the hazards of self-interruption of pregnancy.

B. Control of the infected individual, contacts and environment:

1. Report to local health authority: Obligatory report of epidemics; no individual case report.

2. Isolation: Strict isolation while infectious discharges persist. In patients with Group A streptococcal infection, isolation may be terminated after 24 hours treatment with penicillin, provided therapy is continued for 7–10 days.

3. Concurrent disinfection: Of dressings and discharges.

4. Terminal disinfection: Thorough cleaning; sunning or other treatment of blankets.

5. Quarantine: None.

6. Immunization: None.

7. Investigation of contacts and source of infection: Serologic typing of strains of Group A streptococci is of value in tracing the source of infection.

8. Specific treatment: Penicillin as for other streptococcal infections. Strict aseptic technic must be used in examination, obtaining of cultures or surgical interference since all vaginal manipulations increase the danger of reinfection or the introduction of new organisms.

C. Epidemic measures: The most probable cause of an epidemic of streptococcal infection is a Group A streptococcus and the most likely location is a hospital or maternity home. General asepsis should be strictly enforced. The identity and source of the infecting strain of streptococcus should be determined. Infected attendants or carriers should be treated with penicillin. Other personnel and patients may be given oral penicillin prophylactically (200,000 to 250,000 units twice a day on an empty stomach).

D. International measures: None.

SYPHILIS

A. Venereal Syphilis

1. *Identification.* An acute and chronic relapsing treponematosis characterized clinically by a primary lesion, a secondary eruption involving skin and mucous membranes, long periods of latency, and late lesions of skin, bone, viscera, the central nervous and cardiovascular systems. The primary lesion appears at about 3 weeks as a papule, and after erosion presents a variety of forms, the most distinctive although not the most frequent being an indurated chancre; invasion of the blood precedes the initial lesion; a hard non-fluctuant painless satellite bubo commonly follows. Infection without chancre is fairly frequent. During the next

[745]

4 to 6 weeks, even without specific treatment the chancre begins to involute and the generalized secondary eruption appears, often accompanied by mild constitutional symptoms. Secondary manifestations disappear spontaneously within a few weeks to as long as 12 months, with subsequent clinical latency of weeks to years, often interrupted in early years by recurrence of infectious lesions of skin and mucous membrane or developing lesions of the eye and central nervous system; in later years (5 to 20) by explosive destructive non-infectious lesions of skin, bone and mucosal surfaces. Latency sometimes continues through life, sometimes spontaneous recovery occurs and in other instances and unpredictably late disabling manifestations of cardiovascular, central nervous or other system appear. Actual case fatality is unknown; prenatal infection is frequently fatal, before birth or in infancy. Early acquired syphilis does not result in death or serious disability but the late manifestations shorten life, impair health and limit occupational efficiency.

Primary and secondary syphilis are confirmed by dark field examination of exudates of lesions; in all instances by serologic tests for syphilis through examination of blood or spinal fluid, with treponemal immobilization or agglutination tests to exude biologic false positive reactions.

2. *Etiologic agent.* Treponema pallidum.

3. *Source and reservoir of infection.* Exudates from obvious or concealed moist early lesions of skin and mucous membrane of infected persons; body fluids and secretions (saliva, semen, blood, vaginal discharges) during infectious period.

4. *Mode of transmission.* By direct contact (sexual intercourse, kissing, fondling of children) during primary and secondary syphilis. Transmission through indirect contact with contaminated articles has relatively little significance. Prenatal infection may occur during the first four months of pregnancy through placental transfer of treponemata.

5. *Incubation period.* Ten days to 10 weeks, usually 3 weeks.

6. *Period of communicability.* Variable and not definitely known; during primary and secondary stages and during mucocutaneous recurrence which may occur intermittently during 2–4 years. Extent of communicability through sexual intercourse during early latent period (2–4 years) has not been established; the possibility of inapparent lesions requires that this stage be considered potentially infectious.

7. *Susceptibility and resistance.* Susceptibility is universal; no natural immunity. Infection leads to gradually developing resistance against the homologous strain and to an extent against heterologous strains of treponema; may be overcome by large reinfecting doses or fail to develop by reason of early treatment. Superinfection may produce lesions simulating those of the currently existing stage; in late latency, superinfection has special significance through ability to produce benign late lesions of skin and mucous membrane.

8. *Occurrence.* One of the more frequent communicable diseases; widespread throughout the world and primarily involving young persons between ages 15 and 30 years. The considerable differences in racial incidence are related more to social than to biologic factors.

9. *Methods of control:*

A. Preventive measures. The following are applicable to all venereal diseases: syphilis, chancroid, lyphogranuloma venereum, granuloma inguinale and gonorrhea.

[746]

1. General health promotional measures, health and sex education, preparation for marriage, premarital and prenatal examinations as part of general physical examination. Improvement of social and economic conditions, including recreational facilities.

2. Protection of the community by suppression of commercialized prostitution and of clandestine sexual promiscuity, in cooperation with social and law enforcement agencies; by teaching methods of personal prophylaxis applicable before, during and after exposure; by repeated prenatal serologic examination of all pregnant women.

3. Provision of facilities for early diagnosis and treatment; encouragement of their use through education of the public concerning symptoms of the venereal diseases and modes of spread, and through making these services available irrespective of economic status of the infected person. Intensive case-finding programs, to include interview of patients and tracing of contacts, and repeated mass serologic examination of special groups with known high incidence of venereal disease.

4. An emphasis on control of patients with venereal disease in a transmissible stage should not preclude search for persons past that stage; has value in preventing relapse, congenital syphilis and disability due to late manifestations.

B. Control of the infected individual, contacts and environment:

1. Report to local health authority: Case report is required in all states of the United States and variously in other countries. Reporting in the United States is commonly too incomplete to be a reliable guide to administrative practice. Accurate reporting has increasing value as syphilis declines, as a means to determine the amount of effort to be expended on control activities.

2. Isolation: None; modern therapy limits communicability to 24 hours or less. To avoid reinfection, patients should refrain from sexual intercourse with previous partners not under treatment.

3. Concurrent disinfection: None; care in disposal of discharges from open lesions and articles soiled therewith.

4. Terminal disinfection: None.

5. Quarantine: None.

6. Immunization: None.

7. Investigation of contacts and source of infection: Interview of patients and tracing of contacts are the fundamental features of a program for control of venereal disease. Trained interviewers obtain the best results. The stage of the disease determines criteria for contact tracing: (a) for primary syphilis, all sex contacts of preceding 3 months; (b) for secondary syphilis, those of the preceding 6 months; (c) for early latent syphilis, those of the preceding 1 year provided time of primary and secondary lesions is not established; (d) for late and late latent syphilis, marital partners and children of infected mothers; (e) for congenital syphilis, all members of immediate family.

8. Specific treatment: Penicillin; dosage depends on stage of disease and whether on individual or mass control basis. In general, large amounts should be given initially on the day of diagnosis to assure reasonably effective therapy if the patient fails to return. Consideration should be given to a plan whereby a full course of antibiotic therapy is given as abortive or "preventive" treatment to contacts of patients with proven primary or secondary syphilis.

[747]

C. Epidemic measures: Intensification of measures outlined under 9A and 9B.

D. International measures:

    1. Appropriate examination of groups of adolescents and young adults moving from areas of high prevalence of treponemal infections.

    2. Adherence to agreements among nations (e.g. Brussels agreement) as to records, and provision of diagnostic, treatment and contact interviewing facilities at seaports for foreign seamen engaged in maritime commerce.

    3. Provision for rapid international exchange of information on contacts.

B. NON-VENEREAL SYPHILIS

1. *Identification.* "Endemic syphilis" and bejel, non-venereally transmitted treponematoses, are acute infections, predominantly household diseases characterized clinically by an eruption of skin and mucous membrane, usually without evident initial primary sore. Early skin lesions, indistinguishable from those of venereal syphilis, are macular or papular, often hypertrophic and frequently circinate; mucous patches of the mouth often appear first, soon followed by moist papules in folds of skin and by drier lesions on trunk and extremities. Plantar and palmar hyperkeratoses frequently occur in bejel, often with painful fissuring; a patchy depigmentation and hyperpigmentation of the skin, and alopecia, are common. Inflammatory or destructive lesions of skin, long bones and nasopharynx are late manifestations. Unlike venereal syphilis, the nervous and cardiovascular systems seem rarely to be involved. Case fatality is negligible.

    Serologic tests for syphilis are reactive in the early stages and remain so for many years of latency, gradually tending toward non-reactivity; response to treatment as in venereal syphilis.

2. *Etiologic agent.* Treponema pallidum.

3. *Source and reservoir of infection.* Infected persons; surfaces and exudates of early lesions of skin and mucous membrane.

4. *Mode of transmission.* Direct household or other contact with infectious lesions; common eating and drinking utensils, household crowding under substandard hygienic conditions; flies, lice and fleas are possible factors. Congenital transmission is rare.

5. *Incubation period.* 2 weeks to 3 months, usually about 6 weeks.

6. *Period of communicability.* During the period of moist eruptions of skin and until mucous patches disappear; may extend over several weeks or months.

7. *Susceptibility and resistance.* Similar to venereal syphilis.

8. *Occurrence.* A common disease in local areas; known as endemic syphilis in the Balkans and in Turkey, and as bejel in Eastern Mediterranean regions. The two conditions resemble each other in practically all respects, occurring equally in the two sexes and primarily among infants and young children. An apparently similar syndrome has been reported by other names in various parts of the world, as sibbens in Scotland and radesyke in Scandinavia.

9. *Methods of control.* The considerable decline in overt early venereal syphilis throughout much of the world calls for particular attention to non-venereal treponematoses, not yet under control, including yaws.

A. Preventive measures:

    1. Those of the non-venereal treponematoses. See Yaws 9A.

B. Control of the infected individual, contacts and environment:
 1. Report to local health authority: In selected endemic areas; in most countries not a reportable disease.
 2. See Yaws 9B for Items 2–8, applicable to all non-venereal treponematoses.
C. Epidemic measures: Intensification of preventive and control activities.
D. International measures: See Yaws 9D.

TAENIASIS AND CYSTICERCOSIS

1. *Identification.* Cestode infection of man is manifest in two forms, the one a benign intestinal infection with the adult worm of two species, beef and pork tapeworms, and the other a severe somatic disease (cysticercosis) of many different tissues arising through localization of larvae of the pork tapeworm.

 Clinical manifestations of infection with the adult worm are variable, frequently vague or absent, sometimes nervousness, insomnia, anorexia, loss of weight, abdominal pain, and digestive disturbances. A non-fatal disease. Synonym: beef or pork tapeworm infection. Infection with adult tapeworms is confirmed through identification of proglottides (segments) of the worm or of eggs in feces. Specific diagnosis is through morphological characters of the gravid proglottides (strobia), usually obtained after treatment; obtaining the scolex or head confirms the identification and assures elimination of the worm.

 If eggs of the pork tapeworm are swallowed by man, they will hatch in the small intestine and the larval forms (cysticerci) will develop in the subcutaneous tissues, striated muscles and other regions of the body. Grave consequences can ensue when they localize in heart, eye or central nervous system. Recognition of subcutaneous or somatic cysticercosis is by excision of the larva and microscopic examination. In the presence of cerebral symptoms, somatic cysticercosis strongly suggests cerebral involvement. Roentgen ray examination is helpful in locating calcified cysticeri in the brain and somatic muscles, and in determining the intensity of infection. A chronic disease with ultimate high case fatality.

 Other species, including Hymenolepsis nana, the common dwarf tapeworm, and H. diminuta, and Dipylidium caninum, are relatively rare adult tapeworms of man, have doubtful pathogenicity, but the eggs must be differentiated from taenia eggs.
2. *Etiologic agent.* Taenia saginata, the beef tapeworm of man, intestinal infection with adult worm only; Taenia solium, the pork tapeworm of man, intestinal infection with adult worm and somatic infection with larvae (cysticercosis).
3. *Source and reservoir of infection.* Immediate source of infection for Taenia saginata is the flesh of infected cattle; reservoir is feces of an infected person. For intestinal taeniasis due to Taenia solium the source of infection is the flesh of infected pigs, and the reservoir is eggs in feces of infected persons.
4. *Mode of transmission.* For Taenia saginata, by ingestion of raw or inadequately cooked beef containing the infective larva—a cysticercus. For Taenia solium (1) by ingestion of raw or inadequately cooked pork containing the infective larva (cysticercus) resulting in the development of the adult worm in the intestine; or (2) by direct hand to mouth transfer of eggs in feces, or indirectly through ingestion of food or water contaminated with eggs, resulting in somatic cysticercosis.
5. *Incubation period.* Eight to ten weeks.

6. *Period of communicability.* The adult worm of Taenia saginata is not transmissible from man to man; eggs are disseminated in the environment as long as man harbors the worm in the intestine. Man disseminates eggs of Taenia solium as long as the worm is harbored in the intestine. Transmission of adult worms from man to man is impossible.

7. *Susceptibility and resistance.* Man is universally susceptible. No apparent resistance follows infection.

8. *Occurrence.* Cosmopolitan distribution; particularly prevalent wherever beef or pork is eaten raw or slightly cooked. Incidence is highest in tropical countries and in the Slavic countries of Europe. Where Taenia saginata and Taenia solium co-exist, Taenia saginata is by far the commoner. Infection with T. solium is rare in the United States and Canada.

9. *Methods of control:*

   A. Preventive measures:
   1. Prevention of soil pollution with human feces in rural areas, improvement in barnyard sanitation, and education of the public.
   2. Thorough cooking of beef and pork insures against infection.
   3. Since cysticercosis in cattle is usually a light infection, meat inspection is of limited value; cysticercosis in swine is often intense and meat inspection can eliminate much infective pork from markets but cannot insure against infection.
   4. Immediate treatment of persons harboring adult Taenia solium is essential to prevent human cysticercosis.

   B. Control of the infected individual, contacts and environment:
   1. Report to local health authority: Official report not ordinarily justifiable.
   2. Isolation: None. Patients with T. solium infection should be excluded from food preparation and serving.
   3. Concurrent disinfection: Sanitary disposal of feces; for T. solium rigid sanitation with washing of hands after defecating and before eating.
   4. Terminal disinfection: None.
   5. Quarantine: None.
   6. Immunization: None.
   7. Investigation of contacts and source of infection: Usually not a profitable procedure.
   8. Specific treatment: Oleoresin of aspidium is used most commonly for intestinal taeniasis; successful results have been reported with quinacrine. No specific therapy for cysticercosis.

   C. Epidemic measures: None.
   D. International measures: None.

TETANUS

1. *Identification.* An acute disease induced by toxin of the tetanus bacillus; characterized by painful muscular contractions, primarily of masseter and neck muscles, and secondarily of the trunk; rigidity is sometimes confined to the region of injury. History of injury and known portal of entry sometimes lacking. Much variation in fatality according to age and length of incubation; average about 30–40%. Tetanus neonatorum, usually through infection of the unhealed

umbilicus, appears first as a general illness of the infant, refusal to nurse, stiffness of the jaws, and later rigid convulsions ending almost invariably in death.

2. *Etiologic agent.* Clostridium tetani, tetanus bacillus.

3. *Source and reservoir of infection.* Soil, street dust, and animal feces.

4. *Mode of transmission.* Direct or indirect inoculation of wound.

5. *Incubation period.* Commonly 4 days to 3 weeks, dependent somewhat upon the character, extent, and location of the wound; longer periods have been noted. Subsequent operative interference or local tissue changes may initiate activity of quiescent spores at long intervals after the original wound infection.

6. *Period of communicability.* Not communicable from man to man.

7. *Susceptibility and resistance.* Susceptibility is general. Active immunity is produced by tetanus toxoid, passive immunity by tetanus antitoxin with duration about 10 days.

8. *Occurrence.* World-wide distribution following wound infection, but a relatively uncommon disease. Most frequent in North America among young males and in summer, especially following wounds contaminated with manured soil. The condition is a serious factor in infant mortality where midwives are ignorant or incompetent. A disease of much moment in military practice, now effectively controlled by active immunization.

9. *Methods of control:*

A. Preventive measures:

1. Active immunization with tetanus toxoid is desirable for those likely to be exposed to infection with tetanus; advised in infancy or early childhood, preferably combined with appropriate immunizing agents for protection against pertussis or diphtheria or both (see Diphtheria 9A1). In addition to the initial inoculation with doses and intervals between injections recommended for the particular form of toxoid used, another (reinforcing) dose should be given 8 to 12 months later, and renewal doses at the time of each injury where danger of tetanus exists. Reinjections in the absence of injury should be at intervals no longer than 5 years. It is also important that the person should have with him at all times a record of his inoculation in case of injury. Tetanus toxoid under such conditions has proved a more effective method of prevention than tetanus antitoxin which is not without danger from sensitivity to horse serum; particularly indicated in persons known to be allergic to a wide range of substances and especially to horse serum. Active immunization of pregnant women with tetanus toxoid is recommended in regions where tetanus neonatorum is prevalent; maternally transmitted passive immunity will protect the newborn infant.

2. In the absence of previous active immunization with tetanus toxoid, passive protection by tetanus antitoxin is recommended in regions where tetanus is prevalent, and in all instances where contaminated material may be imbedded in a wound.

3. Removal from wounds of all foreign matter by thorough cleansing, with debridement where applicable.

4. Extension of preventive methods to persons in industry and on farms.

5. Licensing of midwives authorized to attend confinements, with professional supervision and education as to methods, equipment and the technic of asepsis.

B. Control of the infected individual, contacts and environment:
   1. Report to local health authority. Case report required in most states and countries.
   2. Isolation: None.
   3. Quarantine: None.
   4. Immunization: In absence of adequate previous inoculation with tetanus toxoid reinforced by another injection of toxoid at the time of injury, a person who has been so wounded that danger of tetanus exists, should receive a sub-cutaneous injection of tetanus antitoxin, 3,000 units, on the day of the wound. A second injection within 10 days may be desirable in certain instances, but precautions must be taken against developed sensitivity.
   5. Investigation of contacts and source of infection: None; the infecting micro-organism is widespread.
   6. Concurrent disinfection: None.
   7. Terminal disinfection: None.
   8. Specific treatment: Tetanus antitoxin in a single large dose intravenously; penicillin in large doses intramuscularly. Sedation is the important therapeutic consideration.
C. Epidemic measures: Thorough search for inadequacies in technic of sterilization in the uncommon hospital outbreaks; in tetanus of the newborn, rigid inquiry into competence and licensure of attendants at birth.
D. International measures: Active immunization against tetanus is recommended for international travellers.

TOXOPLASMOSIS

1. *Identification.* A protozoan infection which may be acquired prenatally from the mother, or at any time of life postnatally. Prenatal infection acquired during gestation may lead to death of the fetus or to manifestations at birth of chorio-retinitis, cerebral calcification, hydrocephalus or microcephalus, psychomotor retardation or convulsions. Prenatal infection acquired late in gestation may be manifested after birth by fever, jaundice, rash, hepatomegaly, splenomegaly, xanthrochromic spinal fluid and convulsions. The chronic manifestations listed above may develop later. Infections acquired after birth may be mild, with no recognized symptoms, or may be manifested by fever, lymphadenopathy and lymphocytosis lasting a few weeks, or may be severe with a generalized exan-them, jaundice, and cerebral manifestations leading rapidly to death.

   Definitive diagnosis is by microscopic demonstration of Toxoplasma in body tissues or fluids during life or at autopsy; or in laboratory reared albino mice inoculated with such materials. Laboratory diagnostic aids are complement fixation test and methylene-blue dye test of Sabin and Feldman.
2. *Etiologic agent.* Toxoplasma gondii.
3. *Source and reservoir of infection.* The exact source of human infection is not known; the pregnant woman in the primary stage of the infection infects the fetus in utero or possibly during delivery. Rodents, dogs, cats, swine, cattle, sheep, goats and other mammals and birds are reservoirs; a most ubiquitous protozoan parasite.
4. *Mode of transmission.* Unknown; presumably man becomes infected by ingesting excreta from infected animals or by direct contact with them. Congenital in-

[752]

fection is apparently through the placenta. No arthropod vector has been discovered, but certain ticks, infected in the laboratory, have transmitted the infection to experimental animals.

5. *Incubation period.* Unknown; probably from about 2 weeks to several months.

6. *Period of communicability.* Probably not communicable from man to man except during period of gestation through the placenta and possibly during delivery. In animals, probably during acute stage or as long as organisms are excreted in feces, urine or saliva.

7. *Susceptibility and resistance.* Susceptibility in general. Recovery from one attack probably confers permanent immunity.

8. *Occurrence.* World-wide distribution in animals. Serological surveys and recognition of clinical cases also indicate world-wide distribution in man. In some areas 50 percent or more of surveyed groups over 20 years of age have positive serological reactions.

9. *Methods of control:*
   A. Preventive measures:
      1. Avoidance of intimate contact with sick animals and birds, avoidance of tick bites, and keeping premises free from rats and mice may prevent infection. No specific preventive measures are known.
   B. Control of the infected individual, contacts and environment:
      1. Report to local health authority: Official report not ordinarily justifiable.
      2. Isolation: None.
      3. Concurrent disinfection: None.
      4. Terminal disinfection: None.
      5. Quarantine: None.
      6. Immunization: None.
      7. Investigation of contacts and source of infection: In congenital cases, determine antibodies in mother and other members of family; in acquired cases, determine contact with infected animals and history of tick or insect bite.
      8. Specific treatment: In experimentally infected mice and rabbits. Sulfonamides have a prophylactic value, and when administered early during the course of the infection have a curative effect. When combined with pyrimethamine (Daraprim) these compounds have given better results in mouse infections, but little or none in man.
   C. Epidemic measures: Not applicable, a sporadic disease. Community surveys of voluntary reporting by lying-in hospitals for prescribed periods and in particular regions to estimate incidence, and thorough case study to obtain information leading to improved control.
   D. International measures: None.

TRACHOMA

1. *Identification.* A chronic communicable disease of the eye characterized by acute onset with inflammation of the conjunctivae and subepithelial infiltration, followed by granulation and pannus, by capillary infiltration of the cornea and by cicatrization leading to gross deformity of the eyelids, visual disability and possibly blindness.

Laboratory diagnosis is by finding cytoplasmic inclusion bodies, and by cytological changes in expressed follicular material.

A number of forms of chronic conjunctivitis of bacterial origin simulate trachoma and require differentiation.

2. *Etiologic agent.* The virus of trachoma, one of the psittacosis-lymphogranuloma group.

3. *Source and reservoir of infection.* Secretions from the eyes, and mucoid or purulent discharges of nasal mucous membranes of infected persons; tears of such persons also carry the infection.

4. *Mode of transmission.* By direct contact with secretions of infected persons or by indirect contact with materials recently soiled therewith. Flies are vectors in Eastern countries. Carriers have not been demonstrated.

5. *Incubation period.* Five to 12 days as determined by human volunteer experiments.

6. *Period of communicability.* While active lesions are present in the conjunctivae and in the adnexed mucous membranes. After cicatrization is complete, communicability no longer exists, but reactivation of the disease may occur with reappearance of infective discharges.

7. *Susceptibility and resistance.* Susceptibility is general; in all races, affects children more frequently than adults, and females more than males; particularly, persons of unclean habits and those whose eyes are irritated by exposure to sun, wind, and sand. Natural or acquired immunity has not been demonstrated.

8. *Occurrence.* World-wide, but with unequal and varying distribution in different countries and continental areas. High prevalence generally associated with poor hygiene, poor nutrition and crowded living conditions, particularly in dry, dusty areas.

9. *Methods of control:*

A. Preventive measures:

   1. In areas where trachoma is prevalent, careful and systematic examination of the eyes of children, especially school children.

   2. The use in common of toilet articles and towels should be prohibited.

B. Control of the infected individual, contacts and environment:

   1. Report to local health authority: Case report required in most states and countries.

   2. Isolation: The patient should be excluded from school. With proper instruction of patient and family in means of preventing spread, and with adequate treatment of the patient, no need exists for isolation. Children should be excluded from school when active lesions exist and when adequate preventive measures are not practicable.

   3. Concurrent disinfection: Of eye discharges and articles soiled therewith.

   4. Terminal disinfection: None.

   5. Quarantine: None.

   6. Immunization: None.

   7. Investigation of contacts and source of infection: Members of the family, playmates and schoolmates.

   8. Specific treatment: Sulfonamides orally, an initial loading dose and smaller amounts thereafter for about 20 days. After an interval without treatment, the course is repeated. Recent reports indicate the tetracycline antibiotics or chloramphenicol may replace sulfonamides, but further evaluation is necessary.

C. Epidemic measures: None.

D. International measures: None.

TRICHINOSIS

1. *Identification.* An infection arising through invasion of human and animal hosts by larvae (trichinae) of a parasitic nematode, Trichinella spiralis. Clinical disease in man is markedly irregular, severity varying with number of trichinae invading, tissue invaded and physiological state of the host. Sudden appearance of edema of upper eyelids is a common, early, and characteristic sign of clinical trichinosis, usually about the eleventh day of infection and sometimes followed by subconjunctival and retinal hemorrhage, pain and photophobia. Gastrointestinal symptoms may precede or accompany ocular manifestations. Muscle soreness and pain, skin lesions, thirst, profuse sweating, chills, weakness, prostration and rapidly increasing eosinophil count may shortly follow ocular signs. Fever is usual, remittent, and terminates by lysis after about a week; sometimes as much as 104° F. for several days. Respiratory and neurological symptoms may appear in the third to sixth week. Myocardial failure, when it occurs, is between the fourth and eighth weeks. Trichinosis is usually a mild febrile disease.

   Daily study of blood smears for increasing eosinophilia is the most useful diagnostic laboratory procedure. Skin tests, flocculation tests and complement fixation tests may aid diagnosis but are not in themselves conclusive. Search for parasites in feces, blood, spinal fluid and biopsied striated muscle is usually futile.

2. *Etiologic agent.* Trichinella spiralis.

3. *Source and reservoir of infection.* The source of infection is meat of infected animals, chiefly pork and pork products, occasionally wild game. Swine and many wild animals, fox, wolf, bear, polar bear, marine mammals and rats are reservoirs of infection.

4. *Mode of transmission.* Consumption of flesh of animals containing viable trichinae.

5. *Incubation period.* Onset about 9 days after ingestion of infective meat with variations between 2 and 28 days.

6. *Period of communicability.* Not directly transmitted in nature from man to man.

7. *Susceptibility and resistance.* Susceptibility is general. Neither natural nor acquired immunity is known to occur in man; has been demonstrated in experimental animals.

8. *Occurrence.* World-wide, but rare or absent in native populations of the tropics or where swine are fed on root vegetables, as in France. The parasite is particularly widespread in the United States, about one in every six necropsies showing infection; less prevalent in Canada and Mexico. Widely distributed in Germany, Spain, Hungary and the lower Danube countries but prevalence is low. Clinical cases occur more frequently than indicated by morbidity reports; often confused with other illnesses and patients with mild infection do not seek medical aid. No selection by age, sex, race, region, season, or climate except as those effect the eating of insufficiently cooked flesh of infected hogs.

9. *Methods of control:*
   A. Preventive measures:
      1. Inauguration of local and state meat inspection to assure adequate processing of all pork products not under federal inspection and customarily eaten without further adequate cooking by the consumer.
      2. Encouragement of farmers and hog raisers in the use of standard swine sani-

tation practices which will reduce opportunity for trichinal infection in swine, such as burial or other adequate disposal of swine and rat carcasses to prevent hogs from feeding on them; burning, burial, or other adequate disposal of swine offal to prevent feeding of swine or rats; control of rats, particularly on farms and around hog-raising establishments and stockyards; rats probably constitute a minor source of swine trichinosis.

3. Elimination of the current practice of feeding uncooked garbage and offal to swine and the adoption and enforcement of suitable laws and regulations ensuring cooking such material before its consumption by swine. In Great Britain and Canada it is illegal to feed unboiled swill to swine.

4. Cooking of all fresh pork and pork products by the consumer at a temperature and for a time sufficient to allow all parts of the meat to reach at least 65.6° C. (150° F.) (a temperature which allows a good margin of safety) unless established that these meat products have been processed under federal or other official regulations adequate for the destruction of trichinae.

5. Low temperatures maintained in central portions of pork, are believed effective in killing trichina larvae; such as −27° C. (−16° F.) for 36 hours. Storage in home freezers as a safeguard against trichinosis is not to be depended upon.

B. Control of the infected individual, contacts and environment:

1. Report to local health authority: Case report desirably required in most states and countries.

2. Isolation: None.

3. Concurrent disinfection: None.

4. Terminal disinfection: None.

5. Quarantine: None.

6. Immunization: None.

7. Investigation of contacts and source of infection: More likely a community than a case effort.

8. Specific treatment: None.

C. Epidemic measures: Establish the diagnosis. Examine dietary histories and institute epidemiologic study to determine the common food involved. Destroy remainders of food and initiate measures to correct faulty practices responsible.

D. International measures: None.

TRICHOMONIASIS

1. *Identification.* A common non-fatal infection of the genito-urinary tract characterized in women by vaginitis associated with profuse leukorrhea and thin, foamy, yellowish discharge of foul odor. The vaginal mucosa is inflamed, frequently with small petechial punctate hemorrhagic lesions. In men, the infectious agent lives in the prostate, urethra or prepuce, producing neither symptoms nor demonstrable lesion.

   Diagnosis is through identification of the motile parasite by direct and immediate microscopic examination of discharges.

2. *Etiologic agent.* Trichomonas vaginalis, a protozoan.

3. *Source and reservoir of infection.* Vaginal and urethral discharges of infected persons.

4. *Mode of transmission.* By sexual intercourse with infected persons; possibly by contact with contaminated articles.

5. *Incubation period.* Four to twenty days, average seven days.

6. *Period of communicability.* For the duration of the infection.

7. *Susceptibility and resistance.* General and high grade susceptibility.
8. *Occurrence.* In selected areas of the United States the incidence among negroes is twice that of whites. Geographically wide spread, and a frequent disease of all continents and all peoples, primarily of adults, with highest incidence among young girls and women, aged 16 to 35 years.
9. *Methods of control:*
   A. Preventive measures:
      1. Rigid personal hygiene in the use of public toilet facilities.
      2. Avoidance of sexual intercourse with known infected individuals.
   B. Control of the infected individual, contacts and environment:
      1. Report to local health authority: Official report not ordinarily justifiable.
      2. Isolation: None; avoid sexual relations during period of infection and treatment.
      3. Concurrent disinfection: None; the organisms can not withstand drying.
      4. Terminal disinfection: None.
      5. Quarantine: None.
      6. Immunization: None.
      7. Investigation of contacts and source of infection: Marital partner, particularly if a recurrent infection.
      8. Specific treatment: Most infected females respond promptly to chemotherapy with acetarsone, silver picrate or diodoquin.
   C. Epidemic measures: None.
   D. International measures: None.

TRYPANOSOMIASIS, AFRICAN

1. *Identification.* A protozoan disease confined to tropical Africa, characterized in its early stage by fever, intense headache, insomnia, lymph node enlargement (especially posterior cervical), anemia, local edema and rash; and in its later stages by wasting, somnolence and other symptoms due to involvement of the central nervous system. The disease may run a protracted course of several years, or be rapidly fatal within a few months. Synonym: African sleeping sickness.

   Definitive diagnosis in early stages is by finding trypanosomes in the peripheral blood or by lymph node puncture; in late stages, in the cerebrospinal fluid. Inoculation of rats, guinea pigs or monkeys with blood or lymph, or culture on appropriate media, are also used.
2. *Etiologic agent.* Trypanosoma gambiense and T. rhodesiense, both probably varieties of the same species, T. brucei.
3. *Source and reservoir of infection.* Immediate source is infected Tsetse fly. Reservoirs of both gambiense and rhodesiense are the blood of infected persons. Wild game, especially antelopes, and domestic cattle and pigs are the chief animal reservoirs, and may occasionally be the source of human infection.
4. *Mode of transmission.* By the bite of certain species of Glossina, tsetse flies. Four species are mainly concerned, G. palpalis, G. tachinoides, G. morsitans, and G. swynnertoni. In nature, the first two transmit T. gambiense and the latter two T. rhodesiense infections, although in the laboratory many other species are capable of transmitting both infections. The fly is infected by biting an infected person or animal. The parasite develops in the gut and proventriculus of the fly, the cycle requiring 18 days or longer according to temperature and other factors.

[757]

Infection is conveyed by the bite. The metacyclic forms are injected with the salivary gland secretion into the wound made by the proboscis of the fly. Direct mechanical transmission by blood on proboscis of glossina is presumably possible. Once infected, a tsetse fly remains infective for life, up to 3 months; infection is not passed from generation to generation. A few cases of congenital infection in man have been reported.

5. *Incubation period.* Usually 2 to 3 weeks. May be as short as 7 days.

6. *Period of communicability.* As long as the parasite exists in the blood of the infected person; extremely variable in untreated cases; in late as well as in early stages of the disease.

7. *Susceptibility and resistance.* Susceptibility is general, but the African native shows greater resistance than the European, in whom the disease tends to run a more acute course. Some patients recover without symptoms of central nervous system involvement; inapparent infection is known.

8. *Occurrence.* The disease is confined to tropical Africa between 15° N. and 20° S. corresponding to distribution of the tsetse fly. A prevalence of 30 per cent of a population has been demonstrated in some regions. Epidemics tend to occur when the disease is introduced into non-immune populations. In regions where G. palpalis is the principal vector, infection occurs mainly along streams (Gambia, Liberia, Sierra Leone, Gold Coast, Congo, Sudan, Uganda). Where G. morsitans is the principal vector, infection is over wider dry areas (Mosambique, Nyasaland, Rhodesia, Tanganyika).

9. *Methods of control:*

A. Preventive measures:

1. Mass treatment of whole local populations with appropriate chemotherapeutic agents in order to lower index of new infections.

2. Wide and if necessary repeated clearings of bush around villages, along lines of communication, especially streams, near houses and roads. More likely to be successful against G. palpalis than other species.

3. A concentration of the population in relatively large villages.

4. Fly control by all practicable means including use of insecticides with residual effect, trapping, flypaper, and handnets.

5. Destruction of pupae in breeding places.

6. Segregation of big game into game reserves away from human habitation (for G. morsitans).

7. Education of the population as to the mode of spread and methods of prevention.

8. Individual protection can be achieved temporarily by administration of an appropriate chemoprophylactic agent, preferably pentamidine, adult dose 250 mg. intramuscularly, which protects for about six months.

B. Control of the infected individual, contacts and environment:

1. Report to local health authority: In selected endemic areas to obtain records of prevalence and to encourage control measures; not a reportable disease in most countries.

2. Isolation: Patients with trypanosomes in the blood should be protected from bites of tsetse flies; isolation not practicable. Legal restrictions are placed on movement of untreated patients in some countries.

3. Concurrent disinfection: None.

[758]

4. Terminal disinfection: None.
5. Quarantine: None.
6. Immunization: None.
7. Investigation of contacts and source of infection: Should be done in connection with study of infected population groups.
8. Specific treatment: Rhodesiense infection is much more resistant than gambiense to chemotherapy. Before the nervous system is involved, Bayer 205 (antrypol suramin) is used intravenously for both T. gambiense and T. rhodesiense infection.

    Tryparasamide is indicated in late T. gambiense infections. Serious side affects are possible; interrupt treatment if visual disturbances appear. Various combinations of Bayer 205 and tryparsamide are used for possible synergic effect. Melarsen and its derivatives may be useful in tryparsamide-resistant T. gambiense infections. Prognosis in advanced T. rhodesiense infection is poor with all treatment; Mel B and arsobal have been used recently with good effect in both gambiense and rhodesiense infections.

    Pentamidine is effective in early T. gambiense infections, and is practically non-toxic; may be combined with tryparsamide; has not replaced Bayer 205 in treatment of T. rhodesiense infections.

C. Epidemic measures: In presence of an epidemic or in localized areas of high incidence, it may be necessary to move villages from sources of infection to fly-free areas. Other measures as in 9A.
D. International measures: Cooperative efforts of governments in endemic areas should be promoted. An International Bureau for Trypanosomiasis, acting as a clearing center for information, exists in Brazzaville, French Equatorial Africa.

TRYPANOSOMIASIS, AMERICAN

1. *Identification.* A protozoan disease in which the parasite exists in the peripheral blood in the trypanosome form and in muscle and other tissues as leishmania-form bodies. The acute stage, lasting several weeks, is characterized by fever, malaise, enlargement of spleen and liver, and myocardial damage. Other early physical signs are unilateral edema of the eyelids extending to the face with red-purple discoloration of the skin, inflammation and swelling of the lachrymal gland, conjunctivitis and regional lymphadenopathy. The disease may become chronic with encephalopathy or end with gradual myocardial failure; death is uncommon. Many infected persons, especially adults, have few or no clinical manifestations. Synonym: Enfermedad de Chagas.

    Definitive diagnosis is by finding trypanosome forms in the peripheral blood during febrile episodes, or leishmania forms in muscle biopsy; by culture, by inoculation of albino rats, or by xenodiagnosis (feeding non-infected triatomine bugs on the patient and finding characteristic trypanosomes in the gut). A complement fixation test provides presumptive evidence.

    Two other species of trypanosome, T. rangeli and T. ariarii, have been found in blood films of man in Guatemala, Venezuela and Colombia; their distribution in other countries is unknown. They produce no demonstrable clinical disease, and are distinguishable from T. cruzi by morphological criteria.

2. *Etiologic agent.* Trypanosoma cruzi, a hemoflagellate.

[759   ]

3. *Source and reservoir of infection.* Source of infection is a bug; reservoirs include infected persons and a number of domestic and wild animals, such as dogs, cats, wood rats, opossums, and armadillos.

4. *Mode of transmission.* By the fecal material of infected insect vectors; various blood sucking species of Reduviidae (cone-nosed bugs), especially of Triatoma, Rhodnias and Panstrongylus which frequently attack man. Infection may take place through conjunctivae, mucous membranes, abrasions, or wounds in the skin. Probably not transmitted by the actual act of biting; transmission by blood transfusion has been noted.

5. *Incubation period.* About 7 to 14 days.

6. *Period of communicability.* Not directly communicable in nature from man to man; organisms are present in the blood only during the acute, febrile period.

7. *Susceptibility and resistance.* Children, especially infants under 2 years of age, are particularly susceptible.

8. *Occurrence.* The disease has a wide geographic distribution in Central and South America and is highly endemic in some areas. Cases have been found in southern Mexico. No natural infection of man has been reported in the United States but several species of Triatoma have been shown to be carriers of Trypanosoma cruzi in Texas, New Mexico, Arizona, and California, and wild rodents and opossums have been found infected in these areas.

9. *Methods of control:*
   A. Preventive measures:
      1. Construction or repair of dwellings so that they do not afford hiding places for the insect vector or shelter for the wild hosts.
      2. Elimination of infected domestic animals and destruction of the habitations of the wild hosts in known endemic areas.
      3. Use of a bed net in houses infested by the vector.
      4. Systematic attack upon vectors through use of effective insecticides, especially those having residual actions, with hexachlorocyclohexane much used in endemic areas.
   B. Control of the infected individual, contacts and environment:
      1. Report to local health authority: In selected endemic areas; not a reportable disease in most countries.
      2. Isolation: None.
      3. Concurrent disinfection: None.
      4. Terminal disinfection: None.
      5. Quarantine: None.
      6. Immunization: None.
      7. Investigation of contacts and source of infection: Search of bedding and rooms for the vector, and investigation among domestic and wild animals for evidence of infection. Other members of the family should be examined for evidence of infection.
      8. Specific treatment: Bayer 7602 (Ac), a 4-aminoquinoline, gives good results in some cases and has little or no effect in others. Tryparsamide and suramin are ineffective.
   C. Epidemid measures: In areas of high incidence, field surveys to determine distribution and frequency of vectors.
   D. International measures: None.

[760]

APPENDIX D

TUBERCULOSIS

1. *Identification.* A chronic bacterial disease of great importance as a cause of death in nearly all parts of the world. Primary infection frequently goes unnoticed clinically; some patients have fever, vague constitutional symptoms, or roentgenographic evidence of infiltration of the lungs and enlarged tracheobronchial nodes. The course of events thereafter is subject to much variation. Pleurisy with effusion may occur; in some areas, notably the Scandinavian countries, erythema nodosum is common. Some few individuals develop disseminated tuberculosis. Such developments are more likely within the first 6 to 12 months. Usually, however, the lesions heal spontaneously, leaving no residual changes except tuberculin sensitivity and occasionally pulmonary or tracheobronchial node calcifications. Disseminated or extrapulmonary (particularly skeletal) tuberculosis develop more often in infants and in Negroes. In late childhood primary disease is likely to be benign, and in young adults it may resemble, or merge into, pulmonary tuberculosis.

   Pulmonary tuberculosis characteristically has a chronic variable course, with exacerbations and remissions but capable of arrest at any stage. Three stages (minimal, moderately advanced and far advanced) are distinguished, according to extent of lung involvement; activity is determined by progression or retrogression as detected in serial roentgenograms, by presence of tubercle bacilli, and by symptoms. Abnormal roentgen shadows indicative of pulmonary infiltration, excavation, or fibrosis are common in advance of clinical manifestations. Symptoms of cough, fatigue, fever, weight loss, hoarseness, chest pain and hemoptysis and physical signs of dullness and rales are usual features of advanced disease.

   Specific diagnosis is by demonstration of tubercle bacilli in sputum by stained smear, concentration and culture, or animal inoculation. Negative results on microscopic examination of sputum do not rule out tuberculosis; repeated examinations with more sensitive methods are eventually successful in most active cases; gastric washings may be examined where sputum is absent or negative. Tuberculin test is positive in active tuberculosis except in critically ill persons; a negative reaction aids differential diagnosis.

   Extrapulmonary tuberculosis is an early or late result of hematogenous dissemination of tubercle bacilli during the primary phase, as miliary tuberculosis, tuberculosis of bones and joints, central nervous system (tuberculous meningitis), lymphatic glands, and kidneys; or as a complication of pulmonary tuberculosis, involving intestines or larynx. Diagnosis is by isolation of tubercle bacilli from a lesion or exudate (cerebrospinal fluid in meningitis) or by histopathology. In the United States these forms are far less common than pulmonary tuberculosis, and as causes of death are decreasing more rapidly.

2. *Etiologic agent.* Myobacterium tuberculosis, tubercle bacillus. The human type causes nearly all pulmonary tuberculosis, the bovine type a considerable share of extrapulmonary disease, proportions varying according to opportunities for infection.

3. *Source and reservoir of infection.* Respiratory secretions of persons with "open" (bacillary-positive) pulmonary tuberculosis; milk from tuberculous cattle. Patients with extrapulmonary tuberculosis are usually not sources of infection.

[761]

4. *Mode of transmission.* Coughing or sneezing by patients with open pulmonary tuberculosis sets up a cloud of infectious material; minute particles may be inhaled directly or after settling and resuspension as dust. Direct and indirect contact are important; alimentary infection, as by contaminated eating and drinking utensils, is less so. Infection usually results from the continued and intimate exposure that characterizes household relationships; some susceptible family contacts avoid infection for long periods.

Bovine tuberculosis is transmitted by ingestion of unpasteurized milk or dairy products from tuberculous cows, by airborne infection in barns and by handling contaminated animal products.

5. *Incubation period.* From infection to demonstrable primary phase lesions, about 4–6 weeks; from infection to progressive pulmonary or extrapulmonary tuberculosis may be years, with the first 6–12 months most hazardous.

6. *Period of communicability.* As long as tubercle bacilli are being discharged by the patient. Commences when a lesion becomes open (discharges tubercle bacilli) and continues until healed or death occurs. Some patients remain sputum-positive intermittently for years. Degree of communicability depends upon the number of bacilli discharged and hygienic practices of the patient. Chemotherapy, collapse therapy, and pulmonary resection commonly shorten communicability.

7. *Susceptibility and resistance.* Susceptibility is general; highest in children under 3 years, lowest from 3 to 12 years, and intermediate thereafter; greater in aboriginal races than in populations long exposed to the disease; in the undernourished, neglected, and fatigued more than in the well fed and well cared for. Especially prevalent among persons with silicosis or diabetes. The resistance conferred by healed primary infection is difficult to assess, but is not complete.

8. *Occurrence.* Among the most common communicable diseases of man, endemic in practically all populations. In most western nations, incidence and mortality are declining. Age at first infection varies; persons living in cities ordinarily are infected earlier than in rural areas, and children living in household contact with a case are likely to be infected at a comparatively early age. Prevalence of infection and disease varies greatly in different areas; in some places a majority of adults are negative to usual doses of tuberculin. Photofluorographic surveys show prevalence of pulmonary tuberculosis to be low under age 15, rising gradually thereafter, although a large proportion of lesions of older persons are inactive. Prevalence of infection and roentgenographically demonstrable disease vary less with race than does mortality. In the United States, mortality is highest among infants and adult males beyond middle age. Mortality rates commonly reflect the social and economic welfare of a region; in many countries tuberculosis remains an important cause of death, with rates in excess of 100 per 100,000 population per year; in others rates are below 20. Reported cases in the United States show prevalence declining more slowly than mortality; this is attributable to improvements in case-finding, wider use of roentgenograms, and probably altered survivorship.

9. *Methods of control:*

A. Preventive measures:

   1. Education of the public in the danger of tuberculosis, its mode of spread, and methods of control.

   2. Provision of adequate sanatorium facilities for isolation and treatment of active

cases. The minimum number of beds needed per annual tuberculosis death is 2.5 in most communities of the United States.

3. Provision of Roentgenographic and clinical facilities for examination of contacts and suspects, and for clinical supervision and treatment of ambulant patients and those not hospitalized.

4. Public health nursing service for home supervision of patients and to encourage and arrange for examination of contacts.

5. Insuring a safe milk supply, through pasteurization of milk and elimination of tuberculosis among dairy cattle; meat inspection and condemning of all tuberculous carcasses.

6. Measures to limit inhalation of dangerous concentrations of silica dust in industrial plants and mines.

7. Routine Roentgenographic examination of groups who have a higher prevalence of tuberculosis than the general population, such as nurses, medical students, patients and outpatients in general and mental hospitals, and selected groups of industrial workers; also those who constitute a special hazard to others if infected, to include pregnant women and school personnel.

8. Photofluorographic screening of adult populations where feasible; periodic resurveys should be made.

9. The role of BCG vaccination of uninfected persons is still unsettled. In many areas where mortality rates are high and economic resources do not permit a complete control program, mass vaccination of uninfected children and young adults is practiced, but its efficacy is still under evaluation. Vaccination has been advocated for newborn infants in communities with high morbidity, for household contacts of cases, for susceptible racial groups and for persons with unusual exposure by reason of occupation, such as medical and nursing students. In areas where mortality and morbidity from tuberculosis are low, and other control measures are available, the place of BCG vaccination in control of tuberculosis presently appears to be minor.

B. Control of the infected individual, contacts, and environment:

1. Report to local health authority: Obligatory case report in most states and countries. Health departments should maintain a current register of active cases.

2. Isolation: A period of hospital or sanatorium treatment removes a focus of infection from the home, teaches the patient hygienic essentials of tuberculosis control, and increases the chances of recovery. Public health nursing supervision for patients remaining at home, including instruction in personal hygiene; compulsory isolation of those with open tuberculosis who do not observe necessary precautions.

3. Concurrent disinfection: Of sputum and articles soiled therewith, including handkerchiefs, cloths, or paper napkins, and of eating utensils used by patient. Patients should be trained to cover mouth and nose in coughing and sneezing.

4. Terminal disinfection: Cleaning. Wet cleaning of walls and floors and subsequent exposure to sunlight and fresh air.

5. Quarantine: None.

6. Immunization: BCG vaccination of tuberculin negative contacts may be warranted. See Section 9A9.

7. Investigation of contacts and source of infection: All members of the house-

[763]

hold of a newly discovered case and all intimate extra-household contacts should be examined roentgenologically, with particular attention to elderly persons with chronic cough. Annual retesting of tuberculin-negative persons, with intensive study of converters and their contacts, has been effective in some areas in disclosing early lesions, as well as finding previously unrecognized sources of infection.

8. Specific treatment: Most primary infections heal without treatment; if discovered in an active stage in susceptible age and racial groups, antimicrobial drug therapy may be instituted.

Active cases of pulmonary tuberculosis should be in a sanatorium, or on sanatorium regimen of rest followed by graduated resumption of activity. Prompt treatment with antimicrobial drugs is indicated for most cases; choice of regimens is rapidly widening with increasing experience. At present a combination of streptomycin and para-aminosalicylic acid (PAS) is most commonly employed in adults for six months to one year; toxic reactions are to be watched for and in vitro tests made for streptomycin resistance of tubercle bacilli isolated from the patient. Isoniazid is approximately as effective, used alone or in combination with PAS, streptomycin or both. The combination of isoniazid with streptomycin is advisedly reserved for serious situations, in order to avoid development of strains of tubercle bacilli that are resistant to both drugs.

Reversible forms of lung collapse (pneumothorax, pneumoperitoneum and phrenic nerve interruption) are less frequently employed than formerly. Thoracoplasty is selectively indicated. Pulmonary resection to remove diseased lung is used increasingly, as well as the less radical procedure of extrapleural plombage.

In extrapulmonary tuberculosis, medical therapy as described above for pulmonary tuberculosis is combined with specific measures, often surgical, suited to the particular form and type of disease.

In miliary and meningeal tuberculosis treatment should be started immediately with isoniazid by mouth, supplemented by intramuscular streptomycin. In comatose patients, streptomycin may also be given intrathecally. Therapy should be continued at least 6 months.

C. Epidemic measures:

1. Alertness to recognize the occasional cluster of new cases resulting from contacts with an unrecognized infectious case; intensive search for the source of infection in such situations.

D. International measures: None.

TULAREMIA

1. *Identification.* An infectious disease of wild mammals and man; onset is sudden, with chills and fever, the patient usually prostrated and confined to bed. Lymph nodes draining the site of original infection become swollen and tender, and commonly suppurate. Case fatality is about 5%.

Diagnosis is confirmed by inoculation of animals with material from local lesions or with sputum, by isolation of the microorganism bacteriologically and by agglutination reaction. Skin test is less reliable.

2. *Etiologic agent.* Pasteurella tularensis (Bacterium tularense).

APPENDIX D

3. *Source and reservoir of infection.* Many species of wild animals and some domesti-
   cated animals; wild rabbits and hares, woodchuck, coyote, muskrat, opossum,
   tree squirrel, quail, skunk, water rat of Europe (Arvicola emphibus), cat, deer,
   dog, fox, hog, sage hen, and bull snake; also wood ticks.
4. *Mode of transmission.* By bites of infected flies and ticks, and by inoculation of
   skin or conjunctival sac through handling infected animals, as in skinning,
   dressing, or performing necropsies, or by fluids from infected flies, ticks, rabbits,
   and woodchucks. Arthropods directly related to disease in man are the following: one species of deer fly, Chrysops discalis; the wood tick, Dermacentor
   andersoni; the dog tick, Dermacentor variabilis and the Lone Star tick, Amblyomma americanum; and in Sweden the mosquito, Aëdes cinereus. Ingestion
   of insufficiently cooked rabbit meat and drinking contaminated water. Rare
   cases occur from bites of coyotes, skunks, hogs, cats, and dogs, where the mouth
   of the animal was presumably contaminated from eating infected rabbits.
   Laboratory infections are relatively frequent.
5. *Period of incubation.* From 24 hours to 10 days, usually 3 days.
6. *Period of communicability.* Not communicable from man to man. The infectious
   agent may be found in the blood of man during the first 2 weeks of the disease,
   in the lesions of the disease up to a month from onset and sometimes longer.
   Flies are infective for 14 days, ticks throughout their lifetime, about two years.
   Refrigerated rabbits kept constantly frozen at −15° C. (5° F.) may remain
   infective for 3½ years.
7. *Suspectibility and resistance.* All ages are susceptible; permanent immunity follows
   recovery. Through abrasion of the hand or by contact with contaminated
   material, an immune person may acquire a local tularemic papule which harbors
   virulent organisms but causes no notable constitutional reaction.
8. *Occurrence.* Throughout North America, in many parts of continental Europe and
   in Japan; unknown in Australia. Occurs in the United States in every month
   of the year, but especially autumn during the rabbit hunting season.
9. *Methods of control:*
   A. Preventive measures:
      1. Avoid bites of flies and ticks or handling such arthropods when working in
         infected areas during seasonal incidence of bloodsucking flies and ticks.
      2. The use of rubber gloves by persons engaged in dressing wild rabbits wherever
         taken, or when performing necropsies on infected laboratory animals will
         usually prevent occupational infections; employment of immune persons for
         dressing wild rabbits or conducting laboratory experiments. Thorough cooking
         of meat of wild rabbits.
      3. Avoid drinking raw water in areas where the disease prevails among wild
         animals.
   B. Control of the infected individual, contacts and environment:
      1. Report to local health authority: In selected endemic areas (USA); in many
         countries not a reportable disease.
      2. Isolation: None.
      3. Concurrent disinfection: Of discharges from ulcer, lymph nodes, or con-
         junctival sac.
      4. Terminal disinfection: None.
      5. Quarantine: None.

6. Immunization: None.
7. Investigation of contacts and source of infection: Should be undertaken in each case.
8. Specific treatment: Streptomycin, the tetracyclines and chloramphenicol are effective when continued until four to five days of normal temperature.
C. Epidemic measures: Search for sources of infection related to arthropods, to animal hosts and to water. Control measures as thus indicated (see 9A). Interstate or interarea shipment of infected animals or carcasses should be prohibited.
D. International measures: None.

TYPHOID FEVER

1. *Identification.* A systemic infection characterized by continued fever, involvement of lymphoid tissues especially ulceration of Peyer's patches, enlargement of spleen, rose spots on trunk, and diarrhea. Many mild, atypical and often unrecognized infections. A usual case fatality of 10% is reduced to 2–3% by antibiotic therapy. Synonyms: Enteric fever, Typhus abdominalis.

   Typhoid bacilli are found in blood during first two weeks and in feces and urine after second week. Widal reaction becomes positive during second week; O agglutinins more significant than H agglutinins.

2. *Etiologic agent.* Salmonella typhosa, typhoid bacillus. About 30 types can be distinguished by Vi-phage.

3. *Source and reservoir of infection.* Feces and urine of infected persons. Family contacts may be transient carriers; fecal carriers more common than urinary. The carrier state is most common among persons over 40 years of age, especially females; fecal carriers frequently have a typhoid cholecystitis with carrier state, usually permanent unless cholecystectomy is done.

4. *Mode of transmission.* Direct or indirect contact with patient or carrier. Principal vehicles of indirect spread are contaminated water and food, especially milk, milk products and shellfish, usually contaminated by hands of carrier or missed case. Under some conditions, flies are vectors.

5. *Incubation period.* Variable; average 2 weeks, usual range 1–3 weeks.

6. *Period of communicability.* As long as typhoid bacilli appear in excreta; usually from appearance of prodromal symptoms, throughout illness, and for varying periods of time after cessation of symptoms. About 10% of patients will discharge bacilli three months after onset; 2 to 5% become permanent carriers.

7. *Susceptibility and resistance.* Susceptibility is general, although many adults appear to acquire immunity through unrecognized infections; attack rates decline with age after second or third decades. Permanent immunity usually follows recovery. The degree of artificial active immunity conferred by typhoid vaccine is uncertain.

8. *Occurrence.* Widespread throughout world. Endemic in some rural areas of United States, but commonly occurring as sporadic cases and as small contact and carrier epidemics; steadily falling in incidence, particularly in urban areas. Still common in many countries of the Far East, Middle East, eastern Europe, Central and South America, and in Africa.

9. *Methods of control:*
A. Preventive measures:
   1. Protection and purification of public water supplies; construction of safe private supplies.

[766]

2. Sanitary disposal of human excreta.
3. Boiling of milk or pasteurization of milk and dairy products, including cheese.
4. Limitation of collection and marketing of shellfish to those from approved sources.
5. Sanitary supervision of processing, preparation and serving of all foods, especially those that are eaten raw; special attention to provision and use of hand-washing facilities.
6. Persons suffering from diarrhea should be excluded from handling food for public consumption and from handling family food supply if possible.
7. Fly control, control of fly breeding, and protection of foods against fly contamination by screening.
8. Immunization with a vaccine of high antigenicity. The extent of protection conferred by vaccination is under reevaluation. It is current practice to vaccinate persons subject to unusual exposure by reason of occupation or travel, those living in areas of high endemic incidence of typhoid fever, and institutional populations in which maintenance of sanitation is difficult. In the light of present knowledge, periodic reinforcing injections are desirable; except under conditions where risk of exposure is especially great, re-inoculation once in three years is common practice.
9. Discovery and supervision of typhoid carriers; exclusion from handling of foods.
10. Instruction of convalescents and chronic carriers in personal hygiene, particularly as to sanitary disposal of excreta, handwashing after defecation and before eating, and restraint from acting as food handlers.
11. Education of general public and particularly of food handlers concerning sources of infection and modes of transmission.

B. Control of the infected individual, contacts and environment:
1. Report to local health authority: Obligatory case report in most states and countries.
2. Isolation: In flyproof room. Hospital care desirable for patients who cannot command adequate sanitary environment and nursing care at home. Release from supervision by local health authority should be by not less than three negative cultures of feces and urine, at least 24 hours apart and not earlier than one month after onset.
3. Concurrent disinfection: Of feces and urine and articles soiled therewith. In communities with modern and adequate sewage disposal systems, feces and urine can be disposed of directly into sewer without preliminary disinfection.
4. Terminal disinfection: Cleaning.
5. Quarantine: Family contacts should not be employed as food handlers during period of contact nor before repeated negative feces and urine cultures are obtained.
6. Immunization: Administration of typhoid vaccine to family, household and nursing contacts who have been or may be exposed during course of disease.
7. Investigation of contacts and source of infection: Actual or probable source of infection of every case should be determined by search for common and individual sources, unreported cases and carriers, or contaminated food, water, milk or shellfish. Presence of agglutinins in blood of suspected carriers is suggestive of the carrier state. Organisms from patients and carriers should be

typed by phage to determine cases of same type and therefore of presumed common origin.

8. Specific treatment: Chloramphenicol; an initial oral loading dose is followed by oral doses every six hours until temperature is normal, then in smaller doses for a total of 14 days.

C. Epidemic measures:

1. Intensive search for case or carrier who is source of infection.
2. Exclusion of suspected food.
3. Boiling of milk or pasteurization or exclusion of suspected milk supplies or other suspected foods on epidemiologic evidence, pending elimination of cause of contamination.
4. Chlorination under competent supervision of suspected water supply or its exclusion. All water used for drinking must be chlorinated or boiled before use.

D. International measures: Inoculation of international travellers with triple typhoid vaccine (TAB: typhoid, paratyphoid A, paratyphoid B) is advisable for travel in all areas except the United States, Canada, Great Britain and Northwest Europe if not protected through previous attack.

TYPHUS FEVER

A. Epidemic or Classical Typhus (Louse-borne)

1. *Identification.* A rickettsial disease with a history of great epidemics and a continued existence in numerous areas of the world. The onset is variable, often sudden and marked by headache, chills, fever, and general pains; a macular eruption appears on the 5th or 6th day, toxemia is usually pronounced and the disease terminates in rapid lysis after about 2 weeks of fever. In the absence of specific therapy case fatality varies from 10 to 40% in different epidemics and increases with age. Mild infections may occur with eruption evanescent or absent, especially in vaccinated persons. A recrudesence of epidemic typhus fever may occur years after the primary attack (Brill's disease); it differs from the classical type in that it need not be associated with lousiness and is milder, with fewer complications and lower mortality. Synonym: Typhus exanthematicus.

The Weil-Felix reaction with Proteus OX19 is usually positive with serums obtained after the 10th day, the complement fixation test a few days later.

2. *Etiologic agent.* Rickettsia prowazeki, var. prowazeki.

3. *Source and reservoir of infection.* Lice infected by feeding on blood of man with the febrile disease. Man is the reservoir during interepidemic periods. Persons with recrudescent typhus (Brill's disease) can infect their lice and probably serve as foci for new outbreaks in louse infested communities.

4. *Mode of transmission.* Infected body lice, Pediculus humanus, excrete rickettsiae in their feces and usually defecate at the time of feeding. Man is infected by rubbing feces or crushed lice into the wound made by the bite or into superficial abrasions of the skin. Inhalation of dried infective louse feces as dust from dirty clothes may account for some infections.

5. *Incubation period.* From 6 to 15 days, commonly 12 days.

6. *Period of communicability.* Patients are infective for lice during the febrile illness and possibly for 2 or 3 days after the temperature returns to normal. The living louse is infective as soon as it begins to pass rickettsiae in feces; earlier if crushed.

Under favorable conditions, rickettsiae remain viable in the dead louse for weeks. Not communicable from man to man.

7. *Susceptibility and resistance.* Susceptibility is general. The disease in children and in vaccinated adults is mild and may go unrecognized. Attack usually confers permanent immunity.

8. *Occurrence.* In most colder areas of the world where appreciable groups of people live under unhygienic conditions and are lousy. Endemic centers exist in mountainous regions of Mexico and Central and South America, the Balkans and Central and Eastern Europe, North Africa and mountainous areas of Central and South Africa, and most of Asia except the humid tropics. Prior to modern methods of control, epidemics were frequent among military and refugee populations and in areas suffering famine or war.

9. *Methods of control:*

A. Preventive measures:

1. Application by hand or power blower of residual insecticide powder (10% DDT or newer lousicides) at appropriate intervals to clothes and persons of populations living under conditions favoring lousiness. Lice are known to develop DDT resistance; lindane may be substituted as a dusting powder.

2. Improvement of living conditions with provision for frequent bathing and washing of clothing.

3. Individual prophylaxis of persons subject to unusual risk through insecticide applied at appropriate intervals to clothing by dusting or by impregnation; immunization.

B. Control of the infected individual, contacts, and environment:

1. Report to local health authority: Case report universally required by international regulation.

2. Isolation: Not required after proper delousing of patient, clothing, living quarters and household contacts.

3. Concurrent disinfection: Appropriate insecticide powder applied to clothing and bedding of patient and contacts; treatment of hair for louse eggs (nits) with tested chemical agents.

4. Terminal disinfection: If death occurs before delousing, thorough application of insecticides to body and clothing.

5. Quarantine: Exposed lousy susceptibles should be quarantined for 15 days but may be released after application of insecticide with residual effect.

6. Immunization: Of all immediate contacts.

7. Investigation of contacts and source of infection: Every effort should be made to trace the source of infection to direct or indirect contact with a preceding case.

8. Specific treatment: The tetracyclines or chloramphenicol orally in a loading dose followed by daily doses until the patient becomes afebrile (usually 2 days) and for one additional day.

C. Epidemic measures:

1. Delousing: The most important measure for the rapid control of typhus, where reporting has been good and numbers of cases are small, is application of insecticides with residual effect to all contacts. Where infection is known to be widespread, systematic application of residual insecticide to all persons in the community is indicated.

[769]

2. Immunization: Of persons in contact with cases; vaccination may be offered to entire community. The usual vaccines contain rickettsiae grown in yolk sac of developing chick embryo and inactivated by formalin. The vaccine is administered in 2 doses, one week apart; re-inoculation with a single dose every 4 months where danger of typhus persists. For vaccinated persons the risk of infection is reduced, the course of the disease is modified and the case fatality lowered.

D. International measures:

1. Telegraphic notification of WHO and of adjacent countries by governments of the existence of an epidemic of typhus fever.

2. Measures applicable to ships, aircraft and land transport arriving from typhus areas are specified by International Sanitary Regulations (WHO Techn. Rep. Ser., No. 41, Geneva, 1951).

3. International travellers may leave a typhus area without restraint after thorough application of insecticide with residual effect. Vaccination is recommended for all persons entering areas where typhus is present.

B. MURINE TYPHUS (FLEA-BORNE, ENDEMIC)

1. *Identification.* The clinical course resembles that of epidemic typhus but tends to be milder. Case fatality for all ages is about 2%, with prognosis grave in older people.

   The Weil-Felix reaction is usually positive with Proteus OX19 after the 9th day; the complement fixation reaction a few days later. Differential diagnosis from louse-borne typhus is by serologic tests using rickettsial suspensions.

2. *Etiologic agent.* Rickettsia prowazeki, var. typhi (Rickettsia mooseri).

3. *Source and reservoir of infection.* Fleas, commonly Xenophylla cheopis, infected from rats which are the reservoir, Rattus rattus and Rattus norvegicus. The rodent disease is maintained in nature by a rat-flea-rat cycle.

4. *Mode of transmission.* Infected fleas excrete rickettsiae in feces, defecate after sucking blood, and contaminate the fresh skin wound. Inhalation of dried infected flea feces may account for an occasional case.

5. *Incubation period.* From 6 to 14 days, commonly 12 days.

6. *Period of communicability.* Not communicable from man to man.

7. *Susceptibility and resistance.* Susceptibility is general. One attack confers immunity, not always permanent. Murine typhus vaccine (similar to epidemic typhus vaccine) has had field trial but requires further evaluation.

8. *Occurrence.* World wide in areas where men and rats occupy the same buildings. Five thousand cases occurred in the USA in 1945, but numbers are markedly less in recent years. Highest attack rates are in Gulf and South Atlantic seaboard states, mainly during summer months when fleas are abundant. Changes in agricultural practices and increased rat populations of farms make the disease increasingly rural, replacing the former urban distribution centered around feed and grain stores.

9. *Methods of control:*

   A. Preventive measures:

   1. Application of insecticide powders with residual activity (10% DDT or other compounds) to rat runs, burrows, and harborages.

[770]

2. Rodent control measures should be delayed until flea populations have been reduced by insecticides, to avoid temporary increase in cases.

B. Control of the infected individual, contacts and environment:

1. Report to local health authority: Case report obligatory in most states and countries.
2. Isolation: None.
3. Concurrent disinfection: None.
4. Terminal disinfection: None.
5. Quarantine: None.
6. Immunization: None for contacts.
7. Investigation of contacts and source of infection: Search for rodents around premises or home of patient.
8. Specific treatment: As for epidemic typhus.

C. Epidemic measures: In endemic areas with numerous cases, widespread use of DDT has markedly reduced the flea index of rats, and incidence of infection in rats and man. Inoculation with an inactivated R. mooseri vaccine may be useful for limited groups in hazardous occupations but the efficiency of specific therapy eliminates the need for general protection of populations.

D. International measures: None.

YAWS

1. *Identification.* An acute and chronic relapsing non-venereal treponematosis characterized by hypertrophic, granulomatous or ulcerative destructive lesions of the skin, and by destructive and hypertrophic changes in bone. Two to 8 weeks after exposure, a primary lesion appears at the site of inoculation as an ulcer or granulation ("mother yaw"). In several weeks to several months, and often before the initial lesion has healed, mild constitutional symptoms appear, with generalized eruption of papules and granulomatous nodules, often in successive crops and lasting from a few months to several years, eventually developing into typical frambesiaform lesions. Eruptions of soles of the feet ("crab yaws") are common in this and the tertiary stage. The tertiary stage develops after an intervening latency, sometimes a matter of years, with destructive or proliferative lesions of bone and joint, and destructive lesions of skin. Unlike venereal syphilis, seldom involves the central nervous system or viscera; rarely if ever fatal. Synonyms: Frambesia tropica, pian, bouba, parangi and many others.

Serologic tests for syphilis are reactive with the same frequency in yaws as in syphilis, becoming positive during the primary stage, remaining positive during the secondary stage and tending toward non-reactivity after many years of latency, even without specific therapy.

2. *Etiologic agent.* Treponema pertenue.
3. *Source and reservoir of infection.* An infected person; surface and exudates of early skin lesions.
4. *Mode of transmission.* Principally by direct household or other contact with infectious lesions; infrequently by direct contact with contaminated articles; some evidence of vector transmission by a minute fly, Hippelates pallipes; transmission in utero not established.
5. *Incubation period.* From 2 weeks to 3 months, generally 3–6 weeks.

[771]

6. *Period of communicability.* Variable; may extend intermittently over several years while relapsing moist lesions are present; treponemata are not usually found in late ulcerative lesions.

7. *Susceptibility and resistance.* No clear evidence of natural or racial immunity but acquired resistance against homologous strains seems established; resistance against heterologous strains is not disproved. Resistance develops slowly; is relatively weak during the first months or years and may be overcome by large reinfecting doses; later become solid unless suppressed by early treatment. Superinfection in late latency may be manifested by late ulcerative lesions.

8. *Occurrence.* Widely and unevenly distributed; affected by many variables within the physical and social environment. Predominantly a childhood disease but occurs in later life; males outnumber females. Primarily a disease of rural peoples of the tropics and subtropics; the lowest social and economic groups have the highest rates. Particularly common in equatorial Africa, the Caribbean area, parts of India, Ceylon, the Philippines, Burma, Indochina, Indonesia, Thailand and throughout the South Pacific Islands; endemic foci in parts of Brazil, Colombia, Venezuela and the Guianas and in several countries of Central America; sporadic cases occur in North America and Europe from infection contracted elsewhere.

9. *Methods of control.* Venereal syphilis has declined significantly in many areas; the non-venereal treponematoses are a continuing problem. The etiologic agents of all these disorders are morphologically and biologically indistinguishable and the clinical syndromes produced are the result of epidemiologic rather than biologic differences. A controlled situation in syphilis is not to be achieved without control of yaws, bejel, pinta and "endemic syphilis."

A. Preventive measures: The following are applicable to yaws and to other non-venereal treponematoses named above.

    1. General health promotional measures; health education, better sanitation and improved social and economic conditions over a period of years will lead to a lesser incidence.

    2. In endemic areas education of the public about treponematosis; organization of intensive control activities on a community basis, to include analysis of the specific local problem, examination of entire populations, mass treatment of infected persons and contacts, and periodic assessment of results achieved.

    3. Provision of facilities for early diagnosis and treatment on a continuing plan, whereby the mass control campaign (9A2 above) is eventually consolidated into permanent local health services providing early diagnosis and treatment to patients and contact investigation and health education to the community.

    4. Emphasis on control of infectivity should not preclude treatment of disfiguring and incapacitating late manifestations nor the discovery and treatment of latent cases, since many late and latent lesions subsequently become reactivated and possibly infectious.

B. Control of the infected individual, contacts and environment:

    1. Report to local health authority: In selected endemic areas; in many countries not a reportable disease. Differentiation of venereal and non-venereal treponematoses with proper reporting of each has particular importance in evaluation of mass campaigns and in the consolidation period thereafter.

    2. Isolation: None; avoid intimate personal contact until lesions are healed.

[772]

3. Concurrent disinfection: None; care in disposal of discharges and articles contaminated therewith.
4. Terminal disinfection: None.
5. Quarantine: None.
6. Immunization: None.
7. Investigation of contacts and source of infection: All familial contacts should be treated, see 9B8.
8. Specific treatment: Penicillin; for early infectious lesions in adults no less than 1.2 million units of procaine penicillin in oil with 2% aluminum monostearate, proportionately less for children, in one injection; the preventive dose for contacts is not less than half that for early infectious cases.

C. Epidemic measures: At the present time most control activities have to do with hyperendemic situations. The problem is broader than the control of the infected individual and his immediate contacts. In areas of high incidence a broad segment of the population at risk should be given "preventive" or "abortive" treatment, especially children of preschool and school age, where attack rates are commonly high. In areas of lower incidence "preventive" treatment may be restricted to intimate contacts (household and extra-household) regardless of age.

D. International measures:
1. Appropriate examination of groups of adolescents and young adults moving from areas of high prevalence of treponemal infections.

YELLOW FEVER

1. *Identification.* An acute infectious disease of short duration and varying severity. The mildest cases are clinically indeterminate; typical attacks are characterized by sudden onset, fever, headache, backache, prostration, nausea and vomiting. As the disease progresses, the pulse rate slows in relation to temperature and albuminuria is pronounced. Leukopenia appears early, most pronounced about the fifth day. Common hemorrhagic symptoms include epistaxis, buccal bleeding, hematemesis and melena. Jaundice is moderate but post mortem icterus may be pronounced. Case fatality among indigenous populations of endemic regions is less than 5 per cent; for persons of other origin, rates of 30–40% are common.

Laboratory procedures in diagnosis are isolation of virus from blood through animal inoculation; demonstration of antibodies in convalescent serum when absent during the first 4 days; and demonstration of typical histopathological lesions of the liver.

2. *Etiologic agent.* The virus of yellow fever.

3. *Source and reservoir of infection.* The immediate source of infection for man is an infected mosquito; in urban areas the reservoir of infection, and the source of infection for mosquitoes, is an infected person, in forest areas monkeys, marmosets and probably marsupials.

4. *Mode of transmission.* In urban and certain rural areas, by the bite of the mosquito, Aëdes aegypti. In the forests of South America by the bite of forest mosquitoes that include Haemagogus spegazzinii, H. spegazzinii falco, H. capricornii, and Aëdes leucocelaenus. In East Africa, rural and sylvan transmission occurs through the bite of Aëdes simpsoni, A. africanus, and possibly other Aëdes mosquitoes.

[773]

5. *Incubation period.* Three to six days.

6. *Period of communicability.* Shortly prior to onset of fever and for the first three days of illness. Highly communicable where many susceptible persons and abundant vector mosquitoes co-exist. Not communicable by contact from man to man or by fomites. The extrinsic incubation period of Aëdes aegypti varies with temperature, commonly 10 to 14 days. Mosquitoes once infected remain so for life.

7. *Susceptibility and resistance.* Recovery from yellow fever is regularly followed by lasting immunity; second attacks are unknown. Mild, inapparent infections are common in endemic areas. Transient passive immunity in infants born to immune mothers may persist up to six months. In natural infection, antibodies appear in the blood within the first week. Active immunity is induced by inoculation with a suitable vaccine, see 9A3.

8. *Occurrence.* All ages are susceptible; in endemic areas of urban yellow fever with many adults immune, more than half of cases are among children, the ratio of males to females being approximately equal. Jungle yellow fever of tropical America is predominantly a disease of adult males, the 20–40 year age group being most affected. Seasonal incidence follows rainfall and prevalence of local vector mosquitoes; commonest in summer months. In Colombia and part of Brazil the seasonal curve of jungle yellow fever is bimodal. Geographic distribution of urban yellow fever has changed greatly as a result of mosquito control campaigns. In the Americas as a whole, the last case known to be transmitted by Aëdes aegypti was in Brazil in 1942. Outbreaks of urban yellow fever are still reported from Africa. Available evidence indicates that jungle yellow fever is present from time to time in all countries of the mainland of the Americas, from Mexico south to Central and South America, with the exception of Uruguay and Chile where there are no tropical or subtropical forests with monkeys or other susceptible animals.

9. *Methods of control:*

   A. Preventive measures:

   1. Control of Aëdes aegypti breeding is the most important factor in prevention of urban outbreaks of yellow fever and should be undertaken in towns and cities of countries where the disease is endemic. Complete control of urban yellow fever is possible in the Americas since A. aegypti is not a forest mosquito. Permanent protection is not to be had without a permanent control service.

   2. Sylvan or jungle yellow fever, transmitted by forest species of Aëdes and Haemagogus, cannot be controlled by any known anti-mosquito measures. Intensive vaccination programs are effective, particularly when aimed at persons living in rural areas whose daily occupation brings them into forests in yellow fever areas.

   3. Active immunization of all persons necessarily exposed to infection because of residence or occupation is necessary. Two living modified vaccines have had wide acceptance. The one (17-D strain) produces satisfactory immunity after one inoculation. Antibodies appear from 7 to 10 days after vaccination and persist for at least 6 years, probably longer. A vaccine extensively used in West Africa combines living neurotropic yellow fever virus with vaccinia virus, applied once by scarification; effective, but reactions are more frequent and encephalitis is an occasional complication.

[774]

B. Control of the infected individual, contacts and environment:
  1. Report to local health authority: Case report universally required by international regulation.
  2. Isolation: None; prevent access of mosquitoes to patient during first three days by screened sickroom or by spraying quarters with insecticide having residual effect.
  3. Concurrent disinfection: None; home of patient and all houses in vicinity should be sprayed promptly with an insecticide having residual action, such as 5% DDT, benzene hexachloride or chlordane.
  4. Terminal disinfection: None.
  5. Quarantine: None.
  6. Immunization: Family contacts and neighbors of patient not previously immunized should be vaccinated promptly.
  7. Investigation of contacts and source of infection: Inquiry about areas of forest visited by patient 3 to 6 days before onset, to identify foci of jungle yellow fever; observation of all others visiting that tract of forest. Search of premises and place of work for mosquitoes believed capable of transmitting infection. Attention to mild febrile illnesses and unexplained deaths suggesting yellow fever.
  8. Specific treatment: None.
C. Epidemic measures:
  1. Urban or Aëdes aegypti transmitted yellow fever:
    a. Spray interior of all homes in community with residual insecticide, such as DDT or benzene hexachloride.
    b. Application of a larvicide to all water containers of the community; 2% DDT in ethyl alcohol has been used successfully in jars and barrels containing drinking water.
    c. Mass vaccination.
  2. Jungle or sylvan yellow fever:
    a. Vaccination of all persons living near forested areas or entering forests.
    b. Avoidance of forests by unvaccinated individuals, and by vaccinated persons for the first week after vaccination; particularly those tracts of forest where infection has been localized.
  3. In regions where yellow fever may occur, a viscerotome service should be organized to collect for diagnostic purposes small specimens of liver tissue from fatal febrile illnesses of ten days' duration or less; many cases and outbreaks otherwise missed are thereby discovered.
  4. Immunity surveys by neutralization test, of human populations and of primates captured in forested areas, are useful in defining endemic-enzootic areas.
D. International measures:
  1. Telegraphic notifications of WHO and of adjacent countries, by governments, of the existence of an epidemic of yellow fever.
  2. Measures applicable to ships, aircraft and land transport arriving from yellow fever areas are specified in International Sanitary Regulations (WHO Techn. Rep. Ser. No. 41, Geneva, 1951).
  3. Animal quarantine: Quarantine of monkeys and marmosets arriving from yellow fever areas may be required until seven days have elapsed after leaving.

4. International travellers: A valid anti-yellow fever vaccination certificate is required by most countries for travellers into or coming from recognized yellow fever zones of Africa and South America; otherwise, quarantine measures are applicable. The international certificate of vaccination is valid from 10 days after date of vaccination and for 6 years; if revaccinated within that time, from data of that revaccination.

APPENDIX E

Glossary

A

ab-do′men: the belly, the portion of the body between the chest and the pelvis. It contains the stomach, the large and small intestines, the liver, spleen, pancreas, and kidneys, as well as blood vessels, nerves, etc.

a-bor′tion: premature expulsion of the fetus before it is capable of living.

ab′scess: a collection of pus in the body.

ab-sorp′tion: transfer of materials into the blood, *e.g.*, water, food, etc., from the intestinal tract; toxins from an area of infection; drugs, etc., from mucous membranes.

ac-id-o′sis: a condition in which the alkaline reserve of the body is depleted, as in advanced stages of diabetes.

ac′ne: an affection of the skin characterized by small pustules, chiefly on the face.

ad′dict: one who gives himself over to a constant practice.

Add′ison′s disease: a disease due to diminished function of the adrenal glands, marked by weakness, anemia, and yellow pigmentation of the skin; usually due to tuberculosis.

ad′e-ni′tis: inflammation of a gland.

ad′e-noids: collections of lymphoid tissue in the pharynx posterior to the nose; also called the pharyngeal tonsils.

ad′i-pose: fatty.

ad-re′nal glands: also called suprarenal glands; small glands of internal secretion located just above the kidneys.

ad-ren′a-line: the secretion of the adrenal glands.

al-bu′min: a protein found in nearly every animal tissue and fluid.

al-bu′mi-nu′ria: the occurrence of albumin in the urine; usually denotes some disturbance of the kidneys.

al′ka-line: having the properties of an alkali; the opposite of acid.

al′ler-gy: the natural hypersensitiveness of an individual to an antigen.

a-mi′no ac-id: an organic acid containing an NH_2 and a $COOH$ group: the structural element of proteins.

[777]

am′ni-on: the innermost membrane covering the embryo.

an-a′er-o′bic: referring to bacteria which thrive best in the absence of free oxygen or air.

a-ne′mia: deficient quantity or quality of the blood, reducing its capacity to carry oxygen.

an′es-the′si-a: a condition of complete or partial loss of feeling.

an-gi′na: a severe inflammation of the throat; any disease marked by spasmodic suffocative attacks.

an-gi′na pec′to-ris: a painful disease of the heart accompanied by a sense of suffocating contraction in the chest.

an-ky-lo′sis: abnormal immobility of a joint.

an-ti-bi-ot′ic: a drug effective against microorganisms.

an′ti-bod-ies: protective substances in the blood of immune animals.

an′ti-gen: a substance which stimulates the formation of antibodies.

an′ti-sep′tic: a substance which prevents the growth of bacteria.

an′ti-tox′in: an antibody developed against a specific toxin (poison).

ap′o-plex′y: sudden paralysis and loss or diminution of consciousness, usually from a hemorrhage into the brain.

ap-pen′di-ci′tis: inflammation of the vermiform appendix.

ar-te′ri-o-scle-ro′sis: hardening of arterial walls.

ar-thri′tis: inflammation of a joint.

ar′thro-pod: animal with articulated body and limbs, such as insects, etc.

ar-tic′u-lated: joined by a joint.

a-sep′sis: aseptic state; free from harmful organisms, as in surgery.

as-phyx′i-a: unconsciousness or death from lack of oxygen in blood.

as-sim′i-la′tion: the process of absorption of nourishment and transformation of it into tissues.

asth′ma: a disease characterized by difficulty in breathing, a sense of constriction in the chest, cough, and expectoration.

a-stig′ma-tism: visual defect in which light rays are not brought to a proper focus by the unaided eye; due to improper curvature of eyeball.

as-tring′ent: a substance which causes contraction of tissues and arrests discharges.

a-te-lec′ta-sis: partial collapse or incomplete expansion of lung.

at′ro-phy: wasting or diminution in size.

at′ro-pine: a drug extracted from belladonna; remarkable for its power to dilate the pupil of the eye and to arrest secretions.

at-ten′u-at′ed: weakened.

au′di-to′ry: pertaining to hearing.

au′to-in-tox′i-ca′tion: poisoning from toxic substances produced within the body.

au′to-nom′ic: self-controlling.

au′to-nom′ic system: that portion of the nervous system which regulates the action of involuntary muscles, blood vessels, and the organs and glands of the body.

au′top-sy: dissection of a dead body to learn the cause, seat, or nature of disease, or the cause of death: post-mortem examination.

B

ba-cil′lus (pl. bacilli): rod-shaped bacterium.

bac-te′ri-e′mia: bacteria in the blood stream.

bar'bi-tur'ates: various synthetic drugs which produce sedation and sleep.

bar'i-um: a chemical element of the alkaline earth group, which prevents the passage of x-rays.

bar'i-um meal: a suspension of barium in milk that is eaten in order to show by x-ray the passage of food in the digestive tract.

bas'al me-tab'o-lism: the expenditure of energy in the body at rest.

bel'la-don'na: a medicinal extract from the leaves and root of a plant called the "deadly nightshade."

be-nign': harmless.

ber'i-ber'i: a disease due to a deficiency of vitamin B_1 and marked by inflammatory changes in the nerves.

blood pres'sure: the force of the blood in the arteries.

bo'vine: pertaining to a cow.

bot'u-lism: food poisoning caused by the toxin produced by *Bacillus botulinus.*

bron-chi'tis: inflammation of the bronchi.

bron'cho-scope: an instrument for looking into the bronchi.

bron-chos'co-pist: a specialist in the use of the bronchoscope.

bron'chus (pl. bronchi): either of the two main branches of the trachea.

bul'bar polio: poliomyelitis in which area of junction of brain and spinal cord is affected which contains nerve centers of swallowing, breathing, etc.

C

cae'cum (or ce'cum): a pouch which forms the first part of the large intestine.

cal'o-rie: the amount of heat required to raise one gram of water one degree centigrade. A large calorie is the amount of heat required to raise one kilogram of water one degree centigrade.

can'cer: a collection of body tissue cells which reproduce rapidly and without limit until they destroy life; a malignant tumor, which usually gives rise to secondary growths (metastases).

car'bo-hy'drate: an organic chemical compound containing carbon, hydrogen, and oxygen with the hydrogen and oxygen in the same proportion as in water, *i.e.,* two parts of hydrogen to one part of oxygen. Sugars and starches are carbohydrates.

car'bon di-ox'ide: a gas containing one part of carbon and two parts of oxygen; an end product in the burning or oxidation of any carbon compound, a constituent of exhaled air.

car'ci-no'ma: cancers arising from epithelial tissue.

car'i-ous: affected with caries (decay).

ca'se-in: a protein found in milk.

cast: molded, plastic material formed in the cavities of various organs; casts found in the urine come from the kidneys and usually indicate a disease process.

cat'a-ract: opacity of the lens of the eye.

ca-tarrh': an inflammatory infection of a mucous membrane.

ca-thar'tic: a medicine which causes emptying of the bowels.

cell: a unit of life; a minute mass of protoplasm with the power of reproduction and of carrying on vital processes.

cel'lu-lose: the fibrous woody part of vegetable foods.

cer'e-bel'lum: a division of the brain at the base of the skull.

[779]

cer′e-bral: pertaining to the cerebrum, the larger part of the brain.

cer′e-bro-spi′nal: pertaining to the brain and spinal cord.

cer′vix: the neck or necklike part.

Ce-sar′e-an sec′tion: delivery of a child through an incision in the abdominal wall and the uterus.

chan′cre: a venereal sore or ulcer.

chro′mo-somes: the cellular elements regarded as the carriers of hereditary characteristics.

chron′ic: long continued, not acute.

cil′i-a: minute hairlike processes of certain cells.

cil′i-ar′y mus′cle: muscles which regulate the thickness of the lens of the eye.

cir-rho′sis: hardening of an organ due to excessive formation of connective tissue as a result of inflammation.

co-caine′: a drug obtained from coca leaves, used as a local anesthetic, dangerously habit-forming.

coc′cus: a spherical bacterium.

co′de-ine: a drug, related to morphine and derived from opium; relieves pain and is some-what narcotic; carries little if any practical danger of habituation.

co-li′tis: inflammation of the colon.

co′lon: the portion of the large intestine between the caecum and the rectum.

con-gen′i-tal: existing at or before birth.

conges′tion: overfullness of capillaries or other blood vessels in any locality or organ.

con′junc-ti′va: the mucous membrane which covers the front of the eyeball and lines the eyelids.

con-junc′ti-vi′tis: inflammation of the conjunctiva.

con′sti-pa′tion: infrequent and difficult evacuation of the feces.

con-ta′gious: communicable by direct or indirect contact.

con′tra-cep′tion: the prevention of conception, *i.e.,* of pregnancy.

con′va-les′cence: period of recovery from a disease.

cor′ne-a: the transparent portion of the front of the eyeball.

cor′o-nar′y throm-bo′sis: development of obstruction due to a clot in the coronary arteries of the heart.

cor′pus lu′te-um: yellow mass in an ovary in the place of a discharged ovum; produces an internal secretion.

cor′tex: center layer of an organ.

co-ry′za: acute cold in the head with watery discharge.

cre′tin-ism: inherited idiocy with stunted growth and physical deformity caused by deficient thyroid secretion.

D

death rate: ratio of deaths to population, usually expressed as the number of deaths per 1,000 or per 100,000 population.

de-bil′i-ty: weakness, feebleness.

def′e-ca′tion: discharge of the feces.

de-hy′drate: to lose water.

del-e-te′-ri-ous: harmful.

de-lir′i-um: disordered mental state with excitement and illusions.

de-lu′sion: an insanely erroneous belief or fancy.

der'ma-ti'tis: inflammation of the skin.

der'mis: the true skin.

dex'trose: glucose; a single sugar.

di'a-be'tes: diseases which cause a persistent increase of urinary excretion.

di'a-phragm: the muscular septum which divides the thorax and the abdomen.

di-as'to-le: the rest period of the heart between beats during which expansion takes place.

Dick test: skin test with scarlet fever toxin to determine whether one is immune to scarlet fever; redness, called a positive test, indicates susceptibility.

di-ges'tion: process of preparing food for absorption and use by the body.

di-ni'tro-phe'nol: a drug which increases metabolism and causes loss of weight; dangerous.

dis'in-fec'tion: destruction of all organisms and their products capable of producing disease.

dom'i-nant trait: the stronger of mutually antagonistic parental characters.

du'o-de'num: the first part of the small intestine below the stomach.

dys'men-or-rhe'a: painful or otherwise abnormal menstruation.

dys-pep'sia: indigestion.

E

ec-lamp'si-a: a sudden attack of convulsions related to pregnancy.

ec-top'ic pregnancy: pregnancy outside of the uterus, as in the fallopian tube or in the abdomen.

ec'ze-ma: an inflammatory itching disease of the skin.

e-de'ma: swelling due to watery fluids in the body tissues.

e-ma'ci-a'tion: a wasted appearance of the body.

em'bo-lus: a piece of blood clot or other material which is carried by the blood current and lodged in a blood vessel so as to obstruct the circulation.

em'bry-o: a fetus before end of third month.

e-mul'si-fy: to divide fat in solution into minute particles.

en-ceph-a-li'tis: inflammation of the brain.

en-dem'ic: a disease present continuously in an area.

en'do-crine gland: a gland producing a chemical substance which passes directly into the blood stream and affects various functions and organs.

en'do-me'tri-um: the mucous membrane which lines the uterus.

en'e-ma: a liquid injected into the rectum.

en'ter-i'tis: inflammation of the intestine.

en'zyme: a chemical ferment.

e-phed'rine: a synthetic drug similar in its effects to adrenaline.

ep'i-dem'ic: a disease which attacks many persons in the same region at the same time.

ep'i-de'mi-ol'o-gy: the science of the study and control of epidemic diseases.

ep'i-der'mis: the outer layer of the skin.

ep'i-did'y-mis: an elongated mass at the back of the testicle; consists of tortuous tubes leading from the testicle.

ep'i-lep'sy: a nervous disease characterized by paroxysms or fits, occurring at intervals, and attended by sudden loss of consciousness.

ep'i-the'li-um: the cellular tissue which covers surfaces and lines cavities of the body.

e'quine: pertaining to a horse.

er-gos'ter-ol: a substance found in plants and animals which upon exposure to ultraviolet light becomes vitamin D.

e-ryth'ro-cyte: a red blood corpuscle.

e-soph'a-gus or *gullet:* the part of the alimentary canal (digestive tract) between the pharynx and the stomach.

eth'moid: a bone in the base of the skull which forms the roof of the nose. A number of paranasal sinuses are in this bone.

eu-gen'ics: the science of improving the human race through control of offspring.

eu-sta'chi-an tube: a tube between the middle ear and the pharynx.

ex-cre'tion: the elimination of waste products from the body.

ex'oph-thal'mic goiter: a disease characterized by protrusion of the eyes, rapid heartbeat, loss of weight, and overactivity—usually with enlargement of the thyroid.

ex'pi-ra'tion: expulsion of air from the lungs.

F

fal-lo'pi-an tubes: tubelike portions of the uterus which convey the ova from the ovary to the body of the uterus.

fa-tal'i-ty rate: the proportion of persons who die from a disease in relation to the number attacked by that disease; usually expressed in per cent.

fat'ty acids: chemical compounds which combine with glycerine to form fats.

fe'ces: the excreta of the bowels.

fe'mur: thigh bone.

fer'men-ta'tion: a chemical change produced by a ferment.

fe'tus: the unborn child after the end of the third month.

flex: to bend.

flu'o-rine: a chemical element of the chlorine-iodine family.

flu'o-ro-scope: a device used in making x-ray examinations.

fo've-a: a cup-shaped depression.

fu'run-cle: a boil.

G

gan'grene: the dying of tissue due to interference with local nutrition, *e.g.*, cutting off blood supply.

gas'tric: pertaining to the stomach.

gas-tri'tis: inflammation of the stomach.

gas'tro-in-tes'ti-nal: pertaining to the stomach and intestines.

genes: the hypothetical units of which chromosomes are composed; supposedly the carriers of hereditary characteristics.

gen'i-tal: pertaining to reproduction or the sex organs.

ger-i-at'rics: the treatment of diseases of old age.

germ: any microscopic organism, as bacteria or protozoa; may be disease-producing or harmless; also a reproductive cell.

germ plasm: the substance of reproductive cells.

ger'mi-cide: an agent that destroys germs.

gin'gi-vi'tis: inflammation of the gums.

glau-co'ma: a disease characterized by excessive pressure within the eyeball, causing impairment of vision and frequently eventual blindness.

glu'cose: a form of sugar found in many fruits, in the blood, and occasionally in the urine; also called dextrose; a single or simple sugar.

gly'co-gen: a multiple sugar made up of many units of glucose; the form in which sugar is stored in the body, particularly in the liver and muscles.

gly'co-su'ri-a: sugar in the urine.

goi'ter: an enlargement of the thyroid gland.

gon'ad-o-trop'ic: affecting the sex glands.

gon'ad: a sex gland, *e.g.*, the ovary or testis.

gon'or-rhe'a: a contagious inflammatory disease of the genital tract caused by the gonococcus and characterized by a purulent discharge.

Graaf'i-an fol'li-cle: one of the small spherical bodies in the ovary, each of which contains an ovum.

gyn'e-col'o-gy: the science of the diseases peculiar to women.

H

hal-lu'ci-na'tion: perception of objects with no reality, wandering of the mind.

ham'string muscles: muscles on back of thigh.

he'mo-glo'bin: the red pigment of the blood.

he'mo-phil'i-a: a condition in which the clotting time of the blood is prolonged, producing a strong tendency to bleeding, usually hereditary.

hem'or-rhage: the escape of blood from the blood vessels.

hem'or-rhoid: a pile; a swelling formed by dilation of blood vessels at the anus.

ho'mo-sex'ual: sexually attracted by persons of the same sex.

he-red'i-ty: derived from ancestry, transmitted through the germ cells or genes.

her'ni-a: a protrusion of a part or organ through the walls of its cavity; a rupture.

her'o-in: a sedative drug derived from morphine, dangerously habit-forming.

hives: an allergic skin disease with areas of swelling, redness, and itching.

hom'i-cide: the killing of one human being by another.

hor'mone: a chemical substance produced in one organ and carried in the blood to another organ or part of the body where it stimulates functional activity.

hy'brid: an animal or plant bred from two species or races.

hy'giene: science of preserving health.

hy'per-e'mi-a: an excessive amount of blood in some body tissue or organ.

hy'per-gly-ce'mi-a: excess sugar in the blood.

hy'per-o'pi-a: farsightedness.

hy'per-ten'sion: abnormally high blood pressure.

hy-per'tro-phy: increase in the size of an organ.

hy'po-chon'dri-a: a mental disorder characterized by morbid anxiety as to one's health.

hy'po-der'mic: applied beneath or situated under the skin.

hy'po-ten'sion: lowered blood pressure.

I

id'i-o-syn'cra-sy: a peculiarity of constitution or temperament.

il'e-um: the third, last, and longest division of the small intestine.

im-bal'ance: lack of balance between opposing muscles, especially of the eye.

im-mu'ni-ty: state of being protected against a particular disease.

im'pe-ti'go: a skin disease characterized by isolated pustules.

im'po-tence: lacking power, strength, or vigor; chiefly, lacking reproductive power.

in'cu-ba'tion: period of development of an infectious disease to the time of the appearance of symptoms.

in'di-ges'tion: incomplete or difficult digestion.

in-fec'tion: communication of disease from one person to another; implantation of disease from without.

in'fra-red' rays: invisible light rays shorter than the red rays, which produce heat.

in-oc'u-la'tion: the communication of a disease by inserting its virus in the skin or flesh in order to communicate disease, usually in a mild form, and to secure future immunity.

in'or-gan'ic: composed of matter other than animal or vegetable, usually mineral.

in-san'i-ty: a legal term denoting prolonged unsoundness of mental condition; medical term is "psychosis."

in-sec'ti-cide: a preparation that will destroy insects.

in'spi-ra'tion: the inhalation of air into the lungs.

in'su-lin: the active principle of the internal secretion of the islands of Langerhans of the pancreas; employed in treating diabetes.

i'ris: pigmented contractile diaphragm of the eyeball, perforated by the pupil.

i'so-la'tion: separation of persons having an infectious disease.

J

jaun'dice: the presence of bile in the blood, producing a yellow pigmentation of the skin.

je-ju'num: the second portion of the small intestine, between the duodenum and the ileum.

K

ker'a-tin: the nitrogenous base of such tissues as horn, hair, feathers, and so forth.

kid'ney: either of two glandular bodies in the lumbar region which secrete urine.

ky-pho'sis: humpback or hunchback.

L

lac-ta'tion: the secretion of milk.

lac'tose: milk sugar.

lar'ynx: the organ which contains the vocal cords.

le-gu'min-ous: plants the seeds of which are in pods, as peas and beans.

le'sion: any local abnormality: bruise, wound, inflammation, tumor, cavity, etc.

leu'co-cyte: white blood corpuscle.

leu'co-cy-to'sis: increase in white blood cells.

leu'co-pen'i-a: decrease in white blood cells.

lig'a-ment: a tough fibrous band connecting bones or supporting viscera.

li'pase: a ferment which breaks down or digests fats.

lor-do'sis: abnormal forward curvature of the spine, usually in the lumbar region.

lum-ba'go: pain in the lower back.

lymph: the fluid contained in the lymphatic vessels or spaces.

lymph glands: misnomer for lymph nodes.

lymph node: any one of the nodules occurring in the course of the lymphatic vessels; they act as filters for infection and become swollen when inflamed.

lym-phat'ic: pertaining to lymph, or to a lymphatic node or vessel.

lym'pho-cyte: one form of white blood corpuscle.

M

ma-lig'nant: dangerous; tending to produce death.

malt'ase: an enzyme which splits maltose into the single sugar glucose.

malt'ose: a double sugar.

Man-toux' test: the injection of a small amount of tuberculin into the skin; redness, called a "positive" reaction, indicates that one has or has had an infection with the tubercle bacilli.

ma'ri-jua'na: popular name of a poisonous weed, *Cannabis indica,* the dried leaves of which are smoked; a habit-forming drug.

mas'toid: the nipple-shaped bone behind the lower part of the ear.

mas'tur-ba'tion: self-stimulation of one's sex organs.

max'il-lar'y bone: bone on side of the face which bears the upper teeth.

max'il-lar'y si'nus: the air space or paranasal sinus in the maxillary bone.

me'di-an: in the middle.

me-dul'la: marrow or inner substance of an organ.

me-dul'la ob'lon-ga'ta: the lower portion of the brain, continuous with the spinal cord.

mel'an-cho'li-a: a form of insanity characterized by a depression of spirits and gloomy forebodings.

mel'a-nin: dark brown or black pigment in the body.

mem'brane: a thin layer of tissue that covers a surface, *e.g.,* the covering of the lips and lining of the mouth.

me-nin'ges: the three membranes covering the brain and spinal cord.

men'in-gi'tis: inflammation of the meninges.

men'o-pause: the period when menstruation ceases.

men'stru-a'tion: the periodic discharge of blood from the uterus.

me-tab'o-lism: the processes in the body of the building up and the destruction of materials that are used for the production of energy, for growth, and for the replacement of worn-out tissues.

me-tas'ta-sis: transfer of disease from one organ to another.

mi-cro-or'gan-ism: organism that can be seen only with a microscope.

mi'graine: periodic sick headaches.

mis-car'riage: premature birth or expulsion of a fetus after the third month of pregnancy.

mol'e-cule: the smallest possible unit of existence of any compound.

mor'bid: sick or sickly.

mor'phine: the principal alkaloid of opium; relieves pain and produces sleep; habit-forming.

mu-co'sa: a membrane lining the cavities and tubes communicating with the surface of the body and secreting a mucous fluid.

mu'cous: pertaining to or resembling mucus.

mu'cus: the sticky watery secretion of the glands in a mucous membrane that is moistened and protected by it.

my-al'gi-a: muscular pain.

my-o'pi-a: nearsightedness.

myx'e-de'ma: a disease of adults due to insufficient thyroid secretion; characterized by dullness of intellect, slow speech, and coarse skin and hair.

N

nar-cot'ic: a drug that relieves pain and induces sleep; in large doses it causes stupor, coma, or even death.

ne-cro'sis: death of tissues or cells.

ne'o-plasm: an abnormal growth, as a tumor.

ne-phri'tis: inflammation of the kidneys; Bright's disease.

nerve: an elongated bundle of nerve fibers having the ability to transmit nervous stimuli.

neu-ral'gia: nerve pain; pain of a severe, throbbing character along the course or path of a nerve.

neu'ras-the'ni-a: nervous debility from prolonged mental strain, worry, etc.

neu-ri'tis: inflammation of a nerve.

neu-ro'sis: a functional nervous disease; *i.e.,* on; which is dependent upon no evident lesion.

neu-rot'ic: nervous; one who suffers from a functional nervous disorder.

ni'a-cin: the pellagra-preventive portion of the vitamin B complex, nicotinic acid.

nic'o-tin'ic acid: niacin.

ni'tro-gen: a colorless, odorless, gaseous element; constitutes four-fifths of the atmosphere by volume.

no'vo-cain': a local anesthetic drug, not chemically related to cocaine.

nu'cle-us: a small body within a cell; the vital part of the cell.

O

o-bes'i-ty: fatness.

ob-stet'rics: the medical specialty devoted to the care of women during pregnancy and childbearing.

oc'u-lar: pertaining to the eye.

oc'u-list: a physician who is a specialist in the diseases of the eye.

"open case": a patient with lesions of a disease, especially tuberculosis, that discharge germs to the outside.

oph'thal-mol'o-gist: an oculist.

op-ti'cian: one who makes spectacles after a formula prescribed by an oculist.

op'tic: pertaining to vision.

op-tom'e-trist: a person without medical training who fits glasses to correct visual defects.

o'ral: pertaining to the mouth.

or-gan'ic: pertaining to or derived from living organisms; in chemistry, compounds containing carbon; in disease, affecting the structure.

or-tho-pe'dics: correction or prevention of deformities in children or persons of any age.

or-thop'tic: pertaining to securing normal binocular vision, *e.g.,* orthoptic exercises in which ocular muscles are exercised to correct deviations.

o-to-scler-o'sis: a common cause of hearing impairment, due to growth of spongy bone in lining of inner ear.

o'va-ry: the female sex gland in which the ova are formed.

o'vu-la'tion: the formation of eggs in the ovary; the discharge of ova.

o'vum: egg; female reproductive cell.

ox'i-da'tion: combining with oxygen; burning.

P

pan'cre-as: a large elongated gland below the stomach; it secretes a digestive juice that is discharged into the duodenum and acts on all classes of foods; it also produces an internal secretion known as "insulin"; it is called "sweetbreads" when used as food.

pan-dem'ic: a worldwide spread of disease.

pa-pav'er-ine: a drug derived from opium; slightly narcotic, not habit-forming.

pa-ral'y-sis: loss of power of voluntary motion.

par'a-noi'a: a chronic insanity characterized by delusions of persecution.

par'a-site: a plant or animal living on or in some other living organism from which it obtains its food and shelter.

par'a-thy'roids: four small glands of internal secretion lying upon the thyroid; the secretion of these glands controls the metabolism of calcium.

pa-re'sis: a disease of the brain resulting in loss of mental and physical power; it is caused by syphilis.

pa-rot'id: a salivary gland on either side of the head situated below and in front of the ear.

pas'teur-i-za'tion: a treatment of milk to destroy disease-producing organisms.

path'o-gen'ic: causing disease.

path'o-log'i-cal: pertaining to or due to disease.

pe'di-at'rics: a medical specialty dealing with children.

pel-la'gra: a deficiency disease caused by a lack of niacin.

pe'nis: male sex organ.

pep'sin: a ferment of the gastric juice which acts on proteins.

pep'tone: the first stage in the digestion of proteins by pepsin.

per'i-stal'sis: rythmical contraction of the stomach or intestines.

per'i-to-ne'um: membrane lining the abdomen.

per'i-to-ni'tis: inflammation of the peritoneum.

phar'ynx: part of the alimentary canal between the mouth and the esophagus; into it open the mouth, the nose, the eustachian tubes, the esophagus, and the larynx.

phe'nol: carbolic acid.

phe'nol co'ef-fi'cient: the ability of an antiseptic to destroy bacterial life in comparison to a 5 per cent solution of phenol.

phys-i-a'-trist: specialist in physical medicine and rehabilitation.

phys'i-o-log'ic: pertaining to physiology, normal.

phys'i-ol'o-gy: the study of the function of the organs and parts of the body.

pin'e-al: a small pea-shaped endocrine gland located on the under surface of the brain.

pi-tres'sin: an endocrine secretion from the posterior part of the pituitary gland.

pi-tu'i-tar'y: an endocrine gland located under the brain; the so-called "master gland" of the body.

pla-cen'ta: the vascular structure attached to the uterus through which the fetus is nourished.

plas'ma: the fluid portion of the blood.

plate'let: an element of the blood, active in clotting.

pleu'ra: serous membrane lining the chest cavity and covering the lungs.

pleu'ri-sy: inflammation of the pleura.

pneu-mo'ni-a: inflammation of the lungs.

pneu'mo-tho'rax: presence of air or gas in the pleural cavity, causing collapse of the lung.

pol'len: the male fertilizing element of plants and trees.

pol'yp: a grapelike outgrowth of a mucous membrane.

pres'by-o'pi-a: farsightedness due to advancing age.

pro'phy-lac'tic: pertaining to the prevention of disease.

pros'tate: a gland surrounding the neck of the bladder and urethra in the male.

pros'ti-tu'tion: indiscriminate sexual intercourse, especially for hire.

pro'te-in: nitrogenous organic compounds formed by the union of many amino acids.

pro'to-plasm: the substance of cells.

pru-ri'tis: itching.

psy'chic: pertaining to the mind.

psy'cho-neu-ro'sis: a minor mental illness.

psy-cho-path'ic: relating to mental disease; an insane person.

psy-cho'sis: mental illness; a prolonged departure from one's normal standards of thinking, feeling, and acting.

pto'maine: a substance formed during the decomposition of dead animal or vegetable matter.

pty'a-lin: a ferment in saliva which acts on starches.

pu'ber-ty: the earliest age at which one can beget or bear children.

pu-er'per-al sep'sis: infection occurring as a complication of childbirth.

pu'er-pe'ri-um: the period between the termination of labor (childbirth) and the return to normal of the uterus.

pul'mo-nar'y: pertaining to the lungs.

pu'pil: the opening in the center of the iris.

pu'ru-lent: containing or consisting of pus.

pus: the creamy matter produced by an infection; consists chiefly of leucocytes in a serous exudate.

pus'tule: an elevation of the skin filled with pus or serum.

pu'tre-fac'tion: the decomposition of proteins or nitrogenous matter.

py-lo'rus: opening from the stomach into the intestines.

py'or-rhe'a: an infection of the gums around the teeth with the accumulation of pus and final looseness of the teeth.

Q

quar'an-tine: separation of individuals who have been exposed to a communicable disease during the incubation period; the detention of ships coming from infected or suspected ports.

quin'sy: an acute infection of the tonsils with abscess formation.

R

ra'bies: disease commonly known as "hydrophobia."

ra'di-um: a chemical element which gives off emanations similar to x-rays.

re-ces'sive: the weaker of mutually antagonistic inherited characteristics.

rec'tum: the terminal part of the intestine.

re'flex: an action produced by stimulation without necessarily any intervention of consciousness.

re-frac'tion: the determination of refractive errors of the eye and correction of same by glasses.

reg'is-tra'tion a're-a: the states in which the reporting and recording of births, deaths, etc., meets the standards established by the U.S. Bureau of the Census.

re-gur'gi-ta'tion: a reverse flow of food or blood.

re'nal: pertaining to the kidneys.

ret'i-na: the innermost coat lining the eyeball; contains the nerve endings of vision that are stimulated by light.

rheu-mat'ic fe'ver: acute inflammatory rheumatism.

rheu'ma-tism: a disease marked by pains in the joints or muscles, usually recurrent.

rhi-ni'tis: inflammation of the nasal mucous membrane.

roent'gen-ol'o-gist: a physician who specializes in the application of x-rays for diagnosis or treatment.

S

sap'ro-phyt'ic: obtaining nourishment from decaying vegetable matter, not disease-producing.

sar-co'ma: cancer arising from connective tissues.

sca'bi-es: the itch; dermatitis accompanied by intense itching caused by the itch mite.

Schick test: the injection of a small amount of diphtheria toxin into the skin to determine whether one is immune to diphtheria; redness is called a "positive" test and means that one is not immune.

scor-bu'tic: relating to scurvy.

scro'tum: the pouch that contains the testicles.

scur'vy: deficiency disease due to lack of vitamin C; characterized by weakness, bleeding gums, and anemia.

sed'a-tive: an agent that quiets nervous excitement.

se'men: the secretion of testicle, containing sperm.

sem'i-cir'cu-lar can'al: organ of the inner ear that controls equilibrium.

sem'i-nal ves'i-cle: male organ on back of urinary bladder in which semen is stored.

sep'sis: presence of pus-forming germs in blood or tissues.

sep'tic: relating to or caused by sepsis.

sep'ti-ce'mi-a: presence of pathogenic germs or their toxins in the blood.

sep'tum: a thin wall dividing two cavities or masses of tissue.

se'rous: like serum.

se'rum: clear liquid which may be separated from the clot and corpuscles of the blood.

si'nus: a hollow space or cavity.

si'nus, na'sal or *par-a-na'sal:* hollow spaces in bones of head connected with the cavity of the nose.

spasm: a sudden violent involuntary contraction, *e.g.*, of the muscles.

spas'mo-phil'i-a: having a tendency to convulsive seizures.

sperm: male reproductive cell formed in testis.

sper'ma-to-gen'e-sis: the formation of sperm.

spi'ro-chete: a spiral-shaped germ; one type causes syphilis.

staph'y-lo-coc'cus: spherical-shaped bacteria which occur in clusters.

starch: a carbohydrate made of multiple units of glucose.

ste-ap'sin: a fat-digesting ferment of the pancreas.

ste-ril'i-ty: inability to produce young.

ster'i-li-za'tion: destruction of all organisms, saprophytic as well as pathogenic.

ster'ol: a chemical related to the fats.

stim'u-lus: anything that arouses action in a muscle, nerve, or gland.

strep'to-coc'us: spherical shaped bacteria which occur in chains.

sug'ar, sim'ple or *single:* the simplest chemical form of carbohydrate, *e.g.*, glucose.

sug'ar, dou'ble: sugars made up of two units of simple sugar, *e.g.*, cane sugar or beet sugar.

sul'fon-am'ides: the "sulfa drugs," *e.g.*, sulfanilamide, sulfapyradine, sulfadiazine, etc.

su'pra-re'nal: above the kidney; refers to a particular gland of internal secretion; also called the adrenal.

sus-cep'ti-ble: not immune to an infectious disease.

syn'the-sis: processes of building up a compound by union of simpler compounds or its elements.

syn-thet'ic: relating to or made by synthesis.

syph'i-lis: a contagious venereal disease which may affect many tissues and organs.

sys'to-le: contraction of the heart.

T

tes'tis: one of the two male reproductive glands.

tet'a-nus: an infectious disease marked by painful tonic muscular contractions, caused by *Bacillus tetani,* popularly called "lockjaw."

tet'a-ny: a disease resembling tetanus.

the'o-bro'mine: a bitter chemical closely related to caffeine.

ther'a-peu'tic: curative; pertaining to the treatment of disease.

ther'a-py: treatment of disease.

tho-rac'ic: pertaining to the thorax or chest.

throm'bus: a plug more or less completely obstructing a blood vessel.

thy'mus: a gland of internal secretion located above the heart.

thy'roid: a ductless gland in the neck.

thy-rox'ine: the active principle of thyroid secretion.

ton'sil-lec'to-my: removal of the tonsils.

ton'sils: the pair of more or less prominent masses of lymphoid tissue at the back of the mouth.

tox-e'mi-a: blood poisoning; presence in the blood of the poisonous products of any pathogenic germ.

tox'in: a poisonous substance produced by pathogenic germs.

tox'oid: similar to a toxin; a modified toxin used for purpose of immunization.

tra'che-a: the windpipe; the air tube extending from the larynx to the bronchi.

tra-cho'ma: a contagious granular conjunctivitis, caused by a specific germ and tending to cause scars and blindness.

trau'ma: an injury or wound.

Trep'o-ne'ma pal'li-dum: a spiral germ with numerous curves; the causative agent of syphilis.

tryp'sin: the principal protein-digesting enzyme (ferment) of the pancreatic juice.

tu'ber-cle: any mass or small rounded nodule produced by the bacillus of tuberculosis.

tu-ber'cu-lin: a preparation obtained from cultures of the bacillus of tuberculosis.

tu-ber'cu-lo'sis: an infectious disease characterized by the formation of tubercles in the tissues; caused by the bacillus tuberculosis.

tu'mor: swelling; an abnormal mass of tissue, especially one due to morbid growth of tissue not normal to a part.

tur'bi-nate: small bones in the nasal passageways.

tym-pan'ic mem'brane: the eardrum.

U

ul'cer: an open sore, other than a wound.

ul'tra-vi'o-let rays: the invisible rays of light beyond the violet of the visible spectrum.

um-bil'i-cal cord: the cord which connects the fetus to the placenta; includes the blood vessels which carry nourishment and oxygen to the child.

um-bil-i'cus: the navel; the point of entrance of the umbilical cord into the fetus.

u-re'ter: the duct that carries the urine from a kidney to the bladder.

u-re'thra: duct through which urine is discharged from the bladder; and in the male the semen also from the seminal vesicles.

ur'ti-ca'ri-a: hives; an allergic eruption of itching wheals.

u'ter-us: in female mammals an organ for containing and usually for nourishing the young before birth.

V

vac'ci-na'tion: inoculation with a vaccine, to produce an artificial immunity.

vac'cine: any substance used for preventive inoculation.

vac-cin'i-a: cowpox; the disease, usually local and limited to the site of inoculation, induced in man by the inoculation of cowpox virus.

va-gi'na: the genital canal in the female leading from the uterus to the orifice of the genital canal.

var'i-cose: unnaturally swollen, applied especially to veins.

vas'o-mo'tor: nerves controlling the size of blood vessels by constriction and dilation.

vec'tor: an insect which carries disease from the sick to the well.

ve-ne're-al: relating to or resulting from sexual intercourse.

vir'ile: having the qualities of an adult man; capable of procreation.

vir'u-lence: quality or state of being virulent.

vir'u-lent: disease-producing; deadly poisonous.

vi′rus: extremely minute living organisms, too small to be seen by the ordinary microscope; some produce contagious diseases such as measles, mumps, influenza, cowpox, smallpox, rabies, infantile paralysis, etc.

vis′cer-a: the various internal organs of the cavities of the body.

vi′ta-mins: chemical substances present in natural foods and necessary for health.

W

Was′ser-mann test: a blood test for syphilis.

X

xe′roph-thal′mi-a: extreme dryness of the conjunctiva that loses its luster and becomes skinlike in appearance; due to a deficiency of vitamin A.

x′-rays′: roentgen rays; very short ethereal rays which will pass through solid bodies, cause destructive changes in living tissue, and affect a photographic plate.

INDEX

A

Abortion, 431
  contagious, 514
  habitual, 101
Absenteeism, 551
Absorption of foods, 83
Accidents, 26–34
  and alcohol, 201
  automobile, 31
  and community health, 493
  to eyes, 328
  farm, 556
  home, 27
  industrial, 29, 555
Acidosis, 89, 386
Acne, 361
Acromegaly, 381
ACTH, 382, 389, 458
Actinomycosis, 635
Addiction, alcohol, 203
  narcotic, 210–214
Addison's disease, 389
Adenoids, 310, 311
Adrenal glands, 388
Adrenalin, 389
Age, old, 461
  and sickness, 446
Air, bad, 253
  disinfection of, 257
  fresh, 249
  motion of, 253
  outdoor, 254

Air, pollution of, 256
  and tuberculosis, 255
Air-borne infections, 635
Air conditioning, 259
Air pressure, 251
Air sanitation, 541
Alcohol, 199–209
  and accidents, 201
  and athletics, 202
  as medicine, 206
  pros and cons of, 207
  wood, and vision, 331
Alimentary canal, 81
Alkaline foods, 89, 166
Allergic colds, 287
Allergy, 182
American Cancer Society, 582
American Heart Association, 582
American Medical Association, 583
American Public Health Association, 583
American Red Cross, 581
Amino acids, 89
Ancylostomiasis, 636
Anemia, pernicious, 98
Anesthesia for labor, 430
Angina pectoris, 450
Animals and disease, 514
Anthrax, 520, 637
Antibiotics for colds, 304
Antihistamines for colds, 304
Antiseptics, 504
Antitoxin, diphtheria, 271
  tetanus, 277

[793]

[797   ]